CANCER   6

A COMPREHENSIVE TREATISE

RADIOTHERAPY, SURGERY, AND IMMUNOTHERAPY

CANCER 6

A COMPREHENSIVE TREATISE

RADIOTHERAPY, SURGERY, AND IMMUNOTHERAPY

FREDERICK F. BECKER, EDITOR

University of Texas System Cancer Center
M.D. Anderson Hospital and Tumor Institute
Houston, Texas

PLENUM PRESS • NEW YORK AND LONDON

Library of Congress Cataloging in Publication Data

Main entry under title:

Cancer: a comprehensive treatise.

Includes bibliographies and indexes.
CONTENTS: v. 1. Etiology—chemical and physical carcinogenesis.—v. 2. Etiology—
viral carcinogenesis.—v. 3. Biology of tumors—cellular biology and growth. v. 4.
Biology of tumors—Surfaces, Immunology, and Comparative Pathology. v. 5. Chemo-
therapy. v. 6. Radiotherapy, surgery, and immunotherapy.
1. Cancer—Collected works. I. Title. [DNLM: 1. Neoplasms. QZ200 B397c]
RC261.B42   616.9'94'008   74-31196
ISBN 0-306-35206-0 (v. 6)

© 1977 Plenum Press, New York
A Division of Plenum Publishing Corporation
227 West 17th Street, New York, N.Y. 10011

Printed in the United States of America

Contributors

to Volume 6

G. E. ADAMS, Gray Laboratory, Cancer Research Campaign, Mount Vernon Hospital, Northwood, Middlesex HA6 2RN, England. Present address: Division of Physics as Applied to Medicine, Institute of Cancer Research, Sutton, Surrey SM2 5PX, England

J. DENEKAMP, Gray Laboratory, Cancer Research Campaign, Mount Vernon Hospital, Northwood, Middlesex HA6 2RN, England

M. M. ELKIND, Division of Biological and Medical Research, Argonne National Laboratory, Argonne, Illinois 60439

BERNARD FISHER, University of Pittsburgh School of Medicine, Pittsburgh, Pennsylvania 15261

J. F. FOWLER, Gray Laboratory, Cancer Research Campaign, Mount Vernon Hospital, Northwood, Middlesex HA6 2RN, England

ANNA GOLDFEDER, Cancer and Radiobiological Research Laboratory and Laboratory of Experimental Hematology, Department of Biology, New York University, New York, New York 10003

J. U. GUTTERMAN, Department of Developmental Therapeutics, The University of Texas System Cancer Center, M. D. Anderson Hospital and Tumor Institute, Houston, Texas 77030

ERIC J. HALL, Radiological Research Laboratory, College of Physicians and Surgeons of Columbia University, New York, New York 10032

EVAN M. HERSH, Department of Developmental Therapeutics, The University of Texas System Cancer Center, M. D. Anderson Hospital and Tumor Institute, Houston, Texas 77030

ROBERT F. KALLMAN, Department of Radiology, Stanford University School of Medicine, Stanford, California 94305

HENRY S. KAPLAN, Cancer Biology Research Laboratory, Department of Radiology, Stanford University School of Medicine, Stanford, California 94305

v

JOSEPH LOBUE, Cancer and Radiobiological Research Laboratory and Laboratory of Experimental Hematology, Department of Biology, New York University, New York, New York 10003

G. M. MAVLIGIT, Department of Developmental Therapeutics, The University of Texas System Cancer Center, M. D. Anderson Hospital and Tumor Institute, Houston, Texas 77030

MILAN POTMESIL, Cancer and Radiobiological Research Laboratory and Laboratory of Experimental Hematology, Department of Biology, New York University, New York, New York 10003

J. L. REDPATH, Departments of Medical Physics and Radiation Oncology, Michael Reese Medical Center, Chicago, Illinois 60616

S. P. RICHMAN, Department of Developmental Therapeutics, The University of Texas System Cancer Center, M. D. Anderson Hospital and Tumor Institute, Houston, Texas 77030

SARA ROCKWELL, Department of Therapeutic Radiology, Yale University School of Medicine, New Haven, Connecticut 06510

ROBERT J. SHALEK, Department of Physics, University of Texas System Cancer Center, Houston, Texas 77030

Preface

The history of the development of cancer therapy has been marked by a recurring pattern, one of initially exciting and encouraging results as new methods were introduced, followed by dismaying failures. The extremity of the disease and its high mortality have dictated that each means of damaging tumor cells would be rapidly explored and exploited as a mode of therapy, long before the corresponding theory and technique were completely understood and perfected. Thus radiation was used as an antitumor agent almost immediately following recognition of its cytodestructive capability.

Equally constant, following the rapid utilization of new therapeutic methods, has been a period of significant technical improvements. This second aspect of the pattern is also illustrated by the field of radiotherapy. New radiation sources, new methods of dosimetry, use of high-energy radiation, and other new techniques allowed the therapist to better focus upon the tumor and to improve the geometry of exposure. Thus, with each technical advance, the "reach" of radiotherapy was increased and damage to normal tissues was decreased. Inevitably, however, a limit was reached, a point at which clinicians and researchers realized they could go no further without returning to a more fundamental search, one based on the biology of the tumor cell itself.

This then is the third facet of the pattern, wherein technology halts and cell biology must impact. Thus an understanding of cell cycling, of dormancy, of cell repopulation, and of hypoxic influences led to the use of dose fractionation and to sensitization of the tumor cell by chemical agents. Today, the latter holds the greatest promise of any advance in this field and could be the means of taking radiotherapy beyond local control and into the realm of systemic cure.

The newest mode of cancer therapy is immunotherapy. "Newest," of course, as in other areas of medical science, often implies "newly rediscovered," for, in the nonspecific stimulatory modes of immunotherapy we are surely reexpressing the impact of Coley's toxin described many years ago. As a primary mode of therapy, immunotherapy brings the control of metastatic disease into the realm of possibility. As a form of adjuvant therapy, immunotherapy holds great promise as a means of giving surgical manipulation the "reach" of systemic cure and of adding to chemotherapy the finality of cure. But immunotherapy conforms to the pattern of therapeutic intervention in all of its facets. The early reports of tumor regression with cell transfusions, transfer factor, and nonspecific stimulation— the possibility that what was "blocked" could be unblocked—seemed to offer the dazzling promise of a major assault on malignancy. However, the technical limitations of immunotherapy surfaced more rapidly than those of almost any other approach. Certainly, one ancient principle of medical biology had been forgotten, that which reminds us that biological relationships are infinitely complex and infinitely adaptable. The limitations that surfaced were inherent in the complex interface of the tumor and host.

This complexity is awe inspiring, as it reflects both the response of the host to the tumor and the response of the tumor to the host. It appears that at least three factors contribute to this intricate relationship. First, the host may not "see" the tumor if the tumor displays no recognizable differences or if such differences are masked. Second, the response of the host may be intercepted by circulating tumor-cell products; and, third, the host's reponse may be inhibited by means as yet uncertain. These thrusts and counterthrusts resemble a biological version of modern missile warfare.

As humbling as this complexity now appears, as insoluble as this approach to therapy now seems, I, for one, find in its challenge the potential for advances even beyond those which we seek. It appears to me that we may enter an era of immunological manipulation, indeed of host manipulation, with implications for curing a diversity of diseases and for general human improvement. Therefore, as slow as progress has appeared, as limited as is the success of current immunotherapy, the promise remains. It is the purpose of this volume to review the current state of the art and science of cancer therapy (radiotherapy, surgery, and immunotherapy) and to suggest the modalities of the future.

Frederick F. Becker

Houston

Contents

Radiotherapy

Molecular and Cellular Biology of Radiation Lethality

3

M. M. ELKIND AND J. L. REDPATH

Cell Proliferation Kinetics and Radiation Therapy

4

J. DENEKAMP AND J. F. FOWLER

Radiation Effects on Normal Tissues   5

J. F. FOWLER AND J. DENEKAMP

Hypoxic Cell Sensitizers for Radiotherapy   6

G. E. ADAMS

Effects of Radiation on Animal Tumor Models   7

ROBERT F. KALLMAN AND SARA ROCKWELL

High-LET Radiations 8

Eric J. Hall

Stem Cells, Nonproliferating Cells, and Their Kinetics in Normal and Neoplastic Tissues 9

Milan Potmesil, Joseph LoBue, and Anna Goldfeder

Surgery

The Changing Role of Surgery in the Treatment of Cancer   10

BERNARD FISHER

Immunotherapy

Immunotherapy of Human Cancer   11

EVAN M. HERSH, G. M. MAVLIGIT, J. U. GUTTERMAN, AND
S. P. RICHMAN

Radiotherapy

Present Status of Radiation Therapy of Cancer: An Overview

HENRY S. KAPLAN

1. Historical Introduction

The discovery, shortly before the turn of the century, of X-rays by Roentgen, of radioactivity by Becquerel, and of radium by the Curies was promptly followed by the therapeutic application of these new agents, and by 1899 the first cancer, a basal cell epithelioma, had been cured. Thus the entire history of radiation therapy as a treatment modality now encompasses only some 80 years (Case, 1958). The dramatic initial responses observed in the treatment of skin and other superficial neoplasms were so unprecedented that they generated the unrealistic hope that a miraculous cure for cancer had finally been discovered. This naive view was soon followed by an equally unwarranted wave of disillusionment and pessimism when tumor recurrences and injuries to normal tissues began to appear.

The first 25 years of radiation therapy have been likened to the "dark ages" of the discipline. The radiation therapists of that era worked under formidable handicaps. There were no training programs in the new discipline, and virtually

HENRY S. KAPLAN • Cancer Biology Research Laboratory, Department of Radiology, Stanford University School of Medicine, Stanford, California 94305.

all of its early practitioners had been co-opted from other fields such as surgery and dermatology. They did not understand the physical nature of the new and mysterious agents with which they were working, nor did they have any comprehension of their biological effects. They lacked any reliable method with which to measure dose, and had no generally agreed unit of dose. Their equipment was primitive, temperamental, and severely limited in peak energy. Their predominantly surgical heritage led them to adopt treatment techniques involving single, massive exposures, aimed at eradication of tumors in a single treatment, comparable to the extirpation of tumors by surgery (Buschke, 1970). It was thus not surprising that the primary morbidity, and even mortality, of such massive-dose treatment was entirely comparable to that of major surgery at that time. Those patients who survived the immediate postirradiation period, despite impressive initial regression of their tumors, often developed major complications, as well as a high rate of tumor recurrence. Indeed, much of the clinical research of that era was directed toward the description and analysis of a bewildering variety of hitherto unknown forms of tissue injury (Cantril, 1957).

Radiation therapy would soon have been discredited had it not been for the pioneering laboratory and clinical research of the group at the Fondation Curie in Paris, headed by Claude Regaud (Fig. 1). In a classical series of experiments that began in 1919, Regaud and his colleagues showed conclusively that spermatogenesis in the testis could be permanently eradicated by the administration of

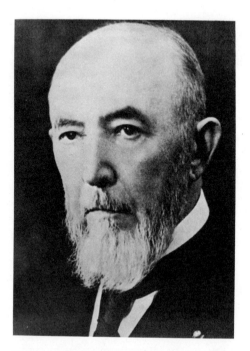

FIGURE 1. Claude Regaud, M.D., Director, Fondation Curie, Paris, 1920–1937.

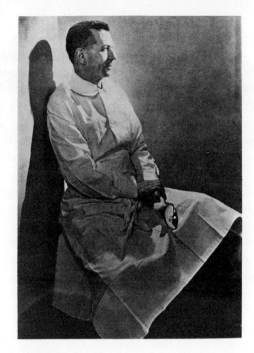

FIGURE 2. Henri Coutard, M.D., Radiotherapist,
Fondation Curie, Paris.

successive daily doses of fractionated radiotherapy, whereas no single massive
dose could elicit the same biological response without concomitantly inflicting
permanent and often intolerable injury to the overlying skin (Regaud, 1922;
Regaud and Ferroux, 1927 a,b). On the hypothesis that the testis, with its very high
rate of cell turnover, might represent a model of a malignant neoplasm, Regaud
suggested that the preferential eradication of spermatogenesis by fractionated
radiotherapy might be mirrored in a similar advantage of this technique,in the
treatment of malignant neoplasms.

He and his colleague, Henri Coutard (Fig. 2), soon applied these techniques of
fractionated radiotherapy to the treatment of patients with a variety of cancers of
the head and neck region. Others adapted this approach to the treatment of
cancer of the cervix uteri. Within a few years, they were able to present 5-year
survival data for a variety of primary cancers of the oral cavity, pharynx, and
larynx which were revolutionary for that era (Regaud *et al.*, 1922; Coutard, 1932,
1938). Equally impressive results began to emerge in the treatment of patients
with cervical cancer. These reports left no doubt that permanent cures of a very
significant fraction of patients with cancers arising in these areas had been
achieved for the first time in history. Accordingly, fractionation of treatment has
become a universally accepted technique in present-day radiotherapy.

Concomitant advances in the technological and physical aspects of the discipline
also occurred in the third decade of this century (*cf.* review by Trout, 1958).

Coolidge introduced the kilovoltage era of radiotherapy by inventing a vacuum X-ray tube capable of operation at energies as high as 200,000 volts (200 kVp). This and other advances made possible the design of apparatus of far greater reliability. Radiological physicists developed quantitative methods for the measurement of radiation dose and collaborated in the definition of the first physical unit of dose, the roentgen. The kilovoltage era was one of great achievement. Substantial cure rates for superficial cancers arising in the skin, the lip, the tonsil, the anterior tongue, the larynx, and the cervix were observed in centers throughout the world.

Nonetheless, the radiotherapists of that era were severely hampered by the physical limitations of dose distribution of 200 kVp X-rays. By about 1940, it had become obvious that beams of higher energy were needed, and soon after World War II several groups of physicists responded to this need with imaginative new approaches to the design of devices of much higher energy. The evolution from the kilovoltage to the "supervoltage" or, more properly, the megavoltage era of radiotherapy has been chronicled by Schulz (1975). The intense neutron fluxes provided by atomic piles enabled the production of radioactive cobalt (^{60}Co) as a cheap, manmade substitute for radium. This artificial radioisotope was first adapted to interstitial and intracavitary therapy. Then, as larger quantities became available, ^{60}Co teletherapy apparatus with beam energies equivalent to those of 3 MeV X-rays was designed. The development of the betatron (Kerst, 1943) and of the linear electron accelerator (Ginzton et al., 1948; Fry et al., 1948) made available for the first time electronic devices capable of yielding beams of very high energy while operating at quite nominal voltages. Linear electron accelerators were soon adapted to medical radiotherapeutic use in England (Howard-Flanders, 1954) and at Stanford University (Ginzton et al., 1957). The successful and remarkably reliable operation of these early machines soon established the linear accelerator as the "work horse" of the megavoltage era of radiotherapy. Such accelerators, as well as cobalt teletherapy units, are now standard equipment in radiation therapy departments throughout the world.

The high-energy X-ray and electron beams generated by these devices liberated radiation therapists from the physical constraints of the kilovoltage era. Megavoltage energy beams produce their maximal ionization at significant depths beneath the skin surface, thus effectively eliminating skin tolerance as a dose-limiting factor. Lateral scatter is also greatly diminished, giving the edges of the beam a knifelike character. Such beams can be used in riflelike fashion in the treatment of very small lesions in the eye, the larynx, and other delicate sites (Kaplan and Bagshaw, 1957). High doses can be safely delivered to tumors in close proximity to vital tissues and organs. Because the penetration of such high-energy beams is substantially greater, it is relatively easy to deliver tumoricidal doses to neoplasms deep within the body, even in very obese patients. The very high beam intensity provided by linear electron accelerators permits their operation at increased target-patient distances, thus permitting quite large fields to be treated, encompassing multiple areas of tumor involvement in contiguity (Kaplan, 1962; Page *et al.*, 1970*a,b*). Taken together, these physical advantages have greatly increased

the versatility and precision of treatment, and have opened the way to entirely new treatment approaches for Hodgkin's disease and other malignant lymphomas (Kaplan, 1972*a*; Schultz *et al.*, 1975; Goffinet *et al.*, 1976). They have also widened the scope of radiotherapy by permitting the definitive treatment of neoplasms such as carcinoma of the prostate (Bagshaw *et al.*, 1965), a widely prevalent cancer which could not be effectively treated with kilovoltage X-rays because of the severe skin reactions induced in the perineal and inguinal regions by such low-energy beams. It has been possible to document the fact that megavoltage radiotherapy has significantly improved the long-term survival and cure rates for several types of deep-seated neoplasms, particularly those arising in the pelvis and in the head and neck regions (Fletcher, 1962; Kaplan, 1965*a*; Earle *et al.*, 1973).

Radiation therapists have also made important clinical contributions by learning to recognize the typical patterns of spread of carcinomas and sarcomas arising in a host of tissues and sites and adapting their therapeutic strategies to the natural history of these neoplasms. Such meticulous and painstaking studies have gradually created the foundations of the modern field of clinical oncology. Concomitantly, acute and chronic complications of treatment were carefully recorded and compiled, gradually yielding a body of data on which present-day concepts of the radiation tolerance of various tissues and organs are based.

With the exception of the pioneering studies of Regaud on fractionation, essentially all of modern radiotherapy has stemmed from a combination of advances on the physical and clinical frontiers of the discipline, while the fundamental radiobiological foundations on which these responses rest remained largely unexplored until about 20 years ago, when the development of a new technique for the clonal cultivation of mammalian cells *in vitro* permitted the quantitative analysis of radiation dose–cell survival relationships, revealing exponential survival curves with an initial "shoulder" region (Puck and Marcus, 1956). The shoulder was later shown by Elkind and Sutton (1960) to be due to recovery from sublethal damage. The lethal effects of ionizing radiation on bacterial and mammalian cells have been shown to be the consequence of strand breakage and other damage produced in chromosomal DNA (Kaplan, 1968*a*). Although enzymatic repair of certain types of strand breakage has been documented (McGrath and Williams, 1966; Town *et al.*, 1973), breaks induced in both strands of the DNA macromolecule appear to be nonreparable (Kaplan, 1966), and are probably the single lesion most directly associated with lethality (Bonura *et al.*, 1975).

In the transition from single to multiple fractionated radiation exposures, several additional important parameters come into play; these include recovery, repair, reoxygenation, repopulation, and redistribution in the cell cycle (Elkind *et al.*, 1968). With the unfolding of these and other aspects of cellular radiobiology relevant to the radiotherapeutic response, radiation therapy now stands at the threshold of a new era in its history, in which substantial gains in the treatment of certain types of cancer may stem from the exploitation of fundamental radiobiological principles.

HENRY S.
KAPLAN

Radiation therapists confine their practice to patients with neoplastic disease. They are clinical oncologists first and are concerned only secondarily with the technical aspects of their own therapeutic modality. They do not hesitate to recommend surgery, chemotherapy, or hormonal treatment instead of irradiation whenever, in their clinical judgment, such alternative treatments would offer more in the management of any given patient. To underscore and emphasize this point, the term "radiation oncology" has come into increasingly widespread use.

The modern care of patients with cancer is increasingly a team effort, involving the expertise of specialists from several different disciplines. Radiotherapy is a consultative discipline, and radiation oncologists see patients in consultation only on referral by other physicians. Referring physicians are often unaware that the consultative assistance of qualified radiation therapists, surgeons, and cancer chemotherapists is freely available to all physicians and their patients throughout the United States through the consultative tumor boards which exist in all hospitals with accredited tumor clinics. Some patients are still referred to radiation oncologists with an implied or explicit commitment by the referring physician regarding the type and extent of the radiation therapy to be employed. Such referrals deprive the patient of the benefit of the independent consultative opinion of the radiation oncologist, and may lead to embarrassment and inappropriate selection of treatment. The referral to the radiation oncologist should be made in such a manner as to elicit his consultative opinion first, after which final decisions concerning treatment may be taken by joint discussion between the referring physician and the radiation oncologist.

In general, it is unwise to initiate a course of radiation therapy for a patient without a definitive tissue diagnosis of a neoplasm. Most patients referred to the radiation oncologist have already had such a diagnosis established by biopsy or by exfoliative cytology and microscopic examination. Sometimes the first biopsy specimen proves to be unsatisfactory for diagnosis or yields an equivocal answer. In such instances, it is best to repeat the biopsy rather than start treatment without a firm diagnosis. There are certain unavoidable, although infrequent exceptions to this general rule involving patients with neoplasms of the brain, eye, pituitary, or other biopsy-inaccessible sites, or patients with superior vena caval obstruction or other acute radiotherapeutic emergencies in whom the biopsy procedure would be life threatening. When patients are referred to a radiotherapy department from some other hospital or town, the radiation oncologist will usually request the biopsy slides, pertinent X-ray examinations, and clinical summary for review at the time of the patient's first visit.

Once the diagnosis is established, an attempt must be made to assess the anatomical extent of disease as meticulously as possible. It is also important to evaluate the general clinical condition of the patient with reference to such factors as age, general debility, previous treatment for the same and/or other neoplasms, presence of coexistent cardiovascular, hepatic, renal, or other life-threatening disease, existence of a second primary neoplasm, and such other clinical informa-

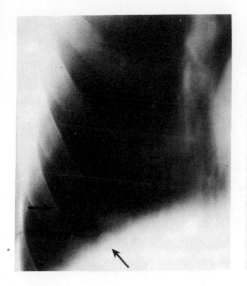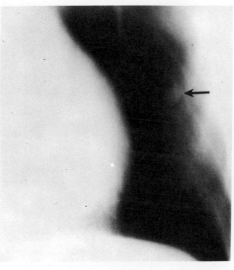

FIGURE 3. Tomogram revealing the presence and location of pulmonary metastases in a patient with testicular carcinoma.

tion as might influence the treatment plan. Since the experienced radiotherapist is first and foremost a clinical oncologist, his knowledge of the natural history and patterns of spread of neoplasms arising in many different primary sites can be expected to focus and expedite the diagnostic workup of each patient.

Clinical evaluation begins with a thorough history and general physical examination. A complete blood count, urinalysis, and serum chemistry panel are routinely obtained; other more specialized biochemical tests which reflect activity of particular types of neoplasms may also be ordered selectively. Radiographic and radioisotopic evaluation is also best performed on a selective basis related to the natural history of the specific neoplasm. Conventional chest radiographs are indicated for many types of neoplasms known to metastasize to the lung and/or to the mediastinal and hilar lymph nodes. When the conventional chest films reveal questionable or suspicious findings, mediastinal or whole-lung tomography (Fig. 3) may assist in their further evaluation. A metastatic survey, which includes roentgenographic examinations of the chest and the most frequently involved portions of the skeletal system, or a radioisotopic bone scan (Fig. 4) is desirable in all patients with malignant neoplasms known to have a proclivity for bloodborne dissemination to bone, such as those arising in the breast and lung. Conversely, the diagnostic workup for patients with carcinoma of the cervix is focused on the detection of invasion and obstruction of the lower urinary and gastrointestinal tract, and thus emphasizes such procedures as cystoscopy, proctoscopy, and intravenous urography. Lymphangiography (Figs. 5 and 6) has proven to be of great practical importance for the detection of occult involvement in the retroperitoneal and pelvic lymph nodes in patients with malignant lymphomas (Castellino *et al.*, 1974) and is now also used increasingly in the assessment of metastasis to pelvic and paraaortic lymph nodes in patients with cancer of the

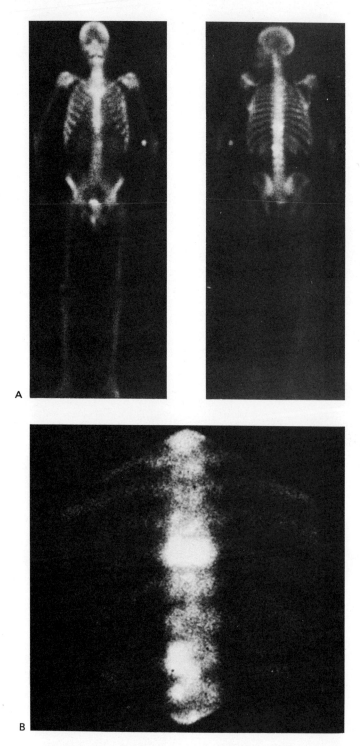

FIGURE 4. Thoracic vertebral metastases revealed by a ^{99m}Tc pyrophosphate bone scan in a patient with carcinoma of the prostate. A: Anterior and posterior whole-body scans. B: Detail of thoracic spine.

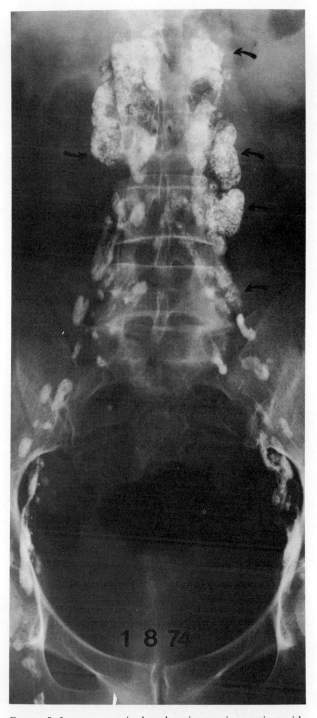

FIGURE 5. Lower extremity lymphangiogram in a patient with Hodgkin's disease, revealing involvement of several lumbar paraaortic lymph nodes (arrows). The involved nodes are enlarged relative to the normal nodes in the iliac chains, and have a typically "foamy," reticulated pattern.

urinary bladder, prostate, ovary, testis, and cervix (Ray *et al.*, 1976; Hintz *et al.*, 1975). Arteriography (Fig. 7) may be extremely helpful in the differentiation of cysts from neoplasms in the kidney, and in detecting soft tissue invasion by malignant osseous, pelvic, and renal tumors.

Surgical procedures other than the initial biopsy are often indicated as part of the diagnostic workup. Patients with lymphomas should have a routine bone marrow biopsy with a Jamshidi or similar cutting needle or trephine (Jamshidi and Swaim, 1971). In Hodgkin's disease and, more selectively, in patients with other types of malignant lymphomas, diagnostic exploration of the abdomen (staging laparotomy), first introduced in the 1960s (Glatstein *et al.*, 1969), has added greatly to our knowledge of the natural history of these neoplasms and has revealed an astonishingly high frequency of occult involvement of the spleen,

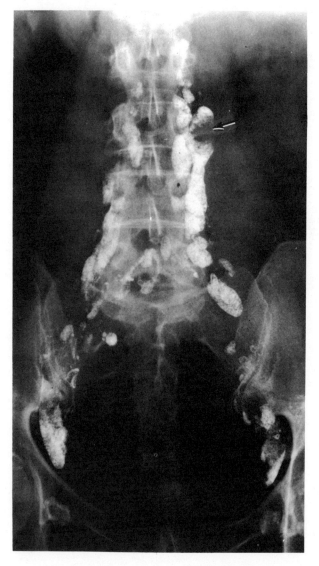

FIGURE 6. Lower extremity lymphangiogram in a patient with carcinoma of the cervix. In addition to the enlargement and filling defects in the lymph nodes near the lateral pelvic border, a common site of metastatis of this tumor, this study has revealed otherwise unsuspected metastasis in the lumbar paraaortic nodes, most evident in the large node just to the left of the third lumbar vertebra, which is partially replaced by a large filling defect (arrow). Lymph nodes at this level are not encompassed by the pelvic radiotherapy fields ordinarily used in carcinoma of the cervix. This metastatic node would have gone undetected, and thus untreated, but for the lymphangiogram.

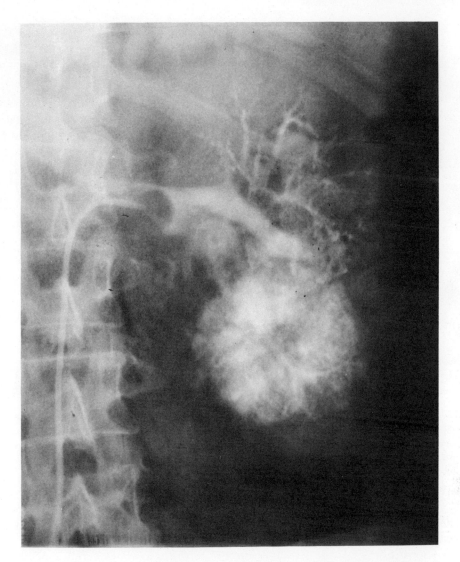

FIGURE 7. Left renal arteriogram, in the venous phase, revealing typical "staining" and vascular distortion due to a large carcinoma replacing the lower half of the kidney. An important additional finding is the filling defect in the left renal vein near the position of the catheter tip, which is due to a metastatic thrombus.

retroperitoneal lymph nodes, mesenteric lymph nodes, liver, and bone marrow (Kaplan *et al.*, 1973*a*; Goffinet *et al.*, 1973*a*). Although certain liver function tests, notably the serum alkaline phosphatase level, have had some usefulness in the detection of hepatic metastasis, radioisotopic scans of the liver, percutaneous liver needle biopsy, laparoscopy with liver biopsy, and biopsy of the liver during direct inspection at laparotomy have, in that order, detected an increasing percentage of occult hepatic metastases. In recent years, new diagnostic procedures such as ultrasound B-scans and computerized axial tomography (Fig. 8) have given promise of adding appreciably to our diagnostic armamentarium in the

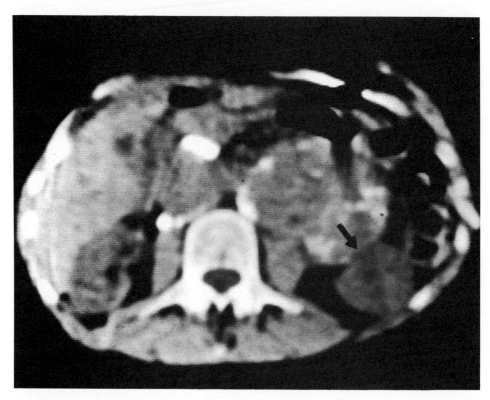

FIGURE 8. Computerized tomographic (CT) scan of the abdominal cavity in a patient with metastatic seminoma. A large retroperitoneal mass may be seen displacing the left kidney (arrow) and distorting the normal outlines of the aorta and other prevertebral structures. Some of the paraaortic nodes are opacified from a previous lymphangiogram. The CT scan assisted the radiotherapist in the selection and positioning of abdominal treatment fields.

assessment of intraabdominal sites of neoplastic involvement. Computerized axial tomography has also revolutionized the detection and delineation of primary and metastatic intracranial neoplasms, and has obviated, to a very large extent, the need for other procedures such as radioisotopic brain scans, cerebral arteriography, pneumoencephalography, and ventriculography.

After the diagnostic workup of the patient has been completed and all the essential information is at hand, it is important to assess the clinical stage of the neoplasm. Clinical staging classifications based on the TNM system have been established by interdisciplinary committees working under the aegis of the International Union Against Cancer and the American College of Surgeons. In the TNM system, the extent of the tumor is separately evaluated with respect to the primary site (T), the regional lymph nodes (N), and the presence or absence of distant metastasis (M). TNM classifications for cancers of several primary sites have now been adopted, extensively field tested, and made available to all interested physicians.* In the case of Hodgkin's disease and other lymphomas, the

* Obtainable from the American Joint Committee for Cancer Staging and End Results Reporting, 55 East Erie Street, Chicago, Illinois, or the International Union Against Cancer, 1200, Geneva, Switzerland.

primary site is usually a lymph node, and there is thus no clear distinction between the T and the N components of the TNM system. Accordingly, other clinical staging classifications have been serially proposed and evaluated; of these, the Ann Arbor Clinical Staging Classification (Carbone *et al.*, 1971) appears to be highly satisfactory for patients with Hodgkin's disease, and is used also for most patients with non-Hodgkin's lymphomas. These clinical staging classifications play a most important dual role: They assist physicians in the selection of appropriate treatment for malignant disease of definable extent, and they facilitate the valid intercomparison of the results of treatment with different modalities and from different institutions.

When the clinical stage of the disease has been established, the radiation oncologist, often acting together with the surgeon and cancer chemotherapist, is then in a position to make a series of crucial decisions concerning management. Such decisions require careful integration of the extent of disease and the general clinical condition of the individual patient with a large body of knowledge relating to prognosis, anticipated response to various forms of treatment, anticipated complication rates, and other relevant clinical considerations. The most vital question to be answered is: Is the extent of the cancer compatible with treatment with curative intent? There is no established lower limit, but, in general, the oncologist tends to think of tumors having a 5-year survival probability in the range of 1–5% as being at or near the lower limits of curability. Thus he will ask whether any modality can still offer the patient such a chance for cure. The risks entailed must then be related to the age and general condition of the patient, any history of prior treatment which might modify or limit tissue tolerance, and other relevant considerations. An intensive treatment program that offers a small chance for permanent cure may be entirely justified for a young, healthy, vigorous adult, and equally inappropriate, despite the presence of a cancer of the same type and extent, in an elderly, frail patient. For these reasons, a correct decision as to whether or not to treat with curative intent is one of the most important judgments that the radiation oncologist must make, and it calls upon the full extent of his background of prior experience and knowledge. Overly aggressive attempts at cure expose incurable patients to needless morbidity, to prolonged and expensive treatment, and sometimes also to distressing complications. Conversely, therapeutic decisions which are unwarrantedly pessimistic deprive the patient who has a small but significant chance for cure of that chance. In some instances, the emotional and psychological outlook of a patient may be relevant to the decision. Some patients, confronted by the knowledge that they have a malignant tumor offering little chance for cure, will strongly prefer an aggressive course of action to be instituted, whereas others will make clear to their physicians that they have lived a long and full life and prefer to be permitted to die in peace.

After it has been decided that a given patient is most appropriately treated with curative intent, the next decision is: What modality or combination of modalities offers the best chance for cure? Here again, the radiation oncologist must call into play a broad body of knowledge concerning all aspects of clinical oncology, including a familiarity with the anticipated results of surgery, chemotherapy, hormone therapy, and other procedures, as compared with those of irradiation. In case of doubt, patients should be referred for consultation by other appropriate specialists, or presented to a multidisciplinary consultative tumor board. Combined-modality treatment is now coming into increasingly widespread use for a spectrum of neoplasms with little or no chance for cure.

Conversely, if the patient, whether by virtue of age, debility, or the extent of the neoplasm, is not an appropriate candidate for treatment with curative intent, the alternative question which must be answered is: Does the patient present symptoms which require palliation? Radiation therapy is extremely effective in the relief of pain, bleeding, compression or obstruction of vital organs, and other distressing symptoms of incurable tumors. Palliative treatment should always be used with discretion and be based on sound clinical indications (Paterson, 1939). It is not true that such treatment may help but cannot harm the patient; injudicious treatment can indeed increase the discomfort of a dying patient, unnecessarily add to the expense of his treatment, or deprive him of precious remaining days or weeks at home. Palliative treatment can appropriately be given to selected asymptomatic patients in whom the impending development of a catastrophic problem such as obstruction of the superior vena cava or a major bronchus or collapse of a vertebra involved by metastatic disease can be anticipated. Patients with severe emotional disturbances relating to their diagnosis of cancer may require limited palliative treatment aimed more at psychotherapy than at inducing remission of the neoplasm. These exceptions aside, however, it is generally wisest to defer palliative treatment of the essentially asymptomatic incurable patient until specific symptoms appear which cannot readily be relieved by simple medication. Such patients should be explicitly followed at periodic intervals, however, to offer emotional support, and it should be made clear to them that appropriate palliative treatment will be made available whenever the need for its use actually arises during the course of their management.

Subsidiary decisions to be made by the radiation oncologist include a choice of high- vs. low-dose palliation. Patients who are otherwise in good general condition and who have severe pain due to localized skeletal metastasis, or distress due to tracheobronchial compression or superior vena caval obstruction, may benefit from relatively intensive treatment aimed at prolonged control of that specific problem, despite the knowledge that other manifestations of metastatic disease will ultimately lead to a fatal outcome. Conversely, patients with multiple, widespread skeletal metastases should usually receive low doses of radiation for the palliation of pain in any given site. It is in these fine nuances of judgment, as well as in the major decisions described above, that the skill and wisdom of the radiation oncologist as a physician can be most effectively displayed.

3. Technical Considerations in Radiotherapy

Most contemporary radiation therapy is carried out with beams of X- or γ-rays. By convention, X- or roentgen rays are the electromagnetic, nonparticulate, ionizing radiation produced by manmade machines, whereas γ-rays emanate from naturally occurring or artificially produced radioactive elements such as radium or cobalt-60, respectively. At the time of their discovery, X-rays were produced only by very-low-energy sources and thus had physical properties which differed appreciably from those of the high-energy γ-rays of radium. In the course of time, megavoltage energy sources such as linear electron accelerators and betatrons provided beams of very-high-energy X-rays having properties essentially indistinguishable from those of the γ-rays of radioactive cobalt (^{60}Co). Accordingly, in the megavoltage energy range, the distinction between X-rays and γ-rays has lost its significance.

Such very-short-wavelength electromagnetic radiations have the capacity to penetrate materials of low atomic numbers such as water or tissue, but are stopped efficiently in materials of high atomic number such as lead. They produce their effects in tissue by virtue of the local deposition of energy in discrete, discontinuous collisionlike events termed "ionizations." In addition to the electromagnetic radiations, a variety of particulate radiations are either in use or are being developed for use in high-energy radiation therapy. These ionizing particles include electrons, protons, deuterons, α-rays (helium nuclei), neutrons, heavy ions, and π^- mesons. Particles characterized by high linear energy transfer (LET) have physical and/or radiobiological properties which differ substantially in certain respects from those of the electromagnetic radiations.

The radiotherapeutic armamentarium includes a wide variety of radiation sources. Intense, highly localized deposition of ionizing radiation may be achieved by the interstitial implantation or intracavitary placement of capsules, needles, tubes, threads, and other devices containing natural or artificial radioactive isotopes (Fig. 9). The physical distribution of such interstitial or intracavitary sources is critical to the achievement of homogeneous dose distributions throughout the tumor volume. The handling of such radioactive sources involves substantial hazards of radiation exposure for the radiation oncologist and supporting personnel. For these reasons, a number of ingenious techniques have been devised to permit the containers to be placed in the tumor initially, and filled with radioactive sources subsequently, when the positions of the implanted devices have been checked and found to be satisfactory. Such "afterloading" techniques have increased the extent of utilization of interstitial and intracavitary devices while at the same time reducing the hazard of occupational radiation exposure (Henschke et al., 1963). Interstitial techniques have been particularly useful in the treatment of a variety of cancers of the oral cavity, oropharynx, and other sites in the head and neck region, and intracavitary techniques have long been used in the management of carcinoma of the cervix and other gynecological neoplasms. Interstitial implantation has also been utilized for the management of cancers of the breast involving the chest wall, of localized carcinomas of the bronchus, and of selected other situations involving neoplasms of limited volume. Radioactive isotopes have been administered intravenously, taking advantage of the phagocytic activity of the reticuloendothelial system to achieve selective localization in the liver, spleen, and/or bone marrow (Kraut et al., 1972). The intralymphatic

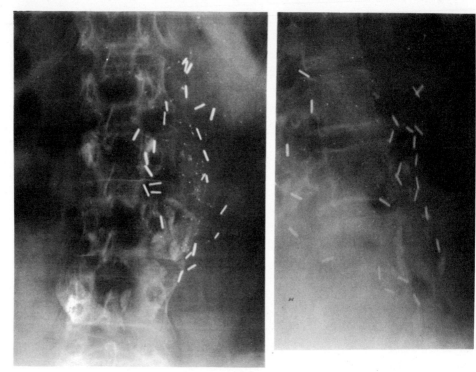

FIGURE 9. Interstitial implant in a patient with an inoperable retroperitoneal soft tissue carcinoma. The tumor was first treated with external megavoltage X-rays to a total dose of 4800 rads. One month later, at a "second-look" exploration, the tumor was partially resected and the unresectable residue of the neoplasm, attached to the aorta and vena cava, was implanted with ^{125}I seeds in Vicryl sutures, which delivered a tumor dose of 14,000 rads (average life 84 days). The patient was asymptomatic at follow-up examination 6 months later. Details of the technique, developed by D. R. Goffinet, M.D., are in preparation.

instillation of radioactive materials has also been tried, but largely abandoned because of excessive variability in the filling of lymph nodes and the problem of nonfilling of lymph nodes too extensively replaced by metastatic deposits. A wide range of radioactive isotopes emitting both β- and γ-rays of a broad spectrum of energies is now available for various types of clinical applications. These include radioisotopes of cobalt (^{60}Co), cesium (^{137}Cs), iridium (^{192}Ir), gold (^{198}Au), and iodine (^{131}I, ^{125}I). In addition, the transuranic element californium (^{252}Cf) has been developed as a source of interstitial neutron irradiation (Schlea and Stoddard, 1965; Hall, 1972).

Superficial X-ray apparatus provides X-rays in the energy range from about 50 to 140 kV, intended primarily for the treatment of dermatological and other relatively superficial lesions. X-ray apparatus operating in the 200–250 kV energy range, now generally referred to as the kilovoltage range, was at one time the standard in radiotherapy, but has been largely superseded in the past 20 years by a number of sources operating in the megavoltage range. Nonetheless, kilovoltage X-rays remain useful for the definitive treatment of lesions of limited depth, as well as for a number of palliative treatment applications. The megavoltage energy range includes all energies above 1 MeV. However, for practical purposes, it begins at the energy of ^{60}Co teletherapy apparatus, which emits homogeneous beams of γ-rays with an energy of about 1.5 MeV, roughly equivalent to that of an X-ray beam with a peak energy of about 3 MeV. Linear electron accelerators (Fig. 10) provide X-ray and/or electron beams in the energy range from 4 to 35 MeV (Karzmark and Pering, 1973). Betatrons are used primarily for electron-beam therapy, and offer beams in the energy range from 20 to nearly 50 MeV. Beams of particulate radiations other than electrons require far more complex and expensive generating sources. Fast-neutron beams of heterogeneous energies and high flux are available from cyclotrons (Fowler *et al.*, 1963; Bewley and Parnell, 1969), and monoenergetic 14 MeV fast-neutron beams of lower flux are provided by neutron generators (Reifenschweiler *et al.*, 1974). π^- meson beams may be provided by proton accelerators (Rosen, 1969), proton synchrotrons (Batho and Kornelsen, 1970), or electron accelerators operating in conjunction with π^- meson spectrometers of specialized design (Boyd *et al.*, 1973; Kaplan *et al.*, 1973*b*). Heavy ions produced by linear accelerators may be accelerated to appropriate

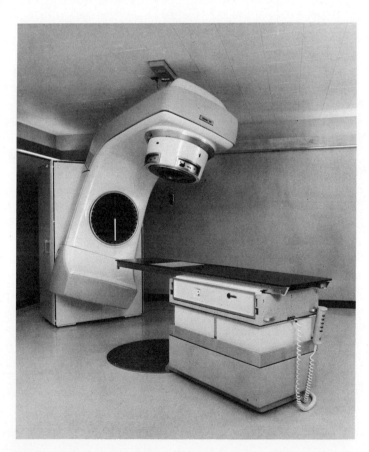

FIGURE 10. Modern 6 MeV linear electron accelerator. Photograph courtesy Varian Associates, Palo Alto, California.

energies in synchrocyclotrons (Tobias *et al.*, 1971). These extremely large, complex, and expensive devices are currently available in only a few major centers in various parts of the world, and are unlikely to become generally available for radiation therapy at the community level.

Measurement of the quantity of ionizing radiation in a beam is a complex and difficult problem, since these highly penetrating radiations cannot readily be captured in calorimeters. The principal physical units used to define quantities of ionizing radiation include a unit of *exposure* dose, the roentgen (R), which is defined with respect to an amount of ionization produced in a standard volume of air, and a unit of *absorbed* dose, the rad, defined as that amount of ionizing radiation which, when absorbed in tissue or tissue-equivalent material, delivers exactly 100 ergs/g. Ionization chambers with selected characteristics may be used to measure the distribution of ionizing energy in "phantoms" of water or tissue-equivalent material, and thus to construct isodose curves (Fig. 11) for electromagnetic and particulate beams of varying energies. The point of maximal ionization of beams of megavoltage energy is at some significant depth below the surface, and is taken as 100% relative to the ionization produced at other depths, both along the central axis of the beam and at various distances lateral to the central axis. Many different sets of isodose curves are required for any given machine, since the patterns change appreciably with the size of the field, and complete sets of curves must encompass all of the possible treatment fields that might be employed in clinical practice. A variety of wedge filters and other compensating devices may be used in selected instances, either to eliminate distortions or asymmetries in the beam or, conversely, to deliberately introduce distortions which will improve the physical distribution of ionizing energy in the irregularly shaped tissue volume occupied by a particular neoplasm. Such special problems must be individually evaluated by radiation oncologists working in collaboration with radiologic physicists and dosimetrists.

Treatment planning ordinarily begins with the delineation by the radiation oncologist of the contour and dimensions of the tumor in relation to the cross-sectional anatomy of the patient, as displayed on body section contour plots (Fig. 12). Tumor localization is achieved by direct visualization of clinically accessible lesions, or with the aid of surgical operative reports, radiographic examinations, and radioactive isotope, computerized axial tomographic, or ultrasound B-scans for more deeply seated lesions. Techniques have now been developed to feed such information into computers in which the isodose contours of a given type of megavoltage energy beam are stored. The computer can then be asked to display the dose distributions that would be achieved by a variety of different treatment techniques, thus facilitating the selection by the radiation oncologist of the optimal technique for the management of a specific patient (Sterling *et al.*, 1965).

Once the technique of irradiation has been decided on, precision in the daily alignment of the beam in relation to anatomical landmarks and to the location of the tumor becomes a critical consideration (Marks *et al.*, 1974). The initial localization of the treatment field in relation to the tumor is often performed on a simulator (Karzmark and Rust, 1972), which mimics the beam geometry of the

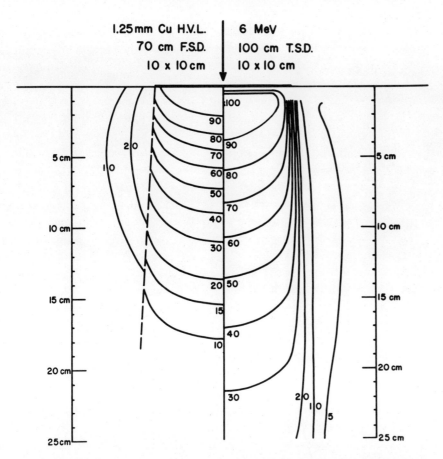

FIGURE 11. Comparison of the isodose curves for 10- by 10-cm fields irradiated with (left) 200 kV X-rays (half-value layer 1.25 mm Cu) vs. (right) 6 MeV linear accelerator X-rays. The penetration of the megavoltage beam to depths of 10 cm or greater is more than twice that of the kilovoltage beam. Note that peak ionization (100%) occurs at a depth of 1.5 cm below the surface with the megavoltage beam, whereas the maximal ionization of the kilovoltage beam is at the surface. Lateral scatter is also sharply reduced with the megavoltage beam.

megavoltage treatment source. A number of techniques have been developed to assure reproducibility of beam alignment during the course of fractionated radiotherapy, including the use of plaster and other types of body casts, specially fitted molds, bite blocks (Karzmark *et al.*, 1975), and mechanical or optical backpointers. Diagnostic X-ray exposures made with the therapeutic beam during the course of treatment provide verification ("port") films which reveal the exact contours of the treatment field in relation to various anatomical landmarks and the known location of the tumor (Fig. 13).

A typical course of fractionated radiotherapy in most radiotherapeutic centers involves three to five treatments per week. Tumor doses are usually delivered at a rate of 800–1000 rads per week to total doses of 3500 to as high as 7500 rads for various types of neoplasms differing in their responsiveness to irradiation. In "split-course" irradiation, treatment is interrupted after approximately 2 weeks to

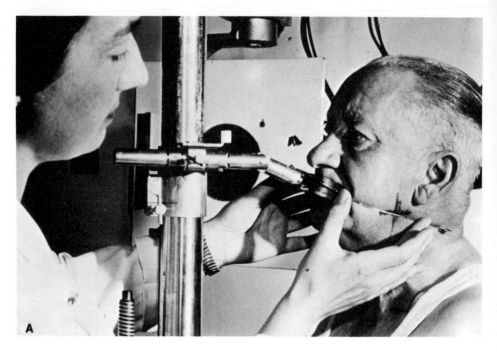

4 MeV 100 cm S.S.D.

Technique: 2 unevenly weighted opposed fields.
Isodose values shown are percent max tumor.

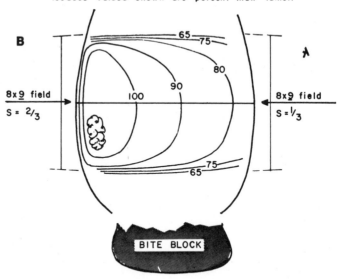

FIGURE 12. A: Dosimetrist using solder wire to obtain a cross-sectional contour of the face and head at the level of the tumor in a patient with a carcinoma of the buccal mucosa. Note that the patient's head is immobilized in the desired treatment position by means of a "bite block" (Karzmark *et al.*, 1975). B: The contour has now been transferred to paper, and the size, shape, and location of the tumor have been carefully drawn in relation to it. A provisional treatment plan involving unequally weighted doses through two opposing lateral fields is being evaluated by examining the overlapping isodose distributions contributed by each of the fields.

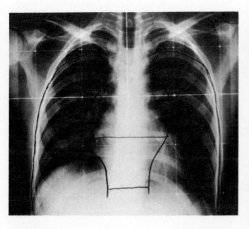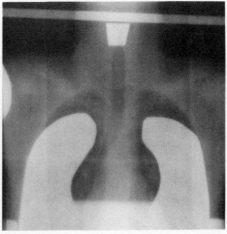

FIGURE 13. Localization film (left) and treatment port verification film (right) of a "mantle" field used in the treatment of a patient with Hodgkin's disease. The outlines of areas to be shielded have been drawn on the localization film by the radiotherapist. Note that the lead blocks shielding the lungs, heart, larynx, and humeral heads are all clearly seen on the verification film, confirming that they have been properly positioned. Details of these alignment procedures have been described by Page *et al.* (1970*a,b*).

permit a rest period of 1–2 weeks, after which treatment is resumed again and carried to completion, sometimes interrupted by one additional rest period. Split-course treatment has been reported to improve normal tissue tolerance and to decrease the hazards of late complications, while yielding substantially similar probabilities of local tumor eradication in several clinical situations (Sambrook, 1964). Certain types of tumors (notably osteogenic and soft tissue sarcomas) are known to have dose–response curves characterized by unusually wide shoulders, indicative of an unusually great capacity for the repair of sublethal damage. In the treatment of such tumors, "paucifractionated" radiotherapy, using large, individual dose increments (on the order of 600–800 rads per treatment) given at intervals of a few days, and a smaller total number of fractions, has recently been explored in conjunction with the use of halogenated pyrimidine analogue radiosensitizers such as 5-bromodeoxyuridine (Goffinet *et al.*, 1975*a*). Total-body irradiation, originally used for the palliative treatment of patients with leukemias and lymphomas in the 1920s, has recently been advocated again for patients with disseminated lymphomas, using total-body doses of 10–15 rads, given two or three times a week to total doses of approximately 150 rads, repeated if necessary after an interval of several months (Johnson, 1975).

Interstitial radiotherapy involves tissue implantation of needles, seeds, wire, or other devices containing radioactive isotopes (Fig. 9). The procedure is performed under local or general anesthesia in the operating room, and the patients are usually hospitalized thereafter for a variable period of time, usually about 1 week. The tumors that can appropriately be treated by this technique are usually of limited volume. The three-dimensional distribution of radiation sources in the tumor volume is highly critical because the radiation dose diminishes rapidly within a few millimeters from each source. Small departures from proper spacing of sources may cause local "hot spots," with ensuing tissue injury and possible necrosis, or "cold spots," in which foci of tumor receive an inadequate dose. Orthogonal radiographs in two planes, made after placement of the interstitial sources, permit the precise location and orientation of each radioactive source to be entered into the computer in relation to coordinates relevant to the tumor volume, and precise calculations of dose distribution can thus be made rapidly (Powers *et al.*, 1966). Similar techniques may be used to compute dose distribution for intracavitary sources in the uterus, vagina, urinary bladder, and other sites.

4. Clinical Responses, Tissue Reactions, and Complications

The responses to radiotherapy of various types of malignant neoplasms differ widely. Highly radiosensitive tumors, such as lymphomas or seminomas, often begin to decrease in size within the first few days after the start of treatment and may have disappeared completely before the end of the treatment course. In contrast, most epidermoid carcinomas and adenocarcinomas exhibit little or no perceptible change during the first 2–3 weeks of a course of fractionated external radiotherapy, and some may exhibit relatively little regression even by its completion. Even in such instances, however, gradual disappearance of tumor may still occur over a period of several weeks following the end of treatment. Tumors containing a relatively dense stroma or islands of avascularity tend to regress more slowly.

During the course of treatment of tumors in visually accessible sites such as the oral cavity or cervix uteri, the adjacent mucous membranes may be seen to develop a radiation reaction, known as a mucositis, during the second or third week of fractionated radiotherapy. Initially, this is manifested as an increase in redness, followed by the appearance of punctate, yellowish-white areas which gradually enlarge and become a confluent pseudomembrane covering substantial areas of the mucosa. Such reactions are accompanied by the development of acute symptoms, such as soreness in the mouth and throat, often accompanied by pain on swallowing and sometimes by hoarseness if the larynx has also been included within the treatment field. Later, patients may complain of dryness of the mouth and loss of the sense of taste. Mucositis often begins to recede during treatment, and normally goes on to complete healing within a few weeks after its completion. Since kilovoltage X-rays produce their maximal effects in the skin, a similar radiation reaction known as an epidermitis appears in the skin of each treated field, usually starting slightly later than the associated mucositis, but progressing through a similar peak of severity near the end of treatment, followed by gradual healing. In reactions of moderate severity, erythema may be the only manifestation, whereas more severe reactions progress to vesicle formation and weeping of the skin surface. In hair-bearing areas of the skin, radiation dose-dependent temporary or permanent epilation may occur. Since megavoltage beams deliver their maximal ionization to significant depths below the skin surface, the dose at the skin surface is often only a small fraction of the dose at the point of maximal ionization, and in most instances there is no visible skin reaction at any time during the entire course of megavoltage radiotherapy. However, when opposing fields are used in regions of the body of lesser thickness, the additive effects of the entrance and exit doses may be sufficient to elicit perceptible erythema, although vesiculation and weeping are seldom seen.

Nausea of varying degree is often experienced by patients during radiotherapy, particularly when the abdominal region is under treatment, and is sometimes accompanied by vomiting. Such symptoms are usually readily relieved by appropriate medication, but may occasionally require interruption of treatment. In the mid- and lower abdomen, large radiation fields may encompass multiple loops of small and large intestine, and as radiation dose increases, diarrhea may develop. Again, this usually responds readily to medication, but may require brief interruption for control. Bleeding associated with diarrhea is a dangerous manifestation, and usually indicates the need for temporary or permanent discontinuation of treatment. Patients are well advised to avoid spicy foods, roughage, and alcohol while gastrointestinal symptoms due to radiotherapy are present. Loss of appetite during radiotherapy is most severe with treatment fields involving the abdomen and may be associated with moderate weight loss during the course of treatment. Both appetite and body weight usually return to normal within the first several weeks after a course of radiotherapy has been completed.

The white blood cell count and platelet count are often reduced during a course of radiotherapy, whereas the red blood cell count seldom falls until an appreciable interval after radiotherapy has been completed, due to the much longer turnover time of the erythrocyte population. Hematological suppression is uncommon when radiotherapeutic fields are small, particularly over the head and neck or thoracic regions, but large fields over the thorax and/or abdomen commonly elicit depression of the white blood cell and platelet counts within the first 2–3 weeks of treatment. When the blood count falls significantly, serial determinations should be made at twice weekly or more frequent intervals to monitor the situation closely. When the white blood cell count falls to less than $1500/mm^3$ or the platelet count to less than $75,000/mm^3$, treatment is usually interrupted and the counts are monitored at frequent intervals until they begin to climb again, at which point treatment can be reinstituted, sometimes at a slightly lower dose rate.

A number of other types of symptomatic reactions do not become manifest until treatment has been completed, and are termed "subacute reactions." In patients treated over the thoracic region, the most frequent subacute reaction is radiation pneumonitis (Carmel and Kaplan, 1976). This may be asymptomatic and discovered only incidentally as a pulmonary infiltrate conforming to the geometry of the treatment field on posttreatment chest radiographs, or may be associated with a dry, hacking, unproductive cough. In more severe instances, this will be associated with shortness of breath and sometimes with fever. In such instances, if appropriate cultures reveal no specific bacterial or fungal organism, and if the pattern of reaction in the lung conforms closely to the outlines of the radiotherapy field, the diagnosis of radiation pneumonitis should be entertained, in which case hospitalization, treatment with steroids, and supportive measures, sometimes including oxygen inhalation, may be indicated. Radiation-induced pericarditis and pancarditis are also important subacute reactions which may follow treatment over most or all of the heart. Many cases are asymptomatic, and are detected only by virtue of cardiomegaly and a positive echocardiogram, whereas others may involve fever, a pericardial friction rub, and signs of cardiac tamponade. Recovery usually occurs promptly with bed rest and diuretic medication, but a small proportion of cases go on to chronic constrictive pericarditis requiring surgical pericardiectomy (Stewart *et al.*, 1967; Carmel and Kaplan, 1976).

When most or all of the liver volume is irradiated to doses in excess of 3000 rads, the syndrome of radiation hepatitis may appear, beginning within a few weeks after completion of irradiation (Ingold *et al.*, 1965). It is characterized by an increase in weight and increase in abdominal girth due to the development of ascites. The liver is usually palpably enlarged and often slightly tender. Elevation of the serum alkaline phosphatase and other abnormal laboratory tests usually indicate the presence of significant abnormalities of liver function. Jaundice is seldom seen. In most instances, the reaction is self-limited and clinical recovery occurs over a period of some months. Radiation nephritis is also a well-established subacute tissue reaction which may occur when both kidneys are irradiated to doses in excess of their tolerance, usually involving total doses on the order of 2500 rads (Luxton, 1953). Patients irradiated over the cervical, supraclavicular, and mediastinal lymph node distribution for Hodgkin's disease or other lymphomas may develop a curious reaction, known as Lhermitte's syndrome, believed to be due to a transient demyelinization of certain pathways in the cervical spinal cord (Jones, 1964). In this subacute syndrome, patients experience a sense of tingling or electric shock in the lumbosacral area, frequently radiating down the lower extremities, and occasionally also experienced in the upper extremities; this sensation is characteristically either brought on or aggravated by flexion of the neck. It is unassociated with motor dysfunction or with late sequelae.

Late reactions and complications following radiotherapy are strongly tissue and dose dependent. Sufficiently high doses of radiation in large segments of the lung may elicit significant pulmonary radiation fibrosis, with diminution of compliance and ventilatory capacity, atelectasis, predisposition to recurrent bouts of pneumonitis, and crippling degrees of pulmonary insufficiency. A small percentage of cases of radiation pericarditis progress to the chronic constrictive state, with engorgement of the liver, pleural effusion, and other typical manifestations which usually require surgical pericardiectomy for relief. Similarly, severe instances of radiation hepatitis may progress to a chronic cirrhosis-like state characterized by chronic ascites and hepatic insufficiency. The occurrence of severe, progressive forms of radiation nephritis, extremely rare now that the possibility of this complication is so well recognized, is associated with intractable renal insufficiency and hypertension. Doses in excess of 4500 rads to the cervical or dorsal spinal cord may produce irreversible transverse myelitis, with paralysis of the lower extremities, loss of sphincter control, and other major neurological dysfunctions (Phillips and Buschke, 1969). It should be stressed that virtually all of these major complications can be avoided by careful dosimetry, treatment planning, and beam alignment during treatment, and that the infrequent instances in which such major complications still occur today can usually be traced to some specific technical error.

Hormonal dysfunction may be induced by radiotherapy. Varying manifestations of hypothyroidism may make their appearance within months or years after radiotherapy which encompasses the lower cervical region anteriorly (Glatstein *et al.*, 1971). If the diagnosis of hypothyroidism is entertained, appropriate laboratory determinations can readily confirm the diagnosis and remedial treatment with thyroid medication eliminates the problem. When both ovaries are irradiated to significant doses in premenopausal women, menopausal symptoms develop soon after the completion of radiotherapy. If the radiation dose has been moderate, menstrual function may recover and symptoms again disappear, but at higher dose levels menopausal symptoms are permanent and may require relief by hormonal medication. Male hormonal function is highly radioresistant, and is ordinarily not affected significantly by doses of radiation capable of inducing either temporary or permanent abrogation of spermatogenesis.

Carcinogenesis may be another late consequence of radiotherapy (Glücksmann *et al.*, 1957). When wide fields are treated, as in the lymphomas or seminoma, secondary leukemias have been reported in a small percentage of patients (Rosner and Grünwald, 1975). An increased incidence of secondary neoplasms has also been reported in patients treated for benign conditions (Palmer and Spratt, 1956; Modan *et al.*, 1974). Secondary sarcomas of the subcutaneous tissues and of bone have occurred as a late manifestation in children treated with kilovoltage X-rays for retinoblastoma (Soloway, 1966), and occasionally in other clinical situations as well (Bloch, 1962; Castro *et al.*, 1967). Thus it is clear that the potential hazards associated with radiation therapy, particularly when carried to critically high doses in certain vital tissues and organs, may indeed be life threatening. Although such late major complications are fortunately infrequent or rare, the knowledge that they can occur should underscore the need for careful judgment in decisions concerning the choice of treatment modality, the selection of treatment doses, and the technically meticulous execution of planned courses of radiotherapy.

5. Contemporary Results of Radiotherapy for Malignant Disease

Radiation therapy has for many years suffered from the unfortunate reputation which it acquired during the "dark ages" in the first three decades of the century. The inadequate treatment techniques of that era accomplished little beyond transient regression of tumors, followed by seemingly inevitable recurrence, leading many physicians to conclude that radiotherapy was useful as a palliative form of treatment but had no curative potential. This erroneous notion became so deeply entrenched that it could not be dispelled by the substantial achievements of the kilovoltage era of X-ray therapy, during which clear-cut evidence of the permanent cure of many cancers of the skin, lip, oral cavity, oral pharynx, larynx, paranasal sinuses, cervix uteri, and selected other primary sites was documented by radiotherapists in many centers. Indeed, vestiges of this long-standing misconception have persisted even into the modern megavoltage era of radiotherapy, during which cure rates have substantially increased, and curative radiotherapy has been extended to several other types of malignant neoplasms which were, for technical reasons, not effectively treatable with the earlier kilovoltage techniques.

The radiation oncologist now can cite an extensive and convincing body of clinical evidence which justifies his use of the term "cure" with the same degree of assurance as the surgeon. Many patients treated 25 or more years ago with kilovoltage X-rays and/or radium for carcinoma of the cervix uteri, or cancers in the head and neck region, have survived into old age with no subsequent manifestation of the tumor, or have died of natural causes with no evidence of persistent neoplasm at autopsy. There can be no question of the appropriateness of the term "cure" in such instances. However, such individual instances suffer from the disadvantage of being anecdotal in nature, and give no clear indication as to the frequency with which curative treatment can be achieved. More meaningful measures of curative potential can be provided only by the systematic, long-term study of large numbers of consecutive, unselected patients with biopsy-proved malignant neoplasms of various types. Analyses of actuarial survival curves based on such large series (Bagshaw *et al.*, 1975; Hintz *et al.*, 1975), as well as studies of the temporal distribution of relapses following radiotherapy (Kaplan, 1968*b*; Weller *et al.*, 1976*a*), have provided unambiguous evidence that radiotherapy can, indeed, yield permanent cure in substantial proportions of patients with malignant neoplasms of various primary sites (Figs. 14 and 15).

Some indication of the improvement in survival which has occurred with the transition from kilovoltage to megavoltage X-ray therapy techniques is provided by comparative data from the literature summarized in Table 1. Five-year survival in patients with cancer of the cervix, which is tantamount to permanent cure, has

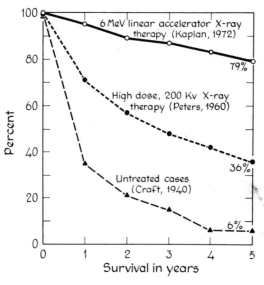

FIGURE 14. Changing prognosis of Hodgkin's disease (all stages) during three therapeutic eras: era of no specific therapy (lowest curve), era of kilovoltage radiotherapy (middle curve), and era of megavoltage radiotherapy (upper curve). From Kaplan (1972*a*).

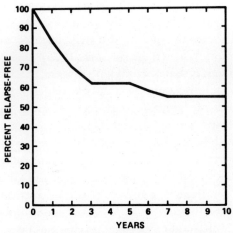

FIGURE 15. Actuarial disease-free survival (62% at 5 years, 55% at 10 years) of a series of 82 patients with carcinoma of the nasopharynx treated with megavoltage radiotherapy. From Hoppe *et al.* (1976).

improved from around 35–45% in the kilovoltage era to approximately 65% with megavoltage radiotherapy (Fletcher, 1971). In cancer of the nasopharynx, there has been a doubling of survival from around 25% to over 50% in the megavoltage radiotherapy era (Hoppe *et al.*, 1976). Similar improvement has been noted in other primary sites in the head and neck region (Weller *et al.*, 1976b; Goffinet *et al.*, 1973b). Cervical lymph node metastasis from these primary sites can also be eradicated by techniques made possible by megavoltage beam energies (Kaplan, 1965a; Hanks *et al.*, 1969; Weller *et al.*, 1976b). Long-term survival in invasive cancer of the urinary bladder has increased from essentially zero to about 30% (Goffinet *et al.*, 1975b). Carcinoma of the prostate represents an example of a

TABLE 1

Improved Survival in Several Types of Cancer with Megavoltage Therapy[a]

Type of cancer	Representative 5-year survival (%)	
	Kilovoltage X-rays	Megavoltage X-rays
Hodgkin's disease	30–35	70–75
Cancer of the cervix	35–45	55–65
Cancer of the prostate	5–15	55–60
Cancer of the nasopharynx	20–25	45–50
Cancer of the bladder	0–5	25–35
Cancer of the ovary	15–20	50–60
Retinoblastoma	30–40	80–85
Seminoma of the testis	65–70	90–95
Embryonal cancer of the testis	20–25	55–70
Cancer of the tonsil	25–30	40–50

[a]Source: Report of the Panel of Consultants on the Conquest of Cancer, U.S. Government Printing Office, Washington, D.C., 1970.

cancer which was essentially untreatable, except for palliation, in the era of kilovoltage X-ray therapy. Today, with the aid of megavoltage radiation therapy, it can be treated with curative intent, and over 60% of such patients survive relapse-free for 5 or more years (Bagshaw *et al.*, 1975). One of the most dramatic examples of improvement is that of Hodgkin's disease, in which 5-year survival in the kilovoltage era was only some 25–30% for patients with all stages of the disease. With the aid of lymphangiography, staging laparotomy, modern megavoltage radiotherapy, and improved chemotherapy, 79% of a series of 1009 consecutive patients with Hodgkin's disease of all stages have survived for 5 years, and 62% for 10 years (Kaplan, 1976). The prognosis of testicular tumors has also improved dramatically. Results were good, even in the kilovoltage era, for the highly radiosensitive seminomas, but have further improved to 85–90% for all stages of seminoma with the advent of megavoltage radiotherapy (Earle *et al.*, 1973). The more radioresistant embryonal carcinomas once had an exceedingly poor prognosis, but are now being treated successfully in over 50% of cases, even after spread to the abdominal lymph nodes has occurred. It is important to stress that most patients with malignant neoplasms who have been successfully treated with megavoltage radiotherapy are not only cured of their neoplasms but also restored to essentially normal functional capacity for work and for the enjoyment of a full, normal span of life, with few or no symptomatically significant sequelae of treatment. These individuals collectively provide an impressive mass of data on long-term survival which attests convincingly to the fact that modern radiotherapy has taken its place firmly alongside of surgery as a major curative modality for cancer.

6. Directions of Future Promise

Despite the impressive achievements of the megavoltage era of radiotherapy, it seems unlikely that substantial further progress will come from continued improvement in dose distribution or in physical techniques of radiotherapy alone. It has thus become important to examine a variety of alternative approaches in a search for new directions of promise.

Combined modalities of treatment are now being explored in a number of clinical situations in which the results with any one form of treatment alone appear to have been pushed to their limits. The rationale for the use of combined radiotherapy and surgery for the management of squamous cell carcinomas arising in the oral cavity and oropharynx, and of their cervical lymph node metastases, has been well stated by Fletcher and Jesse (1962). Preliminary radiotherapy to moderate dose levels may be expected to reduce tumor bulk to levels where subsequent surgical extirpation can be accomplished with greater ease and with substantially less risk of recurrence. Primary colorectal carcinomas are also being treated by preoperative radiotherapy followed by surgery and, in some instances, by subsequent postoperative radiotherapy. "Sandwich" techniques involving preoperative and postoperative radiotherapy with intervening

surgical extirpation of retroperitoneal lymph node chains are being actively
explored in the management of embryonal carcinoma and teratocarcinoma of the
testis, with preliminary reports indicative of improvement in long-term results
(Nicholson *et al.*, 1974). However, in other sites such as primary bronchogenic
carcinoma and carcinoma of the esophagus, attempts to combine radiotherapy
and radical surgery have been disappointing (Collaborative Study, 1969), and
have been largely abandoned.

Radiotherapy is also being used in combination with chemotherapy in an
increasing spectrum of neoplasms. Extremely encouraging results have resulted
from the use of combined-modality therapy in several types of pediatric neoplasms, notably Wilms' tumor, Ewing's tumor, and rhabdomyosarcoma (Benjamin *et al.*, 1974; Pratt *et al.*, 1972; Donaldson *et al.*, 1973; Rosen *et al.*, 1974).
Craniospinal irradiation used in conjunction with intensive chemotherapy has
contributed to the dramatic improvement in prognosis of children with acute
leukemia (Simone *et al.*, 1972). Sequential radiotherapy and combination
chemotherapy have also yielded substantial reduction in relapse rates in advanced
Hodgkin's disease which may ultimately be reflected in improvement in long-term
survival (Moore *et al.*, 1972; Prosnitz *et al.*, 1973; Rosenberg and Kaplan, 1975). As
new chemotherapeutic agents with efficacy against a variety of epithelial neoplasms become available, it seems probable that combined-modality therapy
involving combinations of radiotherapy and chemotherapy or of surgery,
radiotherapy, and chemotherapy will come into increasingly widespread use.
Such combined-modality therapy has a number of potential advantages. It may
permit effective eradication of primary tumors by either surgery or radiotherapy,
coupled with the effective treatment of micrometastases by adjunctive
chemotherapy. In addition, where chemotherapy is effective, at least in part,
against the primary neoplasm, it may permit substantial reductions of
radiotherapeutic dose, and thus sharply decrease the hazard of late tissue injury
and of significant complications.

If effective techniques of specific or nonspecific immunotherapy can be
developed, it is likely that they will also contribute significantly to the long-term
efficacy of radiotherapy, surgery, and chemotherapy. Today, we often succeed in
eradicating nearly all of the cells in a tumor, but, because of the inherent biological
characteristics of tumors, the persistence of 1% or less of the tumor cell population
is sufficient to permit repopulation and recurrence of the neoplasm. If effective
immunotherapy can eradicate that last 1% of the tumor-cell population, it will
improve long-term survival rates obtained by the surgeon, by the radiation
oncologist, and by the cancer chemotherapist. Thus it is likely that immunotherapy will play a supplementary role in the combined-modality approach.

Finally, it seems clear that the principal direction in which radiotherapists can
look for substantial improvement in the efficacy of their own modality is through a
fundamental understanding of radiobiological mechanisms. How does radiation
kill cancer cells? How does it kill normal cells? What are the factors which
determine repair and recovery of normal tissues? Is it possible to influence the
efficiency and reliability of radiotherapeutic eradication of tumor-cell

TABLE 2

Modification of Radiosensitivity

A. Increased yield of irreversible radiochemical lesions
   1. Oxygen
   2. Nitric oxide; organic nitroxides
   3. Metronidazole ('Flagyl'), nitrofurans, Ro-07-0582
   4. High-LET particulate radiations
B. Increased intrinsic sensitivity of target DNA
   1. Halogenated pyrimidine analogues (BUdR, BCdR, IUdR)
   2. Possible potentiation of BCdR by tetrahydrouridine
   3. Purine starvation
C. Inhibition of repair
   1. Hyperthermia
   2. Chemical inhibitors of single-strand-break repair (actinomycin D)
   3. High-LET particulate radiations
D. Partial synchronization in cycle-dependent sensitive states
   1. Fractionated radiotherapy timed to mitotic delay
   2. Colchicine, *Vinca* alkaloid mitotic spindle poisons
E. Differential radioprotection of normal tissues

populations? Studies of cellular and molecular radiation biology during the past 20 years have provided several rational new approaches to the exploitation of radiobiological mechanisms. Table 2 summarizes some of the possible strategies by which one might hope to modify differentially the radiation response of a tumor-cell population relative to that of a normal tissue population. It is essential that a differential effect be obtained; little would be accomplished by increasing the response of both the tumor and the normal tissues to a proportionate extent.

In the presence of oxygen, cells are approximately three times more radiosensitive than they are in its absence. Since it is believed that many tumors contain subpopulations of hypoxic clonogenic cells, the "oxygen effect" may well be clinically relevant (Gray *et al.*, 1953). A number of organic nitroxide, nitrofuran, and related chemical compounds, including the clinically available agent metronidazole (Flagyl), are stable free radicals which can act as oxygen substitutes, and which may, since they are not metabolized, diffuse into hypoxic zones of tumors to replace oxygen in the radiobiological response (Adams *et al.*, 1974; Brown, 1975a). The problem of eradicating hypoxic cells can also be approached through the use of particulate radiations of high linear energy transfer, such as neutrons (Catterall, 1974; Hussey *et al.*, 1974), π^- mesons (Fowler, 1965; Kaplan *et al.*, 1973b), or heavy ions (Tobias *et al.*, 1971), all of which are much less dependent on the presence or absence of oxygen (Barendsen, 1968). However, enthusiasm for these approaches has been dampened by the fact that radiotherapy during hyperbaric oxygen inhalation, initiated about 20 years ago by Churchill-Davidson *et al.* (1957), has not yielded substantial and unambiguous gains (Hall, 1967), probably because the oxygen effect is mitigated by the phenomenon of "reoxygenation" (Van Putten and Kallman, 1968; Suit and Schiavone, 1968; Thomlinson, 1968; Howes, 1969) whereby initially hypoxic tumor cells appear to be recruited into the oxygenated population during the intervals between successive doses of fractionated radiotherapy (Kallman, 1972).

The X-ray sensitization produced by halogenated pyrimidine analogues such as
5-bromodeoxyuridine (BUdR) is due to their incorporation into DNA, thus
changing the inherent radiosensitivity of this target macromolecule (Kaplan,
1970). The mode of action appears to involve the production of a higher yield of
nonreparable types of lesions in such substituted DNA. This approach has clinical
relevance because certain classes of tumors reside in a normal tissue environment
in which there is little cell turnover. The rate of DNA synthesis of such normal
tissues is extremely low. Thus the analogue should be incorporated into the DNA
of the tumor-cell population far more efficiently than into that of the surrounding
normal tissue, leading to differential radiosensitization. Intraarterial BUdR infusion prior to successive radiation treatments has been used in malignant gliomas
(Sano *et al.*, 1968) and osteogenic and soft tissue sarcomas (Goffinet *et al.*, 1975*a*)
with encouraging preliminary results.

The discovery some years ago that radiations produce strand breakage in the
DNA of bacteria and mammalian cells was followed by the recognition that the
more numerous single-strand breaks are highly reparable by normal enzymatic
mechanisms (McGrath and Williams, 1966; Kaplan, 1966; Town *et al.*, 1973).
These enzymatic repair mechanisms can be inhibited by chemical agents (Kaplan,
1972*b*) and by hyperthermia (Ben-Hur *et al.*, 1974). Hyperthermia has the
additional attractive feature of being particularly effective in hypoxic cells (Robinson *et al.*, 1974; Kim *et al.*, 1975). Actinomycin D, a chemical radiosensitizer which
appears to act by inhibiting repair, has significantly improved prognosis in Wilms'
tumor (D'Angio *et al.*, 1959). Continued clinical exploitation of this approach may
thus also hold very substantial promise for the future.

Mitotically active cells exposed to ionizing radiation suffer a mitotic delay in the
G_2 phase of the cell cycle, from which they escape in a partially synchronized state.
Radiosensitivity is known to fluctuate during the cell cycle, and is usually greatest
in mitosis (M) and in early S phase (Terasima and Tolmach, 1963). If one could
succeed in partially synchronizing tumor-cell populations with agents such as
colchicine, or with fractionated radiotherapy timed to sequential periods of
mitotic delay, the time of escape of the tumor-cell population from mitotic arrest
might well differ sufficiently from that of the normal-cell population to permit the
next dose of radiation to be given at strategically timed intervals (Kaplan, 1965*b*;
Brown, 1975*b*). Although this is a very attractive idea in principle, we currently
lack the methods for detecting the time of escape of tumor-cell populations from
mitotic block *in vivo*. Another situation in which unorthodox fractionation
schedules may prove advantageous involves the treatment of sarcomas, the
marked radioresistance of which may be due in large measure to the very wide
shoulders of their dose–survival curves (Reinhold, 1966; Van Putten, 1968). The
use of large dose increments and a smaller number of fractions spaced 3–4 days
apart for the treatment of osteogenic sarcomas has recently been investigated
(Goffinet *et al.*, 1975*a*).

The potentialities of high-LET particulate radiations are also under active
exploration. Fast neutrons, π^- mesons, and heavy ions have substantially different
physical and radiobiological properties than X-rays or electrons. They have a

decreased dependence on oxygen and an increased relative biological efficiency with respect to dose (Barendsen, 1968). In addition, π^- mesons have the advantage that their properties change sharply as they slow down and are captured by atoms in tissue, yielding selective increases in relative biological efficiency at depths which can be selected to match those of the tumor (Fowler, 1965). The efficiency of tumor-cell destruction should thus be differentially enhanced by the use of such radiations. However, the enormous complexity and expense of the machines required to generate clinically useful beams of π^- mesons (Rosen, 1969; Kaplan *et al.*, 1973*b*) or heavy ions (Tobias *et al.*, 1971) may be serious limiting factors in their development and application.

7. *References*

ADAMS, G. E., ASQUITH, J. C., AND WATTS, M. E., 1974, Electron-affinic sensitizers for hypoxic cells irradiated *in vitro* and *in vivo*: Current status, in: *Advances in Chemical Radiosensitization*, pp. 1–12, International Atomic Energy Agency, Vienna.

BAGSHAW, M. A., KAPLAN, H. S., AND SAGERMAN, R. H., 1965, Linear accelerator supervoltage radiotherapy. VII. Carcinoma of the prostate, *Radiology* **85**:121.

BAGSHAW, M. A., RAY, G. R., PISTENMA, D. A., CASTELLINO, R. A., AND MEARS, E. M., JR., 1975, External beam radiation therapy of primary carcinoma of the prostate, *Cancer* **36**:723.

BARENDSEN, G. W., 1968, Responses of cultured cells, tumours and normal tissues to radiations of different linear energy transfer, in: *Current Topics in Radiation Research* (M. EBERT AND A. HOWARD, eds.), pp. 295–356, North-Holland, Amsterdam.

BATHO, H. F., AND KORNELSEN, R. O., 1970, Negative pi-mesons from TRIUMF for radiobiology and radiotherapy. I. Physical aspects, *Phys. Med. Biol.* **15**:141.

BEN-HUR, E., ELKIND, M. M., AND BRONK, B. V., 1974, Thermally enhanced radioresponse of cultured Chinese hamster cells—Inhibition of repair of sublethal damage and enhancement of lethal range, *Radiat. Res.* **58**:38.

BENJAMIN, J. T., JOHNSON, W. D., AND McMILLAN, C. W., 1974, The management of Wilms' tumor: A comparison of two regimens, *Cancer* **34**:2122.

BEWLEY, D. K., AND PARNELL, C. J., 1969, The fast neutron beam from the M.R.C. cyclotron, *Br. J. Radiol.* **42**:281.

BLOCH, C., 1962, Postradiation osteogenic sarcoma: Report of a case and review of literature, *Am. J. Roentgenol.* **87**:1157.

BONURA, T., TOWN, C. D., SMITH, K. C., AND KAPLAN, H. S., 1975, The influence of oxygen on the yield of DNA double-strand breaks in X-irradiated *Escherichia coli* K-12, *Radiat. Res.* **63**:567.

BOYD, D., SCHWETTMAN, H. A., AND SIMPSON, J., 1973, A large acceptance pion channel for cancer therapy, *Nucl. Instrum. Methods* **3**:315.

BROWN, J. M., 1975*a*, Selective radiosensitization of the hypoxic cells of mouse tumors with the nitroimidazoles metronidazole and RO 7-0582, *Radiat. Res.* **64**:633.

BROWN, J. M., 1975*b*, Exploitation of kinetic differences between normal and malignant cells, *Radiology* **114**:189.

BUSCHKE, F., 1970, Radiation therapy: The past, the present, the future; Janeway lecture, 1969, *Am. J. Roentgenol. Radium Ther. Nuc. Med.* **108**:236.

CANTRIL, S. T., 1957, The contributions of biology to radiation therapy; Janeway lecture, 1957, *Am. J. Roentgenol. Radium Ther. Nuc. Med.* **78**:751.

CARBONE, P. P., KAPLAN, H. S., MUSSHOFF, K., SMITHERS, D. W., AND TUBIANA, M., 1971, Report of the Committee on Hodgkin's disease staging, *Cancer Res.* **31**:1860.

CARMEL, R. J., AND KAPLAN, H. S., 1976, Mantle irradiation in Hodgkin's disease: An analysis of technique, tumor eradication, and complications, *Cancer* **37**:2813.

CASE, J. T., 1958, History of radiation therapy, in: *Progress in Radiation Therapy* (F. BUSCHKE, ed.), pp. 1–18, Grune and Stratton, New York.

CASTELLINO, R. A., BILLINGHAM, M., AND DORFMAN, R. F., 1974, Lymphographic accuracy in Hodgkin's disease and malignant lymphoma with a note on the "reactive" lymph node as a cause of most false-positive lymphograms, *Invest. Radiol.* **9:**155.

CASTRO, L., CHOI, S. H., AND SHEEHAN, F. R., 1967, Radiation induced bone sarcomas: Report of five cases, *Am. J. Roentgenol.* **100:**924.

CATTERALL, M., 1974, A report on three years' fast neutron therapy from the Medical Research Council's cyclotron at Hammersmith Hospital, London, *Cancer* **34:**91.

CHURCHILL-DAVIDSON, I., SANGER, C., AND THOMLINSON, R. H., 1957, Oxygenation in radiotherapy. II. Clinical application, *Br. J. Radiol.* **30:**406.

COLLABORATIVE STUDY, 1969, Preoperative irradiation of cancer of the lung: Preliminary report of a therapeutic trial, *Cancer* **23:**419.

COUTARD, H., 1932, Roentgenotherapy of epitheliomas of the tonsillar region, hypo-pharynx, and larynx, *Am. J. Roentgenol.* **28:**313.

COUTARD, H., 1938, Cancer of the larynx: Results of roentgen therapy after five and ten years of control, *Am. J. Roentgenol.* **40:**509.

D'ANGIO, G. J., FARBER, S., AND MADDOCK, C. L., 1959, Potentiation of X-ray effects by actinomycin D, *Radiology* **73:**175.

DONALDSON, S. S., CASTRO, J. R., WILBUR, J. R., AND JESSE, R. H., JR., 1973, Rhabdomyosarcoma of the head and neck in children: Combination treatment by surgery, irradiation, and chemotherapy, *Cancer* **31:**26.

EARLE, J. D., BAGSHAW, M. A., AND KAPLAN, H. S., 1973, Supervoltage radiation therapy of the testicular tumors, *Am. J. Roentgenol.* **117:**653.

ELKIND, M. M., AND SUTTON, H., 1960, Radiation response of mammalian cells grown in culture. I. Repair of X-ray damage in surviving Chinese hamster cells, *Radiat. Res.* **13:**556.

ELKIND, M. M., WITHERS, H. R., AND BELLI, J. A., 1968, Intracellular repair and the oxygen effect in radiobiology and radiotherapy, in: *Frontiers in Radiation Therapy and Oncology* (J. M. VAETH, ed.), pp. 55–87, Karger, Basel.

FLETCHER, G. H., 1962, Supervoltage radiotherapy for cancers of the uterine cervix, *Br. J. Radiol.* **35:**5.

FLETCHER, G. H., 1971, Cancer of the uterine cervix: Janeway lecture, 1970, *Am. J. Roentgenol. Radium Ther. Nucl. Med.* **111:**225.

FLETCHER, G. H., AND JESSE, R. H., 1962, The contribution of supervoltage roentgenotherapy to the integration of radiation and surgery in head and neck squamous cell carcinomas, *Cancer* **15:**566.

FOWLER, J. F., MORGAN, R. L., AND WOOD, C. A. P., 1963, Pre-therapeutic experiments with the fast neutron beam from the Medical Research Council cyclotron. I. The biological and physical advantages and problems of neutron therapy, *Br. J. Radiol.* **36:**77.

FOWLER, P. H., 1965, π^- mesons versus cancer; Rutherford memorial lecture, *Proc. Phys. Soc.* **86:**1051.

FRY, D. W., HARVIE, R. B. R. S., MULLETT, L. B., AND WALKINSHAW, W., 1948, A travelling wave linear accelerator for 4-Mev. electrons, *Nature (London)* **162:**859.

GINZTON, E. L., HANSEN, W. W., AND KENNEDY, W. R., 1948, A linear electron accelerator, *Rev. Sci. Instrum.* **19:**89.

GINZTON, E. L., MALLORY, K. B., AND KAPLAN, H. S., 1957, The Stanford medical linear accelerator. I. Design and development, *Stanford Med. Bull.* **15:**123.

GLATSTEIN, E., GUERNSEY, J. M., ROSENBERG, S. A., AND KAPLAN, H. S., 1969, The value of laparotomy and splenectomy in the staging of Hodgkin's disease, *Cancer* **24:**709.

GLATSTEIN, E., McHARDY-YOUNG, S., BRAST, N., ELTRINGHAM, J. R., AND KRISS, J. P., 1971, Alterations in serum thyrotropin (TSH) and thyroid function following radiotherapy in patients with malignant lymphoma, *J. Clin. Endocrinol. Metab.* **32:**833.

GLÜCKSMANN, A., LAMERTON, L. F., AND MAYNEORD, W. V., 1957, Carcinogenic effects of radiation, in: *Cancer* (R. W. RAVEN, ed.), pp. 497–539, Butterworths, London.

GOFFINET, D. R., CASTELLINO, R. A., KIM, H., DORFMAN, R. F., FUKS, Z., ROSENBERG, S. A., NELSEN, T. S., AND KAPLAN, H. S., 1973a, Staging laparotomies in unselected previously untreated patients with non-Hodgkin's lymphomas, *Cancer* **32:**672.

GOFFINET, D. R., ELTRINGHAM, J. R., GLATSTEIN, E., AND BAGSHAW, M. A., 1973b, Carcinoma of the larynx: Results of radiation therapy in 213 patients, *Am. J. Roentgenol. Radium Ther. Nucl. Med.* **117:**553.

GOFFINET, D. R., KAPLAN, H. S., DONALDSON, S. S., BAGSHAW, M. A., AND WILBUR, J. R., 1975a, Combined radiosensitizer infusion and irradiation of osteogenic sarcomas, *Radiology* **117:**211.

GOFFINET, D. R., SCHNEIDER, M. J., GLATSTEIN, E. J., LUDWIG, H., RAY, G. R., DUNNICK, N. R., AND BAGSHAW, M. A., 1975*b*, Bladder cancer: Results of radiation therapy in 384 patients, *Radiology* 117:149.

GOFFINET, D. R., GLATSTEIN, E., FUKS, Z., AND KAPLAN, H. S., 1976, Abdominal irradiation in non-Hodgkin's lymphomas, *Cancer* 37:2797.

GRAY, L. H., CONGER, A. D., EBERT, M., HORNSBY, S., AND SCOTT, O. C. A., 1953. The concentration of oxygen dissolved in tissues at the time of irradiation as a factor in radiotherapy, *Br. J. Radiol.* 26:638.

HALL, E. J., 1967, The oxygen effect—pertinent or irrelevant to clinical radiotherapy? *Br. J. Radiol.* 40:874.

HALL, E. J., 1972, A comparison of radium and californium 252 using cultured mammalian cells: A suggested extrapolation to radiotherapy, *Radiology* 102:173.

HANKS, G. E., BAGSHAW, M. A., AND KAPLAN, H. S., 1969, Management of cervical lymph node metastasis by megavoltage radiotherapy, *Am. J. Roentgenol. Radium Ther. Nucl. Med.* 105:74.

HENSCHKE, U. K., HILARIS, B. S., AND MAHAN, G. D., 1963, Afterloading in interstitial and intracavitary radiation therapy, *Am. J. Roentgenol. Radium Ther. Nucl. Med.* 90:386.

HINTZ, B. L., FUKS, Z., KEMPSON, R. L., ELTRINGHAM, J. R., ZALOUDEK, C., WILLIAMSON, T. J., AND BAGSHAW, M. A., 1975, Results of postoperative megavoltage radiotherapy of malignant surface epithelial tumors of the ovary, *Radiology* 114:695.

HOPPE, R. T., GOFFINET, D. R., AND BAGSHAW, M. A., 1976, Carcinoma of the nasopharynx: Eighteen years' experience with megavoltage radiation therapy, *Cancer* 37:2605.

HOWARD-FLANDERS, P., 1954, The development of the linear accelerator as a clinical instrument, *Acta Radiol. Suppl.* 116:649.

HOWES, A. E., 1969, An estimation of changes in the proportions and absolute numbers of hypoxic cells after irradiation of transplanted C_3H mouse mammary tumours, *Br. J. Radiol.* 42:441.

HUSSEY, D. H., FLETCHER, G. H., AND CADERAO, J. B., 1974, Experience with fast neutron therapy using the Texas A & M variable energy cyclotron, *Cancer* 34:65.

INGOLD, J. A., REED, G. B., KAPLAN, H. S., AND BAGSHAW, M. A., 1965, Radiation hepatitis, *Am. J. Roentgenol. Radium Ther. Nucl. Med.* 93:200.

JAMSHIDI, K., AND SWAIM, W. R., 1971, Bone marrow biopsy with unaltered architecture: A new biopsy device, *J. Lab. Clin. Med.* 77:335.

JOHNSON, R. E., 1975, Total body irradiation (TBI) as primary therapy for advanced lymphosarcoma, *Cancer* 35:242.

JONES, A., 1964, Transient radiation myelopathy (with reference to Lhermitte's sign of electrical paraesthesia), *Br. J. Radiol.* 37:727.

KALLMAN, R. F., 1972, The phenomenon of reoxygenation and its implications for fractionated radiotherapy, *Radiology* 105:135.

KAPLAN, H. S., 1962, The radical radiotherapy of regionally localized Hodgkin's disease, *Radiology* 78:553.

KAPLAN, H. S., 1965*a*, Current status of radiotherapy for neoplastic disease, *Dis. Mon.* pp. 1–56.

KAPLAN, H. S., 1965*b*, Clinical potentialities of recent advances in cellular radiobiology, in: *Cellular Radiation Biology*, pp. 584–595, Williams and Wilkins, Baltimore.

KAPLAN, H. S., 1966, DNA strand scission and loss of viability after X irradiation of normal and sensitized bacterial cells, *Proc. Natl. Acad. Sci. USA* 55:1442.

KAPLAN, H. S., 1968*a*, Macromolecular basis of radiation-induced loss of viability in cells and viruses, in: *Actions Chimiques et Biologiques des Radiations* (M. HAISSINSKY, ed.), pp. 69–94, Masson, Paris.

KAPLAN, H. S., 1968*b*, Prognostic significance of the relapse-free interval after radiotherapy in Hodgkin's disease, *Cancer* 22:1131.

KAPLAN, H. S., 1970, Radiosensitization by the halogenated pyrimidine analogues: Laboratory and clinical investigations, in: *Radiation Protection and Sensitization* (H. L. MOROSON and M. QUINTILIANI, eds.), pp. 35–42, Taylor and Francis, London.

KAPLAN, H. S., 1972*a*, *Hodgkin's Disease*, Harvard University Press, Cambridge, Mass.

KAPLAN, H. S., 1972*b*, Enzymatic repair of radiation-induced strand breakage in cellular DNA and its chemical inhibition, *Radiology* 105:121.

KAPLAN, H. S., 1976, Hodgkin's disease and other human malignant lymphomas: Advances and prospects: G. H. A. Clowes Memorial lecture, *Cancer Res.* 36:3863.

KAPLAN, H. S., AND BAGSHAW, M. A., 1957, The Stanford medical linear accelerator. III. Application to clinical problems of radiation therapy, *Stanford Med. Bull.* 15:141.

KAPLAN, H. S., DORFMAN, R. F., NELSEN, T. S., AND ROSENBERG, S. A., 1973a, Staging laparotomy and splenectomy in Hodgkin's disease: Analysis of indications and patterns of involvement in 285 consecutive, unselected patients, *Natl. Cancer Inst. Monogr.* **36:**291.

KAPLAN, H. S., SCHWETTMAN, H. A., FAIRBANK, W. M., BOYD, D., AND BAGSHAW, M. A., 1973b, A hospital-based superconducting accelerator facility for negative pi-meson beam radiotherapy, *Radiology* **108:**159.

KARZMARK, C. J., AND PERING, N. C., 1973, Electron linear accelerators for radiation therapy: History, principles and contemporary developments, *Phys. Med. Biol.* **18:**321.

KARZMARK, C. J., AND RUST, D. C., 1972, Radiotherapy treatment simulators and automation: A case for their provision from a cost viewpoint, *Radiology* **105:**157.

KARZMARK, C. J., BAGSHAW, M. A., FARAGHAN, W. G., AND LAWSON, J., 1975, The Stanford "bite-block," a head-immobilization accessory, *Br. J. Radiol.* **48:**926.

KERST, D. W., 1943, The betatron, *Radiology* **40:**115.

KIM, S. H., KIM, J. H., AND HAHN, E. W., 1975, The radiosensitization of hypoxic tumor cells by hyperthermia, *Radiology* **114:**727.

KRAUT, J. W., KAPLAN, H. S., AND BAGSHAW, M. A., 1972, Combined fractionated isotopic and external irradiation of the liver in Hodgkin's disease: A study of 21 patients, *Cancer* **30:**39.

LUXTON, R., 1953, Radiation nephritis, *Q. J. Med.* **22:**215.

MARKS, J. E., DAVIS, M. K., AND HAUS, A. G., 1974, Anatomic and geometric precision in radiotherapy, *Radiol. Clin. Biol.* **43:**1.

MCGRATH, R. A., AND WILLIAMS, R. W., 1966, Reconstruction *in vivo* of irradiated *Escherichia coli* deoxyribonucleic acid; the rejoining of broken pieces, *Nature (London)* **212:**534.

MODAN, B., BAIDATZ, D., MART, H., STEINITZ, R., AND LEVIN, S. G., 1974, Radiation-induced head and neck tumours, *Lancet* **i:**277.

MOORE, M. R., BALL, J. M., JONES, S. E., ROSENBERG, S. A., AND KAPLAN, H. S., 1972, Sequential radiotherapy and chemotherapy in the treatment of Hodgkin's disease: A progress report, *Ann. Intern. Med.* **77:**1.

NICHOLSON, T. C., WALSH, P. C., AND ROTNER, M. B., 1974, Lymphadenectomy combined with preoperative and postoperative cobalt 60 teletherapy in the management of embryonal carcinoma and teratocarcinoma of the testis, *J. Urol.* **112:**109.

PAGE, V., GARDNER, A., AND KARZMARK, C. J., 1970a, Physical and dosimetric aspects of the radiotherapy of malignant lymphomas. I. The mantle technique, *Radiology* **96:**609.

PAGE, V., GARDNER, A., AND KARZMARK, C. J., 1970b, Physical and dosimetric aspects of the radiotherapy of malignant lymphomas. II. The inverted-Y technique, *Radiology* **96:**619.

PALMER, J. P., AND SPRATT, D. W., 1956, Pelvic carcinoma following irradiation for benign gynecological diseases, *Am. J. Obstet. Gynecol.* **72:**497.

PATERSON, R., 1939, Cancer from the point of view of the radiotherapist, *Br. J. Radiol.* **12:**526.

PHILLIPS, T. L., AND BUSCHKE, F., 1969, Radiation tolerance of thoracic spinal cord, *Am. J. Roentgenol. Radium Ther. Nucl. Med.* **105:**659.

POWERS, W. E., SCHNEIDER, A. K., SHUMATE, K., FOTENOS, H., AND GALLAGHER, T., 1966, Evaluation of methods of computer estimation of interstitial and intracavitary dosimetry, *Am. J. Roentgenol. Radium Ther. Nucl. Med.* **96:**59.

PRATT, C. B., HUSTU, H. O., FLEMING, I. D., AND PINKEL, D., 1972, Coordinated treatment of childhood rhabdomyosarcoma with surgery, radiotherapy, and combination chemotherapy, *Cancer Res.* **32:**606.

PROSNITZ, L. R., FARBER, L. R., FISCHER, J. J., AND BERTINO, J. R., 1973, Low-dose radiation therapy and combination chemotherapy in the treatment of advanced Hodgkin's disease, *Radiology* **107:**187.

PUCK, T. T., AND MARCUS, P. I., 1956, Action of X-rays on mammalian cells, *J. Exp. Med.* **103:**653.

RAY, G. R., PISTENMA, D. A., CASTELLINO, R. A., KEMPSON, R. L., MEARES, E., AND BAGSHAW, M. A., 1976, Operative staging of apparently localized adenocarcinoma of the prostate: Results in fifty unselected patients. I. Experimental design and preliminary results, *Cancer* **38:**73.

REGAUD, C., 1922, Influence de la durée d'irradiation sur les effets déterminées dans le testicule par le radium, *C. R. Soc. Biol.* **86:**787.

REGAUD, C., AND FERROUX, R., 1927a, Discordance des effets des rayons X, d'une part dans la peau, d'autre part dans le testicule, par le fractionnement de la dose; diminution de l'efficacité dans le peau, maintien de l'efficacité dans le testicule, *C. R. Soc. Biol.* **97:**431.

REGAUD, C., AND FERROUX, R., 1927b, Influence du "facteur temps" sur la stérilisation des linees cellulaires normales et néoplastiques par la radiothérapie, *Radiophysiol. Radiothér.* **1:**343.

REGAUD, C., COUTARD, H., AND HAUTANT, A., 1922, Contribution au traitement des cancers endolaryngés par les rayons-X, *Xth Int. Congr. Otol.*, pp. 19–22.

REIFENSCHWEILER, O., COLDITZ, J., AND VAN HOUWELINGEN, D., 1974, A neutron tube for radiation therapy, *Medicamundi* **19**:20.

REINHOLD, H. S., 1966, Quantitative evaluation of the radiosensitivity of cells of a transplantable rhabdomyosarcoma in the rat, *Eur. J. Cancer* **2**:33.

ROBINSON, J. E., WIZENBERG, M. J., AND MCCREADY, W. A., 1974, Combined hyperthermia and radiation suggest an alternative to heavy particle therapy for reduced oxygen enhancement ratios, *Nature (London)* **251**:521.

ROSEN, G., WOLLNER, N., TAN, C., WU, S. J., HAJDU, S. I., CHAM, W., D'ANGIO, G. J., AND MURPHY, M. L., 1974, Disease-free survival in children with Ewing's sarcoma treated with radiation therapy and adjuvant four-drug sequential chemotherapy, *Cancer* **33**:384.

ROSEN, L., 1969, The Los Alamos meson factory, *Sci. J.* **5A**:39.

ROSENBERG, S. A., AND KAPLAN, H. S., 1975, The management of stages I, II, and III Hodgkin's disease with combined radiotherapy and chemotherapy, *Cancer* **35**:55.

ROSNER, F., AND GRÜNWALD, H., 1975, Hodgkin's disease and acute leukemia: Report of eight cases and review of the literature, *Am. J. Med.* **58**:339.

SAMBROOK, D. K., 1964, Split-course radiation therapy in malignant tumors, *Am. J. Roentgenol. Radium Ther. Nucl. Med.* **91**:37.

SANO, K., HOSHINO, T., AND NAGAI, M., 1968, Radiosensitization of brain tumor cells with a thymidine analogue (bromouridine), *J. Neurosurg.* **28**:530.

SCHLEA, C. S., AND STODDARD, D. H., 1965, Californium isotopes proposed for intracavitary and interstitial radiation therapy with neutrons, *Nature (London)* **206**:1058.

SCHULTZ, H. P., GLATSTEIN, E., AND KAPLAN, H. S., 1975, Management of presumptive or proven Hodgkin's disease of the liver: A new radiotherapy technique, *Int. J. Rad. Oncol. Biol. Phys.* **1**:1.

SCHULZ, M. D., 1975, The supervoltage story: Janeway lecture, 1974, *Am. J. Roentgenol.* **124**:541.

SIMONE, J., AUR, R., HUSTU, H., AND PINKEL, D., 1972, "Total therapy" studies of acute lymphocytic leukemia in children: Current results and prospects for cure, *Cancer* **30**:1488.

SOLOWAY, H. B., 1966, Radiation-induced neoplasms following curative therapy for retinoblastoma, *Cancer* **19**:1984.

STERLING, T. D., PERRY, H., AND WEINKAM, J. J., 1965, Automation of radiation treatment planning. V. Calculation and visualization of the total treatment volume, *Br. J. Radiol.* **38**:906.

STEWART, J. R., COHN, K. E., FAJARDO, L. F., HANCOCK, E. W., AND KAPLAN, H. S., 1967, Radiation-induced heart disease: A study of twenty-five patients, *Radiology* **89**:302.

SUIT, H. D., AND SCHIAVONE, J., 1968, Effect of a first dose of radiation on the proportion of cells in a mouse mammary carcinoma which are hypoxic, *Radiology* **90**:325.

TERASIMA, T., AND TOLMACH, L. J., 1963, X-ray sensitivity and DNA synthesis in synchronous populations of HeLa cells, *Science* **140**:490.

THOMLINSON, R. H., 1968, Changes of oxygenation in tumours in relation to irradiation, *Front. Radiat. Ther. Oncol.* **3**:109.

TOBIAS, C. A., LYMAN, J. T., CHATTERJEE, A., HOWARD, J., MACCABEE, H. D., RAJU, M. R., SMITH, A. R., SPERINDE, J. M., AND WELCH, G. P., 1971, Radiological physics characteristics of the extracted heavy ion beams of the bevatron, *Science* **174**:1131.

TOWN, C. D., SMITH, K. C., AND KAPLAN, H. S., 1973, Repair of X-ray damage to bacterial DNA, *Curr. Top. Radiat. Res. Q.* **8**:351.

TROUT, E. D., 1958, History of radiation sources for cancer therapy, in: *Progress in Radiation Therapy* (F. BUSCHKE, ed.), pp. 42–61, Grune and Stratton, New York.

VAN PUTTEN, L. M., 1968, Tumor reoxygenation during fractionated radiotherapy: Studies with transplantable mouse osteosarcoma, *Eur. J. Cancer* **4**:173.

VAN PUTTEN, L. M., AND KALLMAN, R. F., 1968, Oxygenation status of a transplantable tumor during fractionated radiation therapy, *J. Natl. Cancer Inst.* **40**:441.

WELLER, S. A., GLATSTEIN, E., KAPLAN, H. S., AND ROSENBERG, S. A., 1976a, Initial relapses in previously treated Hodgkin's disease. I. Results of second treatment, *Cancer* **37**:2840.

WELLER, S. A., GOFFINET, D. R., GOODE, R. L., AND BAGSHAW, M. A., 1976b, Carcinoma of the oropharynx; results of megavoltage radiation therapy in 305 patients, *Am. J. Roentgenol. Radium Ther. Nucl. Med.* **126**:236.

2

Physics of Radiation Therapy

Robert J. Shalek

1. Introduction

Within 6 months after the discovery of X-rays in November 1895 by Roentgen, efforts were made to treat cancer as well as other diseases by the new rays (Brecher and Brecher, 1969). Similarly, radium was tried in the treatment of cancer and other conditions within 3 years after its discovery by Madame Curie in 1898 (Hilaris, 1975). This collaboration among medicine, science, and technology has continued essentially without interruption since. There is probably no way to measure the contribution of physics and engineering to the slow but continued improvement of cure rates in cancer therapy; however, there can be no doubt about the significance of that collaboration. These efforts have resulted in improved sources of ionizing radiation, the definition and measurement of radiation quantity and quality, and the elaboration of systems of radiation dose calculation which permit a knowledgeable application of ionizing radiation to different regions of patients of different sizes and shapes. Development of external-beam radiation treatment initiated by the discovery of X-rays and development of intracavitary and interstitial treatment initiated by the discovery of radium continue to this day.

Although a relationship among radiation dose, control of tumors, and damage of normal tissue was recognized (Strandquist, 1944; Fletcher, 1973), it was not until the general availability of machines emitting high-energy photons in the 1950s and thereafter that the rather critical dependence of clinical result and

Robert J. Shalek • Department of Physics, University of Texas System Cancer Center, Houston, Texas 77030.

radiation absorbed dose was appreciated. Prior to that time, the radiation dose which could be tolerated by the patient was often judged clinically by the skin reaction at the surface of entry; with high-energy X-rays and γ-rays, the maximum absorbed dose is beneath the surface, eliminating simple visual control and necessitating dose control by rather precise calculation or measurement. A much cited reference (Shukovsky, 1970) demonstrates a steep relationship between tumor control probability and radiation dose for T_2–T_3 lesions of the supraglottic larynx from an analysis of clinical results. A dose change of 5% results in a change of tumor control probability from 38% to 62%. This finding, which is likely true to a greater or lesser extent for treatments at other sites, places a demand for careful attention to the many steps of radiation measurement and calculation which occur between definition of the nationl radiation standards and the delivery of a prescribed absorbed dose of radiation to a tumor. During the last 7 years, information has become available on the consistency with which tumor dose prescriptions are fulfilled. The results of the review of radiation measurements and calculations at 174 institutions participating in interinstitutional clinical trials will be discussed. In addition, mention will be made of experimental radiation therapy with neutrons, π^- mesons, and heavy charged particles.

2. Measurement of Radiation

One of the earliest efforts to measure the amount of radiation was in 1903 by F. H. Williams (Brecher and Brecher, 1969). He tried to judge the exposure rate of an X-ray machine by comparing the brightness of a fluorescent screen at different distances from the X-ray target with that caused by a radium source. In the years since, of the many advances, measurement by ionization in gases has been the most important to radiation therapy. The International Commission on Radiation Units (ICRU), which was founded in 1925, has played a prominent role in defining quantities, units, and means of measurement (Taylor, 1966).

Primary radiation standards are maintained by a number of countries including France, Germany, Great Britain, and the United States. These are exposure standards defined by the number of ionizations in a mass of air which are determined from absolute measurements of electrical charge, length, and time; no reference is made to other radiation measurements. These national standards are compared at regular intervals at the Bureau International des Poids et Mesures, BIPM, in Sevres, France, and are thought to be in agreement to better than 0.5%. Other countries maintain secondary standards which are derived by radiation comparison with one of the primary standards. It is probable that some of the primary standards will be absorbed dose standards and will depend on calorimetric methods in the future. In this method, the absorbed dose or energy absorbed in a given mass of material is measured by temperature rise in a defined mass of carbon, aluminum, or lead. Calorimetry is also an absolute method which does not depend on comparison with other radiation measurements.

The dissemination of national standards to users of radiation is achieved by the comparison of field instruments with the standards in a radiation beam. A correction factor is assigned by the standardizing laboratory to the field instrument. The comparison may be between the field instrument and the national standard or a secondary standard maintained at a regional calibration laboratory. Field instruments are ionization chambers with associated charge-measuring systems which are characterized by their reproducible behavior over long periods of time. It is usual to monitor the constancy of field instruments by exposing them to radioactive sources of radiation in defined geometries at regular intervals.

3. Absorbed Dose to the Patient

The definition of quantities and units and the development of national standards and their comparison and distribution have been crucial in achieving some uniformity in the reporting of clinical results of treatment. However, the measurement of radiation emanating from a machine of a radioactive source placed on or in the patient is only the start in knowing the absorbed dose delivered to a tumor. The complications of knowing the extent of a tumor, the distortion of radiation patterns by different intermediate tissues or cavities, and the possible difference between planned and achieved treatment geometry contribute in a major way to the uncertainties in the fulfillment of dose prescription. Calculative systems based on published data have been developed. The organizations of radiotherapists and physicists, as well as the ICRU, have been instrumental in codifying and disseminating information for the measurement and calculation of radiation dose (HPA, 1969; ICRU, 1969, 1972, 1973; AAPM, 1971; Nordic, 1972; Cohen et al., 1972). In addition, most institutions maintain methods for the experimental verification of dose delivered to a patient. Thermoluminescent dosimeters (Cameron et al., 1968) have all but replaced small ionization chambers for measurements on the surface or within body cavities of the patient.

4. External Beam Therapy

X-rays, which were the first source of ionizing radiation for treatment, continue to be a major way of obtaining external beams of radiation and have since been joined by γ-rays from collimated radioactive sources. X-rays are generated when electrons which have been accelerated in a vacuum are caused to strike a target, thus losing a part of their energy as electromagnetic radiation or X-rays. The hot cathode X-ray tube invented by William Coolidge in 1913 (Brecher and Brecher, 1969) was a major step in X-ray technology which permitted the stable operation of these devices. Most of the developments since have been in the means of accelerating electrons. Electric potentials of 200–250 kV generated by transformers and rectifiers continued to be the predominant means of producing external beams until the late 1950s. At that time, cobalt-60 irradiators in large part displaced the X-ray machines then in use. Cobalt irradiators are devices which permit the withdrawal of a collimated beam of high-energy γ-rays (1.1 and 1.3 MeV) from a shielded radioactive cobalt source. These devices provide three significant advantages over the lower-energy X-rays: (1) a greater absorbed dose at depth compared to that at the maximum is achieved; (2) the maximum dose occurs beneath the skin (0.5 cm); (3) approximately equal absorbed dose results in bone, muscle, and fat for the same exposure.

At about the same time, betatrons came into clinical use. These machines accelerate electrons in a circular path through many revolutions. In present clinical betatrons, energies of 5–40 MeV are attained. The electrons may be used directly in therapy or may be allowed to strike a target generating high-energy X-rays. These X-rays are more penetrating than the γ-rays of cobalt-60 and produce greater dose at depth compared to that at the maximum. The electrons, on the other hand, have a lower penetrating capability with a lower absorbed dose to deeper regions, which renders them useful for superficial treatments. The difference in penetrating capability of these radiations is illustrated in Fig. 1.

In the late 1960s and in the 1970s, linear accelerators have become prominent as a means of obtaining electrons for therapy from 4 to 35 MeV and X-rays from 4 to 25 MeV. These devices, which are descended from radar microwave generators developed during World War II, transfer energy from microwaves to electrons in a linear wave guide. The quantity of X-rays from linear accelerators is very much greater than that from betatrons. These devices have become reliable and are becoming a major means of therapy.

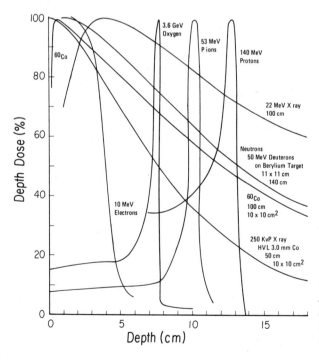

FIGURE 1. Percent depth dose vs. depth for various radiations (Cohen *et al.*, 1972; Koehler *et al.*, 1972; Tobias, 1973; Armstrong *et al.*, 1973).

The aim of radiation treatments is usually to maximize the radiation dose in the tumor volume and to limit the dose to other regions To this end, treatment by multiple beams, moving beams, or beams distorted by wedges or compensators which correct for missing tissue are employed. An example of a calculation for multiple-beam treatment is shown in Fig. 2A, and one for rotational therapy is shown in Fig. 2B. Both of these examples were calculated by computer. Programs and computers for such calculation are now in use in many parts of the world (Stovall and Shalek, 1972).

Energy is transferred to electrons when X-rays, γ-rays, or electrons interact with matter. In tissue, it is the moving electrons which cause the radiobiological effect. Electrons are spoken of as a radiation of low linear energy transfer (LET). That is, the electrons set in motion by the interaction of X-rays, γ-rays, or electrons have a low loss of energy per unit of electron track length. This physical distribution of energy along the electron path has two results of importance clinically. For the energy deposited per unit mass of tissue, there is a low relative biological effectiveness. In addition, the biological effect is greater by a factor of 2 or 3 if molecular oxygen is present in the tissue. It is for these reasons that other types of radiation are being tried in radiation therapy in the hope of increasing the radiation effect on the tumor relative to the effect on surrounding normal tissue (Hall, this volume). Some solid tumors have anoxic foci which are likely to be resistant to radiation of low linear energy transfer, such as that resulting from X-ray, γ-ray, or electron irradiation. With particles of higher linear energy transfer such as those resulting from the interaction of neutrons in tissue, or from charged particles, such as protons or other charged nuclei introduced directly into tissue, the relative radiation sensitivity of anoxic tumor cells is closer to that of normal oxygenated cells. That is, the anoxic tumor cells would more likely be destroyed in a treatment by neutrons than by γ-rays. However, the question is complex, since reoxygenation of cells takes place during protracted treatment (Denekamp and Fowler, this volume). Clinical trials are under way to determine whether neutrons confer a significant advantage over the more conventional radiation treatment (Catterall, 1971; Hussey et al., 1974). The outcome of these trials is not clear at this time.

As shown in Fig. 1, π^- mexons deliver a higher radiation dose at depth than in the tissue between the surface of entry and the depth of the peak. The depth of the peak can be controlled by altering the energy of the entering mesons. In addition to the increased dose in the treatment region, it is a dose delivered by particles of high linear energy transfer resulting from the disintegration of light nuclei by interaction with the pions near the end of the pion track. In this region, then, the absorbed dose results in a high relative biological effect, and the anoxia of some tumor cells is of reduced importance. Thus the treatment region has a higher physical dose, a higher biological effect per unit of dose, and closer response of anoxic and oxic cells than for the irradiated region between the patient's surface and the treatment region (Hall, this volume). All of these factors are favorable to treatment. A negative aspect of treatment with pions is the sharply defined beam, which implies the need for precise knowledge of the tumor location. Despite

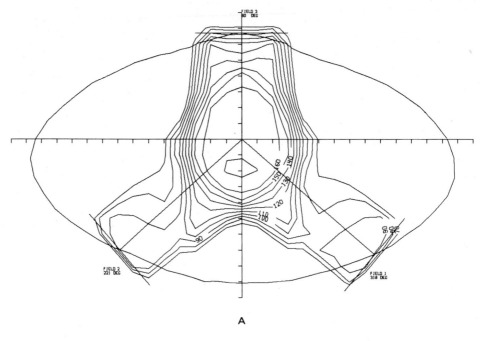

A

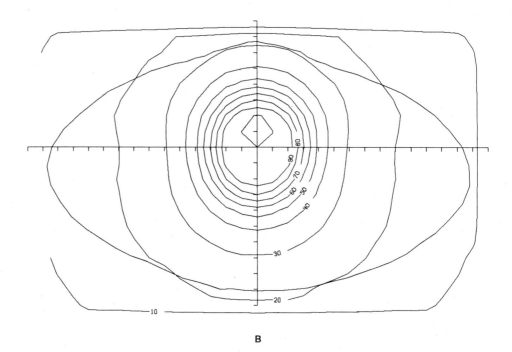

B

FIGURE 2. A: Three-field treatment with $6 \times 8 \, cm^2$ fields at 80 cm from the cobalt-60 source. The numbers represent the relative absorbed dose in the plane defined by the central rays of the treatment fields for 100 units delivered to the maximum of each field. B: Rotational treatment (360°) with a $6 \times 8 \, cm^2$ field. The axis of rotation is located 80 cm from the source. The numbers represent the relative absorbed dose for 100 units delivered to the axis.

theoretical advantages, treatment by π^- mesons will have to be tested against combinations of surgery, chemotherapy, immunotherapy, and conventional radiation therapy. At this time, only a few patients have been treated with pions, and it is too soon to comment whether this complex mode of therapy confers an advantage.

Both neutron and pion therapy require accelerating equipment which is more elaborate and expensive than X-ray or electron therapy. Neutrons for therapy are presently generated by sizable cyclotrons. Pions are generated by very much larger machines of linear or circular design. In both cases, the machines are used primarily for physics experiments unrelated to radiation therapy. In addition to the accelerators for generating these beams, the collimation, shaping, and measurement of the beams have required major effort in the solution of physical problems.

5. Brachytherapy

The delivery of a large radiation dose to a tumor and a small amount of radiation to other regions is favorable in principle. In practice, intracavitary and interstitial radioactive sources do this. This type of therapy is called "brachytherapy," a term from Greek roots meaning short-distance treatment. The sources are either placed in body cavities such as the vagina or introduced as needles directly into the tissue under treatment. By this means, high dose is achieved near the sources and the radiation dose diminishes rapidly with distance away from the sources. Between 1900 and 1920, radium sources were used effectively in the treatment of cancer. During this time, it was recognized that the distribution of radiation dose was a more important parameter of radium treatment than the total quantity of radium present, although the latter remains a consideration. In the 1930s, systems of calculation appeared which permitted the calcultion of a single dose rate representative of an interstitial implant (Quimby, 1932; Paterson and Parker, 1934). In the late 1950s (Nelson and Meurk, 1958; Shalek and Stovall, 1961), computer calculations of complete radiation distributions became available. It is likely, although probably impossible to demonstrate, that the increased information available from computer calculations has been instrumental in the improvement of treatment.

Figure 3 shows the relative absorbed dose at various distances from point sources of radium-226, cesium-137, iridium-192, iodine-125, and californium-252. Despite differences in the type and energy of radiation, the relative absorbed dose patterns from the various sources are remarkably similar. The dose diminishes sharply with distance from the source, mostly because of the geometry, which is the same for all the sources, rather than because of the absorption and scattering of radiation, which differ for the various sources. The combination of sources into arrays for treatment with the resultant distribution of radiation absorbed dose is shown in Fig. 4. An interstitial curved-plane implant is shown.

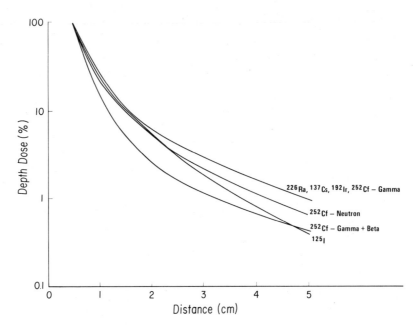

FIGURE 3. Relative absorbed dose in tissue at various distances from point sources of several radioactive isotopes. Replotted from data given by Anderson (1975).

The contour lines are lines of equal dose in the place selected for calculation. For radioactive materials other than radium, the dose distribution patterns would have been similar. Cesium-137 is a widely used substitute for radium because it is less dangerous if a source is broken, its γ-rays are more easily shielded, and it is less expensive. Iridium-192 can be fabricated into thin, flexible wires of any length which are particularly suitable for afterloading; that is, hollow applicators are installed in the patient, and the radioactive wires are installed later, after the surgical, diagnostic X-ray, and initial nursing procedures are completed. After-loading results in less radiation exposure to hospital personnel. Gold-198 and iodine-125, despite widely differing half-lives (2.9 days vs. 60 days), are used for permanent implants which are not removed from the patient. The use is analogous to radon-222 implants, which have been used for over five decades and are still employed to a limited extent. The iodine-125 has a low-energy γ-ray which is easily shielded, thus reducing the radiation exposure to hospital staff during treatments. The californium-252 delivers a mixture of γ-radiation and neutron radiation (Anderson, 1973). As discussed, the neutrons may be more effective against tumors containing anoxic foci. The use of californium-252 is experimental, and increased benefit in treatment has not been demonstrated as yet.

6. Review of Measurement and Calculation Methods

The idea of the review of radiation measurement and calculation procedures by individuals from outside an institution originated in Great Briatin (Spiers and

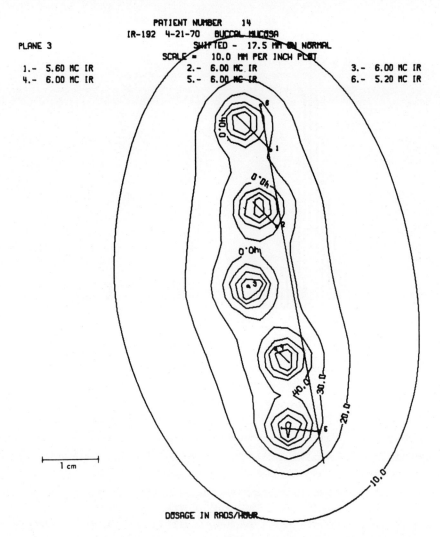

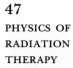

FIGURE 4. Radiation distribution in a plane perpendicular to iridium-192 interstitial sources.

Meredith, 1962). There were five centers which were successfully treating the same type of cancer patient by radiation, but were employing different prescriptions of tumor dose. A team of radiotherapists and physicists reviewed the centers and found that all of them were delivering about the same amount of radiation when differences in specifying and fulfilling the tumor dose were taken into account. Since 1968, a more massive effort has been mounted in the United States to review radiation dose measurement and calculation at institutions participating in interinstitutional clinical trials involving radiation therapy. The results of this review of 174 institutions are shown in Fig. 5. It is seen here that about 88% of the institutions fulfilled the tumor dose prescription to within ±5% as judged by the reviewing physicists. Of those which were outside ±5% agreement, the range was rather large, with the largest discrepancies falling on the side of less radiation

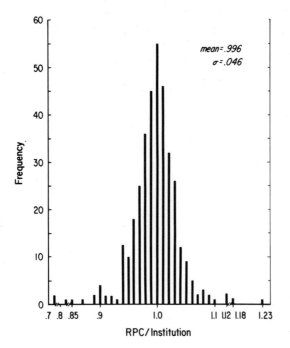

FIGURE 5. For uncomplicated treatments, the frequency of occurrence vs. the ratio of the fulfillment of tumor dose estimated by reviewing physicists to that intended by the institution.

delivered than prescribed. The Radiological Physics Center,* the organization conducting these reviews, cooperates with institutions in suggesting means of resolving discrepancies. The types of measurement and calculative errors have been discussed (Golden *et al.*, 1972). The above comments relate to systematic inconsistencies. The types of measurement and calculative errors have been discussed (Golden *et al.*, 1972). The above comments relate to systematic inconsistencies. However, the dose calculations on individual patients entered into studies are also reviewed. Both levels of review result in greater observed consistency on the part of institutions as time passes.

In the 17 clinical groups which the Radiologica Physics Center serves, there is also, in some instances, review of other aspects of diagnosis and treatment by appropriate specialists, including radiotherapy, pathology, and diagnostic radiology. This type of interaction between groups over specific technical and clinical problems undoubtedly will improve the consistency of diagnosis and treatment of cancer. These interactions may be a major, although unstated result of interinstitutional clinical trials.

7. Conclusion

This chapter has consisted of a brief presentation of the contribution of physics and engineering to radiation therapy. At this time there is intense effort to

* The Radiological Physics Center is sponsored by the American Association of Physicists in Medicine, supported in part by Grant CA10953 from the National Cancer Institute and located at The University of Texas System Cancer Center, M. D. Anderson Hospital and Tumor Institute, Houston, Texas.

improve the accuracy and detail of radiation dose calculations for X-ray, γ-ray, and electron beams. Two-dimensional calculations such as shown in Fig. 2 are usual; one can anticipate expansion to three dimensions, a method which has been demonstrated with computers but which is not now commonly practiced. Treatment with neutron beams and a radioactive neutron emitter used interstitially is under way, and π^- meson therapy has just begun. Treatment with charged heavy particles has been done on a limited scale, but will be done more extensively in the near future.

If the new particles provide an advantage in therapy, it can be anticipated that the demand for physics and engineering support will increase. On the other hand, if the role of radiation therapy in the treatment of cancer decreases or if the magnitude of treatment dose prescriptions decreases as a result of combined treatment with chemotherapy, immunotherapy, and surgery, it is possible that physics in relation to radiation therapy will become custodial, with innovation not expected. The future role of physics in cancer therapy depends on the success of clinical projects which have emerged from techniques in nuclear physics and which are now being or soon will be tested.

8. References

AAPM (American Association of Physicists in Medicine), 1971, Protocol for the dosimetry of x- and gamma-ray beams with maximum energies between 0.6 and 50 MeV, *Phys. Med. Biol.* **16**:379.

ANDERSON, L. L., 1973, Status of dosimetry for ^{252}Cf medical neutron sources, *Phys. Med. Biol.* **18**:779.

ANDERSON, L. L., 1975, Dosimetry in interstitial radiation therapy, in: *Handbook of Interstitial Brachytherapy*, (B. S. HILARIS, ed.), p. 75, Publishing Sciences Group, Acton, Mass.

ARMSTRONG, T. W., ALSMILLER, R. G., JR., AND CHANDLER, K. C., 1973, Calculation of the dose induced in tissue by negatively charged pion beams, *Phys. Med. Biol.* **18**:830.

BRECHER, R., AND BRECHER, E., 1969, *The Rays: A History of Radiology in the United States and Canada*, Williams and Wilkins, Baltimore.

CAMERON, J. R., SUNTHARALINGAM, N., AND KENNEY, G. N., 1968, *Thermoluminescent Dosimetry*, University of Wisconsin Press, Madison, Wis.

CATTERALL, M., 1971, Clinical experience with fast neutrons from the Medical Research Council's cyclotron at Hammersmith Hospital, *Eur. J. Cancer* **7**:227.

COHEN, M., JONES, D. E. A., AND GREENE, D., eds., 1972, Central Axis Depth Dose Data for Use in Radiotherapy, *Brit. J. Radiol.*, Suppl. No. 11.

FLETCHER, G. H., 1973, *Textbook of Radiotherapy*, 2nd ed., Lea and Febiger, Philadelphia.

GOLDEN, R., CUNDIFF, J. H., GRANT, W. H., AND SHALEK, R. J., 1972, A review of the activities of the AAPM Radiological Physics Center in interinstitutional trials involving radiation therapy, *Cancer* **29**:1468.

HILARIS, B. S., 1975, *Handbook of Interstitial Brachytherapy*, Publishing Sciences Group, Acton, Mass.

HPA (Hospital Physicists Association), 1969, A code of practice for the dosimetry of 2 to 35 MV x ray and caesium-137 and cobalt-60 gamma-ray beams, *Phys. Med. Biol.* **14**:1.

HUSSEY, D. H., FLETCHER, G. H., AND CADERAO, J. B., 1974, Experience with fast neutron therapy using the Texas A & M variable energy cyclotron, *Cancer* **34**:65.

ICRU, 1969, *Radiation Dosimetry: X Rays and Gamma Rays with Maximum Photon Energies between 0.6 and 50 MeV*, ICRU Report 14, International Commission on Radiation Units and Measurements, Washington, D.C.

ICRU, 1972, *Radiation Dosimetry: Electrons with Initial Energies between 1 and 50 MeV*, ICRU Report 21, International Commission on Radiation Units and Measurements, Washington, D.C.

ICRU, 1973, *Measurement of Absorbed Dose in a Phantom Irradiated by a Single Beam 9f X or Gamma Rays*, ICRU Report 23, International Commission on Radiation Units and Measurements, Washington, D.C.

50

ROBERT J.
SHALEK

KOEHLER, A. M., PRESTON, A. B., AND PRESTON, W. M., 1972, Protons in radiation therapy, *Radiology* **104**:191.

NELSON, R. F., AND MEURK, M. L., 1958, The use of automatic counting machines for implant dosimetry, *Radiology* **70**:90.

NORDIC, 1972, Procedures in radiation therapy dosimetry with 5 to 50 MeV electrons and Roentgen and gamma rays with maximum photon energies between 1 and 50 MeV, *Acta Radiol (Ther.)* **11**:603.

PATERSON, R., AND PARKER, H. M., 1934, A dosage system for interstitial radium therapy, *Br. J. Radiol.* **7**:592.

QUIMBY, E. H., 1932, The grouping of radium tubes in packs of plaques to produce the desired distribution of radiation, *Am. J. Roentgenol. Radium Ther.* **27**:18.

SHALEK, R. J., AND STOVALL, M., 1961, The calculation of isodose distributions in interstitial implantations by a computer, *Radiology* **76**:119.

SHUKOVSKY, L. J., 1970, Dose, time, volume relationships in squamous cell carcinoma of the supraglottic larynx, *Am. J. Roentgenol. Radium Ther. Nucl. Med.* **108**:27.

SPIERS, F. W., AND MEREDITH, W. J., 1972, Statement of dosage in megavoltage radiation therapy: Recommendations of the faculty of radiologists, *Clin. Radiol.* **13**:163.

STOVALL, M., AND SHALEK, R. J., 1972, A review of computer techniques for dosimetry of interstitial and intracavitary radiotherapy, *Comput. Programs Biomed.* **2**:125.

STRANDQUIST, M., 1944, Studie über die kumulative Wirkung der Röntgenstrahlen bei Fraktiomerung, *Acta Radiol. (Stockholm)*, Suppl. No. 55.

TAYLOR, L. S., 1966, Report to the International Executive Committee of the Eleventh International Congress of Radiology from the International Commission on Radiological Units and Measurements (ICRU), *Health Phys.* **12**:1375.

TOBIAS, C. A., 1973, Pretherapeutic investigations with accelerated heavy ions, *Radiology* **108**:145.

3

Molecular and Cellular Biology of Radiation Lethality

M. M. ELKIND AND J. L. REDPATH

1. Introduction

In the therapy of tumors with radiation and other cytotoxic agents, a primary objective is the differential killing of tumor cells relative to normal cells. Over the years, empirical approaches have had some success; no doubt, some additional widening of the margin between tumor and normal tissue damage can be expected from trial and error. Ultimately, to be able further to improve treatment modes, or to be able to conclude that a given mode has been optimized, a fundamental knowledge of the molecular biology of cell killing is needed.

In Part 2 of this chapter, we review the evidence, largely from studies with microorganisms, in support of DNA and/or DNA–membrane complexes as primary radiation targets. In Part 3, we focus our inquiry on mammalian cells and review the data relative to cell killing that also support DNA or DNA–membrane structures as principal targets. For this purpose damage repair studies will be emphasized both because they illustrate the importance of repair processes in radiation therapy and because they are an effective way of pursuing mechanism. Further, our objectives will be to answer specific questions and to pose hypotheses

M. M. ELKIND ● Division of Biological and Medical Research, Argonne National Laboratory, Argonne, Illinois 60439.   J. L. REDPATH ● Departments of Medical Physics and Radiation Oncology, Michael Reese Medical Center, Chicago, Illinois 60616. By acceptance of this article, the publisher or recipient acknowledges the U.S. Government's right to retain a nonexclusive, royalty-free license in and to any copyright covering the article.

about the where, what, and how of radiation lethality in mammalian cells. Consequently, rather than an overview of all the studies with mammalian cells that may have some bearing on cell killing, we restrict our attention largely to data obtained with a specific mammalian cell system in order to present an internally consistent and coherent story.

2. Radiation Lethality of Prokaryotes

2.1. Evidence Implicating DNA

The central role of DNA in cellular reproduction immediately suggests that radiation damage to this macromolecule could manifest itself in cell death. There is a vast body of evidence in the literature implying that this is so. Terzi (1961), and later Kaplan and Moses (1964), demonstrated a correlation between nucleic acid content and radiosensitivity for a variety of organisms, and Sparrow et al. (1967) observed a similar correlation between chromosome volume and radiosensitivity. The base composition of the DNA in various bacteria has been shown to influence radiosensitivity (Kaplan and Zavarine, 1962), the sensitivity decreasing with increasing adenine-thymine content. This is in contrast to the dependence on base content observed with UV-irradiated bacteria (Haynes, 1962), where the increased sensitivity can be explained by an increased rate of formation of thymine dimers. Action spectra for the effect of UV on a number of simple biological systems containing DNA have recently been shown by Setlow (1974) to correlate fairly closely with the action spectrum of DNA. The fact that bacterial mutants which are DNA repair deficient are more radiosensitive than their repair-proficient counterparts can be considered as evidence that DNA may be a critical radiation target. The increase in sensitivity to both UV and ionizing radiation that is observed when halogenated pyrimidine analogues (e.g., bromodeoxyuridine) are incorporated into the DNA of a variety of organisms supports the importance of DNA as a primary target.

2.2. DNA Lesions and Their Repair

Lesions in DNA can be classified, according to what has been measured thus far, as follows: (1) double-strand breaks, (2) single-strand breaks, (3) base damage, or (4) cross-linking of DNA to DNA or to other molecules. These may be considered to be stable lesions, the precursors of which are unstable free radicals that, in a cellular environment, play an important role in radiation damage modification by various physical and chemical agents (see Section 2.3).

Each of the DNA lesions above may conceivably contribute to cellular inactivation but are thought to do so to widely differing extents. For example, double-

strand breaks are considered by some authors to be nonreparable and therefore
lethal, whereas single-strand breaks usually are thought to be efficiently repaired.
Single-strand breaks can result from several chemical reactions, each of which
yields different end groups (Ullrich and Hagen, 1971; Ward, 1972; Emmerson,
1973; Town *et al.*, 1973*a*). Cross-links have not been studied so extensively as
strand breaks, but there is evidence from bacteriophage that cross-links have an
inactivation efficiency approaching unity (Becker *et al.*, 1977). Base damage has
been implicated in the inactivation by X-rays of bacteriophage (e.g., Blok and
Loman, 1973) and bacteria (Hariharan and Cerutti, 1972, 1974).

Studies of single-strand breaks and their repair received considerable stimulation when McGrath and Williams (1966) introduced a method for releasing DNA
from cells by subjecting them to alkaline hydrolysis (see Section 3.5 for further
discussion of the method). The DNA released in this way is denatured. Also,
breaks result from the OH^- attack of lesions that would not constitute strand
discontinuities under neutral conditions. The repair of single-strand breaks, or
alkali-labile lesions, is enzymatic in nature; radiation chemical processes that
result in the repair of free radicals are noted in the next section.

In bacterial cells, there is evidence for two types of enzymatic repair of
single-strand breaks differing in the enzymes involved, rates of reaction, and
dependence on cellular processes. The slower of the two, the one first observed by
McGrath and Williams (1966), occurs when cells are incubated under conditions
which permit growth. Completion of this repair takes approximately 60 min after
a dose of 20 krads. Recombination-deficient mutants of *Escherichia coli* K12 have
been shown to lack this type of repair process (Town *et al.*, 1973*a*); DNA ligase, an
enzyme which catalyzes the formation of covalent bonds between polynucleotides,
has been inferred to be involved (Dean and Pauling, 1970). The faster of the two
repair processes can occur in buffer and requires about 4 min following irradiation. Through the isolation of *E. coli* mutants deficient in DNA polymerase I, it
has been possible to demonstrate that this is an essential enzyme for this fast,
medium-independent, repair process (e.g., Town *et al.*, 1973*a*).

In addition to the foregoing, other enzymatic processes effective in the rapid
repair of single-strand breaks produced under anoxia have been described (Town
et al., 1973*a*; Serna and Samoylenko, 1975). However, more recent results based
on rapid lysing techniques applied to bacteriophage and bacteria (Johansen *et al.*,
1975*a,b*; Sapora *et al.*, 1975) have shown that the oxygen enhancement ratio
(OER) for single-strand breaks is about 3 even when measured within 100 msec
following irradiation in buffer at 3°C. Using *E. coli* B/r, Fox *et al.* (1976) have
shown the OER for single-strand breaks to be ~3 at 10 msec after irradiation.
These findings support a physicochemical rather than an enzymatic process
underlying the reduced efficiency of strand-break production under anoxia.
Similar conclusions were reached by Palcic and Skarsgard (1975) in studies with
two mammalian cell lines. The OER for single-strand breaks in bacteriophage
DNA has been measured to be 1.0 under conditions where chemical and/or
enzymatic repair processes would be absent (Freifelder, 1966). Consequently,
from the high OER observed under conditions which preclude an involvement of

enzymatic repair—that is, the prompt lysis of bacteria or, in the case of bacteriophage DNA, the rapid lysis of infected cells—it may be inferred that chemical repair occurs under anoxia of lesions that have the potential of producing single-strand breaks. Such repair could reflect the presence of endogenous reducing species such as sulfhydryl compounds. In contrast to the foregoing, Johansen *et al.* (1975*a,b*) demonstrated that rapid, polymerase-dependent repair of single-strand breaks was more effective when cells were irradiated under oxic vs. anoxic conditions and suggested that the lesions differed in the two cases.

Enzymatic repair of DNA double-strand breaks (dsb's) has been reported to occur in *Micrococcus radiodurans*, an extremely radioresistant bacterium (Kitayama and Matsuyama, 1968; Lett *et al.*, 1970; Burrell *et al.*, 1971). Hariharan and Hutchinson (1973) have presented evidence of the repair of double-strand breaks in X-irradiated *Bacillus subtilis*. Using ^{125}I incorporated into the DNA, Krisch *et al.* (1976) studied DNA breakage, repair, and lethality after ^{125}I decay in *rec*$^+$ and *rec*A strains of *E. coli* K12 and demonstrated significant repair of ^{125}I-induced dsb's in *rec*$^+$ but not *rec*A cells. Krasin and Hutchinson (1976) have reported repair of double-strand breaks in X-irradiated *E. coli* by a recombinational process involving a second double helix with the same base sequence. Most of the above workers have observed a 1:1 correlation between unrepaired double-strand breaks and lethality. Evidence for the repair of double-strand breaks in mammalian cells by direct measurement is conflicting (Sawada and Okada, 1970; Painter, 1970; Veatch and Okada, 1969; Lehmann and Ormerod, 1970; Horikawa *et al.*, 1970; Corry and Cole, 1973; Dugle *et al.*, 1976). Disagreements most likely reflect technical difficulties in trying to apply neutral gradient sedimentation techniques similar to those developed by McGrath and Williams (1966) for alkaline conditions. Dugle *et al.* (1976) also report that double-strand breaks are produced in proportion to the square of the absorbed dose, in contrast to the previously reported linear dose relationships (Veatch and Okada, 1969; Lehmann and Ormerod, 1970; Corry and Cole, 1973; Coquerelle *et al.*, 1973).

Interstrand DNA cross-links induced by psoralen plus light treatment of *E. coli* have been shown to be removed in wild-type strains but not in excision- or recombination-deficient strains (Cole and Sinden, 1975). Initial stages of the removal of cross-links in *E. coli* appear to be similar to those of pyrimidine dimer excision, but, because of the different nature of the intermediates produced, it is proposed that the repair process is completed by a different mechanism (Cole *et al.*, 1976). Similar studies have been made with mammalian cells by Ben-Hur and Elkind (1973*a,b*), who showed that, during incubation after exposure to psoralen plus near-UV light, approximately 90% of the covalently bound psoralen disappears from the DNA. These authors also found a correlation between cell killing and the production of cross-links.

The excision repair of damaged thymine residues—an example of repair of base damage—has been reported in bacterial (Hariharan and Cerutti, 1972, 1974; Krisch, 1976) and in mammalian (Mattern *et al.*, 1973) cells, including human lung and skin fibroblasts (Remsen *et al.*, 1976).

Since DNA lesion production and radiation-induced cellular lethality are the results of both direct and indirect effects of radiation, both of these aspects of radiation effects are important in any consideration of physical and chemical modification of radiation damage.

Indirect effects are the result of the reactions of free radicals, created by energy absorption primarily in the intracellular water, with critical target molecules. The damaging free radicals can be either the primary water radicals or secondary radicals formed by reaction of the primary radicals with noncritical cellular components.

The primary water radicals are the hydroxyl radical, OH; the hydrated electron, e_{aq}^-; and the hydrogen atom, H. Of the primary radicals, the hydroxyl radical has been inferred as damaging in a wide variety of biological systems, e.g., DNA (Achey and Duryea, 1974), enzymes (Adams *et al.*, 1972), bacteriophage (Powers and Gampel-Joppagy, 1972), bacterial spores (Powers, 1972), bacteria (Johansen and Howard-Flanders, 1965), and mammalian cells (Chapman *et al.*, 1973). Roots and Okada (1972) have shown OH radicals to play a major role in radiation-induced single-strand break production in mammalian cells. Bonura and Smith (1976) have shown that a significant number of DNA double-strand breaks in irradiated *E. coli* can be suppressed if cells are irradiated in the presence of glycerol; these data probably indicate that OH radicals normally contribute to double-strand breakage. There is evidence that secondary radicals can also interact with DNA in a lethal fashion in bacteriophage (DeJong *et al.*, 1972; Becker *et al.*, 1976).

Direct effects are the result of direct absorption of the ionizing radiation in the critical target molecule. The relative contributions of direct and indirect effects to cellular lethality are still not clearly established but have been estimated at 60% indirect and 40% direct in X-irradiated aerobic mammalian cells (Chapman *et al.*, 1973).

A further parameter of importance to any discussion of physical and chemical modification of radiation damage is time. The time scale for radiobiological events is given in Table 1, from which one can see that a vast range is covered.

TABLE 1
Time Scale for Radiobiological Events

Time interval (sec)	Events
1×10^{-18} to 1×10^{-14}	Energy deposition and ionization
1×10^{-14} to 1×10^{-10}	Formation of primary water radicals
1×10^{-10} to 1×10^{-1}	Primary and secondary radical reactions leading to target lesion production
1×10^{-1} to 1×10^{4}	Enzymatic repair of target lesions
1×10^{2} to 1×10^{6}	Expression of cellular functions

M. M. ELKIND
AND
J. L. REDPATH

2.3.1. *Effect of Dose Rate*

Dose rate is a physical parameter of considerable importance in radiobiology (e.g., Fox and Nias, 1970; Hall, 1972). In recent years, a considerable body of new data using ultra-high dose rates has been published for both prokaryotic and eukaryotic systems. These experiments have been directed toward determining the lifetime of the oxygen-sensitive species in cellular radiobiology. Experiments dealing with the transient nature of this species are discussed here; more general questions relative to the sensitization due to oxygen are discussed in 2.3.3.

Epp and co-workers (see Epp *et al.*, 1976) employed high-tensity pulsed irradiation techniques resulting in average dose rates as high as $\sim 1 \times 10^{12}$ rads/sec. At high dose rates, the radiation chemical depletion of O_2 occurs faster than the diffusion of oxygen back to the critical oxygen-sensitive site(s). The result is that the survival curves obtained in this manner have an initial oxic-type response with dose that goes over to an anoxic response as was originally observed by Dewey and Boag (1959). The dose at which the transition occurs is dependent on the initial oxygen tension, as is evidenced by the experiment of Epp *et al.* (1968) illustrated in Fig. 1. Such curves have also been obtained for mammalian cells (Town, 1967; Nias *et al.*, 1969; Berry *et al.*, 1969; Epp *et al.*, 1972).

Using a double-pulse technique, Epp and co-workers have been able to irradiate bacteria with a first dose large enough to deplete the oxygen and then with a second dose, at various short intervals, in the presence of different oxygen tensions. From measurements of the response to the second dose and a knowledge of the diffusion characteristics of oxygen, they were able to estimate an upper limit

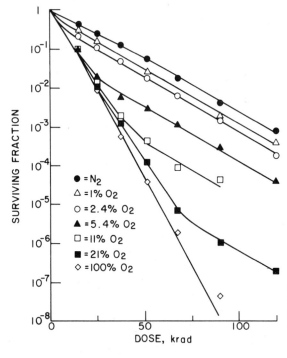

FIGURE 1. Survival curves for *Escherichia coli* B/r irradiated with single 30-nsec pulses of electrons after equilibration with various concentrations of oxygen. Courtesy of Epp *et al.* (1968).

of 0.1 msec for the lifetime of the oxygen-sensitive species in *E. coli* B/r and

Serratia marcescens. This value is lower than the value of 0.5 msec obtained by Michael *et al.* (1973) using a rapid-mixing technique; this is a discrepancy as yet unresolved. Precise information is at present unavailable on the lifetime of oxygen-dependent damage in irradiated mammalian cells. However, an upper limit of ~5 msec may be inferred from the rapid-mixing studies of Shenoy *et al.* (1975a) using Chinese hamster V79 cells.

All the preceding experiments employed cell death as an end point; more than likely, similar data for DNA lesions will become available in due course. Some preliminary data are already available from rapid-mixing studies of suspensions of Chinese hamster V79 cells, sensitization by a factor of 1.6 for single-strand break production being observed when O_2 was added 7 msec after irradiation; a factor of 1.1 was observed if the addition of O_2 was delayed for 50 msec (Agnew *et al.*, 1975). These data are in contrast with those relative to cell death since a factor of 1 was observed if the addition of O_2 was delayed for >5 msec. Discrepancies such as this put in question a close connection between single-strand breaks and lethality, as discussed further in Section 3.9 (see Adams, this volume, for further discussion of the oxygen effect).

2.3.2. Effect of Linear Energy Transfer (LET)

The variation of radiobiological effectiveness of radiations with different rates of linear energy deposition is a subject of considerable practical and theoretical interest (see also Hall, this volume, for a discussion of LET effects). We confine our attention here to the variation of yields of DNA lesions with LET and correlations of such variations with lethality.

The parameter LET is used to describe beams of different radiation quality and is the energy transferred per unit length of track of the ionizing particles; the units frequently used are kilo electron volts per micrometer in unit-density material. If monoenergetic beams are used, track-segment irradiations of cells permit a fairly precise specification of LET. However, many radiation beams consist of particles having a wide spectrum of energies and therefore they can be specified only by some type of average LET. In spite of inherent shortcomings in the use of average LET values, they are widely used to describe radiation quality when intercomparing biological effectiveness.

Most measurements of yields of DNA damage in relation to function have involved DNA extracted from bacteriophage, or the whole bacteriophage. As noted in Section 2.2, four types of DNA lesions have been measured: double-strand breaks, single-strand breaks, cross-links, and nucleotide damage. The relative proportions of these lesions depend on the irradiation conditions, e.g., dilute solution or broth, protectors present or absent. Christensen *et al.* (1972) measured the dependence of the various types of DNA damage on LET for the RF-DNA of bacteriophage ϕX174 irradiated under conditions of predominantly direct action. A summary of their data is shown in Fig. 2; relative contributions of different lesions to inactivation are given in Table 2.

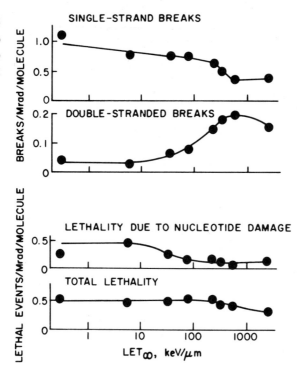

FIGURE 2. Dependence of DNA damage and survival in bacteriophage ϕX174 on linear energy transfer. Courtesy of Barendsen (1974), after the data of Christensen *et al.* (1972).

TABLE 2

Relative Contributions of DNA Lesions to the Inactivation of RF-DNA from Bacteriophage ϕX174 Irradiated under Conditions of Predominantly Direct Action[a]

Radiation	LET (keV/μm)	Lesion	Relative contribution to inactivation
$^2H^{+1}$	5.8	Single-strand breaks	<0.05
		Double-strand breaks	0.07
		Nucleotide damage	0.9
$^{16}O^{+8}$	550	Single-strand breaks	0.3
		Double-strand breaks	0.5
		Nucleotide damage	0.2

[a] From Christensen *et al.* (1972).

Neary *et al.* (1970, 1972) studied the influence of radiation quality and oxygen tension on strand breakage using dry DNA. Their results show that: (1) on the average, one strand break is produced for each energy-loss event; (2) about one in 20 energy-loss events produces a double-strand break; (3) there is only a minor increase of single- and double-strand breaks up to ~ 100 keV/μm; (4) at larger values, the efficiency of production of both types of breaks increases more markedly; and (5) there is no significant effect of oxygen on the production of either single- or double-strand breaks.

The observations of Christensen *et al.* (1972) and of Neary *et al.* (1970, 1972) show little or no increase in double-strand break production with LETs up to

100 keV/μm. This is in contrast to cell killing, which peaks at 20 keV/μm for

bacteria and 100 keV/μm for mammalian cells. Thus it would appear that the
LET dependence of cell killing cannot be attributed mainly to double-strand-
break induction. Judging from the results in Fig. 2, it is even difficult to correlate
any particular DNA lesion with loss of function.

Munson *et al.* (1967) studied the dependence of radiosensitivity on LET with *E.
coli* strains of differing repair capacities. They showed that the radiosensitivity of
repair-proficient (i.e., radioresistant) strains increase with LET to a peak at
~20 keV/μm and then decreased, presumably due to "overkill." On the other
hand, the repair-deficient strains, while always more sensitive than the proficient
strains, showed no increase of radiosensitivity with LET up to 20 keV/μm; above
this value, a decrease was again observed. Thus, in accord with the LET dependence of mammalian cell killing (see Hall, this volume), at maximally effective
LETs repair processes in bacteria are less effective, just as the repair of sublethal
damage (see Section 3.1) becomes minimal in mammalian cells at maximally
effective LETs. Qualitatively, therefore, the results of Munson *et al.* (1967) suggest
that in bacteria there are at least two types of damage: a LET-dependent type, the
repair of which is minimal at maximally effective LETs, and a LET-independent
type that characterizes repair deficient cells. (A further development of these
ideas is to follow presently.)

2.3.3. Oxygen Sensitization

The effect of radiation on living cells is usually enhanced by the presence of
oxygen. The radiation dose required to produce a given effect is about 3 times
greater for hypoxic than for oxic or aerobic cells (see Table 4). This enhancing
factor, called the "oxygen enhancement ratio" (OER), is usually independent of
level of survival for a given type of radiation. The dependence of survival on
oxygen tension is a factor of considerable importance in the radiation treatment of
tumors which may contain cells under a range of oxygen tensions.

Many studies have been carried out to determine the concentration dependence of the oxygen effect in both bacterial and mammalian cells (see Adams, this
volume). The results from both cell types lead to essentially the same answer,
namely, that the concentration of oxygen required to produce a full sensitization is
~2% (~30 μM). The concentration to produce one-half of a full effect, often
referred to as the *K* value (Alper and Howard-Flanders, 1956; Alper *et al.*, 1967),
is somewhat dependent on dose rate, method of irradiation, and LET of the
radiation but is in the range of 0.1–0.7% (1.5–10.5 μm). The concentration of
oxygen in venous blood or lymph is in the range 2.5–5%; therefore, most normal
tissues have oxygen tensions in excess of that required for full sensitization.

In order to exert its sensitizing effect, oxygen must be present during delivery of
the radiation dose. Addition of oxygen even a few milliseconds after irradiation is
less than fully effective. This means that oxygen must interact with a short-lived
lesion on a critical target or with a short-lived species that can interact with a
critical target (see Section 2.3.1).

From Table 3, it may be seen that the OER for single-strand breaks is equal to, or close to, unity for DNA from organisms possessing no repair ability (i.e., bacteriophage B3) or for repair-proficient cells whose repair capability has been compromised by various treatments (e.g., heat in the case of *E. coli* K12 *pol*A1, EDTA in the case of *M. radiodurans*). For repair-proficient bacteria or for bacteriophage irradiated intracellularly, the OER for single-strand-break production is in the range of 2.8–3.3. The OER for lethality in such organisms is similar (e.g., Town *et al.*, 1973*b*). In spite of the foregoing correlation, the connection is not a strong one between single-strand breaks and cell killing. For example, at a 10% survival level, the dose required for *E. coli* K12 *pol*A1 is 2 krads (Town *et al.*, 1973*b*), whereas for *M. radiodurans* it is ~400 krads (Dean and Alexander, 1962), yet the yield of single-strand breaks is about the same in both cases (see Table 3).

In regard to double-strand breaks, however, the correlation with OER and survival is quite good, at least in the instance of *E. coli* K12 W3110. Bonura *et al.* (1975) observed 1.3–1.4 double-strand breaks per D_0 (mean lethal dose) under both oxic and hypoxic conditions; the OERs for strand breakage (Table 3) and survival are almost the same. Thus, in this instance, the implications follow that ~1 double-strand break kills a cell, that double-strand breaks are not repaired, and, since a contribution to break formation probably comes from indirect action (Bonura and Smith, 1976), that both direct and indirect action are affected by oxygen equally.

While the exact mechanism of the oxygen effect is not fully understood, the "repair-fixation" hypothesis of Howard-Flanders (1960) still has general validity. Simply stated, according to this hypothesis, oxygen competes with endogenous

TABLE 3

Effect of Oxygen on the Yield of Single- and Double-Strand Breaks in Various Organisms When Irradiated with Low-LET Radiation

| Organism | Lesion | G-value[a] | | OER[b] | Reference |
		O$_2$	N$_2$		
Bacteriophage B3	Single-strand breaks	4.3	4.3	1.0	Freifelder (1966)
Bacteriophage B3 + histidine (10^{-3} M)		2.5	2.5	1.0	Freifelder (1966)
M. radiodurans + EDTA (2×10^{-3} M)		2.0	2.0	1.0	Dean *et al.* (1969)
E. coli K12 *pol*A1 (52°C pretreatment)		1.76	1.23	1.4	Town *et al.* (1972)
Bacteriophage λ in *E. coli* λ		1.4	0.5	2.8	Boyce and Tepper (1968)
Bacteriophage λ in *E. coli* λ		4.1	1.3	3.2	Johansen *et al.* (1971)
E. coli K12 *pol*A1		1.47	0.44	3.3	Town *et al.* (1972)
M. radiodurans		2.0	0.67	3.0	Dean *et al.* (1969)
E. coli K12 W3110	Double-strand breaks	0.19	0.08	2.4	Bonura *et al.* (1975)

[a] G-value = breaks/100 eV absorbed directly by the DNA.
[b] OER = G_{O_2}/G_{N_2}.

TABLE 4

Rough Correlations among RBE, OER, and Sensitivity to Ultraviolet and Ionizing Radiation for a Series of Strains of E. coli[a]

Strain of E. coli	Anoxic D_0,[d] X-rays (krads)	OER	Relative UV dose, 1% survival	RBE, aerobic $\left(\dfrac{D_0, \text{X-rays}}{D_0, \text{neutrons}} \right)$
B_{2-12}	2.43	1 to 1.2*	1	1.0
B_{S-1}	2.78	1.77	2.4	1.05
K12, AB 2463	2.77	2.08		1.06
B_{S-2}	3.91	2.35	16	
B^b	5.64	2.54		1.17
B_{S-8}	7.5	2.12	15	
B_{S-3}	10.6	2.51	13.1	1.36
B^c	10.3	3.20	137	1.44
B–H	18.8	3.34	160	1.53
B/r	20.8	3.19	200	1.54
K12, AB 1157	20.5	3.52		1.52

[a] From Alper (1971). RBE, relative biological effect; OER, oxygen enhancement ratio.
[b] Incubated at 18°C **after** irradiation.
[c] Incubated at 44°C after irradiation.
[d] D_0, the dose that reduces survival by $1/e$ along the exponential part of a curve.

reducing agents, e.g., sulfhydryls, for a lesion on the target, or an activated intermediate near the target, both being almost certainly free radicals:

$$\text{RH} \overset{x}{\rightsquigarrow} \cdot \text{R}$$

$$\cdot \text{R} + \text{O}_2 \rightarrow \cdot \text{RO}_2 \qquad \text{lethal, lesion fixation}$$

$$\cdot \text{R} + \text{XSH} \rightarrow \text{RH} \qquad \text{nonlethal, lesion repair}$$

$$\cdot \text{R} + \cdot \text{R} \rightarrow \text{RH} + \cdot \text{R}' \qquad \text{partially lethal}$$

For bacteriophage or isolated infectious DNA, the OER for inactivation is generally unity, and in some instances oxygen can even have a small protective effect. Howard-Flanders (1960) showed that if such DNA is irradiated in the presence of a sulfhydryl, an OER of the order of 1.5 is observed. More recently, Van Hemmen *et al.* (1974*a,b*) have shown that irradiation in the presence of cell components other than sulfhydryls can impart an oxygen effect of about the same magnitude, ~ 1.5. However, as pointed out by Alper (1970), the OER for cell survival is generally greater than 1.5 and usually ~ 3 (see Table 4). From this and other evidence to follow, she developed the idea that DNA cannot be the sole target involved in the enhanced lethality due to oxygen.

2.4. DNA–Membrane Targets

On the basis of a variety of radiobiological observations, mainly on bacterial systems, Alper (1963*a,b*, 1970, 1971, 1974) has proposed that DNA as such is only one of two important sites of primary damage; a DNA–membrane target is the second site and the one at which the radiosensitization by oxygen mainly occurs. Alper has designated events that are associated with DNA as "type N" and those associated with the DNA-membrane targets as "type O," with the idea that lesions at both sites could interact to cause cell death. Alper further proposed that the probability that a type-O event would result in lethality is appreciably enhanced by the presence of oxygen during irradiation, whereas the OER for type-N events is small, 1–1.5. Some of the observations on which Alper's hypothesis is based are the following: (1) the low OER for the inactivation of DNA, compared to cell inactivation, even in the presence of radioprotectors such as sulfhydryl compounds (as discussed in Section 2.3.3); (2) the positive correlation between the sensitivity to ultraviolet (UV) light, the sensitivity to X-rays of cells under hypoxia, the magnitude of the OER, and the magnitude of the relative biological effectiveness (RBE) for radiations of increasing LET; and (3) the effect of DNA repair inhibitors on damage registration in bacteria irradiated in the presence and in the absence of oxygen. As mentioned in Section 2.1, the UV killing of cells correlates very closely with DNA being the critical target. Table 4 shows that repair-deficient bacteria exhibit a high UV sensitivity (i.e., a low 1% survival dose), have a high X-ray sensitivity (i.e., small D_0) under anoxia, and have low OERs. These observations are consistent with type-N damage being dominant in such cells. In contrast, UV-resistant strains of bacteria are X-ray resistant under anoxia and exhibit high OER values; this implies a dominant role for type-O damage. Table 4 also shows that the OER values for X-rays directly correlate with aerobic RBEs. This suggests that the increase in effectiveness with linear energy transfer reflects a greater contribution of type-O damage to cell killing (see Section 2.3.2, and the discussion of the results of Munson *et al.*, 1967, therein).

Further support for Alper's two-target model comes from bacterial studies with sensitizers. Using *E. coli* B/r and the repair inhibitor acriflavin, Alper (1963*b*) showed that the postirradiation sensitization of hypoxically irradiated cells was greater than that of cells irradiated in the presence of oxygen. Since acriflavin is known to intercalate between complementary base pairs in DNA, this supports the idea that type-N, or DNA, damage is dominant under hypoxia.

In addition to the foregoing, other more general observations point to the DNA–membrane as an important target. A major component of cellular membranes is lipid, a material which is particularly sensitive to radiation damage in the presence of oxygen (Tappel, 1973; Demopoulos, 1973). Further, there is evidence for an attachment site of DNA and RNA to the cell membrane of bacteria (Jacob *et al.*, 1966; Marvin, 1968; Lark, 1972), and it has been shown that the site of attachment of DNA to the membrane is the location at which DNA replication is initiated and at which old and new DNA strands separate. It is therefore apparent that such a site would be a unique target for radiation damage. Watkins (1970) used lysosome preparations as models with which to study radiation damage to membranes. By monitoring the release of enzymes as a measure of radiation effect, he observed OER values of 5 and greater depending on the enzyme studied. These values are consistent with type-O damage, i.e., a large OER for membrane-associated damage. An interesting further observation, of possible

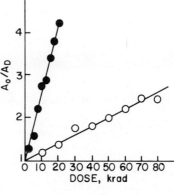

FIGURE 3. Relative amounts of DNA synthesized by DNA–membrane complexes, isolated from irradiated bacteria, plotted against dose (OER = 8). A_0/A_D represents the total amount of DNA synthesized by membrane complexes isolated from unirradiated bacteria (A_0) divided by total amount of DNA synthesized by membrane complexes isolated from irradiated bacteria (A_D); 40 min after irradiation. ●, air gassing; ○, N_2 gassing. Courtesy of Cramp *et al.* (1972).

significance to cellular studies, was the increase in yield of solubilized enzymes from anoxically and oxically irradiated lysosomes with time after irradiation. This effect would not be inconsistent with a postirradiation peroxidation phenomenon similar to that observed by Wills and Wilkinson (1967) with other systems.

The bacterial DNA–membrane complex has been shown to be a radiosensitive site, particularly in the presence of oxygen. This and other evidence of membrane involvement in radiation-induced cellular lethality have come from a variety of approaches. For instance, Cramp *et al.* (1972) studied the effect of ionizing radiation on the DNA-synthetic ability of DNA–membrane complexes isolated from *E. coli* B/r and found an OER of approximately 8 (Fig. 3). This is considerably higher than the OER for intact *E. coli* B/r, that is, an OER of 2–3 depending on the particular experimental conditions.

Petkau and colleagues (Petkau and Chelack, 1974; Chelack *et al.*, 1974) studied the radiobiology of the mycoplasm *Acholeplasma laidlawii* B for indications of membrane involvement. Although this organism does not have a cell wall or an internal membrane, it does have a well-characterized cytoplasmic membrane. Observations of the radioprotection of this organism by cysteine permitted the demonstration that a quantitative relationship exists between the rate of cell inactivation and the sulfhydryl content of the cell membrane. This supports the idea that an important radiation target is located in the membrane in this particular case.

Yet another indication of a relation between altered radiosensitivity and membrane modification has been reported by Shenoy *et al.* (1974, 1975b) and George *et al.* (1975) working with *E. coli* B/r. They correlated the anoxic radiosensitizing effectiveness of the anesthetic procaine HCl with its membrane-interactive properties. The use of membrane-interactive drugs as radiosensitizers has also been explored by Redpath and Patterson (1976). They found the surfactant cetylpyridinium chloride, which contains both a strongly electron-affinic head group and a lipid-directing hydrocarbon chain, to be a potent radiosensitizer of the bacterium *S. marcescens*. Other compounds containing only one of the two moieties were shown to be totally ineffective under comparable conditions. These data have potential importance from clinical radiotherapy of the head and neck region, in that cetylpyridinium chloride is an active ingredient of many mouth-washes and could radiosensitize the oral mucosa.

3. Radiation Lethality of Mammalian Cells

3.1. Damage and Repair Related to Survival

3.1.1. Sublethal Damage

The first mammalian cell survival curve is of interest for historical reasons but also because it set the stage, technically and conceptually, for a number of the advances that followed. In 1956, Puck and Marcus published Fig. 4, the single-cell survival curve of HeLa S3 cells exposed to graded doses of 250 kVp X-rays. This curve had several features of interest. First, in contrast to results with bacteria and yeasts (repair-deficient microorganisms were not known at that time), HeLa cells were very sensitive. The survival curve for doses larger than 125 R, is exponential and is specified by a slope whose reciprocal, D_0, is quite small, about 100–150 R (see caption, Fig. 4). D_0 doses for bacteria were known to be 50–100 times larger. Second, the curve has a shoulder; that is, for small doses the curve bends continuously before becoming exponential (i.e., straight on a semilog plot). Third, the extrapolation number, n, the back-extrapolate to the ordinate of the exponential part of the curve, is 2. It soon became apparent that an association of this last value with a hit multiplicity for cell killing (e.g., two-hit chromosome aberrations) was not justified. Nevertheless, the fact that n was not much larger than unity

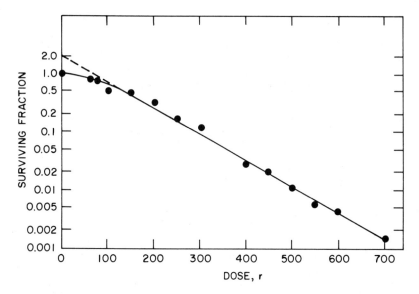

FIGURE 4. Survival curve of HeLa S3 cells (250 kVp X-rays, 100–200 R/min). The dose axis is in units of the roentgen, which, for present purposes, is not significantly different from the unit of absorbed dose, the rad. Courtesy of Puck and Marcus (1956).

implied that HeLa S3 cells had only a small ability to accumulate sublethal damage, in contrast to other cells (see Fig. 5).

With respect to the apparent great sensitivity of HeLa cells—which, in terms of D_0 doses, turned out to be fairly typical of mammalian cells in general—we will comment further in a later section. As for the shoulder or threshold on the survival curve, this led to a line of reasoning in respect to sublethal damage, followed by experimental verification, which was also found to be general for mammalian cells and which we now summarize.

Recognizing that a threshold implies killing as a result of a damage accumulation process, and therefore that a surviving cell is a sublethally damaged cell, Elkind and Sutton (1959, 1960) assumed that: (1) what was true for HeLa cells would apply to other cells as well—for example, to the Chinese hamster cells with which they were working; (2) surviving cells would repair their sublethal damage so that their progeny would not inherit an enhanced radiosensitivity; and (3) the repair of sublethal damage is rapid and might be completed before the first division following irradiation.

3.1.2. Repair of Sublethal Damage, Asynchronous Cells

An example of repair of sublethal damage is shown in Fig. 5. The circles trace the single-dose survival curve, which, although similar in shape to that for HeLa S3 cells, shows a broader shoulder; i.e., $n = 6.8$ and $D_q = 260$ rads, where D_q, the quasi-threshold dose, is the dose intercept of the back-extrapolate of the exponential part of the survival curve. To test for sublethal damage repair, a dose fractionation technique was used. A first dose of 505 rads, followed by graded second doses 2.5 hr later, gave the open squares; 23 hr following the 505 rads, the closed squares were obtained. If the 13% of cells surviving the first dose did not repair their sublethal damage, the fractionation survival curves would be expected to be superimposed on the single-dose survival curve for doses larger than 505 rads. Division in the fractionation interval could, of course, confuse the issue. A first dose of 505 rads confers a delay in division on surviving cells of about 5 hr (Elkind *et al.*, 1963) so that the 2.5-hr curve is not influenced by division. By 23 hr, surviving cells would have divided once. Other factors aside, division could have contributed about a factor of 2 increase in the apparent extrapolation number (because with surface-attached cells, two cells would have to be inactivated to suppress colony formation), and, consequently, division alone is inadequate to explain the value of 6.5 observed. In addition to division, however, there is the partial synchronization that results from the first dose. Because of this, it is not possible to assess the degree of repair by 23 hr, since surviving cells may have reassorted themselves throughout the cell age cycle in a manner different from their original age distribution. (The relevance of this reservation is evident from the material to follow.)

A further complication in the interpretation of dose fractionation data is seen in Fig. 6. Here, the variation in net survival is traced when a given total dose is fractionated. Cells incubated at 37°C (in complete medium) between dose fractions show a pronounced minimum in their two-dose response. The absence of a minimum when cells were at room temperature led to the inference that the two-dose response of asynchronous cells, under conditions that support cell aging and division as well as sublethal damage repair, is due to the combined effects of repair plus progression or cell aging (Elkind *et al.*, 1964*b*; Elkind and Sinclair, 1965). It was reasoned that, since cell aging and division are essentially eliminated at room temperature, the minimum in the curve for 37°C is due to first-dose survivors progressing from a resistant phase—in which they must have been in order to be survivors of the first dose—to a sensitive phase corresponding to the trough. The prompt rise in survival in Fig. 6 is due to repair, and, since the rise is evident even at room temperature, it is clear that repair is appreciably less temperature dependent than cell aging. Further discussion of this point follows.

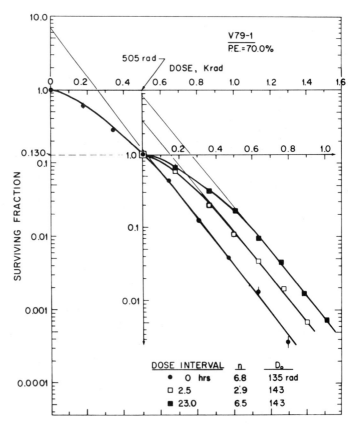

FIGURE 5. Tests for repair of sublethal X-ray damage using asynchronous V79-1 Chinese hamster cells and dose fractionation (50 kVp X-rays, 722 rads/min). The circles trace the single-dose survival curve. The squares refer to dose fractionation; a first dose of 505 rads at 0 time is followed by graded second doses at 2.5 hr and 23 hr. P.E. stands for plating efficiency. From Elkind and Sutton (1960).

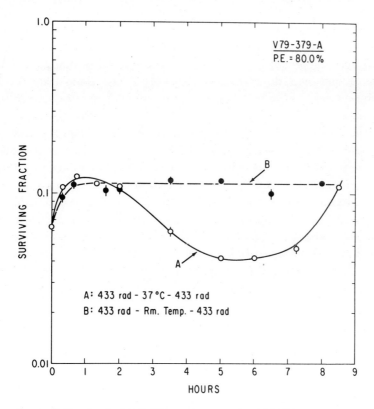

FIGURE 6. Repair of sublethal X-ray damage using V79 Chinese hamster cells, clone V79–379-A (50 kVp X-rays, 722 rads/min). Curve A, cells incubated at 37°C in complete medium between two 433-rad dose fractions; curve B, the same as A except for room temperature (~24°C) between dose fractions. From Elkind *et al.* (1964*a*).

3.1.3. *Repair of Sublethal Damage, Synchronous Cells*

Confirmation of the foregoing comes from studies with synchronized V79 Chinese hamster cells. Sinclair and Morton (1964, 1965) showed: (1) that V79 cells vary in their response to an acute X-ray dose depending on their cell-cycle age; (2) that because of the short G_1 period of these cells, their age–response pattern has a single maximum located in late S; and (3) that the two-dose response of late-S cells at 37°C indicates the effects of both repair and cell aging (see also Elkind and Sinclair, 1965; Elkind *et al.*, 1967*c*).

The foregoing is illustrated in Figs. 7, 8, and 9 from a study by Elkind *et al.* (1966). Using the technique of hydroxyurea treatment to kill cells initially in S and to gather the remainder of an initially asynchronous population at the G_1–S border, the age–response patterns following 542 rads and 1083 rads are traced in Fig. 7. Zero hours corresponds to the G_1–S border, and maximum survival occurs in the latter half of the S phase (Sinclair and Morton, 1964, 1965). The closed squares show that if at $3\frac{1}{2}$ hr the 37°C medium is replaced by 24°C buffer, the cells become progressively more sensitive (1083 rads) even though their aging is apparently stopped (542 rads, no minimum in the curve).

Figure 8 shows the result of dose fractionation sequences started at $3\frac{1}{2}$ hr. For cells in medium at 37°C between dose fractions, the shape of the two-dose curve is similar to that for asynchronous cells (e.g., Fig. 6) and to that for cells at room temperature between dose fractions. Consequently, these data confirm the interpretation that (1) the fractionation response of asynchronous cells is mainly due to that of S cells and (2) the fluctuations in the two-dose response reflect the simultaneous and combined effects of repair of sublethal damage and cell aging.

A comparison of the time courses of repair is approximated by the curves in Fig. 9. Here are plotted the ratios of the two-dose survivals to the equivalent single-dose survivals for cells at 37°C or at 24°C between doses, a comparison that attempts to account for changes due to cell aging in the fractionation interval. The ratios are determined from the two-dose and single-dose survivals at the same times on the abscissa in Fig. 8; that is, for 37°C the single-dose curve is the continuous line (1083 rads) from $3\frac{1}{2}$ hr on, and for 24°C it is the dashed line. Although the data in Fig. 9 suggest that the repair process at 24°C is equally as

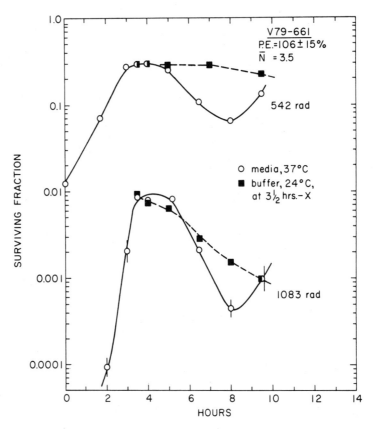

FIGURE 7. Radiation age–response patterns for V79 Chinese hamster cells, clone V79-661 (50 kVp X-rays, 722 rads/min). Cells were synchronized by the hydroxyurea technique (Sinclair, 1965, 1967); consequently, 0 hr corresponds to the G_1-S border. The maximum survivals are for cells in late S and the minimum is for cells in G_2-M-G_1 age interval. $\bar{N}$ is the average multiplicity at the start of the experiment. From Elkind et al. (1966).

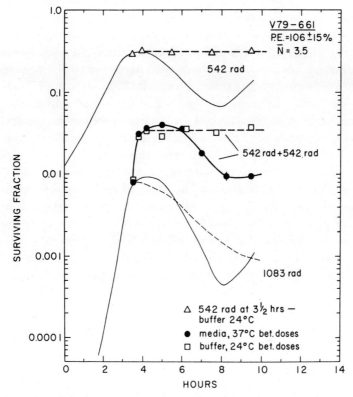

FIGURE 8. Two-dose fractionation responses for Chinese hamster cells obtained in the same experiment as in Fig. 7. From Elkind *et al.* (1966).

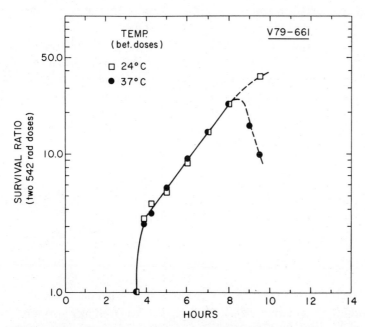

FIGURE 9. Survival ratios of two-dose to single-dose surviving fractions (at the same real times) shown in Fig. 8. From Elkind *et al.* (1966).

rapid as at 37°C, this conclusion must be qualified somewhat. First, there is the enhanced sensitivity with time for cells at 24°C (Fig. 7); consequently, one cannot be confident that this latter dependence should serve as the reference for the 24°C two-dose response. Second, it is known that, following an X-ray dose, surviving cells are delayed in their aging (Elkind *et al.*, 1963); hence, even for cells at 37°C, a progressively increasing phase shift exists between the two-dose and single-dose results. This effect in extreme form is made clear by the last two points for 37°C in Fig. 9. The survival ratio for cells at 37°C beyond 8 hr actually starts to decrease, because the minimum in the two-dose response is displaced to the right due to delay compared to the minimum in the single-dose response (see also Elkind *et al.*, 1967c). The delay in aging also has the effect of causing the 37°C curve to rise more rapidly before 8 hr so that the curve cannot be taken as an accurate indication of the time course of sublethal damage repair. In spite of the foregoing reservations, Fig. 9 shows that repair is rapid, is weakly temperature dependent compared to aging, and is probably not completed in late S cells 4–5 hr after a dose of 542 rads (Elkind *et al.*, 1963). It is quite possible that sublethal damage is not inherited by the progeny of surviving S cells since the latter do not divide for 9–10 hr after they are irradiated.

3.1.4. Summary, Repair of Sublethal Damage

The fractionation studies with Chinese hamster cells just reviewed serve to demonstrate a number of points: (1) Repair of sublethal damage is prompt and weakly dependent on temperature. (2) Cell-cycle aging modulates the two-dose pattern of fractionation response as cells move from phases of resistance, to sensitivity, to resistance, and so on. (3) The results of other studies with fractionation intervals long enough to include the first and second divisions after a first dose (see also Elkind *et al.*, 1961) are consistent with full repair of sublethal damage before the first division is reached. To the foregoing, it should be added that the results of many studies that followed these initial experiments have shown that sublethal damage repair following irradiation with low-LET radiation (e.g., X-rays and γ-rays) apparently is universal. Sublethal damage repair has been demonstrated with a variety of mammalian cells in culture (e.g., see Elkind and Whitmore, 1967; Elkind, 1970), with cells of normal tissues *in vivo* (e.g., Elkind and Withers, 1970), with tumor cells (e.g., Elkind *et al.*, 1968b; Elkind, 1974), and with hypoxic as well as aerobic cells (Elkind *et al.*, 1964a, 1965). Its relevance, therefore, to the treatment of cancer with radiation is clearly established.

3.2. Targets Containing DNA

As we noted in Section 2.1, the genome of a cell has been a favored target for cell killing and other radiation effects in eukaryotes as well as in prokaryotes. Direct evidence for mammalian cells, in support of this presumption, comes from studies involving DNA intercalators, DNA base analogues, and ultraviolet (UV) light.

It is well known that the antibiotic actinomycin D intercalates in, and binds to, duplex DNA selectively (Reich, 1964; Dingman and Sporn, 1965; Ebstein, 1967; Camargo and Plaut, 1967). In fractionation studies with inhibitors of macromolecular synthesis, only actinomycin D was effective in altering the two-dose response of Chinese hamster cells over and above any toxic effects due to the antibiotic (Elkind *et al.*, 1967*b*). In part, this reflects the ability of this antibiotic to introduce damage in cells that is additive to radiation damage, as illustrated in Figs. 10 and 11. These experiments were performed with cells synchronized at the G_1–S border, as already noted, by incubating them with hydroxyurea. Four hours after the removal of the hydroxyurea, they were at their age of maximum radiation resistance, late S. For 0.75 hr on either side of this maximum, cells were incubated in the presence of actinomycin D and then exposed to graded X-ray doses. Although the toxic effect of the actinomycin D by itself increases with concentration, and although a small reduction in D_0 results from the drug compared to cells not exposed to the drug, the main effect is a progressive elimination of the shoulder on the survival curve. A concentration of 0.002 μg/ml

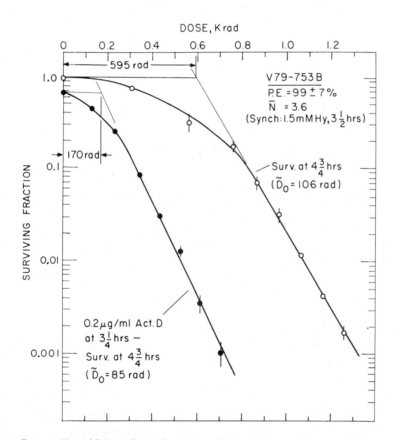

FIGURE 10. Additive effect of actinomycin D damage to X-ray sublethal damage in V79 Chinese hamster S-phase cells, clone V79-753B (50 kVp X-rays, 722 rads/min). The open circles show the survival curve without actinomycin D pretreatment. From Elkind *et al.* (1967*a*).

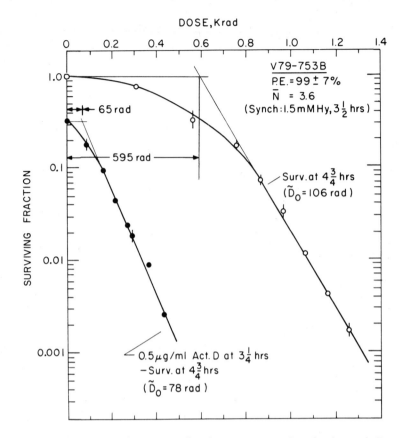

FIGURE 11. Similar to Fig. 10 except for a larger concentration of actinomycin D. From Elkind *et al.* (1967*a*).

$(1.5 \times 10^{-9}\ \mathrm{M})$, which is completely nontoxic, had a small but qualitatively similar effect on the survival curve of late-S cells. Since low concentrations of this antibiotic inhibit only ribosomal RNA synthesis (Perry, 1963), and since other inhibitors of macromolecular synthesis were without effect even though they inhibited ribosomal RNA synthesis quite effectively, it was concluded that actinomycin D damage adds to X-ray damage because of its steric rather than biochemical properties (Elkind *et al.*, 1967*a,b*).

Support for actinomycin D and radiation damage additivity was also obtained by following the time course of the loss of this interaction. Figure 9, for example, shows that over the course of 4 hr or more the damage produced by a first X-ray dose is lost relative to what remains for a second X-ray dose to add to. A similar experiment in which the second X-ray dose was replaced by an exposure to actinomycin D gave a similar result; namely, by 6 hr after an X-ray dose, actinomycin D had little interactive effect (Elkind *et al.*, 1967*c*).

These results with actinomycin D, plus the well-known fact that the nucleus in eukaryotes is much more radiosensitive than the cytoplasm, implicate duplex DNA and possibly its molecular environment as principal sites of radiation damage as well as of the repair of such damage.

3.3. Inhibition of Sublethal Damage Repair

Hyperthermia is a treatment of increasing interest in connection with cancer therapy, because heat by itself is lethal to cells and also because elevated temperatures enhance cell killing by radiation and/or drugs. With respect to enhanced radiation cell killing, hyperthermia has different effects under different conditions of temperature, medium, and duration of treatment. Among these is its effect on repair processes at functional and molecular levels. In this section, we review the influence of mild degrees of heat treatment on the repair of sublethal damage; in later sections, we consider its effect on DNA repair.

3.3.1. Low-Dose-Rate Irradiation

One consequence of the ability of cells to repair sublethal damage between dose fractions should be their ability to effect repair during irradiation if the dose rate and conditions of incubation are favorable. Figure 12 illustrates this with Chinese

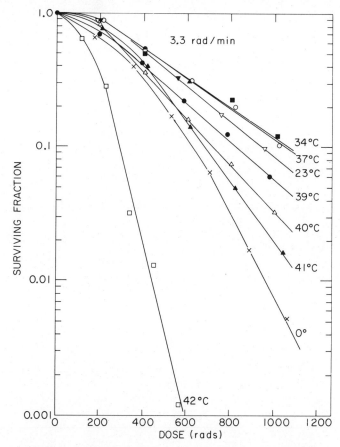

FIGURE 12. Survival dependence on X-ray dose of V79 Chinese hamster cells (clone V79-753B-3M); irradiation was at 3.3 rads/min with 250 kVp X-rays. Cells were suspended in 20% medium in phosphate-buffered saline (which does not support division) at the temperatures shown during irradiation. From Ben-Hur *et al.* (1972).

hamster cells irradiated at a low dose rate while suspended in a medium that does not support division (i.e., 80% phosphate-buffered saline plus 20% medium). Cells irradiated at 0°C survive, as expected, in a manner independent of dose rate. However, as the temperature during irradiation is raised, the survival curve becomes appreciably less steep. (The small difference between 23°C and 37°C is in accord with the weak dependence of sublethal damage repair on temperature as already noted.) For temperatures above 37°C, the survival curves become steeper again, which suggests that repair is adversely affected by hyperthermia.

3.3.2. Hyperthermia and Dose Fractionation

The foregoing expectation is illustrated in the next two figures. Figure 13 illustrates the effect of hyperthermia between doses, compared to 37°C between doses, on cells irradiated at 0°C and at high dose rate. To begin with, the 37°C curve differs from that observed when 100% medium is used because in 20% medium in phosphate-buffered saline cells do not progress toward division; consequently, the minimum in the two-dose response (Fig. 6) is absent. Cells kept at 40°C do not repair as well as at 37°C, and a 2-hr period at 41°C is sufficient to eliminate a survival increase even if the temperature is reduced to 37°C thereafter.

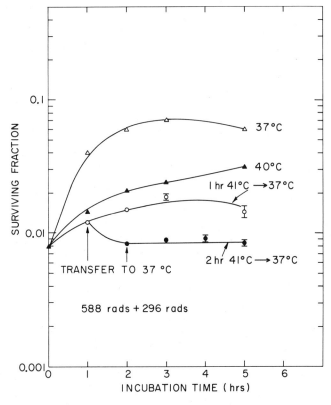

FIGURE 13. Dependence on temperature between dose fractions of the net survival of V79 Chinese hamster cells irradiated at 0°C at 360 rads/min (other details as for Fig. 12). From Ben-Hur *et al.* (1974).

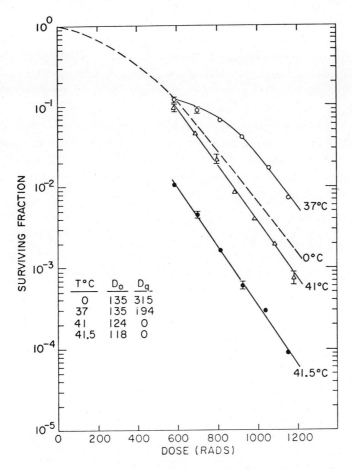

T°C	D_0	D_q
0	135	315
37	135	194
41	124	0
41.5	118	0

FIGURE 14. Fractionation survival curves of V79 Chinese hamster cells incubated at the temperatures shown for 2.5 hr after a first dose of 593 rads (other details as for Fig. 13). Following the first dose, the hyperthermia period by itself reduces survival as shown by the first points on the 41°C and 41.5°C curves. The dashed curve is the single-dose survival curve obtained in another experiment. From Ben-Hur *et al.* (1974).

Figure 14 shows the consequences of hyperthermia on the shape of the fractionation survival curve. Here, too, irradiations were at 0°C and at high dose rate. Although 2.5 hr at 41°C or 41.5°C by itself causes a drop in survival after the first dose of 593 rads, the size of which is temperature dependent, in both cases surviving cells do not repair sublethal damage because the shoulder does not re-form. Thus, in accord with results at low dose rate (Fig. 12), a mild degree of hyperthermia is incompatible with the generation of a renewed ability to accumulate sublethal damage.

3.4. Fluorescent-Light Killing of Cells Containing 5-Bromodeoxyuridine

If part of the thymine in the DNA of a mammalian cell is replaced by bromouracil—as a result, for example, of growing the cells in the presence of

5-bromodeoxyuridine (e.g., Puck and Kao, 1967; Yang *et al.*, 1970)—subsequent exposure to fluorescent light (FL) will kill the cells, inhibit DNA synthesis, and in general produce a gamut of effects associated with DNA damage and cytotoxicity. Since 5-bromodeoxyuridine (BUdR), as an analogue of thymidine, is incorporated into DNA, since the FL exposures by themselves do not produce the effects observed if BUdR is not incorporated, and since debromination of uracil is implicated as the initial step in the lethal process (Wacker *et al.*, 1962), BUdR/FL cell killing ought to be a clear example of a functional change resulting from DNA damage. Debromination of the 5-position of uracil presumably results in a radical which becomes quenched upon abstraction of a hydrogen atom from the vicinity (see Koehnlein and Hutchinson, 1969; Lion, 1972). Preparatory to a discussion of

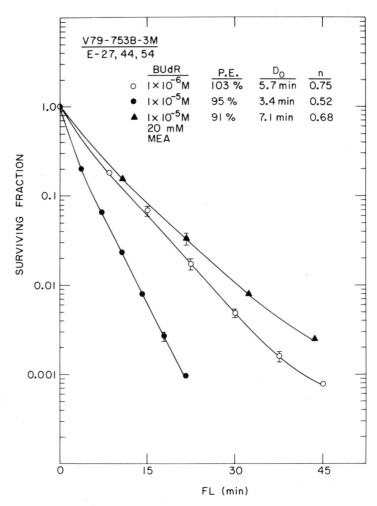

FIGURE 15. Fluorescent-light (FL) inactivation of V79 Chinese hamster cells (V79-753B-3M) grown for 20 hr in the presence of BUdR (lamp F15T8-D Sylvania). D_0 values are derived from the middle parts of the curves. MEA, mercaptoethylamine, was present at the time of exposure for the uppermost curve. From Ben-Hur and Elkind (1972).

the concomitant DNA damage, in this section we show some of the characteristics
of BUdR/FL cell killing.

If V79 Chinese hamster cells are grown for 20 hr in the presence of BUdR, their
subsequent survival curves after exposure to FL (Fig. 15) are characteristically
different from those obtained after ionizing radiation of normal or BUdR-treated
cells (Shipley *et al.*, 1971). The principal qualitative difference is that the curves do
not have a shoulder. In Fig. 15, it is clear that the steepness of the curves reflects
the concentration of BUdR in the medium during the growth period for incorporation. Since asynchronous cells were used, and since 20 hr is not long enough to
uniformly label all cells with BUdR, it is quite reasonable to attribute the changes
in the slope of a given survival curve to different amounts of BUdR incorporation.
Nevertheless, the fact remains that the curves are essentially "single-hit" in
character (i.e., no shoulder), whereas X-ray survival curves are of the damage-
accumulation type.

The uppermost curve in Fig. 15 shows that FL exposure in the presence of the
SH compound mercaptoethylamine (MEA) protects cells with a modification dose
factor of 2.1. This is in accord with the photochemical scheme just described and
the observation that the action portion of the FL spectrum 300–325 nm lies in the
region where BUdR absorbs (Ben-Hur and Elkind, 1972).

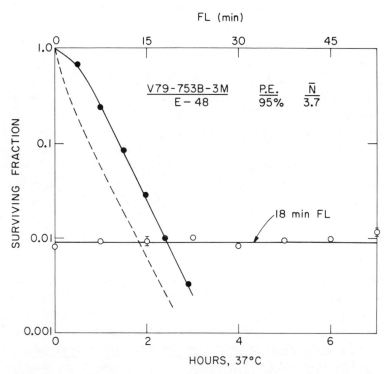

FIGURE 16. Two-dose fluorescent-light (FL) irradiation of V79 Chinese hamster
cells exposed to FL after growth for 20 hr in the presence of 1×10^{-5} M BUdR.
The dashed line estimates the single-cell survival curve derived from the data
points which are for microcolonies of multiplicity $\bar{N} = 3.7$. From Ben-Hur and
Elkind (1972).

The effect of dose fractionation is shown in Fig. 16. In this case, the survival points are for microcolonies of average multiplicity, $\bar{N}$, equal to 3.7; the dashed curve shows the single-cell curve calculated from the observed points. Two 9-min exposures separated by increasing intervals have no effect on the net survival, and, consistent with this, the age–survival pattern was found to be essentially flat through the entire age cycle. Thus, consistent with the lack of a damage-accumulation killing process, dose fractionation does not result in an increase in survival, presumably because surviving cells have no sublethal damage to repair.

3.5. DNA Damage

The presumption from the outset that DNA is the site of damage for the initiation of many of the effects of radiation led to attempts to correlate damage to DNA with changes in cell function. In the decade after the pioneering work of Puck and Marcus (1956), studies of radiation damage in DNA frequently started with the extraction of DNA from the cells or tissues of interest. Since the DNA from unirradiated material usually was about 1×10^7 daltons, very large doses of radiation had to be used in order to detect damage over and above that introduced by the extraction procedure itself. We know today that single-stranded DNA of size 1×10^7 daltons results from irradiating cells with ~ 50 krads; consequently, the early molecular studies amounted to looking for small signals added to a large and frequently not well-controlled starting level.

The change in this state of affairs came about largely as a result of a technical innovation due to McGrath and Williams (1966). They introduced the method of lysing cells on top of a sucrose gradient, eliminating the need for mechanical manipulation of extracted DNA and thus minimizing inadvertent damage. To free the DNA from the cell and from the protein in chromatin, they used alkaline lysis (pH > 12) plus high salt concentrations containing EDTA. This procedure, plus analogous but not as successful methods for extracting duplex DNA on top of neutral sucrose gradients, has led to significant advances in our understanding of the production of lesions in DNA by radiations and other DNA interactive agents.

3.5.1. Single-Strand DNA Breaks Due to Moderate X-Ray Doses

Since various forms of lesions in DNA may yield breaks in the backbone only when chemically attacked at high pH, single-strand breaks more accurately are a mixture of frank breaks and alkali-labile lesions. The estimates of various authors place the proportion of frank breaks to lesions which become breaks at high pH at $1:1$ for hypoxic irradiation and $3:1$ for oxic irradiation (see Lennartz *et al.*, 1973). In addition, even without irradiation, depending on temperature, time, and hydroxide concentration, OH^- attack produces a change in the size range of the DNA until a species of 2–3×10^8 daltons is released (see Elkind and Kamper, 1970, who refer to this species as "main-peak" DNA). Since an average somatic mammalian cell may contain 6×10^{12} daltons, 2–3×10^4 such molecules are contained in a single cell. Moderate doses of X-rays, ~ 1000 rads, give rise to the same DNA

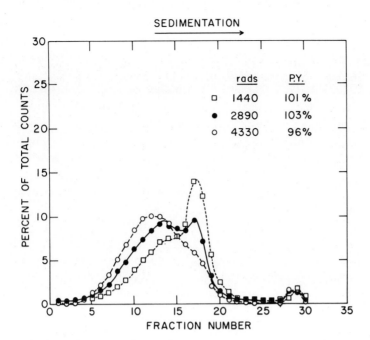

FIGURE 17. Sedimentation (high speed) in an alkaline sucrose gradient of [³H]thymidine-labeled DNA from V79 Chinese hamster cells. Lysis solution: 0.05 M NaOH, 0.95 M NaCl, and 0.01 M Na₂EDTA. Gradient solution: 5–20% sucrose in 0.1 M NaOH, 0.9 M NaCl, and 0.003 M Na₂EDTA. Sedimentation conditions: 38,000 rpm, 60 min, 12°C, and a SW39 rotor. Essentially all of the radioactivity counts placed on a gradient were retrieved in the 30 fractions. From Elkind and Kamper (1970).

species except in a shorter time of lysis. Hence one may infer that OH^- attack results in breaks in the backbone.

A progressive change in sedimenting ability due to increasing doses of X-rays is illustrated in Fig. 17. After 1440 rads, the pattern shows a bulge on the low molecular weight side of the mode, and with increasing doses this bulge grows at the expense of the DNA in the main peak. For 50 kVp X-rays, 49 eV is expended per break. Following irradiation, incubation at 37°C before lysis causes the breaks to disappear rapidly (Elkind and Kamper, 1970), as discussed below; the rate of disappearance is strongly temperature dependent (Elkind and Chang-Liu, 1972a).

3.5.2. Changes in Sedimentation Due to Small X-Ray Doses

Since doses of ~ 1000 rads are required to release the 2–3×10^8 dalton species from Chinese hamster cells, since essentially all of the breaks produced by moderately larger doses (Fig. 17) are repaired in that the DNA returns to 2–3×10^8 daltons, and since essentially all the cells in the population are killed for doses greater than ~ 1000 rads (see Fig. 5), it is difficult to imagine a connection between single-strand damage and cell killing. In order to observe effects due to doses in the physiological range, studies were undertaken involving alkaline lysing conditions that reduce the rate of OH⁻ attack (e.g., lysis at 3°C for 60 min). The results obtained brought to light the fact that the sedimentation of DNA released from mammalian cells is dependent on rotor speed in an unexpected way (Elkind and Kamper, 1970; Elkind, 1971) and is in qualitative agreement with the theory of DNA stretching due to Zimm (1974; see also Rubenstein and Leighton, 1974). In addition Elkind and Kamper showed that small X-ray doses produced a discontinuous change in sedimentation suggestive of a change in configuration.

Figure 18 illustrates the point just noted. Using sedimentation conditions such that the mode of the peak after 1440 rads in Fig. 17 sedimented only to fractions 4–5, Fig. 18 shows the changes induced after high-survival X-ray doses (see Fig. 5). The principal points are the following: (1) with increasing dose, more and more material appears in the position of the main peak (i.e., fractions 4–5); (2) initially, the DNA and lipid ([³H]choline chloride label) cosediment, but in the region of dose corresponding to 60%–25% survival (200–400 rads), this cosedimentation is lost; (3) the lipid material has a density greater than 1.0 g/cm³ and therefore probably contains glycoproteins in addition to lipids; and (4) since a large fraction

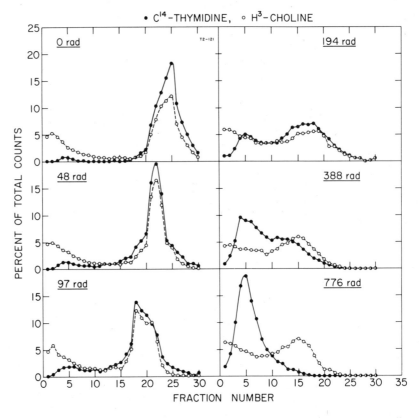

FIGURE 18. Sedimentation (low speed) of material from V79 Chinese hamster cells labeled with [³H]choline chloride and [¹⁴C]thymidine. Cells were irradiated with 250 kVp X-rays and lysed at 3°C for 60 min. Sedimentation: 5000 rpm, 16.25 hr, ~0°C, SW50.1 rotor. From Elkind and Chang-Liu (1972a).

of the lipid label initially cosediments with the DNA, it probably consists of the
nuclear envelope and possibly some of the endoplasmic reticulum as well. (The
lipid–DNA cosedimenting material is called the "complex" to distinguish it from
main-peak DNA; Elkind and Kamper, 1970; Elkind, 1971.) Further studies using
interstrand cross-linking agents (i.e., nitrogen mustard or psoralen plus near-
ultraviolet light) showed that the DNA cosedimenting with the lipid is largely
duplex DNA whereas that in the position of the main peak (fractions 4–5) is
primarily single-stranded DNA (Elkind and Ben-Hur, 1973). (Similar conclusions
were reached by Simpson *et al.*, 1973, and by Cleaver, 1974.)

The following picture has emerged from the foregoing. Because of the size of
the DNA—very likely in the 1×10^9–1×10^{10} dalton range (Elkind, 1971; Elkind
and Chang-Liu, 1972a)—as cells start to lyse under high pH conditions, initially
duplex DNA is released to which the nuclear envelope and structural proteins are
attached, probably at discrete sites. Even though there is mounting evidence for
functional and structural interactions between the nuclear membrane and DNA
(Davies and Small, 1968; Cabradilla and Toliver, 1975, and references therein), it
is likely that most of the envelope is not bound to the DNA but cosediments with it
because of the structural continuity of the envelope itself. Small, high-survival
doses insert breaks in the DNA and the DNA–envelope complex, expediting the
denaturation and the release of single-stranded DNA of average size 2–3×10^8
daltons: the latter is the equivalent of a number of replicons in tandem and may
constitute the "epichromatin" discussed by Stubblefield (1973). A conformational
change involving the relaxation of supercoils (Elkind, 1971; Cook and Brazell,
1975) is also a possibility. Larger doses then proceed to break these single strands
(e.g. Fig. 17). As will be discussed further, repair initially leads to the elimination
of these breaks and therefore to the re-formation of the main peak; further repair
results in a reconstitution of the complex.

3.5.3. Repair of Single-Strand Breaks and the Complex

To see the effect of sequential repair, it is useful to use low-speed sedimentation
(e.g., as in Fig. 18) and doses followed by repair times that enable the sequence to
be observed. In Fig. 19, we consider first the dose dependence of the sequence by
using a fixed repair time of 20 min. In each case, the position of the main-peak
mode value after repair (around fraction 5) indicates whether or not there was a
significant number of breaks in single-stranded DNA. For example, 20 min after
722 rads, the mode value remains at fraction 6 whereas after 8 times that dose,
5780 rads, repair effects a shift from fraction 4 to 6. A smaller but clear shift is
evident after 2890 rads but not after 1440 rads.

The second point evident in Fig. 19 is that repair leads to a re-formation of a
peak near the bottom of the tube as in Fig. 18 for DNA from unirradiated cells.
Thus, after 722 rads, the main peak shrinks in place and the complex re-forms,
indicating the reversal of the dose-dependent resolution of the complex in Fig. 18.
The data also show that in 20 min the amount of complex that re-forms
qualitatively varies inversely with the size of the dose.

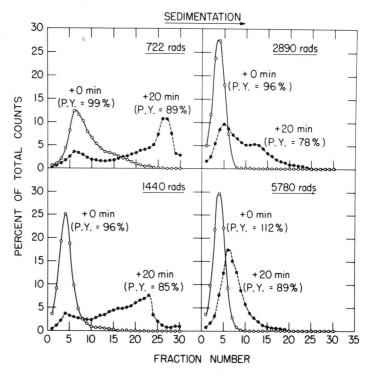

FIGURE 19. Sedimentation (low speed) of DNA from V79 Chinese hamster cells, under conditions similar to those in Fig. 18, showing the effect of a 20-min repair period (complete medium, 37°C). However, in addition to the use of 50 kVp instead of 250 kVp X-rays, these data differ from those in Fig. 18 in that for the upper left and lower right panels the sedimentation was at 6000 rpm instead of at 5000 rpm. From Elkind and Chang-Liu (1972a).

A more complete picture of the time course of the re-formation of the complex is shown in Fig. 20. As in Fig. 19, first the main-peak DNA increases in size (i.e., the mode shifts from 4 to 5) and then, as the amount of main-peak DNA progressively decreases, the complex re-forms. Between 180 min and 360 min, the main peak starts to increase again. After 2890 rads, essentially all the cells are killed; one aspect of the radiopathology of a dying cell is the fragmentation of its DNA illustrated by the change from 180 min to 360 min (e.g., see also Ben-Hur and Elkind, 1974). Lastly, Fig. 21 shows that the re-formation of the complex results in a reassociation of the lipid material with DNA. Consequently, with respect to this property as well, repair results in a reversal of the radiation-induced change.

The results in Figs. 17–21 may be summarized according to the following schemes (Elkind, 1971, 1975a; Elkind and Chang-Liu, 1972a).

1. Damage (increasing doses):

DNA–nuclear envelope complex → main-peak DNA →

degraded main-peak DNA

2. Repair (increasing time after a given dose):

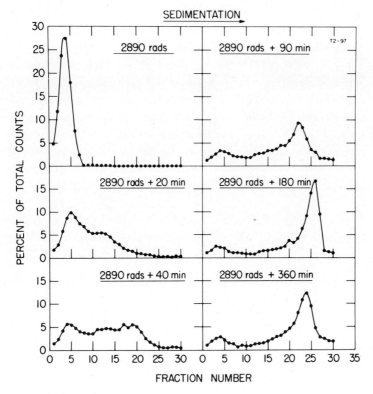

FIGURE 20. Sedimentation (low speed) of DNA from V79 Chinese hamster cells showing the progressive effect of repair. Details as for Fig. 18. From Elkind and Chang-Liu (1972a).

degraded main-peak DNA → main-peak DNA →

DNA–nuclear envelope complex

The first step in scheme 1 involves a conformational change that expedites denaturation (high pH) and results in a species 2–3×10^8 daltons in average size. In scheme 2, single-strand breaks are repaired in strands initially smaller than 2–3×10^8 daltons if the dose was high enough, and this is followed by a conformational change. Interstrand cross-links inhibit the first step in scheme 1 and hasten the second step in scheme 2 (Elkind and Ben-Hur, 1974).

3.6. Hyperthermia and Repair of DNA

As already noted, a principal property of ionizing radiation is its ability to break molecular bonds. On the average, about 60 eV is deposited per energy-loss event when electrons traverse condensed matter (Rauth and Simpson, 1964), which means that bond breakage will accompany almost all energy-loss events. In view of the evidence implicating DNA targets in cell killing, it is natural to inquire if strand scissions in DNA are related to cell killing.

To get at this question, one can look for parallel effects, for example, relative to cell killing and DNA damage and/or the repair of sublethal damage and the repair of DNA breaks. With this approach in mind, the inhibition of sublethal damage repair resulting from hyperthermia is a case in point.

Figure 22 traces the loss of single-strand breaks in cells incubated at either 37°C or 42°C following 5800 rads. Although even 41°C is a high enough temperature to suppress the re-formation of the shoulder of the survival curve of V79 Chinese hamster cells (Fig. 14), at 42°C single-strand breaks are repaired more rapidly over the first 70 min. Ordinarily, a sizable amount of sublethal damage is repaired in 70 min (e.g., Fig. 13). Consequently, one may conclude that hyperthermia does not inhibit the repair of sublethal damage because it slows or inhibits the repair of single-strand breaks. Furthermore, since temperatures greater than 41°C after irradiation reduce single-dose survivals (e.g., in Fig. 14, the first point on the 41.5°C curve is the survival for 593 rads plus hyperthermia only), the results in Fig. 22 suggest that if there is a connection between single-strand breaks and survival, the more rapid the repair of such breaks, the lower the survival.

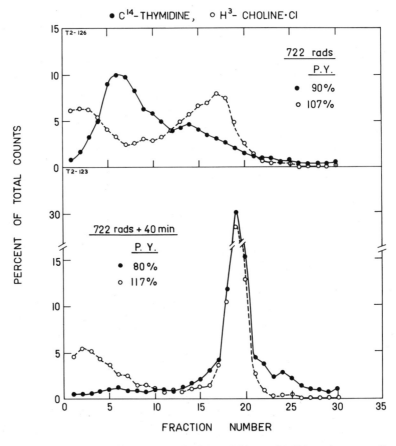

FIGURE 21. Sedimentation (low speed) of material from V79 Chinese hamster cells labeled overnight with the compounds shown. Sedimentation was at 6000 rpm. From Elkind and Chang-Liu (1972a).

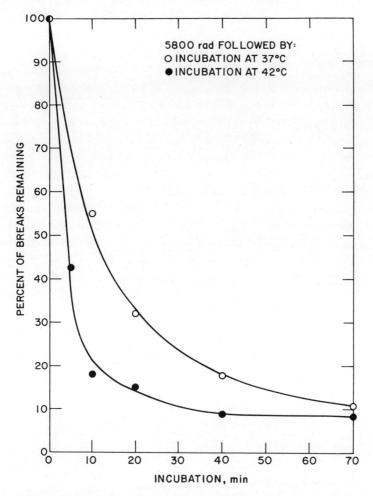

FIGURE 22. Temperature dependence of the loss of single-strand breaks, following 5800 rads, in the DNA of Chinese hamster cells. From Ben-Hur and Elkind (1974).

3.7. DNA Repair after Fluorescent-Light Exposure of BUdR-Containing Cells

A second cell-killing context in which correlations may be sought with DNA damage is the exposure to fluorescent light (FL) of cells labeled with BUdR. First, as noted earlier, unlabeled cells are not affected by the modest FL exposures used (i.e., cells are not killed and DNA breaks are not registered). Second, since no repair of sublethal damage occurs between fractionated exposures (Fig 16), consistent with the exponential character of the killing curve (Fig. 15), one might expect the single-strand breaks which accompany BUdR/FL treatment not to be repaired.

Figure 23 shows the time-dependent loss of single-strand breaks in BUdR-labeled cells following an FL exposure (corresponding to 0.7% survival). The

X-ray data are for an equivalent breakage dose. Thus, even though the BUdR/FL-treated cells do not repair sublethal damage, they do repair single-strand breaks and, in fact, even more rapidly than do cells exposed to an equal-breakage X-ray dose.

The X-ray dose used in Fig. 23 was 20 kR, an X-ray exposure that is clearly supralethal. Compared to ionizing radiation, BUdR/FL DNA damage is much more efficiently registered, as summarized in Fig. 24. Here, in order to compare the breakage effectiveness of FL and X-rays, the doses have been normalized by the respective D_0 doses. This means that the unit of dose, for both types of lethal treatment, is that which reduces survival by the factor $1/e$ as determined from the exponential part of a survival curve. With dose normalized in this way, the triangles show that for cells labeled to two different levels with BUdR, the breakage efficiency is the same, ~ 2 per 2×10^8 daltons per D_0. In contrast, whether or not BUdR-labeled or normal cells are X-irradiated, breaks per D_0 are induced at about 1/50 of the rate for BUdR/FL, ~ 0.04 break per 2×10^8 daltons per D_0. In view of the reasons already noted that indicate that DNA damage is very likely responsible for BUdR/FL killing, from this very large disparity in DNA

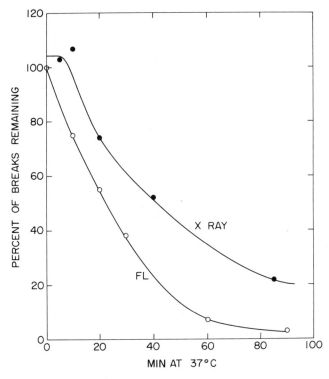

FIGURE 23. Comparison between the rates of loss of single-strand DNA breaks, for equal breakage doses, for BUdR-containing Chinese hamster cells exposed to fluorescent light (FL), and for cells not containing BUdR exposed to X-rays. The FL exposure reduced survival to 0.7%, and the X-ray dose was 20 kR. From Ben-Hur and Elkind (1972).

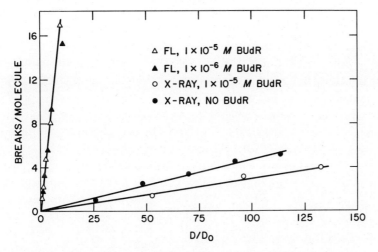

FIGURE 24. DNA single-strand breakage, as a function of dose normalized by the D_0 dose, for fluorescent-light (FL) exposure of cells grown for ~20 hr in BUdR, and for cells X-irradiated with and without prelabeling with BUdR. From Ben-Hur and Elkind (1972).

breakage rates alone, one may conclude that X-ray lethal sites differ from BUdR/FL lethal sites, the sites are the same but the damage is qualitatively different, or both. These possibilities are reasonable; while BUdR/FL lesions are very likely localized to the molecules surrounding the site of debromination, the damage registered by X-rays is not so restricted, and, further, because of the large amount energy deposited per X-ray absorption event, the spectrum of kinds of X-ray lesions could be different from those due to BUdR/FL exposure. (A further discussion of these possibilities follows.)

3.8. Misrepair, a Hypothesis for Radiation Cell Killing

Having reviewed a body of data relative to V79 Chinese hamster cells, which, because they were obtained with one particular cell system, are likely to be internally consistent, it is useful to see to what degree they permit some general questions to be answered.

1. *Is nuclear DNA the sensitive target in respect to cell killing?* Actinomycin D binds to DNA, probably with the ring structure intercalated between complementary base pairs (Waring, 1968). The resulting damage is additive to X-ray damage and *vice versa* (e.g., Figs. 10 and 11 and Elkind *et al.*, 1968a). Further, the normal X-ray response variation through the cell cycle correlates with nuclear DNA synthesis. Hence, while duplex DNA by itself may not be the principal or the only target in a cell, DNA and its structural relationship to its molecular environment (i.e., the nuclear–protein matrix; Berezney and Coffey, 1975; Keller and Riley, 1976), including the nuclear envelope, could be—in view of the helix untwisting that results from intercalation.

2. *Is the repair of sublethal damage the reverse of damage registration?*

Operationally, the answer is yes, since the survival curve returns to its original shape. Further, when the progeny of surviving cells are regrown to establish new populations, the radiation properties of these are very similar to those of the parental population (Elkind and Kano, 1971). In spite of the foregoing, however, evidence is lacking that repair represents a return of the target to the original state at a molecular level (see below).

3.   *Is repair of sublethal damage due to or closely connected with the repair of single-strand lesions in DNA?* Two examples in this chapter require a negative answer (see also Ormerod and Stevens, 1971). First, it was shown that under conditions of hyperthermia, which suppress sublethal damage repair (Fig. 14), the repair of single-strand breaks does occur and is even more rapid than it is at 37°C (Fig. 22). Second, following BUdR/FL treatment which, at a functional level, does not involve sublethal damage accumulation or its repair, DNA single-strand lesions are repaired quite effectively.

4.   *Does a cell survive because its DNA is not hit?* The answer to this must be an unequivocal no! This can be seen from the data summarized in Table 5, where the characteristics of BUdR/FL and X-ray cell killing are compared relative to DNA damage. On a per D_0 basis—that is, for an incremental dose that delivers one additional hit—statistically it is not possible that the cells comprising the $1/e$th fraction of the population that survive that dose do so without suffering any breaks in their DNA. If a particular DNA lesion is responsible for cell killing, on average one of these should be registered per D_0. Thus, for BUdR/FL cell killing, single-strand breaks can be ruled out, although double-strand breaks cannot be, because their incidence, while not measured as yet, is much less. For X-ray cell killing, however, both single- and double-strand breaks are present in very considerable excess. Even if an extreme estimate of 50 single-strand breaks per double-strand break is assumed (see Table 5), it is highly unlikely that a cell would survive with no double-strand breaks registered in it since $e^{-20} \ll e^{-1}$.

5.   *Do surviving cells propagate the DNA damage they contain immediately after they are irradiated?* Similar to damage expressed functionally—e.g., sublethal damage—as one might expect, surviving cells show normal sedimentation patterns when the DNA of their progeny is examined (Elkind, 1975b). Thus, while in general it is technically not possible to examine the time course of DNA repair in

TABLE 5

Comparison of Survival Properties and DNA Damage Induction

	Survival curve	Sublethal damage repair	ssb[a] per D_0	ssb repair	dsb[b] per D_0
BUdR/FL	Exponential	No	~50,000	Yes	≪ ssb[c]
X-rays	Cumulative damage type	Yes	~1,000[d]	Yes	~40[e]

[a] Single-strand breaks (alkali-labile lesions) per cell ($\sim 1 \times 10^{-11}$ g DNA).
[b] Double-strand breaks per cell.
[c] Not measured for mammalian cells but probably much less than the proportion of dsb's to ssb's for X-rays.
[d] Based on $D_0 \approx 100$ rads, ~60 eV per break, and 1×10^{-11} g DNA per cell.
[e] Based on ~25 ssb's per dsb (Elkind, unpublished data); published values for mammalian cells range from ~12 (Corry and Cole, 1968) to ~46 (Lehmann and Ormerod, 1970) ssb's per dsb.

surviving cells shortly after irradiation—in view of the fact that they constitute only a fraction of the population, indeed, a fraction that may be extremely small in a given case—the DNA damage initially registered as breaks is lost, although, of course, changes in the code consistent with replicative ability are not ruled out. Even the cosedimentation of DNA and lipid labels (Fig. 18) is reestablished, which we interpret to imply that the DNA–nuclear envelope structure is reestablished. Thus the excess damage indicated in Table 5 is not found in the progeny of survivors very likely because such damage is incompatible with viability.

6. *Why do cells die?* The damage resulting from ionizing radiation is molecularly nonspecific. In view of the large amount of energy deposited per absorption event, ~ 60 eV, any molecular bond is subject to rupture even if only direct radiation action is considered. The vast initial amount of damage in DNA that is subsequently repaired, in nonsurviving as well as in surviving cells (e.g., Figs. 19–23), supports the inference that evolution has given rise to constitutive repair capabilities in proliferating cells. The enzymes supporting this repair appear to be ubiquitous both with respect to age of cells in their growth cycle (Lohman, 1968) and with respect to cells from different tissues (Lett *et al.*, 1972; Wheeler and Lett, 1974). It is likely that some if not all of the enzymes involved have normal roles to play as, for example, with respect to the DNA ligase-type action that is involved in single-strand repair and semiconservative synthesis. Thus, for reasons at least associated with natural radioactivity and cosmic radiation, nature has endowed us with an efficient radiation repair system(s). As a further example of this, at the level of 10% survival, one in ten cells (or the progeny of one in ten cells) would have to repair ~ 3000 single-strand and ~ 120 double-strand breaks in the course of becoming a survivor. Along with single- and double-strand DNA breaks, it is very likely that lesions are registered in protein and lipid structures associated with DNA. If the latter are vital and their total target size is ~ 0.001 that of the total DNA content (i.e., $\sim 1 \times 10^8$ g per cell), it is possible that one unrepaired event per D_0 in this target kills a cell. However, it seems unreasonable that a DNA or DNA-associated target would be this small, and, consequently, even if DNA alone is not the target, the need for repair for survival seems likely.

Accordingly, the hypothesis is proposed that misrepair is responsible for lethality following ionizing irradiation of repair-competent cells. As just outlined, in the process of surviving, an irradiated cell effects vast amounts of repair which when confined to DNA—e.g., in BUdR/FL killing—at a 10% survival level may involve as many as $\sim 150,000$ single-strand breaks per survivor. Hence what is meant by "misrepair" is that the DNA assumes a configuration or composition incompatible with viability, even though in terms of sedimentation properties the DNA may appear to be repaired. Since sedimentation measurements have limited resolution, a small proportion of breaks remaining open and undetected cannot be ruled out. These may also be considered as due to misrepair if they result from changes in the DNA that accompany the repair of other breaks.

Misrepair is a familiar concept with respect to phenotypic change, which, of course, implies viability. In view of the apparent requirement for large amounts of repair to effect survival, the proposal here, however, is that a low frequency of misrepair, of one or more of the lesions produced by ionizing radiation, leads to cell death. For example, in the instance of BUdR/FL lethality, per D_0 an average of only one in $\sim 50,000$ single-strand breaks would have to be misrepaired, and in the instance of X-rays one in 40 double-strand breaks would suffice. Clearly, the misrepair that is being invoked would be an event of low probability.

7. *What causes misrepair and what is misrepaired?* As discussed, DNA breaks are not found in surviving cells; presumably, the repair of at least such lesions is required for survival in view of the unlikelihood that a cell would survive with a large burden of DNA damage. Lesions evident as DNA breaks, under alkaline (or neutral) sedimentation conditions, may involve damage in structures in addition to the linear continuity of the duplex. The reasonableness of this reflects, to begin with, the packaging and organizational requirements (for replication and segregation) of ~ 3 m of DNA in a nucleus ~ 7 μm in diameter, but also the fact that small, high-survival doses of X-rays produce a conformational change in the DNA in view of the discontinuities in the sedimentation patterns observed (Figs. 18–21). These small doses also eliminate the cosedimentation of DNA and lipid, but, as in the instance of strand breaks, incubation after irradition reestablishes this cosedimentation (Fig. 21). A transition in sedimentation pattern similar to that observed with high-survival doses of X-rays is also observed with high-survival doses of actinomycin D, and this antibiotic also inhibits the re-formation of the DNA–lipid complex when incubation follows both treatments (Elkind and Chang-Liu, 1972b). In view of the fact that relative to cell killing, actinomycin D damage is additive to X-ray damage (Figs. 10 and 11), the misrepair hypothesis is directed at the conformational change effected by small doses of X-rays in addition to the misrepair of DNA single- and double-strand lesions as such.

As for single-strand breaks following X-rays, actinomycin D does not appear to interfere with their repair (Sawada and Okada, 1970; Ormerod and Stevens, 1971; Elkind and Chang-Liu, 1972b). Consequently, it is proposed that each increment of duplex untwisting, concomitant with actinomycin D intercalation, increases the probability of misrepair of the DNA superstructure—perhaps a DNA–lipid structure at the nuclear envelope—even though cosedimentation of DNA and lipid is reestablished and single-strand breaks in main peak DNA are repaired.

Damage additivity at the level of cell killing has also been observed between ultraviolet light and X-rays (Han and Elkind, 1976). The principal DNA photolesion induced by ultraviolet light is the intrastrand pyrimidine dimer. Dimer formation results in a small amount of twisting of the strand plus local denaturation (Hagen *et al.*, 1965; Salgnik *et al.*, 1967). Consequently, rather than specific unwinding of the helix due to intercalation, the feature of actinomycin D action that is identified as responsible for additivity with X-ray damage is strand distortion in general.

3.9. *General Features of Mammalian Cell Killing and Summary*

Part 3 of this chapter has consisted of a review in some depth of those experiments performed with a single mammalian cell system to explore the where,

what, and how of cell killing. A major emphasis was placed upon mechanisms of
repair—at functional and molecular levels—with the underlying assumption that
if the reversal of damage could be understood, insights would emerge about the
specifics of damage registration. With the aid of Fig. 25, it is appropriate to
summarize the picture as developed.

The left side of the figure schematizes functional changes associated with
irradiation. In analogy with atomic and molecular energy level diagrams, this is a
damage level diagram for a mammalian cell initially in a "ground state," top line. A
dose of radiation delivered in a period of time short relative to biochemical
(repair) and biological (cell aging) time scales displaces a cell downward into the
damage domain. If the dose is large enough, the damage it receives will be
potentially lethal. In time, after irradiation, the cell's repair machinery attempts to
cope with the damage; simultaneously, the damaged molecules and structures are
called upon to function. If the competition between repair and fixation, for a
given amount of damage, favors repair, a cell may survive and in so doing repair
its sublethal damage. Changes in postirradiation assay or treatment conditions
may result in enhanced cell killing (e.g., due to hyperthermia) or enhanced
survival (e.g., delayed plating of plateau-phase cells; Hahn and Little, 1972). Of
course, the level of damage can be modified at a physicochemical level, as
described in Part 2, depending on the oxygen tension in the cell or its content of
SH or other sensitizing or protecting molecules that interact with the short-lived
species produced in the target molecules and/or their aqueous surroundings.

In parallel with the foregoing, the right side of Fig. 25 is a schematic of damage
to DNA and the nuclear envelope (see also Ormerod and Lehmann, 1971) or the
nuclear matrix. Here, too, a competition sets in in time after exposure. As indicated
in Table 1, the time scale for the latter competition would be from a fraction of a

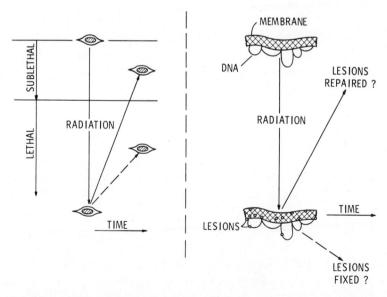

FIGURE 25. Schematic representations of cell killing (left) and DNA damage
(right). See text for discussion.

second to hours. Repair of DNA, or DNA superstructures including membrane complexes, is successfully accomplished in surviving cells, very likely as a necessary condition for survival. Misrepair of the latter processes could be the reason for lesion fixation. The balance between lesion repair and lesion fixation would depend on dose and the assay conditions following exposure as for survival.

The representations in Fig. 25 and the misrepair hypothesis described are consistent with Alper's hypothesis of type-O and type-N damage (i.e., membrane-associated DNA damage and strand lesions, respectively; Alper, 1963a,b, 1970, 1971, 1974), as well as with the observations of Cole and co-workers relative to the penetration dependence of the inactivation of mammalian cells with low-energy electrons (Cole, 1965; Zermeno and Cole, 1969) and variable-energy α-particles (Datta et al., 1976). In a general way, Fig. 25 is also in accord with the work of Cramp et al. (1972) with bacterial DNA-membrane complexes, although, in contrast to bacteria, in mammalian cells not all DNA–membrane attachments may be sites of DNA synthesis (Wise and Prescott, 1973; Comings and Okada, 1970, 1973). Relative to the misrepair hypothesis, a contribution to cell killing that may come from DNA double-strand breaks is not in conflict with the view that an unrepaired double-strand break results in cell death, since the persistence of one or a few of these per cell is beyond the detection limit of sedimentation analysis. However, that double-strand breaks must be repaired should be evident from the data in Table 5, a point supported by recent evidence of double-strand break repair in prokaryotes (see Section 2.2) and in conflict with what has been a commonly held view that a double-strand break is lethal because there is no way for DNA continuity to be maintained in order for repair to proceed.

The report that Chinese hamster cells do not repair double-strand breaks in the first 3–4 hr after irradiation (Dugle et al., 1976) is in accord with the latter view. To fit this observation with the evident need for surviving cells to repair ~ 40 double-strand breaks per D_0, one must assume that such repair occurs slowly, so that in the period during which Dugle and co-workers looked for repair of double-strand breaks little if any repair had occurred.

It should be evident that a fundamental understanding of radiation mammalian cell killing depends critically on a more complete understanding of nuclear DNA—its molecular organization in chromatin, its relationship to the nuclear envelope, its superstructure, its replication, and its segregation. The point may well have been reached where advances in our understanding of the imbalances due to radiation may be dependent on advances in our understanding of the normal biology of the nucleus.

ACKNOWLEDGMENTS

The writing of this chapter was supported in part by the U.S. Energy Research and Development Administration and in part by the National Cancer Institute via Grant CA-13307.

ACHEY, P., AND DURYEA, H., 1974, Production of DNA strand breaks by the hydroxyl radical, *Int. J. Radiat. Biol.* **25**:595.

ADAMS, G. E., REDPATH, J. L., CUNDALL, R. B., AND BISBY, R. H., 1972, The use of free radical probes in the study of mechanisms of enzyme inactivation, *Isr. J. Chem.* **10**:1079.

AGNEW, D. A., STRATFORD, I. J., and ADAMS, G. E., 1975, Sensitization of single-strand breaks, *Cancer Res. Campaign, Gray Lab. Ann Rep.*, p. 93.

ALPER, T., 1963*a*, Lethal mutations and cell death, *Phys. Med. Biol.* **8**:365.

ALPER, T., 1963*b*, Effects on irradiated organisms of growth in the presence of acriflavine, *Nature (London)* **200**:534.

ALPER, T., 1970, Mechanisms of lethal radiation damage to cells, in: *Proceedings of the Second Symposium on Microdosimetry* (Stresa, Italy, 1969) (H. G. EBERT, ed.), pp. 5–36, Euratom, Brussels.

ALPER, T., 1971, Cell death and its modification: The roles of primary lesions in membranes and DNA, in: *Biophysical Aspects of Radiation Quality*, pp. 171–184, I.A.E.A., Vienna.

ALPER, T., 1974, Observations relevant to the mechanism of RBE effects in the killing of cells, in: *Biological Effects of Neutron Irradiation*, pp. 133–147, I.A.E.A., Vienna.

ALPER, T., and HOWARD-FLANDERS, P., 1956, Role of oxygen in modifying the radiosensitivity of *E. coli* B, *Nature (London)* **178**:978.

ALPER, T., MOORE, J. L., AND SMITH, P., 1967, The role of dose-rate, irradiation technique and LET in determining radiosensitivities at low oxygen concentrations, *Radiat. Res.* **32**:780.

BARENDSEN, G.W., 1974, Relative biological effectiveness and biological complexity, in: *Proceedings of the Fourth Symposium on Microdosimetry* (Verbania-Pallanza, Italy, 24–28 Sept. 1973) (J. BOOZ, H. G. EBERT, R. EICKEL, AND A. WAKER, eds.), EURATOM Report EUR 5122 d-e-f, pp. 235–252.

BECKER, D., REDPATH, J. L., AND GROSSWEINER, L. I., 1977, *Radiat. Res.*, in press.

BEN-HUR, E., AND ELKIND, M. M., 1972, Damage and repair of DNA in 5-bromodeoxyuridine labelled Chinese hamster cells exposed to fluorescent light, *Biophys. J.* **12**:636.

BEN-HUR, E., AND ELKIND, M. M., 1973*a*, DNA cross-linking in Chinese hamster cells exposed to near UV light in the presence of 4,5′,8-trimethylpsoralen, *Biochim. Biophys. Acta* **331**:181.

BEN-HUR, E., AND ELKIND, M. M., 1973*b*, Psoralen plus near ultraviolet light inactivation of cultured Chinese hamster cells and its relation to DNA cross-links, *Mutat. Res.* **18**:315.

BEN-HUR, E., AND ELKIND, M. M., 1974, Thermally enhanced radioresponse of cultured Chinese hamster cells: Damage and repair of single-stranded DNA and a DNA complex, *Radiat. Res.* **59**:484.

BEN-HUR, E., BRONK, B., AND ELKIND, M. M., 1972, Thermally enhanced radiosensitivity of cultured Chinese hamster cells. *Nature (London) New Biol.* **238**:209.

BEN-HUR, E., ELKIND, M. M., AND BRONK, B. V., 1974, Thermally enhanced radioresponse of cultured Chinese hamster cells: Inhibition of repair of sublethal damage and enhancement of lethal damage, *Radiat. Res.* **58**:38.

BEREZNEY, R., AND COFFEY, D. S., 1975, Nuclear protein matrix: Association with newly synthesized DNA, *Science* **189**:291.

BERRY, R. J., HALL, E. J., FORSTER, D. W., STORR, T. H., AND GOODMAN, M. J., 1969, Survival of mammalian cells exposed to X-rays delivered at ultra high dose rates, *Br. J. Radiol.* **42**:102.

BLOK, J., AND LOMAN, H., 1973, The effects of γ-irradiation in DNA, *Curr. Top. Radiat. Res. Q.* **9**:165.

BONURA, T., AND SMITH, K. C., 1976, The involvement of indirect effects in cell killing and double-strand breakage in γ-irradiated *Escherichia coli* K12, *Int. J. Radiat. Biol.* **29**:293.

BONURA, T., TOWN, C. D., SMITH, K. C., AND KAPLAN, H. S., 1975, The influence of oxygen on the yield of DNA double-strand breaks in X-irradiated *Escherichia coli* K12, *Radiat. Res.* **63**:567.

BOYCE, R. P., AND TEPPER, M., 1968, X-ray induced single-strand breaks and joining of broken strands in super infecting λ DNA in *Escherichia coli* lysogenic for λ, *Virology* **34**:344.

BURRELL, A. D., FELDSCHREIBER, P., AND DEAN, C. J., 1971, DNA-membrane association and the repair of double breaks in X-irradiated *Micrococcus radiodurans*, *Biochim. Biophys. Acta* **247**:38.

CABRADILLA, C. D., AND TOLIVER, A. P., 1975, S-phase dependent forms of DNA nuclear membrane complexes in HeLa cells, *Biochim. Biophys. Acta* **402**:188.

CAMARGO, E. P., AND PLAUT, W., 1967, The radioautographic detection of DNA with tritiated actinomycin D, *J. Cell. Biol.* **35**:713.

CHAPMAN, J. D., REUVERS, A. P., BORSA, J., AND GREENSTOCK, C. L., 1973, Chemical radioprotection and radiosensitization of mammalian cells growing *in vitro*, *Radiat. Res.* **56**:291.

M. M. ELKIND
AND
J. L. REDPATH

CHELACK, W. S., FORSYTH, M. P., AND PETKAU, A., 1974, Radiobiological properties of *Acholepasma laidlawii* B, *Can. J. Microbiol.* **20**:307.

CHRISTENSEN, R. C., TOBIAS, C. A., AND TAYLOR, W. D., 1972, Heavy-ion-induced single- and double-strand breaks in ϕX-174 replicative form DNA, *Int. J. Radiat. Biol.* **22**:457.

CLEAVER, J. E., 1974, Sedimentation of DNA from human fibroblasts irradiated with ultraviolet light: Possible detection of excision breaks in pigmentosum cells, *Radiat. Res.* **57**:207.

COLE, A., 1965, The study of radiosensitive structures with low voltage electron beams, in: *Cellular Radiation Biology*, pp. 267–271, Williams and Wilkins, Baltimore.

COLE, R. S., AND SINDEN, R. R., 1975, Repair of cross-linked DNA in *Escherichia coli*, in: *Molecular Mechanisms for Repair of DNA, Part B* (P. C. HANAWALT AND R. B. SETLOW, eds.), pp. 487–495, Plenum Press, New York.

COLE, R. S., LEVITAN, D., AND SINDEN, R. R., 1976, Removal of psoralen interstrand cross-links from DNA of *Escherichia coli*: Mechanism and genetic control, *J. Mol. Biol.* **103**:39.

COMINGS, D. E., AND OKADA, T. A., 1970, Association of chromatin fibers with the annuli of the nuclear membrane, *Exp. Cell Res.* **62**:293.

COMINGS, D. E., AND OKADA, T. A., 1973, DNA replication and the nuclear membrane, *J. Mol. Biol.* **75**:609.

COOK, P. R., AND BRAZELL, I. A., 1975, Supercoils in human DNA, *J. Cell Sci.* **19**:261.

COQUERELLE, T., BOPP, A., KESSLER, B., AND HAGEN, U., 1973, Strand breaks and 5′ end-groups in DNA of irradiated thymocytes, *Int. J. Radiat. Biol.* **24**:397.

CORRY, P. M., AND COLE, A., 1968, Radiation-induced double-strand scission of the DNA of mammalian metaphase chromosomes, *Radiat. Res.* **36**:528.

CORRY, P. M., AND COLE, A., 1973, Double strand rejoining in mammalian DNA, *Nature (London) New Biol.* **245**:100.

CRAMP, W. A., WATKINS, D. K., AND COLLINS, J., 1972, Effects of ionizing radiation on bacterial DNA-membrane complexes, *Nature (London)* **235**:76.

DATTA, R., COLE, A., AND ROBINSON, S., 1976, Use of track-end alpha particles from [241]Am to study radiosensitive sites in CHO cells, *Radiat. Res.* **65**:139.

DAVIES, H. G., AND SMALL, J. V., 1968, Structural units in chromatin and their aventation on membranes, *Nature (London)* **217**:1122.

DEAN, C. J., AND ALEXANDER, P., 1962, Sensitization of radioresistant bacteria to X-rays by iodoacetamide, *Nature (London)* **196**:1324.

DEAN, C. J., AND PAULING, C., 1970, Properties of a deoxyribonucleic acid mutant of *Escherichia coli*: X-ray sensitivity, *J. Bacteriol.* **102**:588.

DEAN, C. J., ORMEROD, M. G., SERIANNI, R. W., AND ALEXANDER, P., 1969, DNA strand breakage in cells irradiated with X-rays, *Nature (London)* **222**:1042.

DEJONG, J., LOMAN, H., AND BLOK, J., 1972, Inactivation of biologically active DNA by radiation-induced phenylalanine radicals, *Int. J. Radiat. Biol.* **22**:11.

DEMOPOULOS, H. B., 1973, The basis of free radical pathology, *Fed. Proc.* **32**:1859 (and references therein).

DEWEY, D. L., AND BOAG, J. W., 1959, Modification of the oxygen effect when bacteria are given large pulses of radiation, *Nature (London)* **183**:1450.

DINGMAN, C. W., AND SPORN, M. D., 1965, Actinomycin D and hydrocortisone: Intracellular binding in rat liver, *Science* **149**:1251.

DUGLE, D. L., GILLESPIE, C. J., AND CHAPMAN, J. D., 1976, DNA strand breaks, repair, and survival in X-irradiated mammalian cells, *Proc. Natl. Acad. Sci. USA* **73**:809.

EBSTEIN, B. S., 1967, Tritiated actinomycin D as a cytochemical label for small amounts of DNA, *J. Cell Biol.* **35**:709.

ELKIND, M. M., 1970, Damage and repair processes relative to neutron (and charged particle) irradiation, *Curr. Top. Radiat. Res.* **7**:1.

ELKIND, M. M., 1971, Sedimentation of DNA released from Chinese hamster cells, *Biophys. J.* **11**:502.

ELKIND, M. M., 1974, Recovery, reoxygenation, and a strategy to improve radiotherapy, in: *The Biological and Clinical Basis of Radiosensitivity* (M. FRIEDMAN, ed.), pp. 343–372, Charles C. Thomas, Springfield, Ill.

ELKIND, M. M., 1975a, Damage-repair studies of the DNA from X-irradiated Chinese hamster cells, in: *Molecular Mechanisms for Repair of DNA* (P. C. HANAWALT AND R. B. SETLOW, eds.), pp. 689–698, Plenum Press, New York.

ELKIND, M. M., 1975b, unpublished findings.

ELKIND, M. M., AND BEN-HUR, E., 1974. DNA damage in mammalian cells and its relevance to lethality, in: *Proceedings of the Fourth Symposium on Microdosimetry* (Verbania-Pallenza, Italy, 24–28 Sept. 1973) (J. BOOZ, H. G. EBERT, R. EICKEL, AND A. WAKER, eds.), EURATOM Report EUR 5122 d-e-f, 1974.

ELKIND, M. M., AND CHANG-LIU, C. M., 1972a, Repair of a DNA complex from X-irradiated Chinese hamster cells, *Int. J. Radiat. Biol.* **22**:75.

ELKIND, M. M., and CHANG-LIU, C. M., 1972b, Actinomycin D inhibition of repair of a DNA complex from Chinese hamster cells, *Int. J. Radiat. Biol.* **22**:313.

ELKIND, M. M., AND KAMPER, C., 1970, Two forms of repair of DNA in mammalian cells following irradiation, *Biophys. J.* **10**:237.

ELKIND, M. M., AND KANO, E., 1971, Radiation-induced age–response changes in Chinese hamster cells: Evidence for a new form of damage and its repair, *Int. J. Radiat. Biol.* **19**:547.

ELKIND, M. M., AND SINCLAIR, W. K., 1965, Recovery in X-irradiated mammalian cells, in: *Current Topics in Radiation Research*, Vol. 1 (M. EBERT AND A. HOWARD, eds.), pp. 165–220, North-Holland, Amsterdam.

ELKIND, M. M., AND SUTTON, H. A., 1959, X-ray damage and recovery in mammalian cells in culture, *Nature (London)* **184**:1293.

ELKIND, M. M., AND SUTTON, H. A., 1960, Radiation response of mammalian cells grown in culture. I. Repair of X-ray damage in surviving Chinese hamster cells, *Radiat. Res.* **13**:556.

ELKIND, M. M., AND WHITMORE, G. F., 1967, *The Radiobiology of Cultured Mammalian Cells*, Gordon and Breach, New York.

ELKIND, M. M., and WITHERS, H. R., 1970, Sublethal damage repair and its role in the radiation response of cell renewal systems, in: *Pathology of Radiation* (C. C. BERDJIC, ed.), pp. 86–97, Williams and Wilkins, Baltimore.

ELKIND, M. M., SUTTON, H. A., AND MOSES, W. B., 1961, Postirradiation survival kinetics of mammalian cells grown in culture, *J. Comp. Cell Physiol.* **58**:113 (Suppl. 1).

ELKIND, M. M., HAN, A., AND WOLZ, K., 1963, Response of mammalian cells grown in culture. IV. Dose dependence of division delay and postirradiation growth in surviving and nonsurviving Chinese hamster cells, *J. Natl. Cancer Inst.* **30**:705.

ELKIND, M. M., ALESCIO, T., SWAIN, R. W., MOSES, W. B., AND SUTTON, H., 1964a, Recovery of hypoxic mammalian cells from sub-lethal X-ray damage, *Nature (London)* **202**:1190.

ELKIND, M. M., WHITMORE, G. F., AND ALESCIO, T., 1964b, Actinomycin D: Suppression of recovery in X-irradiated mammalian cells, *Science* **143**:1454.

ELKIND, M. M., SWAIN, R. W., ALESCIO, T., SUTTON, H., AND MOSES, W. B., 1965, Oxygen, nitrogen, recovery, and radiation therapy, in: *Cellular Radiation Biology*, pp. 442–461, Williams and Wilkins, Baltimore.

ELKIND, M. M., SUTTON-GILBERT, H. A., AND MOSES, W. B., 1966, unpublished data.

ELKIND, M. M., KAMPER, C., MOSES, W. B., AND SUTTON-GILBERT, H., 1967a, Sublethal-lethal radiation damage and repair in mammalian cells, *Brookhaven Symp. Biol.* **20**:134.

ELKIND, M. M., MOSES, W. B., AND SUTTON-GILBERT, H., 1967b, Radiation response of mammalian cells grown in culture. VI. Protein, DNA and RNA inhibition during the repair of X-ray damage, *Radiat. Res.* **31**:156.

ELKIND, M. M., SUTTON-GILBERT, H., MOSES, W. B., AND KAMPER, C., 1967c, Sub-lethal and lethal radiation damage, *Nature (London)* **214**:1088.

ELKIND, M. M., SAKAMOTO, K., AND KAMPER, C., 1968a, Age-dependent toxic properties of actinomycin D and X-rays in cultured Chinese hamster cells, *Cell Tissue Kinet.* **1**:209.

ELKIND, M. M., WITHERS, H. R., AND BELLI, J. A., 1968b, Intracellular repair and the oxygen effect in radiobiology and radiotherapy, *Front. Radiat. Ther. Oncol.* **3**:55.

EMMERSON, P. T., 1973, X-ray damage to DNA and loss of biological function: Effect of sensitizing agents, in: *Advances in Radiation Chemistry*, Vol. 3 (M. BURTON AND J. L. MAGEE, eds.), pp. 209–270, Wiley, New York.

EPP, E. R., WEISS, H., AND SANTOMASSO, A., 1968, The oxygen effect in bacterial cells irradiated with high intensity pulsed electrons, *Radiat. Res.* **34**:320.

EPP, E. R., WEISS, H., DJORDJEVIC, B., AND SANTOMASSO, A., 1972, The radiosensitivity of cultured mammalian cells exposed to single high intensity pulses of electrons in various concentrations of oxygen, *Radiat. Res.* **52**:324.

EPP, E. R., WEISS, H., AND LING, C. C., 1976, Irradiation of cells by single and double pulses of high intensity irradiation: Oxygen sensitization and diffusion kinetics, *Curr. Top. Radiat. Res. Q.* **11**:201.

FOX, M., AND NIAS, A. H. W., 1970, The influence of recovery from sublethal damage on the response of cells to protracted irradiation at low dose-rate, *Curr. Top. Radiat. Res. Q.* **7**:71.

FOX, R. A., FIELDEN, E. M., AND SAPORA, O., 1976, Yield of single-strand breaks in the DNA of *E. coli* 10 msecs after irradiation, *Int. J. Radiat. Biol.* **29**:391.

FREIFELDER, D., 1966, DNA strand breakage by X-irradiation, *Radiat. Res.* **29**:329.

GEORGE, K. C., SHENOY, M. A., JOSHI, D. S., BHATT, B. Y., SINGH, B. B., AND GOPAL-AYENGAR, 1975, Modification of radiation effects on cells by membrane binding agents—Procaine HCl, *Br. J. Radiol.* **48**:611.

HAGEN, U., KECK, K., KORGER, H., ZIMMERMAN, F., AND LUCKING, T., 1965, Ultraviolet light inactivation of the priming ability of DNA in the RNA polymerase system, *Biochim. Biophys. Acta* **95**:418.

HAHN, G. M., AND LITTLE, J. B., 1972, Plateau-phase cultures of mammalian cells: An *in vitro* model for human cancer, *Curr. Top. Radiat. Res.* **8**:39.

HALL, E. J., 1972, Radiation dose-rate: A factor of importance in radiobiology and radiotherapy, *Br. J. Radiol.* **45**:81.

HAN, A., AND ELKIND, M. M., 1976, Cell cycle dependent interaction of damage due to ionizing and nonionizing radiation in Chinese hamster cells, *Radiat. Res.* **67**: 586.

HARIHARAN, P. V., AND CERUTTI, P. A., 1972, Formation and repair of gamma-ray induced thymine damage in *Micrococcus radiodurans*, *J. Mol. Biol.* **66**:65.

HARIHARAN, P. V., AND CERUTTI, P. A., 1974, Excision of damaged thymine residues from gamma-irradiated poly (dA-dT) by crude extracts of *Escherichia coli*, *Proc. Natl. Acad. Sci. USA* **71**:3532.

HARIHARAN, P. V., AND HUTCHISON, F., 1973, Neutral sucrose gradient sedimentation of very large DNA from *Bacillus subtilis*. II. Double-strand breaks formed by gamma ray irradiation of the cells, *J. Mol. Biol.* **75**:479.

HAYNES, R. H., 1962, Reciprocal sensitization of *E. coli* by ionizing and UV radiation, *Radiat. Res.* **16**:562.

HORIKAWA, M., NIKAIDO, O., TANAKA, T., NAGATA, H., and SUGAHARA, T., 1970, Comparative studies on the rejoining of DNA strand breaks induced by X-irradiation in mammalian cell lines *in vitro*, *Exp. Cell. Res.* **63**:325.

HOWARD-FLANDERS, P., 1960, Effect of oxygen on the radiosensitivity of bacteriophage in the presence of sulphydryl compounds, *Nature (London)* **186**:485.

JACOB, F., RYTER, A., AND CUZIN, F., 1966, On the association between DNA and membrane in bacteria, *Proc. Roy. Soc. (London)* **164**:267.

JOHANSEN, I., AND HOWARD-FLANDERS, P., 1965, Macromolecular repair and free-radical scavenging in the protection of bacteria against X-rays, *Radiat. Res.* **24**:184.

JOHANSEN, I., GURVIN, I., AND RUPP, W. D., 1971, The formation of single-strand breaks in intracellular DNA by X-rays, *Radiat. Res.* **48**:599.

JOHANSEN, I., BOYE, E., AND BRUSTAD, T., 1975a, Radiation induced strand breaks and time scale for repair of broken strands in superinfecting phage λ DNA in *Escherichia coli* lysogenic for λ, in: *Fast Processes in Radiation Chemistry and Biology* (G. E. ADAMS, E. M. FIELDEN, AND B. D. MICHAEL, eds.), pp. 267–274, Institute of Physics and Wiley, London.

JOHANSEN, I., BRUSTAD, T., AND RUPP, W. D., 1975b, DNA strand breaks measured within 100 milliseconds of irradiation of *Escherichia coli* by 4 MeV electrons, *Proc. Natl. Acad. Sci. USA* **72**:167.

KAPLAN, H. S., 1966, DNA strand scission and loss of viability after X-irradiation of normal and sensitized bacterial cells, *Proc. Natl. Acad. Sci. USA* **55**:1442.

KAPLAN, H. S., AND MOSES, L. E., 1964, Biological complexity and radiosensitivity, *Science* **145**:21.

KAPLAN, H. S., AND ZAVARINE, R., 1962, Correlation of bacterial radiosensitivity and DNA base composition, *Biochem. Biophys. Res. Commun.* **8**:432.

KELLER, J. M., AND RILEY, D. E., 1976, Nuclear ghosts: A nonmembranous structural component of mammalian cell nuclei, *Science* **193**:399.

KITAYAMA, S., AND MATSUYAMA, A., 1968, Possibility of the repair of double-strand scissions in *Micrococcus radiodurans* DNA caused by gamma rays, *Biochem. Biophys. Res. Commun.* **33**:418.

KOEHNLEIN, W., AND HUTCHINSON, F., 1969, ESR-studies of normal and 5-bromouracil-substituted DNA of *Bacillus subtilis* after irradiation with ultraviolet light, *Radiat. Res.* **39**:745.

KRASIN, F., AND HUTCHINSON, F., 1976, Repair of DNA double-strand breaks by recombination, *Radiat. Res.* **67**:534.

KRISCH, R. E., 1976, Lethality and double-strand scissions from ^{14}C delay in the DNA of microorganisms, *Int. J. Radiat. Biol.* **29**:249.

KRISCH, R. E., KRASIN, F., AND SAURI, C. J., 1976, DNA breakage, repair and lethality after ^{125}I decay in rec[+] and rec A strains of *Escherichia coli*, *Int. J. Radiat. Biol.* **29**:37.

LARK, K. G., 1972, Evidence for the direct involvement of RNA in the initiation of DNA replication in *Escherichia coli* 15T[−], *J. Mol. Biol.* **64**:47.

LEHMANN, A. R., AND ORMEROD, M. G., 1970, The replication of DNA in murine lymphoma cells. I. Rate of replication, *Biochim. Biophys. Acta* **217**:268.

LENNARTZ, M., COQUERELLE, T., AND HAGEN, U., 1973, Effect of oxygen on DNA strand breaks in irradiated thymocytes, *Int. J. Radiat. Biol.* **24**:621.

LETT; J. T., CALDWELL, I., AND LITTLE, J. G., 1970, Repair of X-ray damage to the DNA in *Micrococcus radiodurans*: The effect of 5-bromodeoxyuridine, *J. Mol. Biol.* **48**:395.

LETT, J. T., SUN, C., AND WHEELER, K. T., 1972, Restoration of the DNA structure in X-irradiated eucaryotic cells: *In vitro* and *in vivo*, in: *Molecular and Cellular Repair Processes* (R. F. BEERS, JR., R. M. HERRIOTT, AND R. C. TILGHMAN, eds.), pp. 147–158, Johns Hopkins University Press, Baltimore.

LION, M., 1972, Mechanism of sensitization to UV radiation by 5-Br-uracil substituted DNA, *Isr. J. Chem.* **10**:1151.

LOHMAN, P. H. M., 1968, Induction and rejoining of breaks in the deoxyribonucleic acid of human cells irradiated at various phases of the cell cycle, *Mutat. Res.* **6**:449.

MARVIN, D. A., 1968, Control of DNA replication by membrane, *Nature (London)* **219**:485.

MATTERN, M. R., HARIHARAN, P. V., DUNLAP, B. E., AND CERUTTI, P. A., 1973, DNA degradation and excision repair in γ-irradiated Chinese hamster ovary cells, *Nature (London) New Biol.* **245**:230.

McGRATH, R. A., AND WILLIAMS, R. W., 1966, Reconstruction *in vivo* of irradiated *Escherichia coli* deoxyribonucleic acid; the rejoining of broken pieces, *Nature (London)* **212**:534.

MICHAEL, B. D., ADAMS, G. E., HEWITT, H. B., JONES, W. B. G., AND WATTS, M. E., 1973, A post-effect of oxygen in irradiated bacteria: A submillisecond fast mixing study, *Radiat. Res.* **54**:239.

MUNSON, R. J., NEARY, G. J., BRIDGES, B. A., AND PRESTON, R. J., 1967, The sensitivity of *Escherichia coli* to ionizing particles of different LET's, *Int. J. Radiat. Biol.* **13**:205.

NEARY, G. J., SIMPSON-GILDEMEISTER, V. F. W., AND PEACOCKE, A. R., 1970, The influence of radiation quality and oxyen on strand breakage in dry DNA, *Int. J. Radiat. Biol.* **18**:25.

NEARY, G. J., HORGAN, V. J., BANCE, D. A., AND STRETCH, A., 1972, Further data on DNA strand breakage by various radiation qualities, *Int. J. Radiat. Biol.* **22**:525.

NIAS, A. H. W., SWALLOW, A. J., KEENE, J. P., AND HODGSON, B. W., 1969, Effects of pulses of irradiation on the survival of mammalian cells, *Br. J. Radiol.* **42**:553.

ORMEROD, M. G., AND LEHMANN, A. R., 1971, The release of high molecular weight DNA from a mammalian cell (L5178Y), *Biochim. Biophys. Acta* **228**:331.

ORMEROD, M. G., AND STEVENS, U., 1971, The rejoining of x-ray-induced strand breaks in the DNA of murine a lymphoma cell (L5178Y), *Biochim. Biophys. Acta* **232**:72.

PAINTER, R. B., 1970, Repair of DNA in mammalian cells, *Curr. Top. Radiat. Res. Q.* **7**:45.

PALCIC, B., AND SKARSGARD, L. D., 1975, Absence of ultrafast processes of repair of single-strand breaks in mammalian DNA, *Int. J. Radiat. Biol.* **27**:121.

PERRY, R. P., 1963, Selective effects of actinomycin D on the intracellular distribution of RNA synthesis in tissue culture cells, *Exp. Cell. Res.* **29**:400.

PETKAU, A., AND CHELACK, W. S., 1974, Radioprotection of *Acholeplasma laidlawii* B by cysteine, *Int. J. Radiat. Biol.* **25**:321.

POWERS, E. L., 1972, The hydrated electron, the hydroxyl radical, and hydrogen peroxide in radiation damage in cells, *Isr. J. Chem.* **10**:1199.

POWERS, E. L., AND GAMPEL-JOBBAGY, Z., 1972, Water-derived radicals and the radiation sensitivity of bacteriophage T_7, *Int. J. Radiat. Biol.* **21**:353.

PUCK, T. T., AND KAO, F. T., 1967, Genetics of somatic mammalian cells. V. Treatment with 5-bromodeoxyuridine and visible light for isolation of nutritionally deficient mutants, *Proc. Natl. Acad. Sci. USA* **58**:1227.

PUCK, T. T., AND MARCUS, P. E., 1956, Action of X-rays on mammalian cells, *J. Exp. Med.* **103**:653.

RAUTH, A. M., AND SIMPSON, L. A., 1964, The energy loss of electrons in solids, *Radiat. Res.* **22**:643.

REDPATH, J. L., AND PATTERSON, L. K., 1976, Radiosensitization of *Serratia marcescens* by cetyl-pyridinium chloride: Evidence for membrane-associated events, *Radiology* **118**:725.

REICH, E., 1964, Actinomycin: Correlation of structure and function of its complexes with purines and DNA, *Science* **143**:684.

REMSEN, F., HARIHARAN, P. W., AND CERUTTI, P. A., 1976, Excision repair of monomeric, ring-saturated thymine damage in human cells, *Radiat. Res.* **67**:514.

ROOTS, R., AND OKADA, S., 1972, Protection of DNA molecules of cultured mammalian cells from radiation-induced single-strand scissions by various alcohols and SH compounds, *Int. J. Radiat. Biol.* **21**:329.

RUBENSTEIN, I., AND LEIGHTON, S. B., 1974, The influence of rotor speed on the sedimentation behavior in sucrose gradients of high molecular wieght DNA's, *Biophys. Chem.* **1**:292.

SALGNIK, R. I., DREVICK, V. F., AND VASYUNIA, E. A., 1967, Isolation of ultraviolet-denatured regions of DNA and their base composition, *J. Mol. Biol.* **30**:219.

SAPORA, O., FIELDEN, E. M., AND LOVEROCK, P. S., 1975, The application of rapid lysis techniques in radiobiology. I. The effect of oxygen and radiosensitizers on DNA strand break production and repair in *E. coli* B/r, *Radiat. Res.* **64**:431.

SAWADA, S. AND OKADA, S., 1970, Rejoining of single-strand breaks of DNA in cultured mammalian cells, *Radiat. Res.* **41**:145.

SERNA, F. R., AND SAMOYLENKO, I. I., 1975, The effect of temperature shock on the yield of gamma-induced single-strand breaks in bacterial DNA, *Biochem. Biophys. Res. Commun.* **67**:1415.

SETLOW, R. B., 1974, The wavelengths in sunlight effective in producing skin cancer: A theoretical analysis, *Proc. Natl. Acad. Sci. USA* **71**:3363.

SHENOY, M. A., SINGH, B. B., AND GOPAL-AYENGAR, A. R., 1974, Enhancement of radiation lethality of *E. coli* B/r by procaine HCl, *Nature (London)* **248**:415.

SHENOY, M. A., ASQUITH, J. C., ADAMS, G. E., MICHAEL, B. D., AND WATTS, M. E., 1975a, Time resolved oxygen effects in irradiated bacteria and mammalian cells: A rapid mix study, *Radiat. Res.* **62**:498.

SHENOY, M. A., GEORGE, K. C., SINGH, B. B., AND GOPAL-AYENGAR, A. R., 1975b, Modification of radiation effects in single cell systems by membrane-binding agents, *Int. J. Radiat. Biol.* **28**:519.

SHIPLEY, W. U., ELKIND, M. M., AND PRATHER, W. B., 1971, Potentiation of X-ray killing by 5-bromodeoxyuridine in Chinese hamster cells: A reduction in capacity for incurring sublethal damage, *Radiat. Res.* **47**:437.

SIMPSON, J. R., NAGLE, W. A., BECK, M. D., AND BELLI, J. A., 1973, Molecular nature of mammalian cell DNA in alkaline sucrose gradients, *Proc. Natl. Acad. Sci. USA* **70**(12, 1):3660.

SINCLAIR, W. K., 1965, Hydroxyurea: Differential lethal effects on cultured mammalian cells during the cell cycle, *Science* **150**:1729.

SINCLAIR, W. K., 1967, Hydroxyurea: Effect on Chinese hamster cells grown in culture, *Cancer Res.* **27**:297.

SINCLAIR, W. K., AND MORTON, R. A., 1964, Recovery following X-irradiation of synchronized Chinese hamster cells, *Nature (London)* **203**:247.

SINCLAIR, W. K., AND MORTON, R. A., 1965, X-ray and ultraviolet sensitivity of synchronized Chinese hamster cells at various stages of the cell cycle, *Biophys. J.* **5**:1.

SPARROW, A. H., UNDERBRINK, A. G., AND SPARROW, R. C., 1967, Chromosomes and cellular radiosensitivity. I. The relationship of D_0 to chromosome volume and complexity in seventy-nine different organisms, *Radiat. Res.* **32**:915.

STUBBLEFIELD, E., 1973, The structure of mammalian chromosomes, in: *International Review of Cytology* (G. H. BAURNE and J. F. DANIELLI, eds.), pp. 1–60, Academic Press, New York.

TAPPEL, A. L., 1973, Lipid peroxidation damage to cell components, *Fed. Proc.* **32**:1870.

TERZI, M., 1961, Comparative analysis of inactivation efficiency of radiation on different organisms, *Nature (London)* **191**:461.

TOWN, C. D., 1967, Effect of high dose-rates on survival of mammalian cells, *Nature (London)* **215**:847.

TOWN, C. D., SMITH, K. C., AND KAPLAN, H. S., 1972, Influence of ultra fast repair processes (independent of DNA polymerase I) on the yield of DNA single-strand breaks in *Escherichia coli* K12 X-irradiated in the presence or absence of oxygen, *Radiat. Res.* **52**:99.

TOWN, C. D., SMITH, K. C., AND KAPLAN, H. S., 1973a, Repair of X-ray damage to bacterial DNA, *Curr. Top. Radiat. Res. Q.* **8**:351.

TOWN, C. D., SMITH, K. C., AND KAPLAN, H. S., 1973b, The repair of DNA single-strand breaks in *E. coli* K12 X-irradiated in the presence or absence of oxygen, *Radiat. Res.* **55**:334.

ULLRICH, A., AND HAGEN, U., 1971, Base liberation and concomitant reactions in irradiated DNA solutions, *Int. J. Radiat. Biol.* **19**:507.

VAN HEMMEN, J. J., MEULING, W. J. A., VANDER SCHANS, G. P., AND BLEICHRODT, J. F., 1974a, On the mechanism of sensitization of living cells towards ionizing radiation by oxygen and other sensitizers, *Int. J. Radiat. Biol.* **25**:399.

VAN HEMMEN, J. J., MEULING, W. J. A., AND BLEICHRODT, J. F., 1974*b*, Radiosensitization of biologically active DNA in cellular extracts by oxygen: Evidence that the presence of SH compounds are not required, *Int. J. Radiat. Biol.* **26**:547.

VEATCH, W., AND OKADA, S., 1969, Radiation-induced breaks of DNA in cultured mammalian cells, *Biophys. J.* **9**:330.

WACKER, A., MENNINGMANN, H. D., AND SZYBALSKI, W., Effects of visible light on 5-bromouracil labelled DNA, *Nature (London)* **196**:685.

WARD, J. F., 1972, Mechanisms of radiation-induced strand break formation in DNA, *Isr. J. Chem.* **10**:1123.

WARING, M. J., 1968, Drugs which affect structure and function of DNA, *Nature (London)* **219**:1320.

WATKINS, D. K., 1970, High oxygen effect for the release of enzymes from isolated mammalian liposomes after treatment with ionizing radiation, in: *Advances in Biological and Medical Physics* (J. H. LAWRENCE AND J. W. GOFMAN, eds.), pp. 289–305, Academic Press, New York.

WHEELER, K. T., AND LETT, J. T., 1974, On the possibility that DNA repair is related to age in non-dividing cells, *Proc. Natl. Acad. Sci. USA* **71**:1862.

WILLS, E. D., AND WILKINSON, A. E., 1967, The effect of irradiation on lipid peroxide formation in subcellular fractions, *Radiat. Res.* **31**:732.

WISE, G. E., AND PRESCOTT, D. M., 1973, Initiation and continuation of DNA replication are not associated with the nuclear envelope in mammalian cells, *Proc. Natl. Acad. Sci. USA* **70**:714.

YANG, S. J., HAHN, G. M., AND VAN KERSEN-BAX, I., 1970, Effects of light on viability and DNA synthesis of mammalian cells preincubated in media containing brominated pyrimidines, *Photochem. Photobiol.* **11**:131.

ZERMENO, A., AND COLE, A., 1969, Radiosensitive structure of metaphase and interphase hamster cells as studied by low-voltage electron beam irradiation, *Radiat. Res.* **39**:669.

ZIMM, B. H., 1974, Anomalies in sedimentation. IV. Decrease in sedimentation coefficients of chains at high fields, *Biophys. Chem.* **1**:279.

4

Cell Proliferation Kinetics and Radiation Therapy

J. Denekamp and J. F. Fowler

1. Introduction

Radiation can perturb the cell proliferation kinetics of a population, and the cell kinetics can itself influence the response of the cell population to any further dose of radiation. These mutual interactions are of importance in the response of tumors and normal tissues to fractionated irradiation.

The differences in cell proliferation kinetics that distinguish a tumor from its normal tissue of origin also influence its response to the therapy aimed at eradicating it. The growth of a normal or malignant tissue can be characterized by the intermitotic or cell-cycle time, the growth fraction, and the rate of cell loss (Fig. 1). If all cells in a population are dividing (i.e., GF = 1.0), and there is no loss of cells, the tissue will increase in volume in a time equal to the cell-cycle time. If only a fraction of the cells are in the division cycle, the doubling time of the population will obviously be longer than the mean cell-cycle time. This may result from differentiation of some cells or from nutrient deficiencies. In most adult normal tissues, there is no net growth since the production rate of new cells is exactly balanced by a loss of other cells. Thus there is no such thing as a "doubling time," and the birth rate of new cells is the important quantity. However, a "potential doubling time" can be expressed, this being the time taken for as many extra cells to be produced as are initially present in the tissue. If the loss rate equals the birth rate, we have the steady-state condition of constant volume, which is typical of normally renewing tissues in the adult. It is the absence of this exact balance that

J. Denekamp and J. F. Fowler • Gray Laboratory, Cancer Research Campaign, Mount Vernon Hospital, Northwood, Middlesex HA6 2RN, England.

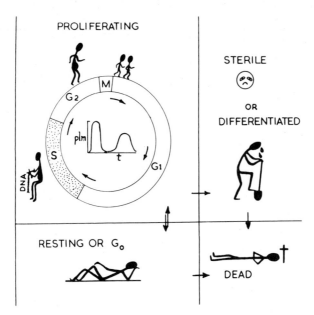

FIGURE 1. Model of tumor growth. Cells in growth fraction can be seen in mitosis or can be identified by labeling with DNA precursors. Nonproliferating cells may be sterile, differentiated, resting, nutritionally starved, or dead. Cells may be lost by exfoliation or by death and resorption. Redrawn from Begg (1975).

results in tumor growth. It may be caused by a reduction in the cell loss rate, an increase in the growth fraction, a shorter cell-cycle time, or a combination of these three.

Most animal tumors are characterized by cell-cycle times shorter than those of the normal tissue of origin, or by having a higher growth fraction. This shortening of T_C appears to result mainly from a reduction in the length of the postmitotic G_1 phase; the duration of mitosis is relatively constant, although the G_2 phase and sometimes the S phase are somewhat longer in tumors than in normal tissues.

Most systemic cancer chemotherapy is aimed at killing dividing cells and usually kills cells in a particular phase, e.g., cells at mitosis or cells in DNA synthesis. Such drugs may be either "cycle specific" or "phase specific" because they act only on those cells which are in cycle or in a particular phase. Therefore, the cell-cycle time and the growth fraction of the tumor cells relative to *any* dividing normal cells in the body are of importance for chemotherapy, because the drugs will reach most of the tissues in the body. The critical toxicity of most chemotherapeutic drugs results from extensive cell killing in rapidly proliferating normal cells, such as those in the bone marrow or in the intestine. In radiotherapy, by contrast, the treatment is given to a well-localized volume. Thus, although the action of radiotherapy is greatest on proliferating cells, whether malignant or not, it is only the cells in the irradiated volume that need to be considered. For primary tumors, this always includes the tissue of origin, the supporting connective tissue with its vasculature, and the overlying epidermis. Other organs may also be within the irradiated field in certain circumstances.

The influence of cell kinetic parameters on the processes occurring between radiation dose fractions can most readily be considered in relation to the four R's of radiobiology: repair, redistribution, reoxygenation, and repopulation.

Small doses of radiation, such as those used clinically, are mainly absorbed as 103
CELL
PROLIFERATION
KINETICS AND
RADIATION
THERAPY sublethal injury, which can be repaired by the cell if time is allowed to elapse before the next irradiation. It is not possible to predict the extent of repair of sublethal radiation injury in any cell from kinetic parameters, but certain tumors have been shown to have a lower repair capacity than normal tissues. Cells *in vitro* which are not in the cell cycle or which are hypoxic have been shown to have a reduced ability to repair sublethal damage. Rapidly dividing cells, however, are unlikely to exhibit slow repair or repair of potentially lethal damage, and this slow repair may be the important time component in fractionated radiotherapy.

Cells in certain phases of the cell cycle are more sensitive to radiation and are more readily killed, leaving a partially synchronized population whose sensitivity will change as it becomes redistributed around the cell cycle. Although the potential exists for using this difference in sensitivity to increase the therapeutic gain, the information necessary to plan such a strategy is formidable and is unlikely to be available for a long time to come.

Hypoxic cells exist in many tumors because of the imbalance between tumor-cell production and vascular proliferation. Normal tissues, by contrast, are adequately vascularized and seldom contain hypoxic cells. Any hypoxic cells are of great importance in the response to radiotherapy because they are 2–3 times more resistant to conventional forms of radiation than well-oxygenated cells. This makes the tumor cells more difficult to eradicate than normal tissue cells. The proportion of hypoxic cells depends on the proliferation characteristics of an individual tumor, as does the improvement in oxygen status, termed "reoxygenation," of these cells between successive doses.

Accelerated proliferation occurs in normal tissues as a response to cell depletion, presumably via some homeostatic feedback mechanism. This repopulation replaces lost cells and can make the normal tissues more tolerant to subsequent doses. However, accelerated proliferation can be slow to occur in some normal tissues, and it can also occur in certain tumors.

An understanding of the quantitation of these four factors in the different normal tissues of the body and in different tumors would obviously aid the rational planning of improved fractionation schedules.

2. Response to Single Doses of Radiation

The response of any cell population, whether normal or malignant, to a dose of radiation follows a well-known pattern. Initially, there is a delay in the progress of cells around the cell cycle (mitotic delay), which is proportional to the radiation dose administered and is also proportional to the cell-cycle time. The cells accumulate in the premitotic G_2 phase, and are blocked from entry into mitosis (Mottram, 1913; Mottram *et al.*, 1926). A delay of approximately one-tenth of a cell cycle is induced for each 100 rads administered, at least up to doses of 1000 rads (Elkind *et al.*, 1963; Whitmore *et al.*, 1967; Doida and Okada, 1969). In rapidly growing tissues such as intestinal epithelium, or cells *in vitro*, this is close to 1 hr delay per 100 rads (Lesher and Bauman, 1968). In more slowly dividing tissues such as skin it is about 7 hr delay per 100 rads, and in very slowly dividing tissues such as liver, kidney, and lung the mitotic delay would be expected to be even longer (Brown, 1970; Hegazy and Fowler, 1973; Denekamp, 1975).

Second, the radiation damage is expressed in dividing cells as a loss of their proliferative capacity. Most cells die at a mitosis subsequent to the radiation-induced mitotic delay (Elkind *et al.*, 1963). At high doses (1000–2000 rads), cells die at the first postirradiation division, but after smaller doses some die at a second or third division. There are a few notable exceptions to the rule of radiation death occurring at mitosis, e.g., lymphocytes, which can die a more rapid interphase death without any attempt at mitosis. For most somatic cells, however, the expression of radiation damage is delayed until mitosis is attempted. After 1000 rads, this may occur within 12 hr in the intestine, within 4–5 days in skin, and presumably not for many weeks in tissues with very long turnover times such as liver, lung, and kidney (Denekamp, 1975). Since most tissues consist of a variety of cells with different proliferation rates, the expression of radiation damage is likely to occur at different times in the different cell compartments. Organ function may be impaired either when the majority of cells have died or when a critical subpopulation has started to express its damage. For this reason, it has been suggested that radiation damage in many organs may have a common pathway of expression in the form of endothelial cell death. Endothelial cells have a very slow turnover time of 2–4 months as measured by simple tritiated thymidine uptake studies (Tannock and Hayashi, 1972). It is not clear whether this is due to a prolonged cell cycle in all the cells, or to only a few cells having a short cell-cycle time. If all the cells have a long cycle, the abortive postirradiation divisions would be expected to occur at 2–4 months, and this corresponds to the time of expression of radiation damage in some tissues, e.g., lung (Phillips, 1966, 1969). Death of endothelial cells, causing a failure to repopulate the endothelium locally, can lead to blood clots forming on the denuded basement membrane, occlusion of the capillary, and a loss of blood flow to the area served by that capillary. This will result in parenchymal cell death if a collateral supply is not available. Because of this interrelationship, it is difficult to determine whether parenchymal cell death in slowly dividing tissues is a primary or a secondary event.

2.1. Sensitivity through the Cell Cycle

The sensitivity of cells to a dose of radiation varies with the cells' age within the cell cycle (Fig. 2). Cells are often most resistant in late-S phase, are most sensitive in mitosis, and have intermediate sensitivities in G_1 and early S (Sinclair and Morton, 1963; Terasima and Tolmach, 1963; Whitmore *et al.*, 1965). Since DNA synthesis and mitosis are of relatively invariant length, the proportion of cells in the different phases varies with the duration of the cell cycle. A small single dose of radiation will preferentially kill the most sensitive mitotic cells, which may

105

CELL
PROLIFERATION
KINETICS AND
RADIATION
THERAPY

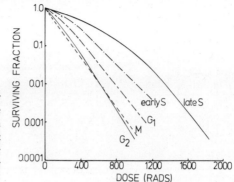

FIGURE 2. Cell survival curves for Chinese hamster cells irradiated at various stages of the cell cycle after synchrony induced by mitotic harvest. Cells in mitosis show an exponential response and are most sensitive. Cells in late-S phase have a large shoulder and are most resistant. Redrawn from Sinclair (1968).

constitute up to 5% of a rapidly dividing tissue such as intestine, or less than 0.1% of a slowly dividing tissue such as lung or liver. With increasing dose, the cells of intermediate sensitivity are killed, and a partially synchronized population of cells in the more resistant phases is left. This population can become further synchronized by the mitotic delay process, i.e., by the accumulation of cells in the G_2 premitotic block. The response to a second dose of radiation will thus depend on the extent of this synchrony and the position to which the cells have progressed.

2.2. Hypoxic Cells in Tumors

The degree of oxygenation at the time of irradiation is the most potent modifier of radiation response known. Cells irradiated under well-oxygenated conditions are approximately 3 times more sensitive than cells which are short of oxygen, i.e., hypoxic (Gray *et al.*, 1953; Alper and Howard-Flanders, 1956; Deschner and Gray, 1959). Such hypoxic cells seldom exist in well-organized normal tissues because the vasculature is sufficiently well developed to supply all cells with an adequate amount of all nutrients, including oxygen. In tumors, however, the rate of production of tumor cells may exceed the maximum rate of production of new blood vessels (Thomlinson and Gray, 1955; Tannock, 1968, 1970). The tumor cells push the capillaries apart, and intercapillary distances become too great for maintenance of an adequate supply of nutrients. Cells at the maximum distance from the blood vessels get very little oxygen, because it is metabolized by the intervening respiring cells. In many tumors, a characteristic histological pattern is observed in which necrosis develops at about 150 μm from the capillaries. Thomlinson and Gray (1955) correlated this appearance of necrosis with the calculated oxygen diffusion distance. They estimated that one to two cell layers bounding the necrotic zone could be radiobiologically resistant because of their low oxygen content (Fig. 3). They argued that if the tumor continued to grow, these cells would traverse the boundary into the necrotic zone. But if they were provided with a better oxygen supply, after the more radiosensitive oxic cells near the capillary had been killed with a noncurative dose of radiation, they could then repopulate the tumor.

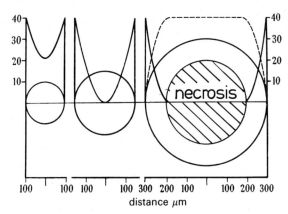

FIGURE 3. Schematic representation of the development of hypoxia and necrosis in a cylinder of tumor cells as it increases in diameter. The oxygen tension (vertical axis = partial pressure of oxygen in mm Hg) falls with increasing distance from peripheral blood vessels. When the cord diameter reaches about 150 μm, some cells have a sufficiently low [O_2] to be radioresistant. At even larger sizes, a necrotic center develops, with hypoxic cells bordering it. After Thomlinson and Gray (1955).

Most experimental tumors have been shown to contain a significant proportion of hypoxic cells, often 10–20% (Table 1). These radioresistant cells can, in animals, be made more sensitive by using hyperbaric oxygen during irradiation, by using densely ionizing radiations, or by administering oxygen-mimicking chemicals before the irradiation. These three approaches are currently being tested in clinical trials as means of overcoming the problem of hypoxic radioresistance (e.g., Henk and Smith, 1973; Dische, 1974; Catterall et al., 1975; Thomlinson et al., 1976; Urtasun et al., 1976).

Thomlinson (1971) has shown in several types of rat tumor that the benefit of hyperbaric oxygen in sensitizing the tumors to radiation varies systematically with the volume doubling time (Fig. 4). In rapidly growing tumors he obtained a high degree of sensitization, but with more slowly growing tumors this advantage was progressively reduced. Five of the six tumors in his series were soft tissue sarcomas, which are likely to have longer cell-cycle times as a cause of their slow volume growth (Denekamp, 1970, 1972). It is possible that slow-growing sarcomas

TABLE 1
Hypoxia in Experimental Tumors

Tumor	Percent hypoxic cells	References
Mouse sarcoma	50	Hewitt and Wilson (1961)
Mouse lymphosarcoma	1	Powers and Tolmach (1963)
Mouse adenocarcinoma	21	Clifton and Briggs (1966)
Mouse sarcoma	15	Van Putten and Kallman (1966)
Rat rhabdomyosarcoma	15	Reinhold (1966)
Mouse squamous carcinoma	18	Hewitt et al. (1967)
Mouse mammary carcinoma	20–25	Suit and Maeda (1967)
Mouse mammary carcinoma	7	Howes (1969)
Mouse osteosarcoma	14	Van Putten (1968a)
Mouse mammary carcinoma	18–21	Kallman et al. (1970)
Rat fibrosarcoma	17	Thomlinson (1971)
Mouse sarcoma	12	Hill et al. (1971)
Mouse mammary carcinoma	1–17	Fowler et al. (1975)
Mouse sarcoma	10–50	McNally (1975)
Mouse mammary carcinoma	6	Denekamp et al. (1976)

107

CELL
PROLIFERATION
KINETICS AND
RADIATION
THERAPY

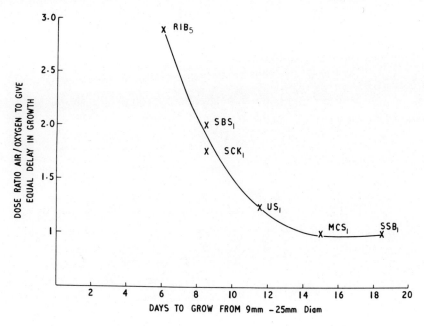

FIGURE 4. Sensitization of tumor cells by hyperbaric oxygen breathing as a function of growth rate for six different rat tumors. The ratio of X-ray dose given in air or under hyperbaric oxygen to achieve the same level of damage may be a measure of the hypoxic fraction. This ratio is highest for the rapidly growing sarcomas RIB5 and SBS1, is intermediate for the kidney carcinoma SCK1, and falls toward unity for the slow-growing sarcomas US1, MCS1, and SSB1. From Thomlinson (1971).

(but not carcinomas) may constitute one group where the cell birth rate is sufficiently slow for an adequate vascular supply to be maintained. These tumors may be exceptional in that they would contain no hypoxic cells. Slow-growing carcinomas differ in that their slow growth is mainly due to extensive cell loss balancing the rapid cell production (Denekamp, 1970, 1972).

3. Response to Fractionated Irradiation

The factors which influence the response to a single dose of radiation are clearly related to the proliferation kinetics. However, radiation therapy is seldom administered as a single dose. More often it is given as a series of small fractions, often 5 times a week for 4–6 weeks. In this way it has been found that more effective tumor ·destruction can be achieved with less extensive normal tissue damage. Since no consistent differences in radiation response of normal or malignant cells cultured *in vitro* have been identified, the reason for the advantage of fractionated treatment *in vivo* may lie in the physiological mechanisms which act upon cells *in vivo* and are absent *in vitro*.

Four main radiobiological processes have been identified as important in fractionated radiotherapy, as mentioned in the introduction:

1. Reassortment around the cell cycle.
2. Repopulation of surviving cells.
3. Reoxygenation of hypoxic cells.
4. Repair of sublethal radiation damage.

The first three of these are obviously related to the cell proliferation characteristics, and certain aspects of repair may be related also.

3.1. Reassortment

After a first dose of radiation, cells which have been partially synchronized by preferential killing in the more sensitive phases of the cell cycle progress around the cell cycle and accumulate in a premitotic G_2 block. During this progression, their sensitivity varies according to the phase of the cycle through which they are passing (Sinclair and Morton, 1963; Whitmore *et al.*, 1965; Denekamp *et al.*, 1969). Since tumors and their normal tissue of origin often have different cell-cycle times, this variation in sensitivity could in theory be used to plan the timing of subsequent doses of radiation, for example, to hit tumor cells in a sensitive mitotic phase while normal cells were in a resistant late-S phase. Although in principle this could give a large differential effect, even if the treatments were only partially optimized (Hahn, 1968*a*, 1975), the information required for such planning is formidable. A detailed knowledge of the cell-cycle parameters of the tumor cells and of all the normal cells in the irradiation field is necessary, together with a knowledge of their differential sensitivities in the different cell-cycle phases. Since after many years of study this is not yet available for any single animal transplantable tumor, it seems unlikely that it could be determined for an individual patient sufficiently rapidly to tailor the treatment for that patient's therapy. Furthermore, if regulatory mechanisms alter the kinetic parameters of either the normal tissue or the tumor during a course of fractionated therapy, the problems and the necessary information would be compounded.

Withers (1975a) has pointed out another aspect of the reassortment in relation to cell kinetic parameters. In a rapidly cycling cell population, progression of the partly synchronized population will result in a redistribution of cells throughout the cell cycle; the average radiosensitivity will increase relative to that of the resistant survivors at the end of the first dose. In slowly cycling populations, however, the cells may remain in their resistant state between fractions. This could result in an apparently greater radioresistance of slowly dividing tissues relative to rapidly cycling cells, i.e., of many slowly dividing normal tissues relative to tumors.

An alternative method of utilizing differential cell-cycle sensitivity is by means of drugs which will induce a synchrony of cells just prior to each radiation dose. In more rapidly dividing tumor populations, vincristine, methotrexate, or some other mitotic-arrest agent could be used to accumulate cells in a sensitive mitotic phase before irradiation. In a more slowly dividing normal tissue, the number of cells accumulated in mitosis would be small, and there could be a net gain in tumor damage relative to normal tissue damage. However, as yet, clinical trials with methotrexate and radiotherapy have shown no clear gain, and there is some doubt about the benefit from such synchronizing treatments (Tubiana *et al.*, 1975).

109

CELL
PROLIFERATION
KINETICS AND
RADIATION
THERAPY

3.2. Repopulation

In normal tissues, there is a finely balanced homeostatic mechanism such that a significant drop in cell numbers below the normal level is compensated for by means of an increased rate of cell production. This increased production may occur in three ways: (1) from a shortening of the cell-cycle time, as in the small intestine and skin (Lesher *et al.*, 1966, 1975; Hegazy and Fowler, 1973; Denekamp *et al.*, 1976); (2) from an increased growth fraction, by inducing some resting G_0 cells to enter the division cycle, as in the liver; or (3) by a delay in the rate of loss of cells along the pathway of differentiation, for example, an extra division in the amplification process of cell production in the bone marrow or the small intestine (Lord, 1975; Lamerton, 1966). This recognition of cell depletion and compensatory proliferation is characteristic of most normal tissues, and it is the loss of this exact balance that characterizes cancer. The growth of a tumor results from the rate of production of cells exceeding the rate of loss. It has been postulated that the ability to recognize cell depletion is also lost with malignancy and that compensatory proliferation will not follow cell depletion in tumors (Lajtha and Oliver, 1962; Ellis, 1969), but this has been shown to be untrue in some tumors (Hermens and Barendsen, 1969; Van Peperzeel, 1970).

3.2.1. Repopulation in Normal Tissues

Accelerated proliferation in response to injury can be very rapid when the injury results in immediate cell destruction such as from mechanical trauma, incision, or burns caused by caustic chemicals (Fowler and Denekamp 1976). Shortly after such injuries to skin, within 6–48 hr, a wave of DNA-synthesizing and mitotic cells is observed near the site of cell death. The compensation appears to occur when cell damage has been recognized, and, since the expression of radiation damage is usually delayed until a subsequent mitosis, the compensatory proliferation after radiation injury is also delayed. In skin, for example, the proliferation kinetics does not alter for at least 1 week after either a single dose or the start of repeated doses that will each kill a substantial proportion of the cells (Denekamp *et al.*, 1969, 1976; Denekamp, 1973; Hegazy and Fowler, 1973). Thus a course of radiation therapy as usually administered over a period of 4–7 weeks will not induce proliferation in skin in the first week, but will induce a more rapid proliferation in the second and third weeks as more and more cell depletion is recognized (Fig. 5). More rapidly dividing tissues such as intestine will respond earlier (Lesher *et al.*, 1975; Withers and Elkind, 1969; Chen and Withers, 1972), but more slowly dividing tissues such as lung, liver, kidney, muscle, nervous tissue, and vascular and connective tissue are unlikely to express their cell death during the course of therapy and hence are unlikely to show increased proliferation rates until after the therapy has been completed (Denekamp, 1975).

J. DENEKAMP
AND
J. F. FOWLER

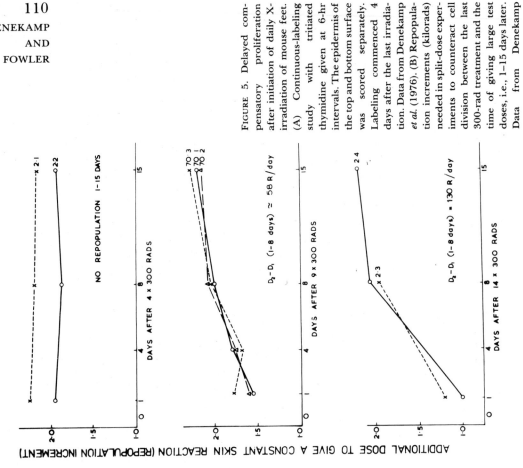

FIGURE 5. Delayed compensatory proliferation after initiation of daily X-irradiation of mouse feet. (A) Continuous-labeling study with tritiated thymidine given at 6-hr intervals. The epidermis of the top and bottom surface was scored separately. Labeling commenced 4 days after the last irradiation. Data from Denekamp et al. (1976). (B) Repopulation increments (kilorads) needed in split-dose experiments to counteract cell division between the last 300-rad treatment and the time of giving large test doses, i.e., 1–15 days later. Data from Denekamp (1973).

3.2.2. *Repopulation in Tumors*

111

CELL
PROLIFERATION
KINETICS AND
RADIATION
THERAPY

Tumor cells often have a shorter cell cycle or potential doubling time than the normal tissue of origin (Table 2). Thus the radiation-injured malignant cells will attempt to divide sooner than the normal cells and will express their lethal damage by an abortive division. A number of studies have been performed to determine whether the cells in X-irradiated tumors can show a compensatory increased proliferation rate. These are summarized in Table 3. Only two out of the ten solid tumors studied have shown a shortened cell-cycle time after irradiation (Hermens and Barendsen, 1969; Van Peperzeel, 1970). Six others have shown no change in T_C (Denekamp and Thomlinson 1971; Tubiana *et al.*, 1968; Nelson *et al.*, 1976), whereas the last two have shown an elongated cell cycle (Brown, 1970; Szczepanski and Trott, 1975). In the rhabdomysarcoma studied by Hermans and Barendsen, the response was associated with changes in density of cells per unit volume. When the cell density decreased as dead cells were lost, the cell cycle shortened to a value similar to that which characterized an earlier phase of the tumor growth (Hermens and Barendsen, 1969). This change of cell cycle is also demonstrated by ascites tumors of different ages, again corresponding to different cell densities.

The other main mode of increase in cell production rate is by increasing the number of cells in the growth fraction. This results from an active stimulus in normal tissues, but it seems more likely in tumors to result from an improvement in their nutritional milieu. The death of some of the well-oxygenated, radiosensitive cells lying between the vasculature and the surviving cells will reduce the rate of utilization of nutrients and increase the diffusion pathlengths. Previously starved or hypoxic cells can then gain access to an adequate nutritional supply and

TABLE 2

Comparison of Cell-Cycle Times of Normal Tissues and Tumors Derived from Them

| Tissue of origin | Cell-cycle time (hr) | | Reference |
	Normal	Tumor	
Mouse skin	100–150[a]	32	Dörmer *et al.* (1964)
			Hegazy and Fowler (1973)
Rabbit skin	125–750	21	Rashad and Evans (1968)
Hamster cheek pouch epithelium	140–170[a]	11–21[a]	Reiskin and Mendelsohn (1964)
			Brown (1970)
Mouse mammary gland	64	15–33[a]	Bresciani (1965)
			Mendelsohn (1965)
			Denekamp (1970)
Mouse forestomach	28–55[a]	8–12[a]	Frankfurt (1967*a,b*)
Human cervix	100–600	15[a]	Iliya and Azar (1967)
			Bennington (1969)
Mouse cervix	23[a]	26[a]	Hasegawa *et al.* (1976)

[a]Obtained from percent labeled mitoses (PLM) curves, or other estimate of T_C. All other values are derived from the 1 hr labeling index (LI) and the duration of S phase (T_S), and are really potential doubling times. If the growth fraction is less than unity, T_C will be shorter than the value shown.

J. DENEKAMP
AND

J. F. FOWLER

TABLE 3

Proliferation Changes after Irradiation in Experimental Tumors

Tumor type	Cell-cycle time (hr)	Growth fraction (GF %)	Cell loss %	References
Hamster buccal carcinoma	Increased 11→13	—	—	Brown (1970)
Rat rhabdomysarcoma	Decreased 25.5→12.5[a] 18.5→11.5[b]	Decreased 30→25 then increased	Increased 60→140	Hermens and Barendsen (1969)
Mouse NCTC fibrosarcoma	No change 17.5→17.5	—	—	Tubiana *et al.* (1968)
Mouse adenocarcinoma	Decreased 14.5→11	Increased 87→100	Decreased 33→0	Van Peperzeel (1970)
Mouse mammary carcinoma	No change 16→15	No change 37→40	No change 70→76	Denekamp and Thomlinson (1971)
Rat fibrosarcoma RIB5	No change 13.2→12.8	Increased 45→57	Increased 0→64	Denekamp and Thomlinson (1971)
Rat fibrosarcoma SSO	No change 20.5 → 20.5	Increased 48→55	Increased 0→64	Denekamp and Thomlinson (1971)
Rat fibrosarcoma SSB1	No change 39→39	Decreased 60→43	Increased 25→68	Denekamp and Thomlinson (1971)
Mouse adenocarcinoma	Increased 13.6→19	Increased 25→50	—	Szczepanski and Trott (1975)
Mouse mammary carcinoma	No change 19.3→18.5	Decreased 70→50	Increased 60→76	Nelson *et al.* (1976)

[a] Center of tumor.
[b] Periphery of tumor.

can reenter the cell cycle. An increase in the growth fraction has been observed in five of the tumors studied (Table 3).

An increased rate of tumor growth could also result from a reduction in the rate of cell loss after irradiation. Although some workers have reported more rapid volume doubling rates in lung tumors after irradiation (Van Peperzeel, 1970; Malaise *et al.*, 1972), this is unusual, and most studies have demonstrated slower growth and an increased rate of cell loss (Table 3).

If proliferation occurs between successive radiation treatments, more dose is, of course, necessary to reduce the population to a particular level. Accelerated proliferation increases this dose even further. Any increased proliferation of normal tissue cells will therefore protect that tissue against excessive damage. Extending treatment times to take advantage of this gain is useful only if the normal tissue proliferation rate, stimulated or otherwise, exceeds the rate of production of tumor cells (Lajtha and Oliver, 1962). This difference is unlikely to occur except in the most rapidly dividing normal tissues such as intestinal epithelia, skin, and mucosa (Denekamp, 1975). Many of the critical normal tissues in clinical radiotherapy, including vascular endothelium, divide slowly and are therefore unlikely to increase their proliferation rate before the end of therapy.

3.3. Hypoxia and Reoxygenation

113

CELL
PROLIFERATION
KINETICS AND
RADIATION
THERAPY

The development of radioresistant hypoxic cells in tumors is due to the imbalance between the rate of production of tumor cells and of new vascular endothelium to line the capillaries feeding them. The exact proportion of hypoxic cells differs in different tumors, but most fall within the range of 5–20% (Table 1). Tumors which are rapidly producing new cells (i.e., all carcinomas and those sarcomas which are rapidly growing) are likely to have hypoxic cells present, whereas in slow-growing sarcomas the vascular supply may develop in step with the tumor volume and no hypoxic cells result (Thomlinson, 1971; Denekamp, 1970).

Differences in proliferation patterns of human tumors with different histologies have also been found in the studies of Malaise *et al.* (1973, 1975). They have divided human tumors into five categories, and they conclude that the proliferation pattern differs in the different groups (Table 4) but that it is more likely to reflect growth fraction variations then cell cycle or cell loss. They found very high cell-loss factors in the squamous carcinomas and somewhat lower values in the mesenchymal sarcomas, in agreement with the animal data (Denekamp, 1970). The response to therapy also varies with the proliferation characteristics and is directly related to the kinetics, in particular, to the rate of cell loss (Malaise *et al.*, 1975).

The nutritional deprivation that is common in tumors does not arise in normal tissues and there are few avascular tissues apart from the lens of the eye and mature cartilage. Because of the resistance of hypoxic tumor cells to radiation, they are more likely to survive a dose of radiation. After large doses of 1–2 krads, hypoxic cells may comprise almost 100% of the surviving tumor cells. Thomlinson (1968) first drew the hypothetical model shown in Fig. 6. This demonstrates the development of hypoxic cells as the first nucleus of cells outgrows its vascular bed and then the suddenly increased proportion of hypoxic cells among the survivors after irradiation. Several alternative fates are then possible for these surviving hypoxic cells. They may remain hypoxic and eventually die of the nutritional deprivation, in which case they are of no importance to the animal bearing the tumor. The tumors could then be sterilized by a dose of radiation just big enough to kill all the well-oxygenated cells. Alternatively, they may gain access to an

TABLE 4

Mean Kinetic Parameters and Radiosensitivity of Human Tumors[a]

Histology	Doubling time (days)	Labeling index (%)	Growth fraction (%)	Cell loss (ϕ) (%)	Average cure dose (krads)
Embryonal tumor	27	30	90	93	2.5–3.0
Malignant lymphoma	29	29	90	93	3.5–4.5
Mesenchymal sarcoma	41	4	11	68	>8.5
Squamous cell carcinoma	58	8	25	89	6.0–7.0
Adenocarcinoma	83	2	6	71	6.0–8.0

[a] From Malaise *et al.* (1975).

J. DENEKAMP
AND
J. F. FOWLER

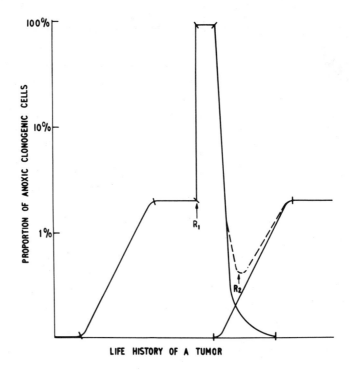

FIGURE 6. Tumor reoxygenation: model of the proportion of hypoxic clonogenic cells in a tumor as it grows, and after treatment with radiation. At very small sizes, the vasculature is adequate, but a characteristic proportion of hypoxic cells develop as the tumor outgrows its blood supply. After a large single dose of radiation, R_1, most of the survivors will be the resistant hypoxic cells. Their oxygenation status will improve (see text) until regrowth of the tumor results in a further increase in the hypoxic fraction. The tumor will be most sensitive to a subsequent dose of radiation R_2 at the time when there are fewest hypoxic cells. After Thomlinson (1968).

improved nutritional supply and may grow up to repopulate the tumor and cause a local recurrence (Thomlinson and Craddock, 1967). This improvement in supply may occur in any of three ways:

1. The cells damaged by the radiation progress more slowly around the cell cycle for a few hours, so their metabolic rate may be slightly reduced and therefore the diffusion pathlength of oxygen may be increased.
2. When the damaged cells die at a subsequent mitosis, they cease to respire and the oxygen can diffuse further.
3. When the dead cells are removed from the tumors by autolysis and phagocytosis, the previously hypoxic survivors will come closer to the blood vessels and the intercapillary distances will be reduced.

All these processes will lead to a *reoxygenation* of the hypoxic cells. This makes them more dangerous to the animal because they can cause tumor regrowth, but it also makes them about 3 times more sensitive to subsequent radiation doses. This process of reoxygenation is shown as a falling proportion of hypoxic cells in Fig. 6. 115

CELL
PROLIFERATION
KINETICS AND
RADIATION
THERAPY

Any surviving cells will regrow within the tumor, however, and intercapillary distances will eventually increase again, so that the original hypoxic fraction may be reestablished (Thomlinson, 1968). The timing of subsequent doses of radiation is therefore critical in terms of these reoxygenation patterns, and this timing is likely to vary from tumor to tumor.

The detailed and time-consuming studies needed to determine the reoxygenation kinetics have been performed on only six different types of animal tumors. These are summarized in Fig. 7. They include three sarcomas and three carcinomas. All six tumors showed an immediate increase in hypoxic fraction after irradiation as the more sensitive oxygenated cells were lethally injured. The hypoxic fraction fell within the first 24 hr in all but one of the tumors at a time when the sarcomas were continuing to increase in size. Thus shortened intercapillary distances could not be the cause of the reoxygenation for all of them. Reoxygenation could, however, result from reduced oxygen metabolism and increased diffusion pathlengths. A 30% reduction in oxygen utilization was observed in the rat tumor RIB5 at 18 hr after a large single dose of X-rays (Evans and Thomlinson, personal communication). In tumor RIB5, this initial phase of reoxygenation was superseded after 24 hr; the tumors became more hypoxic, probably as a result of the cells being pushed beyond the new diffusion length by the continued expansion of the tumor (Thomlinson, 1971). Only after 48 hr did

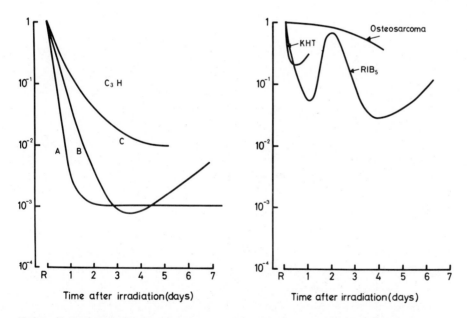

FIGURE 7. Reoxygenation kinetics for six experimental tumors. Normalized proportion of hypoxic cells as a function of time after irradiation. The three rapidly shrinking carcinomas (left) show very extensive reoxygenation, whereas the three sarcomas (right) show much less effective reoxygenation. The second phase of reoxygenation in RIB5 occurs at the time when the tumor shrinks. A, B, and C are for C3H mammary carcinomas from Fowler *et al.* (1975), from Howes (1969), and from Howes' calculations on data from Suit and Maeda (1967). KHT data from Kallman (1972), RIB5 from Thomlinson (1971), and osteosarcoma from Van Putten (1968*b*).

this tumor start to shrink, and the shrinkage was accompanied by a second phase of reoxygenation, presumably due to reduced intercapillary distances. Delayed shrinkage is characteristic of soft tissue sarcomas in experimental animals (Fig. 8), and this may be the reason for the poor reoxygenation in all three sarcomas in Fig. 7. Carcinomas, on the other hand, are characterized by rapid shrinkage after large single doses of radiation, often being appreciably smaller within 24 hr after irradiation (Fig. 9). Thus the shrinkage phase and the early phase of reduced oxygen consumption will occur simultaneously, and reoxygenation should be more extensive. This has indeed been observed in the three carcinomas shown in Fig. 7, and in none of the sarcomas. The rapid shrinkage after irradiation in carcinomas and its absence in sarcomas seem to correlate with the rates of cell loss in the tumor before irradiation. When mitotic delay is induced by the radiation, the tumors showing a high cell-loss factor shrink rapidly because the loss is no longer balanced by production. Thus both the development of hypoxic cells and the rate of reoxygenation between successive treatments are closely related to the proliferation kinetics of the constituent tumor cells. This is summarized in Table 5.

New forms of therapy such as different fractionation schemes, hyperbaric oxygen, high-LET radiations, and electron-affinic sensitizers, as described in the next chapter (Fowler and Denekamp, this volume), are likely to be most effective on tumors which have a large proportion of hypoxic cells, and in which this

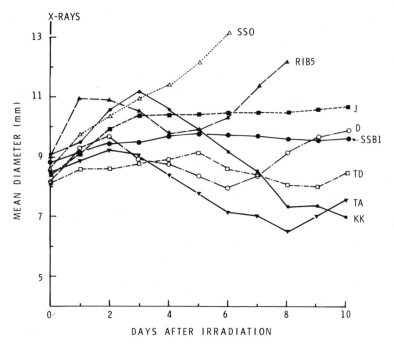

FIGURE 8. Growth curves for eight different experimental sarcomas after irradiation with 1.5–2 krads at day 0 (i.e., when they were between 8 mm and 10 mm diameter). All the tumors showed continued growth before they regressed. From Denekamp (1972).

117

CELL
PROLIFERATION
KINETICS AND
RADIATION
THERAPY

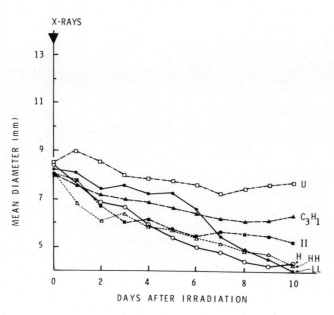

FIGURE 9. Growth curves for six different experimental carcinomas after irradiation with 1.5–2 krads. Five of the groups of mice showed regression within 24 hr of irradiation. From Denekamp (1972).

TABLE 5

Differences between Kinetic Properties and Radiation Response of Experimental Sarcomas and Carcinomas

	Sarcomas	Carcinomas
Growth rate, T_D	Fast	Slow
Cell-cycle time	Varies with T_D	Invariant
Cell-loss rate	Low or none	Very high
Shrinkage after irradiation	Delayed	Immediate
Hypoxic cells	May be absent in *slow* sarcomas	Present
Reoxygenation pattern	Ineffective	Extensive and rapid
Benefit from HPO, high LET, or sensitizers	Probable	Possibly none

proportion remains high throughout a course of fractionated therapy. The very rapidly shrinking tumors which can develop effective reoxygenation soon after the initiation of therapy, and perhaps also very slowly growing sarcomas which may have no hypoxic cells, would be expected to show no improvement over what is obtained with existing treatments. Since these forms of therapy may have to be restricted to certain tumors for reasons of economy, rapidly growing sarcomas or any other slowly shrinking tumors seem likely to benefit most. The choice of rapidly shrinking tumors for clinical trials could demonstrate no advantage of the new methods, because the wrong tumors are treated, not because the new treatment would be generally ineffective.

3.4. Repair Processes

3.4.1. Repair of Sublethal Injury

It has long been known that the killing effects of radiation on cell populations are not linear with dose. Cells are capable of absorbing some radiation energy as sublethal damage, and it is only if large enough doses are given that the sublethal damage is converted to a lethal injury. This sublethal damage is reparable if the cell is left for some hours before the rest of the dose is administered (Elkind and Sutton, 1959). Thus cell survival curves exhibit inefficient regions at low doses, often called a "shoulder," before exponential cell killing is demonstrated. This shoulder is reestablished when the dose is fractionated; the shoulder is approximately repeated for each fraction if sufficient time is allowed to elapse for full repair to occur. It is commonly believed that this involves enzymatic repair of damaged macromolecules at an intracellular level. However, cell contact and extracellular phenomena may influence this repair process. The shoulder is often small for cells *in vitro* (150–300 rads) (e.g., Elkind and Sutton, 1959), whereas for cells *in vivo* (Withers, 1967; Emery *et al.*, 1970; Withers and Elkind, 1969; Chen and Withers, 1972; Wara *et al.*, 1973), or grown as multicellular spheroids with intimate desmosome-like cell junctions (Durand and Sutherland, 1972), much larger shoulders can be demonstrated, suggesting higher capacity for absorbing radiation injury as sublethal reparable damage. Rapid repair (within a few hours) has been observed in tissues as unlike as intestine, skin, and lung, with a similar magnitude of repair capacity and a similar time course. There is some evidence that the rate of repair is slower in tumor cells than in normal cells (Hill and Bush, 1976). Hence 3-hr intervals between fractions are being tested clinically to inflict more damage on the tumor while allowing for full repair in the normal tissue.

Differences in the capacity to repair sublethal injury appear to exist between normal tissues and some solid tumors in mice. The repair capacity appears to be smaller in at least four tumors than in lung, intestine, or skin, although it is exceedingly difficult to measure with accuracy, and more data are required before we can generalize (Denekamp, unpublished). This could result from less intimate cell contact in tumors, or from a reduced repair capacity in starved or hypoxic cells (Hahn, 1968b). If it is true that tumor cells have smaller repair capacity, then multiple fractions of radiation are, of course, advantageous. The logical extension is several small fractions each day, or continuous irradiation at a low dose rate, as provided by interstitial implants or intracavitary radium treatments.

3.4.2. Repair of Potentially Lethal Damage (PLD)

It has been observed in many systems that postirradiation conditions such as the presence or absence of an adequate supply of nutrients can modify the expression of radiation injury. Thus damage that is potentially lethal can be expressed under one set of conditions, but not under another (Alper and Gillies, 1958; Hahn and Little, 1972; Hahn *et al.*, 1972; Little *et al.*, 1972; Shipley *et al.*, 1975). This repair seems to occur best in starved, nondividing populations, as if PLD can be repaired only when the cell is not actively engaged in the division cycle. Thus the extent to which potentially lethal injury is expressed may depend on the nutritional status of the cells and could be greater in the starved cells in tumors which are distant from the capillaries than in dividing, nutritionally privileged cells.

3.4.3. Slow Repair

The third repair process has been identified by three groups, Van den Brenk *et al.* (1974) and Reinhold and Buisman (1975) looking at two different capillary end points and Field *et al.* (1976) looking at mouse death resulting from lung irradiation. Van den Brenk and Reinhold found a very slow repair process in capillary endothelium (half-time about 1 week) if they delayed the stimulus for endothelial proliferation which was necessary to cause the radiation damage to be expressed. This time scale was very similar to that observed by Field and Hornsey using two-dose experiments on lethality from lung damage, when the interval between two doses was varied over 1–40 days. Slow repair, like repair of potentially lethal damage, may depend on slow cell turnover, in that rapid proliferation will cause the damage to be expressed before it has been repaired. In the three systems just mentioned it seems most unlikely that proliferation is involved, since the mitotic and labeling indices are very low and the time of expression of the cell death is very much delayed. It may be this slow repair, rather than proliferation in normal tissues, that allows the addition of more radiation dose in an extended course of fractionated radiotherapy to achieve the maximum tumor damage without exceeding a given level of normal tissue injury. A repair process would give a time factor similar to the exponent in Ellis's NSD formula or Kirk's CRE formula (Ellis, 1969; Kirk *et al.*, 1971), whereas delayed proliferation would give a quite different time–dose relationship (see Fowler and Denekamp, this volume). Nevertheless, slow repair has as yet been inadequately investigated and its nature is not clear.

4. Cell Proliferation Studies

It is obvious that the proliferation characteristics of both normal and malignant cells can have a profound effect on their response to radiation therapy. However, methods of manipulating the therapy to take advantage of the proliferation differences are as yet in their infancy. A brief summary of tumor and normal tissue kinetic studies follows.

4.1. Solid-Tumor Kinetics

A large body of information is now available on the detailed proliferation characteristics of a wide range of experimental tumors in animals. Most of these

studies have been performed on transplantable solid tumors grown subcutaneously in the mouse or rat (see review by Steel, 1972). Many of the tumors have been
induced by chemical carcinogens or by viruses, and have been passaged through
many (often hundreds) of generations. Such passaging must inevitably result in a
selection of the most competent cells, probably those with the fastest proliferation
rates, and may also result in gross immunological differences between the host and
the tumor cells, particularly if they are not maintained in strictly isogeneic
animals. Also, the induction of tumors with single doses or a few repeated
applications of strong carcinogens may not bear any relationship to "spontaneous" tumors in man (Hewitt *et al.*, 1976). Although some human tumors, e.g., in
the lung or bladder, are known to be induced by chemicals, the induction is by
prolonged exposure to the carcinogen, not by a single application, and these
tumors may not evoke such a strong immune response as the induced animal
tumors. With these reservations in mind, some generalizations can be made about
the animal tumor data.

4.1.1. Volume Doubling Times

Most rodent tumors are quite rapidly growing, if estimated by external diameter
or volume measurements. Some transplantable tumors will grow from a few cells
to a tumor burden that will kill the animal within 2–3 weeks. Most of the tumors
have volume doubling times between 1 and 3 days, and it is exceptional to find a
rodent tumor with a doubling time longer than 1 week. These times are all much
faster than for most human tumors (Steel and Lamerton, 1966; Malaise *et al.*,
1975), but this is inevitable since tumors with a volume doubling time of weeks or
months could not easily arise within the 2–3 year life span of a mouse. Most of the
rapidly growing tumors are of mesenchymal origin, being either lymphosarcomas
or soft tissue sarcomas. Although tumors of epithelial origin (carcinomas) can also
show rapid growth, they tend to be more slowly growing, often with doubling
times of 3–7 days (Denekamp 1970, 1972; Steel, 1972). A similar difference
between the volume doubling time of sarcomas and carcinomas has been observed
in humans (Fig. 10).

4.1.2. Cell-Cycle Times

The volume doubling time characterizing a tumor results from the balance of cell
production, cell differentiation, and cell loss. The cell production rate depends on
the cell-cycle time and the growth fraction. The parameters may change within a
given tumor as it increases in size, since most animal tumors show a progressively
slower growth as they get larger. It is often stated that human tumors exhibit
exponential growth even over a long period of time (Collins *et al.*, 1956; Steel and
Lamerton, 1966) rather than the progressive slowing that is characteristic of
animal tumors (Mayneord, 1932; Laird, 1964). With the limited accuracy of
human tumor volume measurements, it is difficult to exclude either possibility.

The most variable phase of the cell cycle is the G_1 phase, which is also the most
difficult to measure experimentally, since it depends on identifying a second wave

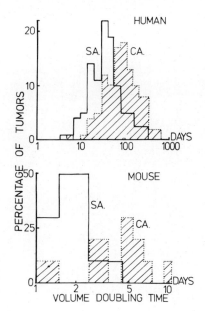

121

CELL
PROLIFERATION
KINETICS AND
RADIATION
THERAPY

FIGURE 10. Histograms of the doubling times of sarcomas and carcinomas for human tumors (from Charbit *et al.*, 1971) and for 20 mouse tumors used by Denekamp. In both species, the sarcomas are more rapidly growing than the carcinomas, with a mean volume doubling time about one-third as long as the mean for the carcinomas. Human tumors grow about 30 times more slowly than mouse tumors, approximately in the ratio of the hosts' life spans.

of labeled mitoses. Because the variation in phase durations obscures the second wave and since there is room for considerable variation in a long cell cycle, the second wave in tumors is often highly damped (Steel, 1972). Four examples are shown in Fig. 11. For RIB5 and SSO, with short cell-cycle times, there are distinct second waves. For C3HCa and SSB1, one with a short T_C and a big spread and the other with a long T_C and a moderate spread, the second wave is much less well defined (Denekamp, 1970).

It has been noted by Steel (1972), who has analyzed many such sets of data using a computer model, that the second wave is always less well defined in spontaneous tumors, or those which have undergone fewer transplants, than in the serially transplanted animal tumors. This indication of greater variability is what would be expected if a selection system is operating by repeated passage. The cell-cycle time in a range of mouse and rat carcinomas, with volume doubling times between 1 and 10 days, shows remarkably little variation (Denekamp, 1970). Most of these tumors have mean T_C values between 12 and 20 hr, with the notable exception of Mendelsohn's C3H mammary tumor (1965). A similar short T_C is found in the majority of the rapidly growing sarcomas, which have volume doubling times of 2 days or less. In three slow-growing sarcomas, however, the cell-cycle time is much longer and is consistent with T_C being the main determinant of tumor volume doubling time in all the sarcomas (Fig. 12). In the carcinomas, by contrast, the main determinant of overall growth rate appears to be the cell loss factor as shown below.

4.1.3. Growth Fraction

There are several ways of estimating the growth fraction using autoradiographic techniques, but none of them gives good precision in tumors, partly because of the

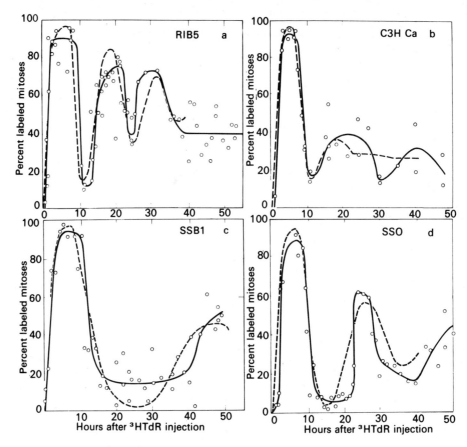

FIGURE 11. Percent labeled mitoses curves after injection of tritiated thymidine to measure the cell-cycle time in four experimental tumors. Tumors RIB5 and SSO show well-defined second waves. The second waves in tumors SSB1 and C3H Ca are less well defined because of the greater variability of cell-cycle times within the population. Solid lines are fitted by eye; dashed lines are computer fitted. Redrawn from Denekamp (1970).

great inhomogeneities of labeling in different areas of the tumor and the consequent difficulty in determining a representative average value (Denekamp and Kallman, 1973; Begg, 1971). Some estimates of GF are shown in Fig. 13. These values certainly have no greater accuracy than ± 10% and may sometimes be less accurate than that. Figure 13 shows that there is no clear difference in the GF of experimental carcinomas and sarcomas. There is also remarkably little variation

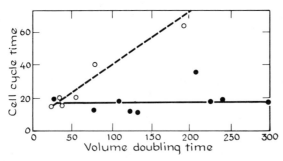

FIGURE 12. Cell-cycle time (hours) for 15 experimental tumors. The carcinomas (●) show little variation in cell-cycle time over a tenfold variation in growth rate; the sarcomas (○) show a longer cell-cycle time in the slowly growing tumors. From Denekamp (1970).

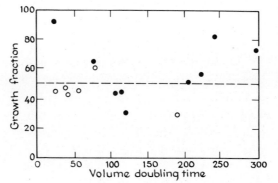

123

CELL
PROLIFERATION
KINETICS AND
RADIATION
THERAPY

FIGURE 13. Growth fraction estimates for 15 experimental tumors as a function of their volume doubling time. There is no consistent variation in doubling time with differing growth rates. From Denekamp (1970).

over a wide range of volume doubling times, and a GF of 40–60% would include most of the tumors. There is, however, a slight tendency to lower GF values at long doubling times among the sarcomas, but this tendency is too small to play a major role in determining the rate of tumor growth. The fact that many tumors have a GF of 40–60%, in spite of wide variations in the degree of differentiation, may be a reflection of the nutritional failure that leads to fewer cells in the growth fraction at progressively greater distances from the capillaries. This was observed in the detailed study by Tannock (1968) of a corded mammary carcinoma: no change in T_C was seen with increasing distance from the capillary, but the labeling index fell, indicating a reduction in the growth fraction. This relatively constant 50% growth fraction in many tumors may correspond to the similar narrow range of hypoxic fractions (often 10–20%) resulting also from inadequate vascularity.

The cells which are not in the division cycle may be either differentiated, as in many fibrosarcomas, squamous carcinomas, and adenocarcinomas, or inherently sterile, or else simply so starved of nutrient that they are out of the cycle. It is cells in the last category that are most dangerous during tumor therapy, because they may reenter the cell cycle as soon as they rediscover an adequate nutrient supply. While they are in a dormant state, they may be radioresistant, either because of hypoxia or because of their ability to repair potentially lethal damage. They are also resistant to cycle-specific chemotherapeutic agents. However, they will become more sensitive to all cytotoxic therapy, both chemical and radiation, if they reenter the cell cycle before the end of treatment.

4.1.4. Cell-Loss Factor

Since the rate of cell production exceeds the rate of volume doubling in a tumor, it is apparent that many of the cells which are born do not persist within the tumor volume; they are lost either by exfoliation, by lymphatic or hematogenous dissemination as viable cells, or by death within the tumor followed by lysis and removal. This cell loss cannot be measured directly, nor can its exact mode of operation be studied, although it can be estimated from the loss of [125]IUdR after this has been incorporated into the cells' DNA (e.g., Porschen and Feinendegen, 1971; Dethlefson, 1971; Begg, 1976). It is more usually estimated from the discrepancy between cell production and net growth, using the formula devised by Steel (1968):

$$\phi = 1 - T/T_D$$

In this way, a cell-loss factor ϕ is estimated. If this is unity, it corresponds to no net growth, i.e., one cell is lost for each new cell born. If it is 0.50, it means that half the *additional* cells being born into the system are being lost from the tumor volume. Values of ϕ ranging from 0 to greater than 90% have been found in solid tumors. Some fast-growing tumors, particularly sarcomas, have no discrepancy between production rate and loss rate; for them, ϕ equals 0. At intermediate growth rates, ϕ values of 25–50% are often found (Denekamp, 1970, 1972; Steel, 1972). In the slow-growing carcinomas, however, very high cell-loss factors of 70–95% are usually found. The few slow-growing sarcomas studied show significant but much lower cell-loss factors (Fig. 14). Thus, again, there seems to be a difference between the growth patterns of sarcomas and carcinomas. The sarcomas derive from normal connective tissue structures, which have no cell loss or production in the adult animal unless in response to wounding. This no-loss characteristic seems to be retained by the malignancies arising from them. Carcinomas, on the other hand, arise from epithelial structures, which are constant-turnover tissues in which production is normally exactly balanced by cell loss. In the carcinomas arising from these epithelial tissues, a high-loss pattern is often retained, perhaps due to an inbuilt, limited life span for each cell (Denekamp, 1970).

As was mentioned earlier, the carcinomas shrink rapidly after irradiation, possibly as a result of mitotic delay halting cell production and allowing the normal rate of cell loss to be revealed (Fig. 9). This rapid shrinkage appears to correlate with extensive reoxygenation after large radiation doses, in contrast to the slowly shrinking and poorly reoxygenating sarcomas (Table 5).

The importance of cell loss in spontaneous tumors may be even greater than in serially transplanted tumors. Steel has shown a progressive reduction in cell loss in some tumors with successive transplantation (Steel *et al.*, 1971; Steel, 1972). In the human tumors which have been studied autoradiographically, most of which are superficial squamous carcinomas, high cell-loss factors have also been observed, often being 90–95% (e.g., Bennington, 1969; Tubiana, 1971; Malaise *et al.*, 1975; Bresciani *et al.*, 1974; Bresciani and Nervi, 1976).

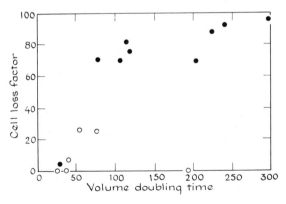

FIGURE 14. Cell-loss factor as a function of volume doubling time. The slow-growing carcinomas all exhibit high cell-loss factors. The sarcomas, by contrast, have low or zero cell-loss factors. From Denekamp (1970).

125

CELL
PROLIFERATION
KINETICS AND
RADIATION
THERAPY

Tumor growth is influenced to varying extents in different tumor types by the processes of cell loss, the intermitotic time, and the growth fraction. In carcinomas, the main determinant seems to be the cell-loss factor since the cell-cycle time and the growth fraction do not vary much. Soft tissue sarcomas have lower cell-loss factors and their growth rate is markedly influenced by the intermitotic time. The artifact of serial transplantation, resulting in a tighter distribution of cell-cycle times and perhaps in lower values of cell-loss factor ϕ, may affect the commonly used sarcomas more than the carcinomas because these tumors have undergone more serial passages, sometimes many hundreds (e.g., Denekamp, 1972). The artifact of strong immunogenicity is also likely to affect the sarcomas more than the carcinomas since they are often carcinogen induced, whereas many of the carcinomas studied result from the mammary tumor virus.

4.1.5. Tumor Size

It is well known that the volume doubling time of solid tumors increases with increasing tumor size. This can be shown as a smoothly bending curve when plotting log volume against time or as a straight line when plotting diameter against time (Fig. 15). Tumor growth curves can often be fitted by a Gompertz function, i.e., by an exponential growth curve with an exponential slowing component (Laird, 1964). This slowing of growth may be due to an elongation of the cycle, to an increased rate of cell loss, or to a reduced growth fraction. Since many animal tumors develop massive areas of necrosis at large sizes, the proliferating population may be reduced to focal areas or even to a rim around the edge of the tumors. Some tumors develop cores of differentiated cells, or of collagen or reticulin fibers, or "pearls" of keratinizing cells. If these products of differentiation occupy less volume than the cells producing them would, it will also look like cell loss (Denekamp, 1970; Tannock, 1969). Thus studies of tumors at different sizes need to include these factors of changing proportions of viable (proliferating and differentiated) to necrotic tissue, and also changes in the proportion of stroma to parenchyma.

Frindel *et al.* (1967) studied the changes in the kinetics of the mouse fibrosarcoma NCTC with increasing size. They found very little change in T_C over the range 0.01–2.0 g. There was a change in the growth fraction, and the fourfold

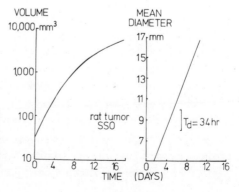

FIGURE 15. Tumor growth curves (an example from the rat tumor SSO). The gradual decrease in growth rate as the tumor increases in size is obvious in the plot of log volume against time. When mean diameter is plotted against time, this is shown as a straight line.

decrease in growth rate was due to this and to increased cell loss. Simpson-Herren (1974), Hermens (1973), and Watson (1976) all found increases in the cell-cycle time in older tumors, together with decreased growth fraction and increasing cell loss. Studies on aging in ascites tumors have shown that the most obvious feature is a much greater elongation of the cell cycle, mainly due to an increase in the S phase. This is accompanied by a reduction in GF and an increase in ϕ (Lala, 1968; Tannock, 1969; Frindel *et al.*, 1970; Dombernowsky and Hartmann, 1972). The situation in ascites tumors is more like that of cells grown in suspension culture than that in solid tumors. The cells have no fixed anatomical relationship to the vasculature, but are freely floating in the ascitic fluid and only periodically come into intimate contact with the nutrient supplied via the mesenteric capillaries. With such an intermittent supply, all cells seem to continue to progress through the cell cycle, but the rate is determined by the frequency of nutritional contact, which is inversely related to cell density. In solid tumors, by contrast, the cells which are close to the nutrient supply progress through the cycle. These cells that are nutritionally deprived, either at the greatest distance from the capillaries in young tumors or throughout the tumor as the vasculature progressively fails in some larger tumors, seem to have a much lower probability of proliferating, and the growth fraction decreases (Tannock, 1968), and/or the cell-cycle time elongates toward the center of the tumor (Hermens and Barendsen, 1967).

4.1.6. Tumor Site

Most animal tumor studies are performed on transplanted tumors grown from subcutaneous implants of tumor fragments or of a cell suspension. These implants have to derive a blood supply from the subcutaneous vascular bed and then have to create a space for themselves by local infiltration or by stretching the overlying tissues. While this model is convenient for experimentation because it is accessible for external measurement, it is unlike most human tumors. Carcinomas generally arise at a surface, e.g., skin or intestine, where cell loss may occur by exfoliation. Tumors arise in sites with very different mechanical properties, e.g., in lung, in bone, or within the skull. Sometimes the spontaneous tumor uses the vasculature of the normal tissue by infiltration rather than by evoking a totally new vasculature as in a subcutaneous implant. Infiltration is also shown by some experimental lymphomas, which will not grow as round, isolated spheres when implanted subcutaneously, but rather form a diffuse and ill-defined infiltrate into the subcutaneous tissue. The reasons for these different patterns of growth are not clear, but they may relate to differences in the tumor angiogenesis factor produced by different tumors (Folkman, 1974).

Tumors transplanted into subcutaneous tissues which have previously been heavily irradiated grow more slowly, presumably because of vascular insufficiency in the stroma (Hewitt and Blake, 1968). No change in T_C or GF was observed in two studies of tumors implanted into previously irradiated sites, but the rate of cell loss was in each case higher than in tumors grown in normal unirradiated sites (Clifton and Jirtle, 1975; Denekamp, unpublished).

127

CELL
PROLIFERATION
KINETICS AND
RADIATION
THERAPY

Secondary tumors in patients often occur in lymph nodes (an unlikely site to prosper if they are antigenic) and in lungs. Tumors in lungs have very little resistance to expansion, have a well-developed vasculature on which to draw, and are closer to the oxygen and nutritional supply than most normal tissues in the body. However, even in this site, necrosis develops because of an inadequate vasculature (Thomlinson and Gray, 1955). There are few studies in the literature where the growth of tumors in different sites has been compared. In mice, more rapid growth of metastases sometimes occurs in regional lymph nodes that in the primary implant from which they have seeded, and which has been treated with radiation. However, no kinetic information is available. More rapid growth of lung metastases relative to the primary tumor has been observed by several workers, by Simpson-Herren *et al.* (1974) in mice and by Charbit *et al.* (1971) and Bresciani and Nervi (1976) in man. Bresciani and Nervi found that the metastases retained many of the characteristics of the primary tumor, but the cell-loss factor was somewhat reduced and the spread of cell-cycle times was smaller. Van Peperzeel (1970) studied mouse tumor growing subcutaneously and in the lungs, and she found similar doubling times and labeling indices. Simpson-Herren *et al.* (1974) found distinctly different kinetics in the lung tumors relative to the subcutaneous tumors, but this may relate to the smaller size of the tumors in the lungs.

4.2. Changes in Tumor Kinetics after Irradiation

There have been a number of detailed studies of the changes in proliferation kinetics in experimental tumors after irradiation, as described earlier and summarized in Table 3. The dose of radiation and the time at which the studies were made differed in each publication, and only two studies included several different times within the same tumor (Hermens and Barendsen, 1969; Szczepanski and Trott, 1975). Six of the ten studies have shown no change in T_C after irradiation, although of course transient changes could have been missed in some of these studies. Changes in GF have been observed in most of the tumors. Some authors have found an increased GF, others a reduction, and yet others no change. The presence of doomed and dying cells makes it even harder to measure GF in irradiated tumors than in control tumors, and at early times the response of the small number of surviving clonogenic cells will be masked by the lethally damaged but not yet dead cells. An increased growth fraction seems very likely in the tumors which are limited by their vasculature, since the nutritional supply improves after irradiation, as can be demonstrated by reoxygenation of hypoxic cells.

All but one study have shown a continued high cell-loss factor, sometimes for many weeks after irradiation. This presumably reflects the delayed removal of cells killed by the radiation. A vascular supply is necessary to remove the products of dead cells, and, since this is inadequate in tumors, it also serves as an inadequate, slow, refuse disposal system. Most workers observe a slower growth rate in irradiated tumors of the same size, although studies on lung metastases have shown accelerated growth, i.e., faster volume doubling rates in irradiated tumors than before irradiation in both mice and men (Malaise *et al.*, 1972; Van Peperzeel, 1970, 1972). This is seldom, if ever, observed in subcutaneous tumors.

Some radiobiologists argue that only a small fraction of the cells in a tumor are capable of indefinite proliferation (i.e., are stem cells), and any study of the tumor as a whole may be misleading. While this may be true, such "stem cells" cannot be studied at present since they are not morphologically identifiable.

4.3. Normal Tissue Kinetics: Changes after Irradiation

Unlike systemic chemotherapy, where the most rapidly dividing tissues limit the dose of cycle-specific cytotoxic drug that can be used for any cancer, radiotherapy is usually localized, and it is only the tissue included in the beam that is at risk. If a primary tumor is irradiated, the tissue of origin is likely to be in the beam. This usually has a·slower proliferation rate than the tumor derived from it, with the exception of tumors of the intestine, where reduced cell loss causes the tumor growth. The tumor is also characteristically less differentiated than the tissue of origin, and this may be reflected in a difference in GF.

The cell-cycle time varies enormously in different normal tissues. It is known in detail for several rapidly dividing tissues, but no detailed information is available for the very slowly dividing tissues.

4.3.1. Intestine

The intestinal epithelium constitutes the fastest-turnover system in the body, with a mean T_C of 10–12 hr (Lesher *et al.*, 1966). Most of the cells in the crypts are in DNA synthesis, and differentiation occurs as the cells progress out onto the villus. The small intestine is sensitive to single doses of radiation, resulting in death at 4–5 days if the whole body is irradiated with about 1000 rads, but it has a high capacity for repair of sublethal injury (even within 10 min), and also compensates rapidly by accelerated proliferation as the damage is recognized rapidly. The intestine is therefore much less sensitive to fractionated irradiation if it is given over an extended time (Lesher *et al.*, 1975). During compensatory proliferation, the cell cycle is reported to shorten to an astonishing 6 hr (Lesher and Banman, 1969). Proliferation has been studied by split-dose techniques as well as by autoradiography (Withers, 1975*b*). The timing of the compensatory acceleration varies with the preirradiation cycle time, being fastest in the jejunum and less fast in the stomach and colon (see review, Denekamp, 1975). Similarly, the speed of proliferation (i.e., T_C accelerated) is also different in the different regions, as is summarized in Fig. 16.

4.3.2. Bone Marrow

The bone marrow has also been thoroughly investigated, and the role of a common stem cell, with progeny committed to various forms of differentiation, has been well documented (IAEA Symposium, 1968; Lord, 1975; Till, 1976;

129

CELL
PROLIFERATION
KINETICS AND
RADIATION
THERAPY

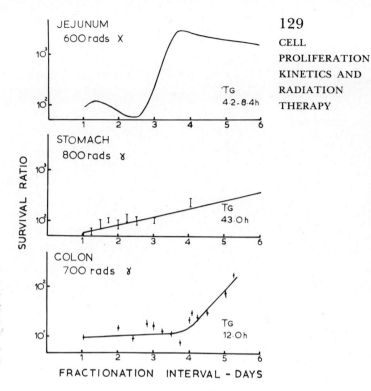

FIGURE 16. Accelerated proliferation in jejunum, stomach, and colon after irradiation with doses of 600–800 rads. The proliferation is shown by the increased surviving fraction if two doses are separated by an interval varying between 1 and 6 days. The doubling time, T_G, derived from these data is shown on each graph. Data from Withers *et al.*, reviewed by Denekamp (1975).

Trentin, 1976). The cell-cycle times of the different stages of differentiating amplification compartments have been estimated. Because of the prolonged transit time through a series of amplification stages and because of the life span of the differentiated cells in the bloodstream, death from whole-body irradiation does not occur until about 20 days in small animals, although the tissue is more sensitive than the small intestine (see Fowler and Denekamp, this volume). This sensitivity probably relates to the relative lack of repair capacity, and consequently the dose that can be tolerated does not increase much with fractionation. Because of the lack of a "shoulder," blood cells and particularly peripheral lymphocytes, among the differentiated cells of the hemopoietic system, respond to very low doses of only a few rads or tens of rads. These cells are exceptional in that they can undergo interphase death, which can occur rapidly. After irradiation, some compensatory proliferation can be induced, partly by a shortening of T_C, but largely by increasing the number of divisions within the amplification series, i.e., before differentiation (Lord, 1976; IAEA Symposium, 1968).

4.3.3. Skin

The relationship between kinetic parameters and radiation response can readily be demonstrated in skin. Mouse skin has a cell-cycle time of 4–5 days for the basal layer and a transit time of 10–15 days through the superficial two or three layers of differentiating cells (Hegazy and Fowler, 1973). Skin can tolerate quite high doses of radiation, but the tolerance dose is ultimately determined by the size of the irradiated field, since small areas can be repopulated from the peripheral un-irradiated cells. Desquamation occurs after 2000–3000 rads and occurs at 15–20 days in accord with the transit time through the differentiating layers (Hegazy and Fowler, 1973; Fowler *et al.*, 1965; Fowler and Denekamp, 1976). Skin which has been stimulated before irradiation, e.g., by plucking, develops a reaction earlier, and skin with more superficial layers, e.g., that of pig or man, develops a reaction later (Fig. 17). Large doses cause considerable mitotic delay, followed by extensive cell death in the basal layer, but the rate of progression of cells into the more superficial layers is unchanged, at least for several days (Etoh *et al.*, 1975). Eventually, the lack of cell production results in a significant lack of basal layer cells, and this may be the signal for more rapid compensatory proliferation (Fowler and Denekamp, 1976). The proliferative response is thus delayed about 1–2 weeks after single large doses or after starting multiple small doses of radiation. After surgical or mechanical wounding, however, a deficit is recognized immediately and proliferation is faster, within 24 hr.

The level of cell depletion affects the rate of compensatory proliferation and in skin the cell-cycle time can shorten from its control value of $4\frac{1}{2}$ days down to 2 days after moderate damage, or to 18–24 hr after severe depletion (Denekamp, 1973; Denekamp *et al.*, 1976). This delayed compensatory response is unusual: it does not occur after surgical injury or after chemical or mechanical trauma, where a rapid response is elicited because the cells express their damage quickly. The other form of injury producing the delayed response is that of a deep thermal burn involving the dermis (Winter, 1971). After the initial lag, compensatory proliferation will commence during a course of daily fractions of radiation and

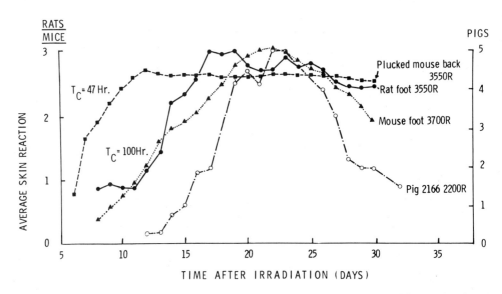

FIGURE 17. Time course of erythema and desquamation of the epidermis in four different situations. The skin reactions develop between 8 and 15 days for rat feet and mouse feet, as can be predicted from the cell-cycle time and the transit time through the differentiated layers. The reactions develop faster in skin which has been stimulated by plucking and more slowly in pig skin, where the transit time is longer because there are more superficial layers.

can even become sufficiently effective to heal the radiation-induced desquamation
even though daily irradiation at the same level is continuing (Field *et al.*, 1975).
This corresponds to the mucosal or epithelial healing that is sometimes observed
during prolonged clinical radiotherapy.

131

CELL
PROLIFERATION
KINETICS AND
RADIATION
THERAPY

4.3.4. Slowly Dividing Tissues

Most of the organs of the body have a slow rate of turnover in the adult animal
(Cameron, 1970). The labeling index is less than 1% in kidneys, lungs, liver,
muscle, spinal cord, bladder, etc. (Unger and Gidali, 1971). As would be expected
from the pattern seen in intestine, bone marrow, and skin, the radiation reaction
in these tissues is also correspondingly slow, and often no change is observed for
6–12 months or more, in both mice and men. The expression of the injury may be
precipitated by some other form of trauma which induces a proliferative
response, e.g., partial hepatectomy or unilateral nephrectomy. As the cells
attempt to divide, the latent radiation damage is expressed because the divisions
are abortive. Thus mechanical, chemical, or surgical intervention into an area
irradiated many months or even years earlier can give rise to sudden and
unexpected necrosis as the latent damage is expressed. Since compensatory
proliferation in most rapidly renewing tissues does not occur until the cell
depletion has been recognized, rapid compensation during the course of 4–7
weeks of therapy is extremely unlikely in these slow tissues, and no increase in
proliferative indices has been observed (Unger and Gidali, 1971; Tannock and
Hayashi, 1972). The fact that an increasing dose can be given without increasing
the damage as the overall time is prolonged is more likely to be a result of a slow
repair process than of proliferation in these slow tissues. In addition to the lack of
proliferation between fractions in slow tissues, there may be a lack of redistribution around the cell cycle. This would also result in a gradual increase in the
radioresistance with successive doses, as cells in the more sensitive phases of the
cell cycle are killed first.

5. Conclusions

Cell proliferation kinetics influences the response of a cell population to radiation,
either as a single dose or as a fractionated course.

1. The position of a cell within the cell cycle influences its sensitivity to a single
dose of radiation and results in a partial synchrony of resistant survivors. These
progress through stages of different radiosensitivities at a rate that depends on the
cell-cycle time. This gives the potential for optimum scheduling of doses, to
maximize tumor sensitivity while minimizing normal tissue damage. The detailed
information needed for this is not yet available. Slowly dividing or nondividing
cells may become more resistant to subsequent fractions if they fail to progress
through the cell cycle.

2. The repair capacity of a cell depends on its nutritional state, its oxygenation, and its proliferative state. Cells which are in the nonproliferative fraction may be less capable of repairing sublethal injury, but more capable of repairing potentially lethal damage or of exhibiting slow repair. The growth fraction in experimental tumors is relatively constant and probably results from inadequate nutrition due to the imbalance of tumor-cell and endothelial-cell proliferation.

3. Hypoxic cells develop in tumors, probably at the limit of oxygen diffusion from the inadequate blood supply. These hypoxic cells are very resistant to radiation. If fractionated radiation is used, the hypoxic cells may reoxygenate and become more sensitive to subsequent doses. The pattern of reoxygenation relates to the preirradiation cell-loss rate and to the shrinkage rate after irradiation. It appears to be more effective in carcinomas than in sarcomas. Methods of overcoming hypoxia are most likely to help with slowly shrinking tumors.

4. Compensatory proliferation between successive radiation doses can offset the damage caused by each dose. This compensation develops rapidly in intestinal epithelium, develops more slowly in skin, and probably does not occur within a course of radiotherapy in the very slowly dividing tissues such as lung, liver, and kidney. The onset of compensatory proliferation requires the recognition of a cell deficit for its initiation, and this is delayed until the cell attempts to divide in most tissues. Tumor cells can also increase their growth rates after the initiation of therapy, either by a shortening of the cell cycle time or by an increased growth fraction as their nutritional milieu improves.

ACKNOWLEDGMENTS

The authors take pleasure in thanking Dr. Adrian Begg for permission to use Fig. 1 and Dr. R. H. Thomlinson for permission to use Figs. 3, 4, and 6.

6. References

ALPER, T., AND GILLIES, N. E., 1958, "Restoration" of Escherichia coli strain B after irradiation: Its dependence on suboptimal growth conditions, J. Gen. Microbiol. 18:461.

ALPER, T., AND HOWARD-FLANDERS, P., 1956, The role of oxygen in modifying the radiosensitivity of E. coli B, Nature (London) 178:978.

BEGG, A. C., 1971, Kinetic and histological changes of a serially transplanted mouse tumour, Cell Tissue Kinet. 4:401.

BEGG, A. C., 1975, Ph.D. thesis, London.

BEGG, A. C., 1977, Cell loss from several types of murine solid tumour, measured in situ using ^{125}I-iodo-deoxyuridine or tritiated thymidine, Radiat. Res. 69 (in press).

BENNINGTON, T. C., 1969, Cellular kinetics of invasive squamous carcinoma of the human cervix, Cancer Res. 29:1082.

BRESCIANI, F., 1965, A comparison of the cell generative cycle in normal, hyperplastic and neoplastic mammary gland of the C3H mouse, in: Cellular Radiation Biology, pp. 547–557, Williams and Wilkins, Baltimore.

133

CELL
PROLIFERATION
KINETICS AND
RADIATION
THERAPY

BRESCIANI, F., AND NERVI, C., 1976, Growth kinetics in human squamous carcinoma, in: *Growth Kinetics and Biochemical Regulation of Normal and Malignant Cells, Proceedings of the 29th Annual Symposium on Fundamental Cancer Research,* Houston, in press.

BRESCIANI, F., PAOLUZI, R., BENASSI, M., NERVI, C., CASALE, V., AND ZIPARO, E., 1974, Cell kinetics and growth in squamous cell carcinomas in man, *Cancer Res.* **34:**2405.

BROWN, J. M., 1970, The effect of acute X-irradiation on the cell proliferation kinetics of induced carcinomas and their normal counterpart, *Radiat. Res.* **43:**627.

CAMERON, I. L., 1970, Cell renewal in the organs and tissues of the non-growing adult mouse, *Tex. Rep. Biol. Med.* **28:**203.

CATTERALL, M., SUTHERLAND, I., AND BEWLEY, D. K., 1975, First results of a randomised clinical trial of fast neutrons compared with X- or gamma rays in treatment of advanced tumours of the head and neck, *Br. Med. J.,* p. 653.

CHARBIT, A., MALAISE, E. P., AND TUBIANA, M., 1971, Relation between the pathological nature and the growth rate of human tumors, *Eur. J. Cancer* **7:**307.

CHEN, K. Y., AND WITHERS, H. R., 1972, Survival characteristics of stem cells of gastric mucosa in C3H mice exposed to local gamma irradiation, *Int. J. Radiat. Biol.* **21:**521.

CLIFTON, K. H., AND BRIGGS, R. C., 1966, Quantitative radiosensitivity studies of solid carcinomas *in vivo*: Methodology and effect of anoxia, *J. Natl. Cancer Inst.* **36:**965.

CLIFTON, K. H., AND JIRTLE, R., 1975, Mammary carcinoma cell population growth in pre-irradiated and unirradiated transplant sites, *Radiology* **117:**459.

COLLINS, V. P., LOEFFLER, R. K., AND TIVEY, H., 1956, Observations on growth rates of human tumours, *Am. J. Roentgenol.* **76:**988.

DENEKAMP, J., 1970, The cellular proliferation kinetics of animal tumours, *Cancer Res.* **30:**303.

DENEKAMP, J., 1972, The relationship between the "cell loss factor" and the immediate response to radiation in animal tumours, *Eur. J. Cancer* **8:**335.

DENEKAMP, J., 1973, Changes in the rate of repopulation during multifraction irradiation of mouse skin, *Br. J. Radiol.* **46:**381.

DENEKAMP, J., 1975, Changes in the rate of proliferation in normal tissues after irradiation, in: *Radiation Research: Biomedical, Chemical and Physical Perspectives* (O. NYGAARD, H. I. ADLER, AND W. K. SINCLAIR, eds.), pp. 810–825, Academic Press, New York.

DENEKAMP, J., AND HARRIS, S. R., 1976, Studies of the processes occurring between two fractions in experimental mouse tumours, *Int. J. Radiat. Oncol. Biol. Phys.* **1:**421.

DENEKAMP, J., AND KALLMAN, R. F., 1973, *In vitro* and *in vivo* labelling of animal tumours with tritiated thymidine, *Cell Tissue Kinet.* **6:**217.

DENEKAMP, J., AND THOMLINSON, R. H., 1971, The cell proliferation kinetics of four experimental tumours after acute X-irradiation, *Cancer Res.* **31:**1279.

DENEKAMP, J., BALL, M. M., AND FOWLER, J. F., 1969, Recovery and repopulation in mouse skin as a function of time after X-irradiation, *Radiat. Res.* **37:**361.

DENEKAMP, J., STEWART, F. A., AND DOUGLAS, B. G., 1976, Changes in the proliferation rate in mouse skin after irradiation: Continuous labelling studies, *Cell Tissue Kinet.* **9:**19.

DESCHNER, E. E., AND GRAY, L. H., 1959, Influence of oxygen tension on X-ray induced chromosomal damage in Ehrlich ascites tumour cells irradiated *in vitro* and *in vivo*, *Radiat. Res.* **11:**115.

DETHLEFSON, L. A., 1971, An evaluation of radio iodine-labelled 5-iodo-2-deoxyuridine as a tracer for measuring cell loss from solid tumours, *Cell Tissue Kinet.* **4:**123.

DISCHE, S., 1974, The hyperbaric oxygen chamber in the radiotherapy of carcinoma of the uterine cervix, *Br. J. Radiol.* **47:**99.

DOIDA, Y., AND OKADA, S., 1969, Radiation induced mitotic delay in cultured mammalian cells L5178Y, *Radiat. Res.* **38:**513.

DOMBERNOWSKY, P., AND HARTMANN, N. R., 1972, Analysis of variations in the cell population kinetics with tumour age in the L1210 ascites tumour, *Cancer Res.* **32:**2452.

DÖRMER, P., TULINIUS, H., AND OEHLERT, W., 1964, Untersuchungen über die Generationszeit, DNA Synthesezeit und Mitosedauer von Zellen der hyperplastischen Epidermis und des Plattenepithelcarcinomas der Maus nach MCA, *Z. Krebsforsch.* **66:**11.

DURAND, R. E., AND SUTHERLAND, R. M., 1972, Effects of intercellular contact on repair of radiation damage, *Exp. Cell Res.* **71:**75.

ELKIND, M. M., AND SUTTON, H., 1959, X-ray damage and recovery in mammalian cells in culture, *Nature (London)* **184:**1293.

ELKIND, M. M., HAN, A., AND VOLZ, K. W., 1963, Radiation response of mammalian cells grown in culture. IV. Dose dependence of division delay and postirradiation growth of surviving and non-surviving Chinese hamster cells, *J. Natl. Cancer Inst.* **30**:705.

ELLIS, F., 1969, Dose, time and fractionation, a clinical hypothesis, *Clin. Radiol* **20**:1.

EMERY, E. W., DENEKAMP, J., BALL, M. M., AND FIELD, S. B., 1970, Survival of mouse skin epithelial cells following single and divided doses of X-rays, *Radiat. Res.* **41**:450.

ETOH, H., TAGUCHI, Y. H., AND TABACHNICK, J., 1975, Movement of beta-irradiated epidermal basal cells to the spinous-granular layers in the absence of cell division, *J. Invest. Dermatol.* **64**:431.

FIELD, S. B., MORRIS, C., DENEKAMP, J., AND FOWLER, J. F., 1975, The response of mouse skin to fractionated x-rays, *Eur. J. Cancer* **11**:191.

FIELD, S. B., HORNSEY, S., AND KUTSUTANI, Y., 1976, Effects of fractionated irradiation on mouse lung: A phenomenon of slow repair, *Br. J. Radiol.* **49**:700.

FOLKMAN, J., 1974, Tumor angiogenesis factor, *Cancer Res.* **34**:2109.

FOWLER, J. F., AND DENEKAMP, J., 1976, Regulation of epidermal stem cells, in: *Stem Cells of Renewing Cell Populations* (A. B. CAIRNIE, P. K. LALA, AND D. G. OSMOND, eds.), pp. 117–134, Academic Press, New York.

FOWLER, J. F., LINDOP, P. J., BERRY, R. J., KRAGT, K., AND ELLIS, R. E., 1965, Split dose experiments on skin reactions in mice, *Int. J. Radiat. Biol.* **9**:241.

FOWLER, J. F., SHELDON, P. W., BEGG, A. C., HILL, S. A., AND SMITH, A. M., 1975, Biological properties and response to X-rays of first generation transplants of spontaneous mammary carcinomas in C3H mice, *Int. J. Radiat. Biol.* **27**:463.

FRANKFURT, O. S., 1967*a*, Mitotic cycle and cell differentiation in squamous cell carcinomas, *Int. J. Cancer* **2**:304.

FRANKFURT, O. S., 1967*b*, Cell proliferation and differentiation in the squamous epithelium of the forestomach of the mouse, *Exp. Cell Res.* **46**:603.

FRINDEL, E., MALAISE, E. P., ALPEN, E., AND TUBIANA, M., 1967, Kinetics of cell proliferation of an experimental tumour, *Cancer Res.* **27**:1122.

FRINDEL, E., VASSORT, F., AND TUBIANA, M., 1970, Effects of irradiation on the cell cycle of an experimental ascites tumour of the mouse, *Int. J. Radiat. Biol.* **17**:329.

GRAY, L. H., CONGER, A. D., EBERT, M., HORNSEY, S., AND SCOTT, O. C. A., 1953, The concentration of oxygen dissolved in tissues at the time of irradiation as a factor in radiotherapy, *Br. J. Radiol.* **26**:638.

HAHN, G. M., 1968*a*, Possible improvements in differential cell killing by cell cycle modulation, *Br. J. Radiol.* **41**:239.

HAHN, G. M., 1968*b*, Failure of Chinese hamster cells to repair sublethal damage when x-irradiated in the plateau phase of growth, *Nature (London)* **217**:741.

HAHN, G. M., 1975, Modification of cell killing by precise timing of x-irradiation, in: *Proceedings of the Madison Conference on the Time–Dose Relationships in Clinical Radiotherapy* (W. CALDWELL AND D. D. TOLBERT, eds.), pp. 153–159, University of Wisconsin, Madison, Wis.

HAHN, G. M., AND LITTLE, J. B., 1972, Plateau-phase cultures of mammalian cells: An *in vitro* model for human cancer, *Curr. Top. Radiat. Res. Q.* **8**:39.

HAHN, G. M., ROCKWELL, S. C., KALLMAN, R. F., AND FRINDEL, E., 1972, Repair of potentially lethal damage in tumour cells X-irradiated *in vivo*, *Radiat. Res.* **51**:523.

HASEGAWA, K., MATSUURA, Y., AND SHIMPEI, T., 1976, Cellular kinetics and histological changes in experimental cancer of the uterine cervix, *Cancer Res.* **36**:359.

HEGAZY, M. A. H., AND FOWLER, J. F., 1973, Cell population kinetics and desquamation skin reactions in plucked and unplucked mouse skin. II. Irradiated skin, *Cell Tissue Kinet.* **6**:587.

HENK, J. M., AND SMITH, C. W., 1973, Unequivocal clinical evidence for the oxygen effect, *Br. J. Radiol.* **46**:146.

HERMENS, A. F., 1973, Variations in the cell kinetics and the growth rate in an experimental tumor during natural growth and after irradiation, Ph.D. thesis, Radiobiological Inst. T.N.O., Rijswijk, the Netherlands.

HERMENS, A. F., AND BARENDSEN, G. W., 1967, Cellular proliferation patterns in an experimental rhabdomyosarcoma in the rat, *Eur. J. Cancer* **3**:361.

HERMENS, A. F., AND BARENDSEN, G. W., 1969, Changes in cell proliferation characteristics in a rat rhabdomyosarcoma before and after X-irradiation, *Eur. J. Cancer* **5**:173.

HEWITT, H. B., AND BLAKE, E. R., 1968, The growth of transplanted murine tumours in pre-irradiated sites, *Br. J. Cancer* **22**:808.

135

CELL
PROLIFERATION
KINETICS AND
RADIATION
THERAPY

HEWITT, H. B., AND WILSON, C. W., 1961, Survival curves for tumor cells irradiated *in vivo*, *Ann. N.Y. Acad. Sci.* **95**:818.

HEWITT, H. B., CHAN, D. P. S., BLAKE, E. R., 1967, Survival curves for clonogenic cells of a murine keratinising squamous carcinoma irradiated *in vivo* or under hypoxic conditions, *Int. J. Radiat. Biol.* **12**:539.

HEWITT, H. B., BLAKE, E. R., AND WALDER, A. S., 1976, A critique of the evidence for active host defence against cancer, based on personal studies of 27 murine tumours of spontaneous origin, *Br. J. Cancer* **33**:241.

HILL, R. P., AND BUSH, R. S., 1977, Repair and reoxygenation in a transplantable murine sarcoma, *Radiat. Res.* **70** (in press).

HILL, R. P., BUSH, R. S., AND YEUNG, P., 1971, The effect of anaemia on the fraction of hypoxic cells in an experimental tumour, *Br. J. Radiol.* **44**:299.

HOWES, A. E., 1969, An estimation of changes in the proportion of hypoxic cells after irradiation of transplanted C3H mouse mammary tumours, *Br. J. Radiol.* **42**:441.

ILIYA, F. A., AND AZAR, H. A., 1967, Radioautographic studies in neoplasia of uterine cervix, *Am. J. Obstet. Gynecol.* **99**:515.

INTERNATIONAL ATOMIC ENERGY AGENCY SYMPOSIUM AT MONACO, 1968, *Effects of Radiation on Cellular Proliferation and Differentiation*, IAEA, Vienna.

KALLMAN, R. F., 1972, The phenomenon of reoxygenation and its implications for fractionated radiotherapy, *Radiology* **105**:135.

KALLMAN, R. F., JARDINE, L. J., AND JOHNSON, C. W., 1970, The effects of different schedules of dose fractionation on the oxygenation status of a transplantable mouse sarcoma, *J. Natl. Cancer Inst.* **44**:369.

KIRK, J., GRAY, W. M., AND WATSON, E. R., 1971, Cumulative radiation effect. 1. Fractionated treatment regimes, *Clin. Radiol.* **22**:145.

LAIRD, A. K., 1964, Dynamics of tumor growth, *Br. J. Cancer* **18**:490.

LAJTHA, L. G., AND OLIVER, R., 1962, Cell population kinetics following different regimes of irradiation, *Br. J. Radiol.* **35**:131.

LALA, P., 1968, Cytokinetic control mechanisms in Ehrlich ascites tumour growth, in: *Effects of Radiation on Cellular Proliferation and Differentiation*, IAEA, Vienna.

LAMERTON, L. F., 1966, Cell proliferation under continuous irradiation, *Radiat. Res.* **27**:119.

LESHER, S., AND BAUMAN, J., 1968, Recovery of reproductive activity and the maintenance of structural integrity in the mouse intestinal epithelium after single dose whole-body ^{60}Co gamma ray exposures, in: *Effects of Radiation on Cellular Proliferation and Differentiation*, IAEA, Vienna.

LESHER, S. AND BAUMAN, J., 1969, Cell kinetic studies of the intestinal epithelium: Maintenance of the intestinal epithelium in normal and irradiated animals, *Natl. Cancer Inst. Monogr.* **30**:185.

LESHER, S., LAMERTON, L. F., SACHER, G. A., FRY, R. J. M., STEEL, G. G., AND ROYLANCE, P. J., 1966, Effect of continuous gamma irradiation on the generation cycle of the duodenal crypt cells of the mouse and rat, *Radiat. Res.* **29**:57.

LESHER, S., COOPER, J., HAGEMAN, R., AND LESHER, J., 1975, Proliferative patterns in the mouse jejunal epithelium after fractionated abdominal X-irradiation, *Curr. Top. Radiat. Res. Q.* **10**:229.

LITTLE, J. B., HAHN, G. M., FRINDEL, E., AND TUBIANA, M., 1972, Repair of potentially lethal radiation damage *in vitro* and *in vivo*, *Radiology* **106**:689.

LORD, B. I., 1975, The control of cell proliferation in haemopoetic tissue, in: *Radiation Research: Biomedical, Chemical, and Physical Perspectives* (O. NYGAARD, H. I. ADLER, AND W. K. SINCLAIR, eds.), pp. 826–833, Academic Press, New York.

LORD, B. I., 1976, Stem cell reserve and its control, in: *Stem Cells of Renewing Cell Populations* (A. B. CAIRNIE, P. K. LALA, AND D. G. OSMOND, eds.), pp. 165–180, Academic Press, New York.

MALAISE, E. P., CHARBIT, A., CHAVAUDRA, N., COMBES, P. F., DOUCHEZ, J., AND TUBIANA, M., 1972, Change in volume of irradiated human metastases—investigation of repair of sublethal damage and tumour repopulation, *Br. J. Cancer* **26**:43.

MALAISE, E. P., CHAVAUDRA, N., AND TUBIANA, M., 1973, The relationship between growth rate, labelling index, and histological type of human solid tumours, *Eur. J. Cancer* **9**:305.

MALAISE, E. P., CHAVAUDRA, N., PÊNE, F., RICHARD, J. M., AND TUBIANA, M., 1975, Cell proliferation kinetics and growth rate of the irradiated human tumors, in: *Radiation Research: Biomedical, Chemical, and Physical Perspectives* (O. NYGAARD, H. I. ADLER, AND W. K. SINCLAIR, eds.), pp. 850–856, Academic Press, New York.

MAYNEORD, W. V., 1932, On a law of growth of Jensen's rat sarcoma, *Am. J. Cancer* **16**:841.

McNally, N. J., 1975, The effect of an hypoxic cell sensitizer on tumour growth delay and cell survival: Implications for cell survival *in situ* and *in vitro*, *Br. J. Cancer* **32**:610.

Mendelsohn, M. L., 1965, The kinetics of tumor cell proliferation, in: *Cellular Radiation Biology*, Williams and Wilkins, Baltimore.

Mottram, J. C., 1913, On the action of beta and gamma rays of radium on the cell in different states of nuclear division, *Arch. Middlesex Hosp.* **30**:98.

Mottram, J. C., Scott, G. M., and Russ, S., 1926, On the effects of beta rays from radium upon division and growth of cancer cells, *Proc. R. Soc. London Ser. B* **100**:326.

Nelson, J. S. R., Carpenter, R. E., and Durboraw, D., 1976, Mechanisms underlying reduced growth rate in C3HBA mammary adeno-carcinomas recurring after single doses of X-rays or fast neutrons, *Cancer Res.* **36**:524.

Phillips, T. L., 1966, An ultrastructural study of the development of radiation injury in the lung, *Radiology* **87**:49.

Phillips, T. L., 1969, Observations on heart, lung and kidney after 500–4500 rads from 1 hour to 1 year, in: *Carmel Conference on Time–Dose Relationships in Radiation Biology as Applied to Radiotherapy*, pp. 194–199, BNL 50203 (C–57).

Porschen, W., and Feinendegen, L. E., 1971, *In vivo* determination of RBE factors of 15 MeV neutrons for different biological effects in normal tissues and sarcoma 180, using cell labelling with [125]IUdR, in: *Radiobiological Applications of Neutron Irradiation*, pp. 121–134, IAEA, Vienna.

Powers, W. E., and Tolmach, L. J., 1963, A multicomponent X-ray survival curve for mouse lymphoma cells irradiated *in vivo*, *Nature (London)* **197**:710.

Rashad, A. L., and Evans, C. A., 1968, Radioautographic study of epidermal cell proliferation and migration in normal and neoplastic tissues of rabbits, *J. Natl. Cancer Inst.* **41**:845.

Reinhold, H. S., 1966, Quantitative evaluation of the radiosensitivity of cells of a transplantable rhabdomyosarcoma in the rat, *Eur. J. Cancer* **2**:33.

Reinhold, H. S., and Buisman, G. H., 1975, Repair of radiation damage to capillary endothelium, *Br. J. Radiol.* **48**:727.

Reiskin, A., and Mendelsohn, M. L., 1964, A comparison of the cell cycle in induced carcinoma and their normal counterpart, *Cancer Res.* **24**:1131.

Shipley, W. U., Stanley, J. A., Courtenay, V. D., and Field, S. B., 1975, Repair of radiation damage in Lewis lung carcinoma cells following *in situ* treatment with fast neutrons and gamma rays, *Cancer Res.* **35**:932.

Simpson-Herren, L., Sanford, A. H., and Holmqvist, J. P., 1974, Cell population kinetics of transplanted and metastatic Lewis lung carcinoma, *Cell Tissue Kinet.* **7**:349.

Sinclair, W. K., 1968, Cyclic X-ray responses in mammalian cells *in vitro*, *Radiat. Res.* **33**:620.

Sinclair, W. K., and Morton, R. A., 1963, Variations in X-ray response during the division cycle of partially synchronised Chinese hamster cells in culture, *Nature (London)* **199**:1158.

Steel, G. G., 1968, Cell loss from experimental tumours, *Cell Tissue Kinet.* **1**:193.

Steel, G. G., 1972, The cell cycle in tumours: An examination of data gained by the technique of labelled mitoses, *Cell Tissue Kinet.* **5**:87.

Steel, G. G., and Lamerton, L. F., 1966, The growth rate of human tumours, *Br. J. Cancer* **20**:74.

Steel, G. G., Adams, K., and Hodgett, J., 1971, Cell population kinetics of a spontaneous rat tumour during serial transplantation, *Br. J. Cancer* **25**:802.

Suit, H. D., and Maeda, M., 1967, Hyperbaric oxygen and radiobiology of a C3H mouse mammary carcinoma, *J. Natl. Cancer Inst.* **39**:650.

Szczepanski, L. V., and Trott, K. R., 1975, Post-irradiation proliferation kinetics of a serially transplanted murine adenocarcinoma, *Br. J. Radiol.* **48**:200.

Tannock, I. F., 1968, The relation between cell proliferation and the vascular system in a transplanted mouse mammary tumour, *Br. J. Cancer* **22**:258.

Tannock, I. F., 1969, A comparison of cell proliferation parameters in solid and ascites Ehrlich tumors, *Cancer Res.* **29**:1527.

Tannock, I. F., 1970, Population kinetics of carcinoma cells, capillary endothelial cells and fibroblasts in a transplanted mouse mammary tumor, *Cancer Res.* **30**:2470.

Tannock, I. F., and Hayashi, S., 1972, The proliferation of capillary endothelial cells, *Cancer Res.* **32**:77.

Terasima, T., and Tolmach, L. J., 1963, Variations in several responses of HeLa cells to X-irradiation during the division cycle, *Biophys. J.* **3**:11.

Thomlinson, R. H., 1968, Changes of oxygenation in tumours, in: *Frontiers of Radiation Therapy and Oncology*, Vol. 3 (G. Vaeth, ed.), pp. 109–21, Karger, Basel.

137

CELL
PROLIFERATION
KINETICS AND
RADIATION
THERAPY

THOMLINSON, R. H., 1971, The oxygen effect and radiotherapy with fast neutrons, *Eur. J. Cancer* **7**:139.

THOMLINSON, R. H., AND CRADDOCK, E. A., 1967, The gross response of an experimental tumour to single doses of x-rays, *Br. J. Cancer* **21**:108.

THOMLINSON, R. H., AND GRAY, L. H., 1955, The histological structure of some human lung cancers and the possible implications for radiotherapy, *Br. J. Cancer* **9**:539.

THOMLINSON, R. H., DISCHE, S., GRAY, A. J., AND ERRINGTON, L. M., 1976, Clinical testing of the radiosensitizer Ro-07-0582. III. Response of tumours, *Clin. Radiol.* **27**:167.

TILL, J. E., 1976, Regulation of hemopoietic stem cells, in: *Stem Cells of Renewing Cell Populations* (A. B. CAIRNIE, P. K. LALA, AND D. G. OSMOND, eds.), pp. 143–156, Academic Press, New York.

TRENTIN, J. J., 1976, Hemopoietic inductive micro-environments, in *Stem Cells of Renewing Cell Populations* (A. B. CAIRNIE, P. K. LALA, AND D. G. OSMOND, eds.), pp. 255–264, Academic Press, New York.

TUBIANA, M., 1971, Review article: The kinetics of tumour cell proliferation and radiotherapy, *Br. J. Radiol.* **44**:325.

TUBIANA, M., FRINDEL, E., AND MALAISE, E., 1968, The application of radiobiologic knowledge and cellular kinetics to radiation therapy, *Am. J. Roentgenol.* **102**:822.

TUBIANA, M., FRINDEL, E., AND VASSORT, F., 1975, Critical survey of experimental data on an *in vivo* synchronization by hydroxyurea, *Recent Results Cancer Res.* **52**:187.

UNGER, E., AND GIDALI, J., 1971, Autoradiographic studies on ^{3}H-thymidine incorporation in the liver and kidneys of irradiated mice, *Strahlentherapie* **141**:354.

URTASUN, R., BAND, P., CHAPMAN, J. D., FELDSTEIN, M. L., MIELKE, B., AND FRYER, C., 1976, Radiation and high dose metronidazole (Flagyl) in supratentorial glioblastomas, *N. Engl. J. Med.* **294**:1364.

VAN DEN BRENK, H. A. S., SHARPINGTON, C., ORTON, C., AND STONE, M., 1974, Effects of X-radiation on growth and function of the repair blastema (granulation tissue). II. Measurements of angiogenesis in the Selye pouch in the rat, *Int. J. Radiat. Biol.* **25**:277.

VAN PEPERZEEL, H. A., 1970, Patterns of tumor growth after irradiation: A comparative study in men, dogs and mice, Ph.D. thesis, University of Amsterdam.

VAN PEPERZEEL, H. A., 1972, Effects of single doses of radiation on lung metastases in man and experimental animals, *Eur. J. Cancer* **8**:665.

VAN PUTTEN, L. M., 1968a, Tumour reoxygenation during fractionated radiotherapy; studies with a transplantable mouse osteosarcoma, *Eur. J. Cancer* **4**:173.

VAN PUTTEN, L. M., 1968b, Oxygenation and cell kinetics after irradiation in a transplantable osteosarcoma, in: *Effects of Radiation on Cellular Proliferation and Differentiation* (*Proceedings of the Monaco Symposium*), pp. 493–505, IAEA, Vienna.

VAN PUTTEN, L. M., AND KALLMAN, R. F., 1966, Oxygenation states of a transplantable tumor during fractionated radiotherapy, *J. Natl. Cancer Inst.* **40**:441.

WARA, W. M., PHILLIPS, T. L., MARGOLIS, L. W., AND SMITH, V., 1973, Radiation pneumonitis; a new approach to the derivation of time dose factors, *Cancer* **32**:547.

WATSON, J. V., 1976, The cell proliferation kinetics of the EMT6/M/AC mouse tumour at four volumes during unperturbed growth *in vivo*, *Cell Tissue Kinet.* **9**:147.

WHITMORE, G. F., GULYAS, S., AND BOTOND, J., 1965, Radiation sensitivity throughout the cell cycle and its relationship to recovery, in: *Cellular Radiation Biology*, pp. 423–431, Williams and Wilkins, Baltimore.

WHITMORE, G. F., TILL, J. E., AND GULYAS, G. S., 1967, Radiation induced mitotic delay in L cells, *Radiat. Res.* **30**:155.

WINTER, G. D., 1971, The poor healing of burns, in: *Research on Burns* (P. MATHER, T. L. BARCLAY, AND Z. KONICKOVA, eds.), pp. 614–619, Huber, Bern.

WITHERS, H. R., 1967, Recovery and repopulation *in vivo* by mouse skin epithelial cells during fractionated irradiation, *Radiat. Res.* **32**:227.

WITHERS, H. R., 1975a, Cell cycle redistribution as a factor in multifraction irradiation, *Radiology* **114**:199.

WITHERS, H. R., 1975b, Iso-effect curves for various proliferative tissues in experimental animals, in: *Proceedings of the Madison Conference on Time–Dose Relationships in Clinical Therapy* (W. CALDWELL AND D. D. TOLBERT, eds.), pp. 30–38, University of Wisconsin, Madison, Wis.

WITHERS, H. R., AND ELKIND, M. M., 1969, Radiosensitivity and fractionation response of crypt cells of mouse jejunum, *Radiat. Res.* **38**:598.

5

Radiation Effects on Normal Tissues

J. F. FOWLER AND J. DENEKAMP

1. Introduction

Radiotherapy and surgery are the two most successful forms of treatment for localized neoplasms, each having a high cure rate in certain sites but a low cure rate in others. If the tumor is accessible and no vital structures are involved, surgery is the treatment of choice. The radiotherapist therefore tends to treat the more inaccessible tumors, or those with vital structures in close juxtaposition. Both surgery and radiotherapy are treatments of localized disease. Systemic chemotherapy is the main method of treatment for widely disseminated cancer, but whole-body or regional irradiation is sometimes used prophylactically, for example, in leukemia (brain) or osteosarcoma (lungs). Hyperthermia is also being used more extensively.

All these treatments are limited in their efficacy by the normal tissues which are inevitably included in the treatment volume: tissues close to the tumor for surgery and for radiotherapy, and all the tissues in the body for systemically administered drugs.

All localized tumors are potentially curable with radiation, but the dose necessary to achieve that cure may leave such a high level of normal tissue injury that it is fatal, or it makes the quality of life unacceptable. Therefore, the radiotherapist cannot select the dose appropriate for curing the tumor; instead, he selects the dose which will give a small but finite probability of intolerable radiation damage to the normal tissue, i.e., the tolerance dose. Radiotherapy depends on a

J. F. FOWLER AND J. DENEKAMP ● Gray Laboratory, Cancer Research Campaign, Mount Vernon Hospital, Northwood, Middlesex HA6 2RN, England.

knowledge of the tolerance doses for different normal tissues. This knowledge has been acquired empirically during 80 years of clinical practice, but quantitative data are still sparse. The further improvement of radiotherapy is therefore limited by our understanding of the ways in which normal tissues respond, for example, to changes in the overall treatment time, the way the doses are divided within that time, and the effect of various drugs and different types of radiation. A better understanding of these responses could lead to substantial improvements in radiation therapy, however, and they are currently under investigation in laboratory animals. For any new technique to be advantageous over conventional methods of treatment, it must be shown to have a "therapeutic gain." Its efficiency of killing malignant cells must be increased *without* a correspondingly increased effect on normal tissues. Thus data on normal tissues and tumors must be obtained concurrently, whether in laboratory animals or in the clinic, although the dose that will be administered clinically will be determined by the normal tissue response.

The scientific understanding of radiation tolerance levels, based on relevant radiobiological studies, is still in its infancy. In this chapter, we shall try to correlate what is known clinically with the available radiobiological data that have been obtained relatively recently.

Normal tissue tolerance differs for different organs. It also varies if the whole organ, instead of only a part of it, is included in the radiation field. The tolerance dose is affected by the severity of the malignant erosion of normal structures, the functional status of the irradiated tissues, the need for a cosmetic result, and the patient's willingness to tolerate any disability or morbidity. These facts are well known by radiotherapists, and they adjust the prescribed doses accordingly, using their clinical experience.

Some of the early pioneers were quick to observe that the sensitivity of various tissues seemed to be related to the proliferative activity of the tissue, i.e., the number of mitotic cells. This led to the "law" of Bergonie and Tribondeau (1906) that tissues with high mitotic indices responded more readily to X-rays. By "readily," however, the early workers meant "sooner," and this criterion inevitably reflects the cellular turnover rate of the tissues rather than the number of cells killed by the irradiation.

The timing of the radiation treatments was studied very early in the history of radiotherapy, but the superiority of fractionated radiotherapy was not universally accepted for many years. Krönig and Friedrich (1918) and Seitz and Wintz (1920) advocated a single dose of radiation for malignant tumors. However, the techniques of Coutard (1932) and Baclesse (1958), who used a very prolonged overall treatment time with many small doses of equal size, up to 30–50 dose fractions in 6–10 weeks, have prevailed. These fractionation schemes were based on some radiobiological data: for example, the rabbit skin erythema experiments of Krönig and Friedrich, and the testis weight-loss experiments of Regaud and Ferroux (1937). However, the interpretation of their results which led to the clinical fractionation schemes was not valid—for example, the assumption that tumors would respond like testicles. Nevertheless, the current widespread practice is to give daily treatments of 200–300 rads per day, 5 times a week for 3–8 weeks.

In later years, the clinical allowances for sensitivity or tolerance for the various tissues, using the conventional fractionation schemes, were developed to a fine art. There are a number of standard textbooks (e.g., Paterson, 1948; Fletcher, 1973; Moss *et al.*, 1973) and conference proceedings (e.g., Vaeth, 1972) for reference, and these show a considerable agreement between the tolerance doses that are recommended in different countries. The difference between the dose given by a conservative radiotherapist and that given by an aggressive radiotherapist seldom exceeds 15%. This is an indication of how sharp the dose response is and how well the tolerance levels are known for existing schedules of treatment.

The early studies, using low-energy (orthovoltage) radiation, were often limited by skin reaction, both as an acute response and as a delayed dermal response. The advent, in the 1950s, of supervoltage machines such as ^{60}Co units, linear accelerators, and betatrons allowed a sparing of the superficial layers, because the maximum dose is deposited at least several millimeters below the surface. While somewhat larger tumor doses can now be achieved because of the better depth-dose distributions, and a significant improvement in cure rates at some sites has evolved (Table 1), the tolerance of the deeper tissues has not permitted dramatically greater total doses to be administered.

Since so much is known from clinical practice, it is pertinent to ask why radiobiological information on an animal other than man is at all necessary. The present knowledge, being empirical, is restricted to conventional fractionation schemes, using conventional forms of radiation. While this achieves good local success in many sites, there are still many patients who fail to respond adequately, and a modified form of treatment is obviously necessary for them. In order to modify the treatment, the reasons for failure must be understood. Radiobiological studies on tumors and normal tissues can be used to elucidate the factors controlling the response to single doses and to fractionated doses of conventional radiation, to new forms of radiation, and to combinations with chemotherapy, immunotherapy, or surgery. By this means, the harmful sequelae that sometimes follow a change in clinical practice may be avoided. Changes in treatment should be based on a scientific understanding of the various factors involved in the response of cells and organized tissues to radiation, not on inspired guesswork.

In vitro studies have enabled us to list the factors which can affect the radiosensitivity of cells. These factors* are discussed in detail in other chapters in this volume (e.g., Denekamp and Fowler; Elkind). *In vitro* studies have shown there to be no consistent difference in radiosensitivity between malignant cells and normal cells. However, the radiosensitivity of certain tumors such as lymphomas has been shown to result from a low capacity for absorbing radiation as nonlethal damage,

---

* These include the extrapolation number n, which is related to the ability to accumulate and repair sublethal injury; D_Q, the "quasi-threshold dose," which is proportional to n; D_0, the inverse slope, or efficiency per rad, of the exponential killing process; and the state of oxygenation and the stage in the proliferation cycle. In addition, intercellular contact and postirradiation changes of milieu can alter the cellular radiosensitivity.

TABLE 1

Five-Year Survival from Several Types of Cancer Treated with Radiotherapy

Type or site of cancer	Approximate representative 5-year survival (%)	
	1950–1955	1970–1975
Hodgkin's disease, all stages	35	60
Early		80
Late		50
Cancer of cervix, all stages	50	60
Stage I		90
Stage II		65
Stage III		40
Stage IV		10
Cancer of nasopharynx, all stages	30	60
Stage T1		85
Stage T2		70
Stage T3		50
Stage T4		30
Cancer of breast, all stages	50	50
Early		80
Late		20
Cancer of bladder, all stages	20	30
Stage T1, T2		40
Stage T3		25
Stage T4		6
Cancer of prostate	10	60
Brain tumors	20	30
Testicular tumors		
Seminoma	—	90
Teratoma	—	25

i.e., a small shoulder or D_Q, and also a sensitive response, i.e., a low value of D_0. Similarly, cells derived from radioresistant melanomas have shown a resistance to low doses, resulting from a larger capacity to absorb radiation as reparable sublethal damage (see Fig. 1). Unfortunately, the radiosensitivity of the tumor

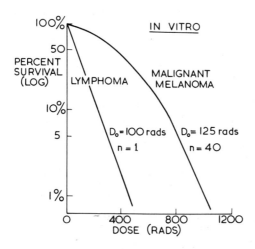

FIGURE 1. Curves relating the proportion of surviving, replicating cells to X-ray dose for malignant melanoma or lymphoma cells in tissue culture. The upper curve shows a "shoulder," i.e., reduced cell-killing efficiency at low doses.

may relate closely to the sensitivity of the normal tissue of origin; e.g., lymphoma and bone marrow are both sensitive, as are seminomas and the normal testis.

2. Dose–Response Curves

Radiobiology has developed from a qualitative study of radiation effects into one of the most quantitative areas of biological research. Radiation doses in tissues can be measured very accurately (±2%), and wherever dose–effect relationships can be studied an increased incidence of any form of damage for an increase in absorbed dose can be demonstrated. *In vitro* studies are usually devoted to studying the loss of proliferative capacity as judged by the ability of individual surviving cells to form colonies or clones of at least 50 cells by rapid cell division in dishes. In these experiments, the environment and metabolic state of the cells can be manipulated easily and the basic parameters controlling radiation sensitivity have been elucidated (e.g., Elkind *et al.*, 1965).

Radiobiological studies on tumors are of three basic types: (1) measurements of delay in regrowth to a particular size; (2) measurements of the proportion of tumors cured locally by various doses; or (3) measurements of cell survival obtained by irradiating *in vivo*, then removing the tumor, breaking it up into a single-cell suspension, and assaying the cells' proliferative capacity, either *in vitro* or by further growth in recipient mice. All these techniques yield dose–response curves so that different forms of treatment of the tumors can be compared quantitatively. The first two techniques necessitate local irradiation and are like clinical radiotherapy in that normal tissue injury will be evoked. The quantitative study of cell survival can be more precise and does not always require localized irradiation. However, the response of tumors assayed in this way is often not the same as for cells in similar tumors left *in situ* (McNally, 1972, 1975).

Normal tissue studies fall into three groups: (1) lethality studies, (2) measurements of altered function or morphology, and (3) cell survival assays.

2.1. Lethality Studies in Animals

Animals can be killed by radiation if the tolerance dose to any critical organ is exceeded. Whole-body irradiation results in death due to damage in the most rapidly renewing organs. If a whole-body dose of 700–900 rads is given to mice, the animals will survive for 2 or 3 weeks, but will succumb before 30 days to infection because their bone marrow, which was depleted by the radiation, has failed to supply enough lymphocytes to combat the normal level of microbial infection. The response is not a sharp step-function, as is shown in Fig. 2. As the X-ray dose increases, the number of animals that die increases. At somewhat higher doses (1000–1500 rads), the animals do not survive 20–30 days, but instead they die at 3–5 days because of the denudation of the intestinal epithelium. This less sensitive tissue (i.e., it needs a higher dose) responds at an earlier time because

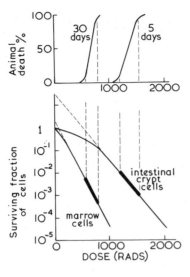

FIGURE 2. Proportion of mice killed by single doses of X-rays to the whole body by 5 days or between 5 and 30 days. The lower part shows the corresponding cell survival curves. Cells of the intestinal crypts are more radioresistant than stem cells in the marrow, but their transit time through the differentiated compartment is much shorter so that depopulation of the tissue, leading to death, occurs sooner in gut than in marrow. After Alper (1973).

of its more rapid proliferation characteristics (see previous chapter by Denekamp and Fowler). Again, a dose–response curve can be established by varying the dose level and scoring the proportion of survivors (Fig. 2).

Similar dose–response relationships can be established for other organs, e.g., esophagus, lung, and kidney, if the radiation dose is increased still further and if the more sensitive intestine and bone marrow are "spared" by shielding (Fig. 3). The time at which death occurs from the expression of radiation damage in these different organs depends on the turnover time of critical cells within the organ. Slowly dividing tissues respond later than rapidly dividing tissues, so the most rapidly renewing organs are usually the critical ones in whatever volume is irradiated. Lethality studies are obviously not directly relevant to clinical radiotherapy, because they record much more gross injury than that occurring

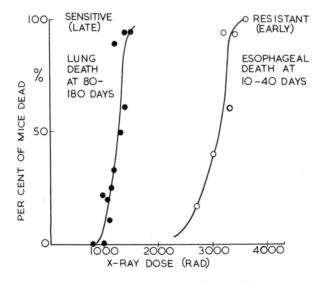

FIGURE 3. Proportion of mice killed by single doses of X-rays to the thorax only by 40 days (esophageal death) or between 80 and 180 days (lung death). As in Fig. 2, the more radiosensitive tissue expresses its radiation damage later. From Field and Hornsey (personal communication).

from present clinical treatment. They do, however, give useful information on relative tissue sensitivities and time scales.

2.2. Functional Tests

Dose–response curves can also be obtained if a functional test is performed that can be given an arbitrary grading. The most commonly used system is the gross response of skin scored as erythema, desquamation, and ulceration. Using this technique, the acute response, within the first few weeks, or the delayed response, after several months, can be measured, and "average skin reactions" can be plotted as a function of dose in order to compare different forms of treatment (Fig. 4). Skin has been used, because of its accessibility and ease of scoring, to obtain many of the radiotherapy-oriented radiobiology data that are available on both animals and patients. The effects of oxygen, of different fractionation schemes, of different qualities of radiation, and of combined modalities (e.g., radiation plus drugs, plus hyperthermia, or plus surgery) have been studied. Two approaches are used: the scoring of reaction on an arbitrary scale (Fig. 4) or the scoring of the percent of animals showing a particular level of damage (i.e., the ED_{50}, or effective dose to produce a given level of damage in 50% of the animals).

Other normal tissue functional or morphological end points include paraplegia after irradiation of the spinal cord, kidney malfunction as tested by renographs or by ^{86}Rb uptake, bone healing and callus formation after a fracture, necrosis of rodent tails, vascular changes, and testis weight loss. These all give dose–response curves that may possibly be related to the morbidity observed in clinical practice, if

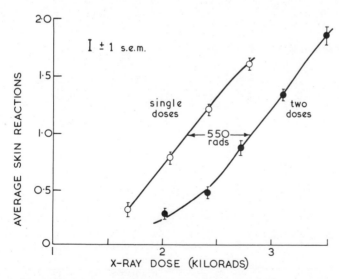

FIGURE 4. Average skin reaction in groups of six mice over the period 8–30 days after single doses (left-hand curve) or two equal doses given 24 hr apart (right-hand curve) of 250 kV X-rays. The dose increment of 550 rads necessary to counteract repair of sublethal injury in 24 hr is shown.

differences in tissue turnover rates between small animals and patients can be taken into account. However, most of these techniques are slow and expensive to perform and information from them is sparse.

2.3. Cell Survival Clonal Assays

In recent years, a number of *in vivo* cloning techniques have been developed for normal tissues. The first of these was the spleen colony assay for surviving bone marrow cells, assayed in the irradiated animal itself (endogenous colonies) or in another recipient mouse (exogenous colonies) (Till and McCulloch, 1961, 1963). This test assays for colony-forming units (CFUs), which may represent the multipotent, noncommitted precursor stem cell for all the different blood cells.

Withers (1967) developed an assay for cell survival of individual skin cells. Small test areas were defined and isolated from the rest of the skin by a heavily irradiated moat of dead cells. Surviving cells grow up as visible clones after 2–3 weeks (Fig. 5). This had enabled more quantitative studies of skin to be performed, which have confirmed the previous assumption that gross skin reactions, where desquamation and ulceration are scored, are a result of depletion of the proliferating basal layer.

Further work by Withers and Elkind (1969, 1970) has extended this cloning technique to studies of the small intestine (jejunum), the stomach (Chen and Withers, 1972), and the colon (Withers, 1971), and also to studies of the testis (Withers *et al.*, 1974). In each case, small colonies produced by the proliferation of

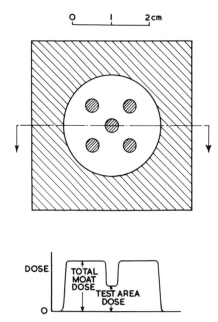

FIGURE 5. Pattern of irradiation required for the skin colony assays (Withers, 1967). A circular area of dorsal skin in the mouse 2.5 cm in diameter is irradiated by low-energy X-rays which do not damage the internal organs. Five small "islands" of skin are shielded against this ulcerating "moat" dose. They are then irradiated with the test dose of irradiation so that only about one cell survives in each island. In those islands containing at least one surviving cell, a macroscopic colony will be seen about 3 weeks later. Thus cell survival curves can be constructed for epithelial cells *in vivo*.

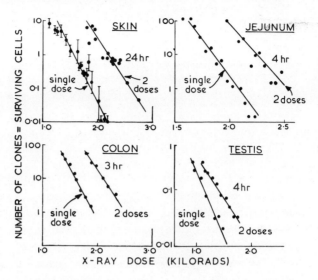

FIGURE 6. Cell survival curves (strictly "island survival curves") obtained in four tissues in the mouse by methods devised by Withers, modified from that in Fig. 5. For the three tissues other than skin, the whole organ was irradiated and the number of clones in the organ at a set time later was determined microscopically. Skin: clones per square millimeter. Jejunum and colon: clones per circumference of a section. Testis: clones per tubule. After Withers and colleagues (see text).

surviving cells are scored, either in histological sections or with the naked eye, as viable islands in a sea of heavily irradiated cells. While these techniques allow cell survival to be measured (Fig. 6) and are a useful tool for comparing gross responses with cell survival, they seldom have a direct application in the field of clinical radiotherapy; i.e., they cannot be applied in patients.

2.4. Clinical Studies

Most of the tests used to obtain dose–response curves in the laboratory cannot be directly applied to patients in the clinic. The most relevant tests, i.e., the functional, nondestructive experiments, are more difficult to use experimentally and the dose–response relationships are less well defined. This perhaps makes it all the more surprising that clinical tolerance doses are as well known empirically as they seem to be. Much of the information was obtained in an anecdotal form by many individual therapists throughout the world, each of whom quickly decided which dose levels killed his patients or produced unacceptable late normal tissue injury and should therefore be avoided. Unfortunately, there is a lack of controlled studies of a large homogeneous series of patients treated with a range of doses, and therefore few clinical dose–response curves for normal tissue damage exist. Few radiotherapists are willing to accept, let alone exceed, 5–10% complications due to normal tissue injury, although it is obvious that a finite level of morbidity must be weighed against the increased cure rate that would accompany it (Mendelsohn, 1969; Paterson, 1948; Rubin and Casarett, 1972), as indicated in Fig. 7.

If the incidence of normal tissue complications is to be kept desirably low, a large series of cases is necessary before a statistically significant dose–response curve for normal tissue damage can be established. This is difficult to achieve in any one department within a reasonable length of time, and multicenter trials, although difficult, are essential. *More than one dose level needs to be used in each type of*

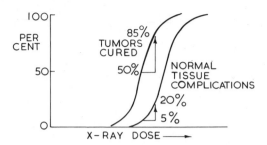

FIGURE 7. Proportions of patients cured and patients with normal tissue complications increase with total dose (schematic representation). Both curves have a similar sigmoid nature. It is possible to obtain a large increase in cures for a modest increase in risk of complications at certain dose levels. However, starting from higher dose levels, the risk of complications rises steeply for little increase in tumor cure probability.

treatment. At the present time, however, information about either tumor response or normal tissue complications at several dose levels, using a given treatment schedule, is exceedingly rare. The clearest data available are those from Morrison (1975) for bladder complications and local control, Shukovsky (1970) for local control of cancer of the supraglottic larynx, and Shukovsky and Fletcher (1973) for local control of cancer of the tonsillar fossa. The probability of local control of carcinomas of the bladder followed almost the same dose–response curve as that found by Shukovsky for both the supraglottic larynx and the tonsillar fossa, for the same values of NSD (nominal standard dose) above 1800 rets (rad equivalent therapy). At the highest levels of dose used, equivalent to 2100 rets, the local control rates were 81% and 86% for bladder and throat cases, respectively.

Morrison found that an increase of 10%* in dose caused the complication rate to rise from 7% to 20%, and local control of tumors to rise from 59% to 69% (see Fig. 8). Only complications of major severity were included: intestinal obstructions, fistula formation, bladder contracture, and hemorrhage. The complication rates in similar cases of bladder treatment from six other authors agreed well with Morrison's own series. This type of clinical information, where tumor response and the associated complication rates are compared quantitatively at several levels of radiation dose, is required to enable the potential gain of radiotherapy to be assessed in relation to the risks (Stewart and Jackson, 1975).

Radiotherapists and hospital physicists aim at narrow limits of precision in their doses because of the relatively sharp boundary between little normal tissue damage and severe normal tissue damage. An increase of 10% in radiation dose may be detected clinically in the first one or two patients treated, by the unusually

* From 5550 to 6100 rads in 25 fractions in 35 days.

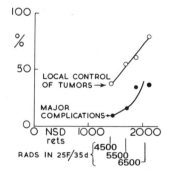

FIGURE 8. Proportion of bladder tumors locally controlled, and of major normal tissue complications, as the total dose is increased. After Morrison (1975).

high acute reactions. This is less likely to be true for a 10% reduction in dose, unless a brisk early reaction is normally being produced with the conventional treatments. A change of 5% is unlikely to be clinically detected in any one patient, although this has sometimes been claimed.

An example of an unintended increase in effective radiation dose occurred in one series of treatments for breast cancer when the fractionation was changed from five sessions per week to three per week, in the same overall time of 8 weeks. This was an effective increase in dose of about 13%. The proportion of patients in whom the cancer was controlled rose from 75% to 88%, but the proportion with chest wall necrosis rose from 5% to 18%. In this example, the numbers saved from recurrence were equal to the numbers of those who suffered chest wall necrosis (Montague, 1968; Shukovsky, 1974). In some types of normal tissue injury, surgical repair is possible, whereas a recurrence of tumor is fatal.

3. Time of Expression of Damage

A better understanding of the development of radiation injury in various tissues is still evolving; it includes the concepts of cell killing and of tissue recovery both by repair of damaged cells and by proliferation of surviving cells. The time course of radiation injury in the renewing tissues can be logically explained by cell kinetic considerations. Other types of injury which are not obviously proportional to cell killing are poorly understood. These include edema, fibrosis, very late effects, and injury to nonproliferating or slowly proliferating tissues. Relationships between the early, acute tissue reactions and late injury are still the subject of much discussion and research, and the role of vascular injury is particularly debatable.

3.1. Phases of Radiation Response

In most tissues, there are at least two or three phases of radiation response: a transient response during therapy, an early acute phase, and a delayed or chronic phase (see Table 2). The exact timing of these phases varies considerably from one tissue to another. There may be a transient early response during the course of therapy resulting from increased permeability of the blood vessels, leading to local edema. This is followed by the main acute phase, due to the death of proliferating cells within the tissue. This death of cells usually occurs at mitosis, with a few notable exceptions such as lymphocytes which can die an earlier interphase death. The loss of proliferating cells is manifested in a loss of tissue function at some later time when the proliferating cells fail to replenish the mature differentiated cells as they are lost in the normal wear-and-tear process. This loss of parenchymal cells characterizes the tissues that respond within 1 or 2 months after irradiation, e.g., skin, buccal mucosa, and intestinal epithelium. More slowly responding tissues show changes in the blood vessels and fibrosis at about the same time as parenchymal cell damage occurs, i.e., with onset at 6–8 months. It is then very

TABLE 2[a]

Organ	Transient during therapy	Early injury	Late injury
Small intestine	Diarrhea, colic, malabsorption	6 mo–1 yr, obstruction	1–11 yr, obstruction may require surgery
Colon and rectum	Diarrhea, colic	6–12 mo, diarrhea, necrosis	2–3 yr, slow stenosis, fibrosis, and induration
Stomach	Anorexia plus nausea, reduced acidity	1–2 mo, superficial ulcers	Chronic atrophic gastritis
Esophagus	Pain on swallowing	—	1–5 yr, stenosis
Oral mucosa	Mucositis, moist desquamation	2–3 mo, atrophy	6 mo–1 yr, fibrosis 1–5 yr+, ulcers, deep necrosis, atrophy
Skin	Erythema, desquamation	6–8 wk, desquamation plus healing pigmentation	6 mo–5 yr, atrophy, ulcers, deep fibrosis
Lung	Pneumonitis at end	0–3 mo, pneumonitis	8 mo–2 yr, fibrosis
Kidney	None	6–12 mo, nephrosclerosis	1.5–>3 yr, chronic radiation nephritis with vascular sclerosis
Liver	Changed liver function (rose bengal scan)	—	7 mo–1 yr, changed liver function
Ureters	None	—	1–2 yr, fibrosis and obstruction
Bladder	Cystitis	—	7–8 mo, contraction-yr+, atrophic ulcers
Spinal cord	None unless tumor present	Edema, compression, pain if tumor is present	Transverse myelitis: 6–12 mo, reversible 1–2 yr, paraplegia
Brain	Edema	6 mo–1 yr, reversible effects	1–2 yr, necrosis
Heart	None	—	1–2 yr, pericarditis
Major blood vessels	None	Arterial fibrosis	Seldom seen unless involved with tumor
Eyes	None	—	>2 yr, cataract even at low doses

[a] With acknowledgment to Rubin and Casarett (1968) and Urtasun (personal communication).

difficult to determine which cells are responding primarily to the radiation damage and whether any of the damage to parenchymal cells is secondary to vascular damage. Increased permeability of the capillaries may lead to edema, and ultimately to fibrosis. It has been suggested that this may be a common pathway of late damage in many slowly dividing tissues.

The central role of vascular injury has been questioned on the basis of the different tolerance levels for different organs: if they were all responding because of vascular damage, it would seem likely that they should have similar tolerance levels. However, different tissues will have different reserve capacities for a collateral blood supply if some of the capillaries are occluded. Attempts to identify microscopically (with both the light and the electron microscope) the exact sequence of cell degeneration in the lungs and in the kidneys suggest that vascular changes precede the deposition of collagen and the loss of parenchymal cells

(Phillips and Margolis, 1972; Glatstein, 1973). However, this is still an area of
debate based on inadequate experimental information.

The time course of damage to certain organs in the mouse can be well explained
by the proliferation characteristics of the tissues where they are known. Figure 9
shows the initial depletion of basal skin cells which occurs soon after irradiation
because, although cell division ceases, the movement of cells into the more
superficial differentiating compartments continues. This loss of cells does not
cause a failure of tissue function, i.e., desquamation and ulceration, until the
superficial layers have all been removed by the normal wear-and-tear processes,
corresponding to the normal transit time of the cells through the differentiating
layers. In the mouse, cells are being produced with a cycle time of 5 days, and there
are two or three superficial layers on the dorsum. Radiation-induced desquamation is expressed, commencing at 10–15 days. The skin reaction is healed by
proliferation of the surviving basal cells, or, after very high doses, by migration of
cells from the adjacent undamaged epidermis. This reparative proliferation does
not start for several days, until some loss of basal cells has been recognized (Fowler
and Denekamp, 1976). In the skin of some animals, although not in mice, a quite
separate late wave of injury develops after high doses, starting at 4–6 months. This
has been attributed to damage to the vasculature leading by way of nutritional
failure to secondary damage to the basal layer cells. Another form of late damage
that can be scored in mouse feet is the late deformity, seen as loss of nails, toes, or
even larger portions of the foot. This correlates extremely well with the early skin
reactions for a whole variety of treatments, and it seems probable that it is directly
related to the extent of epidermal depletion in the early phase (Field, 1969; Brown
and Probert, 1975; Denekamp, unpublished).

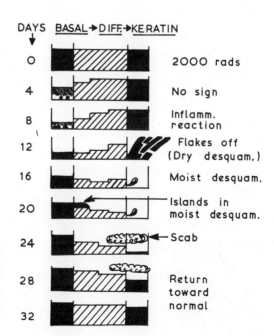

FIGURE 9. Time course of skin reactions
after irradiation. The deficit in cell production caused in the basal layer (on left) pro-
gresses through the granular and spinous
layers to cause dry desquamation of the
existing keratin (on right), followed by moist
desquamation until repopulation from surviving basal cells replenishes the epithelium.

By analogy, the response of other organs or tissues can be interpreted in terms of depeletion of differentiated functional cells. The whole-body death due to intestinal injury occurs in mice at 3–5 days. This relates directly to the transit time of cells from the proliferative regions in the crypts of Lieberkühn to their eventual loss into the lumen from the tips of the villi. When cell production in the crypts stops after irradiation, cells continue to move up onto the surface of the crypt, the crypt gradually shrinks and becomes denuded of epithelium, and the mouse dies of fluid loss across the intestinal wall leading to electrolyte imbalance. This occurs rapidly because the transit time of the differentiating cells is only 2 days. Nevertheless, higher doses are required to cause this mode of injury than to damage bone marrow (Fig. 2), because of the greater capacity for absorption and repair of sublethal radiation injury in gut cells relative to bone marrow cells. This greater capacity is evidenced by larger dose increments needed to counteract repair if the radiation is given as two fractions spaced apart by a few hours rather than as a single dose (Hornsey and Vatistas, 1963; Withers and Elkind, 1969). It means that the intestinal cells require larger doses than marrow cells for a given proportion to be killed. This distinction between speed of response on the one hand and cellular radiosensitivity on the other was not appreciated in the early days of radiotherapy.

Although bone marrow responds to total-body irradiation at lower doses than the gut, its damage is not expressed until later, again because of the longer transit time through the maturation compartments of the limiting lymphocytes, granulocytes, and platelets. By 10–20 days in the mouse, the white blood count has fallen so low that the animal is unable to combat any bacterial infection and dies a rather complex death. Thirty days is usually chosen as the end time for assessing how many mice will survive a given whole-body irradiation procedure. The corresponding time for human patients exposed to whole-body irradiation is 50–60 days.

Similarly, for esophagus and lung, after irradiation of the thorax the time of expression of injury relates to the proliferation characteristic of the tissue, not to the absolute cellular radiosensitivity (Fig. 3). The lung is the more sensitive organ, but death does not occur until 3–6 months after irradiation in mice because of the long cell-cycle time and the consequent delay in mitotic death. It is not clear whether, in lungs, this death is due primarily to capillary endothelial cells (Phillips *et al.*, 1972) or to "type 2 surfactant producing cells" (Van den Brenk, 1971), but none of the lung cells is known to have a rapid turnover. In the esophagus, however, which required higher doses of radiation to cause injury than does the lung, death in mice occurs at 20–30 days. This is again in accord with the maturation time of the epithelial cells and the time at which depletion of the surface keratinized cells would be expressed; it is similar to the time of skin desquamation.

From these and other tissue studies, the general model shown in Fig. 10 can be proposed. The animal will die, or the tissue function be grossly impaired, only if the differentiated cells fall below a critical level. For rapidly dividing and maturing cells, the cell depletion will be registered quickly, and compensatory proliferation

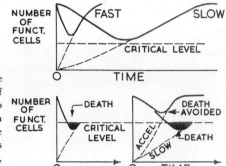

FIGURE 10. Depopulation of functioning cells at some time after irradiation, depending on the rate of turnover (cell loss) in that organ. The time, and also the level, of maximum depopulation depends on how soon the surviving cells can repopulate the tissue. Death will occur if the number of such cells falls below a certain critical level. At the bottom right, the avoidance of death by accelerated proliferation is illustrated.

will be stimulated rapidly. The surviving cells will then repopulate the tissue and may or may not succeed in repopulating it before the critical depletion has occured, depending on the amount of cell killing of the stem cells. In the slowly proliferating tissues, cell depletion will be registered slowly, but cell loss will also be slow. Compensatory proliferation may be delayed, but when it occurs it has more scope for acceleration than in tissues which normally proliferate faster. In both cases, the success in repopulating the tissue before a critical level of depletion is reached depends on the extent to which the proliferation can be accelerated.

Thus both the time of appearance of damage and the dose required to produce it may depend on the cell-cycle time, the transit time of differentiating cells, and the time of onset of compensatory proliferation. Furthermore, the critical level of depletion will differ from one organ to another. In some tissues, e.g., kidney and liver, a loss of 50% of the functional capacity may not impair the ability of that individual to cope with *normal* body functions, because there is a reserve functional capacity. It may, however, affect the ability to cope with extra work, and this may explain why late radiation injury can be precipitated by some nonspecific external stress. In summary, the organ sensitivity depends on the following:

1. The cell survival characteristics of the constituent cells, both parenchymal and stromal, i.e., the D_0 and n, the state of oxygenation, and the position in the cell cycle.
2. The critical population size at which organ function fails.
3. The reserve functional capacity of the organ.
4. The fraction of the organ that is irradiated.
5. The time at which compensatory proliferation is initiated and the rate at which it can replace cells in the differentiated compartment.
6. The overall treatment time and the way the dose is distributed within it.
7. The structural nature of the organ, e.g., its mechanical ability to swell when edematous (not easy in brain or kidney).
8. The reserve capacity of its vasculature.

J. F. FOWLER
AND
J. DENEKAMP

3.2. Late Effects in Radiotherapy

Many critical organs show little or no acute reaction. The histological nature of the radiation injuries that occur months to years after irradiation is described in detail by Rubin and Casarett (1968), and some are listed in Table 2. However, we are ignorant of many of the important aspects of the pathogenesis and radiobiology of late effects. In particular, we are unable to give a reliable early prediction of late damage in any individual case or how it is affected by fractionation, by the time between radiation courses if retreatment is necessary, and by the use of radiation with various drugs.

What is commonly observed at about the time functional defects occur is the gradual disappearance of cells in both the vascular components of an organ and the functioning parenchymal cells. Although the primary injury in some of these organs may be to the capillary network and small arterioles, it is also clear that primary loss of functioning cells, such as the tubule cells of the kidney, also occurs. Quantitative information on the relative importance of cell loss in these two compartments is lacking. The importance of other tissue changes, such as edema or the formation of fibrin and collagen, is also poorly understood. Assay systems for late injury are few and are, of necessity, time consuming.

In some tissues and for certain time–dose schedules, the severities of acute and late reactions are parallel and may be, to some extent, interactive, as mentioned above for acute desquamation and late deformity in the feet of rodents, and as found also for acute desquamation and ultimate necrosis of the tails of rats and mice. However, this is not necessarily the case for other tissues. At the extremes of short treatments and of very protracted schedules, the dissociation between acute and late injury would be expected to be most obvious, particularly if repopulation plays a part in the early response but not in the late damage. It is unwise, therefore, to assume that in new radiation therapy modalities, acute reactions can be used to predict late effects. Therefore, even preclinical trials and early pilot studies may take several years to complete because late effects have to be awaited.

Another aspect of late injury that has not been extensively studied is the residual injury from an earlier course of radiation therapy and its effect on both the acute and late injuries following a second course of radiation therapy. Ellis (1969) suggested that restitution of normal tissues does not continue significantly beyond about 100 days, in which case the residual injury would remain large. Results of the few animal experiments done, which are on skin of the mouse foot, show an amount of residual injury varying between 40% (Brown and Probert, 1975) and 10% (Denekamp, 1975) after 6 months, but these data should probably not be generalized.

4. A Comparison of Human Tissue Radiosensitivities with Those of the Experimental Animal

The main problem in comparing experimental data with clinical data is that the experimental animal treatments have too often used single doses, with some notable exceptions, whereas the clinical treatments are with fractionated, extended treatments. However, an intercomparison of relative tissue sensitivities seems a useful exercise, in order to see whether rodent response bears any relationship to the human response.

In 1972, Rubin and Casarett published a table of clinical radiation tolerance doses for most of the normal tissues in the body, irradiated five times a week at 200 rads per session. They list *minimal injurious doses* (TD$_{5/5}$, the dose leading to a 5% probability of incidence at 5 years) and *maximimal injurious doses* (TD$_{50/5}$, the dose giving an expectation of 50% incidence at 5 years). Because of uncertainties in the interpretation of clinical data or inadequate numbers of cases, broader ranges than strictly 5% or 50% were quoted, namely a "1- to 5-percent level" and a "25- to 50-percent level."

The standard set of radiotherapy conditions are assumed to be supervoltage therapy (1–6 MeV), fractionation using five daily fractions of 200 rads each per week, and treatment completed in 2–8 weeks, depending on the total dose, at 1000 rads per week. These values are shown in Table 3 and in diagrammatic form in Fig. 11. Rubin and Casarett emphasized that these doses represented their own "personal value system in decision making," although they are summarized from and consistent with data from a large number of radiotherapy centers. There have been few changes since then. The values in the table have been acquired over

TABLE 3
Radiation Tolerance Doses[a,b]

Organ	Injury	TD$_{5/5}$	TD$_{50/5}$	Whole or partial organ (field size or length)	References[c]
Class I organs: radiation lesions are fatal or result in severe morbidity					
Bone marrow	Aplasia, pancytopenia	250	450	Whole	Bond *et al.*[2]
		3,000	4,000	Segmental	Rubin *et al.*[19,21]
Liver	Acute and chronic hepatitis	2,500	4,000	Whole	Ingold *et al.*[6]
		1,500	2,000	Whole strip	Kraut *et al.*,[8] Tefft[24]
Stomach	Perforation, ulcer hemorrhage	4,500	5,500	100 cm^2	Friedman[4]
Intestine	Ulcer, perforation, hemorrhage	4,500	5,500	400 cm^2	Friedman[4]
		5,000	6,500	100 cm^2	Roswit *et al.*[17] Palmer[15]
Brain	Infarction, necrosis	6,000	7,000	Whole	Kramer *et al.*[7]
		7,000	8,000	25%	Lindgren[10]
Spinal cord	Infarction, necrosis	4,500	5,500	10 cm	Phillips and Buschke[16] Wara *et al.*[26]
Heart	Pericarditis and pancarditis	4,500	5,500	60%	Newton[14] Stewart and Fajardo[23]
Lung	Acute and chronic pneumonitis	3,000	3,500	100 cm^2	Gish *et al.*[5] Lokick *et al.*[11]
		1,500	2,500	Whole	Wara *et al.*[26]
Kidney	Acute and chronic nephrosclerosis	1,500	2,000	Whole (strip)	Kraut *et al.*,[8] Tefft[24]
		2,000	2,500	Whole	Kunkler *et al.*[9] Luxton and Kunkler[12]
Fetus	Death	200	400	Whole	Rugh[22]

(Continued)

TABLE 3 (*cont.*)

Organ	Injury	TD$_{5/5}$	TD$_{50/5}$	Whole or partial organ (field size or length)
Class II organs: radiation lesions result in moderate to mild morbidity (a fatality is exceptional)				
Oral cavity and pharynx	Ulceration, mucositis	6,000	7,500	50 cm^2
Skin	Acute and chronic dermatitis	5,500	7,000	100 cm^2
Esophagus	Esophagitis, ulceration	6,000	7,500	75 cm^2
Rectum	Ulcer, stricture	6,000	8,000	100 cm^2
Salivary glands	Xerostomia	5,000	7,000	50 cm^2
Bladder	Contracture	6,000	8,000	Whole
Ureters	Stricture	7,500	10,000	5–10 cm
Testes	Sterilization	100[d]	200[d]	Whole
Ovary	Sterilization	200–300	625–1,200	Whole
Growing cartilage, bone (child)	Growth arrest, dwarfing	1,000 / 1,000	3,000 / 3,000	Whole / 10 cm^2
Mature cartilage, bone (adult)	Necrosis, fracture, sclerosis	6,000 / 6,000	10,000 / 10,000	Whole / 10 cm^2
Eye				
Retina		5,500	7,000	Whole
Cornea		5,000	>6,000	Whole
Lens		500	1,200	Whole or part
Endocrine glands				
Thyroid	Hypothyroidism	4,500	15,000	Whole
Adrenal	Hypoadrenalism	>6,000	—	Whole
Pituitary	Hypopituitarism	4,500	20,000–30,000	Whole
Peripheral nerves	Neuritis	6,000	10,000	10 cm^2
Ear				
Middle	Serous otitis	5,000	7,000	Whole
Vestibular	Ménière's syndrome	6,000	7,000	Whole
Class III organs: radiation lesions mild, transient, and reversible or result in no morbidity				
Muscle (child)	Atrophy	2,000–3,000	4,000–5,000	Whole
Muscle (adult)	Fibrosis	6,000	8,000	Whole
Lymph nodes and lymphatics	Atrophy, sclerosis	5,000	>7,000	Whole node
Large arteries and veins	Sclerosis	>8,000	>10,000	10 cm^2
Articular cartilage	None	>50,000	>500,000	Joint surface (mm^2)
Uterus	Necrosis, perforation	>10,000	>20,000	Whole
Vagina	Ulcer, fistula	9,000	>10,000	Whole
Breast (child)	No development	1,000	1,500	Whole
Breast (adult)	Atrophy, necrosis	>5,000	>10,000	Whole

[a] From Chapter I, Committee on Self-evaluation and Testing: *SET R.T.1: Radiation Oncology*, American College of Radiology, 1975, by courtesy of P. Rubin, Series Editor.

[b] TD$_{5/5}$ is the dose, given as approximately five "daily" 200-rad doses each week, which would cause 1–5% of normal tissue complications at 5 years. TD$_{50/5}$ is the dose likely to cause between 25% and 50% complications.

[c] References in the *SET R.T.1* chapter referred to.

[d] 5 rads/day scattered radiation (Rubin, personal communication).

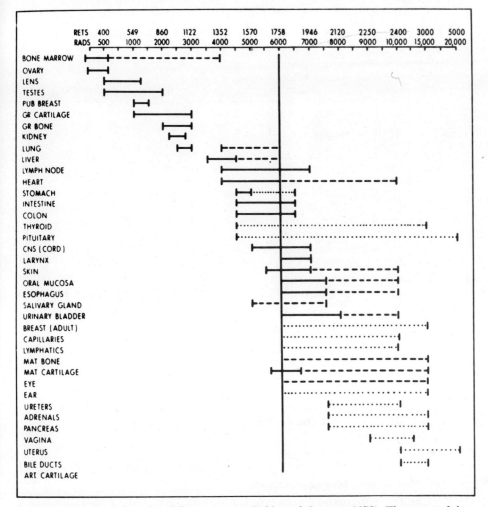

FIGURE 11. Tolerance doses for different organs (Rubin and Casarett, 1972). The range of doses expected to cause between 5% and 50% of serious normal tissue complications by 5 years ($TD_{5-50/5}$) is shown as the total dose in rads, given at 5×200 rads each week. The corresponding nominal standard doses in rets are also given (see Section 6.1.1). They are not simply proportional to total dose. Dashes: part of organ shielded. Dots: few data.

many years of clinical experience with the "standard daily" fractionation schedules. When the dose to the whole or a large segment of an organ in the treatment field approaches the $TD_{5/5}$ level, shielding is recommended to exclude the structure if it is vital. The doses have all been converted by the use of the Ellis "nominal standard dose" formula into rets in Fig. 11 to make an intercomparison of radiosensitivities easier (see Section 6.1.1). The level of tolerance indicated for the different organs in patients will vary in terms of the pain and discomfort that can be tolerated in different sites, but all these tolerance levels are likely to represent less severe injury than the studies in mice.

Table 4 shows certain selected organs in which dose levels to produce particular levels of injury can be compared in rodents and in man, for single doses to the

TABLE 4

Comparison of Radiosensitivities of Various Tissues in Man and Mouse and Labeling Indices in Mice

Tissue	LD_{50}, mouse (single dose, rads)	$TD_{50/5}$, man (rets)	LI, mouse (%)
Bone marrow	~ 700	~300	<10
Small intestine	~1100	1400–1850[a]	20
Lung	1300	1000–1150	< 1
Kidney	1800	900–1100	< 1
Spinal cord	2500	1600–1950	<0.1
Esophagus	3000[b]	1750–2050	5

[a] This value is high because of proliferation.
[b] This value is high, possibly because of hypoxia in anesthetized mice (Field and Hornsey, personal communication).

animals and for the nominal standard dose (NSD) for the clinical data. An average labeling index (LI) for each tissue in mice is also shown. A rough correlation appears to exist in the mouse, higher LD_{50} values being required for local irradiation of the more slowly proliferating tissues. However, the mouse data are for single doses. There is no correlation of mouse LI with the tolerance dose in man; all the human data are for prolonged fractionation where repair of sublethal cellular injury becomes a major factor in addition to proliferation.

5. Analysis of Clinical Tolerance Levels

If the estimates of clinical tolerance doses in Table 3 are arranged by dose level as in Fig. 11, some interesting observations follow:

1. Even at doses of 1000–2000 rads (administered over 1 or 2 weeks), there are some tissues which are totally ablated. For example, the bone marrow would be sterilized by whole-body doses of less than 500 rads in man. The ovary would be sterilized by less than 1000 rads and the testis by less than 2000 rads. The developing breast, growing bone, and growing cartilage would be severely damaged. The lens of the eye would form progressive cataracts at doses between 500 and 1400 rads. The fetus, like the adult, if totally exposed to even lower doses than 1000 rads in 1 week, would be killed. These are all tissues where there are a small number of stem cells feeding a larger amplifying and differentiating compartment, and these stem cells presumably cannot be replaced. Local doses greater than 2000 rads might, however, be required to completely arrest growing bone or cartilage and to prevent localized regions of injured bone marrow from being repopulated from distant unirradiated marrow.

2. In the 2000–4500 rad range, i.e., moderate therapy doses in 2–4 weeks, a small probability of severe injury exists if a portion of the lung or liver is exposed. Lung, liver, and kidney are very vulnerable to these doses if the whole organ is irradiated. Lung is affected at dose levels similar to those affecting the kidney if all

of both lungs is treated beyond 2500 rads in $2\frac{1}{2}$ weeks. The heart is vulnerable when its entire volume is treated, but more resistant if a part of it is shielded. Lymph nodes are sensitive in this dose range, and atrophy of developing muscles can occur, although adult muscle is more resistant.

3. In the 4500–7000 rad range (in 4–7 weeks), some severe injury will occur (1–5%) in a variety of epithelial structures including stomach, small intestine, colon, skin, oral mucosa, esophagus, rectum, salivary glands, and urinary bladder. The thyroid and pituitary glands, the spinal cord and brain, and the larynx all become a problem in this dose range. Complications in these tissues will increase very steeply with dose within this range of doses, as is shown in Fig. 8.

4. At the highest levels exposed in clinical radiation therapy (up to 7500 rads in about 7 weeks or equivalent), there are still some radioresistant structures: ureters, uterus, vagina, adult breast, adult muscle, bile ducts, and articular cartilage. Cartilage appears to be among the most radioresistant of all tissues, perhaps because it is partly hypoxic due to its lack of incorporated blood vessels.

While these clinical tolerance levels can be listed in groups, the radiobiological studies necessary to explain them are as yet incomplete. The sensitive tissues listed in category 1 above have small capacities to accumulate and repair sublethal injury (ovary, testis, and bone marrow) and/or they have a limited number of irreplaceable stem cells feeding a large differentiated population. The tumors deriving from these sensitive normal tissues often show a greater sensitivity to radiation than other tumors.

Most of the epithelial tissues fall in the category of moderately sensitive tissues. These are mostly renewal tissues which can respond rapidly to proliferative demands (excluding the heart). They will tolerate much larger doses if only a part of their volume is treated, presumably because of migration of cells in from adjacent unirradiated areas, and also because of the reserve functional capacity of the unirradiated portions.

The number of radioresistant organs is fairly small, and unfortunately they are usually in a field containing other more sensitive tissues. The reasons for their radioresistance is not understood. It is not always true that the organs with the longest turnover times, i.e., the lowest labeling and mitotic indices, are the most resistant organs (see Table 3), although the most sensitive organs are those which proliferate fast.

6. Changes in Therapeutic Modalities

The main reason for wishing to understand the biological processes controlling the tolerance dose to different organs is in order to modify existing forms of therapy or to introduce entirely new forms of treatment. Four areas of change will be discussed below, namely, changes in fractionation schedules, methods to overcome the hypoxic resistance of some tumor cells without inflicting additional damage on the normal tissues, the use of various cytotoxic drugs with radiotherapy, and methods designed to take advantage of the differences in proliferating characteristics between tumors and normal tissues, e.g., synchronizing agents or BUdR.

6.1. Fractionation Schedules

One of the most obvious changes to consider in radiotherapy appears to be that of the fractionation schedule. It involves no new equipment and no drug toxicity. In attempts to gain more effect on the tumor with no worse effect on normal tissues, nonstandard schedules are currently being tested which range from two or three doses per day, each of about 100 rads, to weekly doses of about 600 rads each (Dutreix, 1975; Ellis, 1974). These extremes use, respectively, more dose fractions (up to 84) or fewer fractions (e.g., 6) in overall times that are not as divergent as would be the case with "daily" doses.

Curable cases are never treated with very small numbers of fractions (such as two or three) in only a few days, except for small superficial skin lesions. In radiotherapeutic practice, a standard schedule may unintentionally become nonstandard if a gap in treatment exceeding a few days has to be introduced or if a "daily" fractionation schedule cannot be achieved because of machine failure or because the patient is not well enough to attend regularly for treatment. The problems of selecting suitable total doses for nonstandard fractionation schedules have led to several well-known time–dose–fraction-number schemes. The best known of these are the nominal standard dose (NSD) of Ellis (1969) and the cumulative radiation effect (CRE) of Kirk et al. (1971). They are both in use in many centers to prescribe modified doses for clinical application when the overall time or fraction number is changed. Although some authors have reported inadequacies in these formulas, they appear to be useful for modest changes in fraction number or overall time. The most serious divergences reported clinically appear to be for two fractions per week, where the NSD formula suggests doses which have been found to be too high (Jardine et al., 1975; Bates, 1975; Hockly and Sealy, 1977).

Other ways of arriving at dose estimates for normal tissue tolerance with nonstandard fractionation schedules are due to Cohen and Kerrick (1951), Fowler and Stern (1963), Dutreix et al. (1973), and Douglas and Fowler (1975). All these are empirical formulas based on available experimental or clinical data. Only Cohen's model attempts to incorporate a fairly full set of biological factors; for some of these parameters, values have to be assumed.

When multiple sessions of irradiation are delivered at intervals greater than a few hours, a larger dose is necessary to achieve the same level of damage. This is mainly due to the accumulation and repair of sublethal radiation injury. Some examples are given in Table 5, which includes less conventional fractionation schemes as well as the North American practice of 1000 rads each week in five sessions of 200 rads. Both the number of fractions (repair) and the overall time (repopulation) have an effect on the total dose that can be tolerated. Figure 12a shows the way that total dose increases with number of fractions for the clinical

TABLE 5
Some Typical Radiotherapy Doses Delivered in Multiple Fractions for Treatments of Larynx and Pharynx[a]

10 fractions in 3 weeks	4500 rads
15 fractions in 3 weeks	5000 rads
20 fractions in 4 weeks	5500 rads
18 fractions in 6 weeks	5750 rads
30 fractions in 6 weeks	6500 rads

[a] These are maximum tissue doses normally considered tolerable in each schedule. They are often reduced depending on the size of the treated area and the type of normal tissue irradiated.

tolerance dose for late skin changes. Figure 12b shows results for a constant number of fractions plotted against overall time. Most of the clinical data were obtained with five or six fractions per week, so it was not possible to separate the effect of fraction number and overall time without further information (Fowler and Stern, 1963).

In 1963, Fowler and Stern concluded that the effect of changing overall time was less than that of changing fraction number, and this was confirmed by experiments in pig skin, as shown in Fig. 13 (Fowler *et al.*, 1963). Five fractions in 4 days required an 80% increase in total dose relative to a single dose, to compensate for the repair of sublethal injury after each of the fractions. Increasing the overall time from 4 to 28 days, still using five fractions, required only a 17% increase in dose to compensate for proliferation.

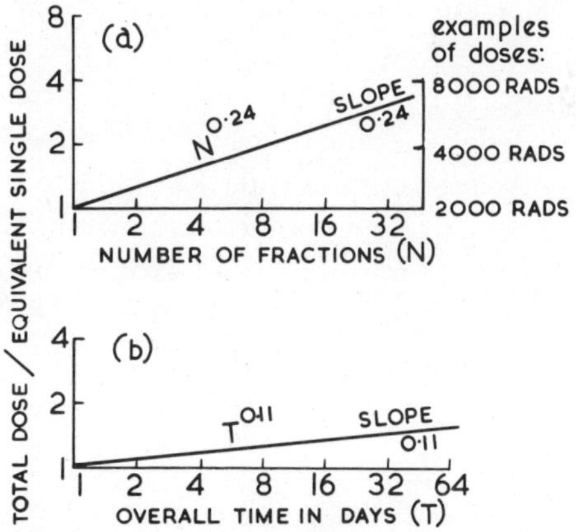

FIGURE 12. Total X-ray dose given in several equal fractions, relative to the single dose, required to produce the same level of normal tissue damage. (a) Constant overall time. (b) Constant number of fractions. After Ellis (1969).

FIGURE 13. Experimental data for skin reactions on the flank of pigs, plotted as in Fig. 12a. The extra dose required when the overall time to give five fractions was increased from 4 to 27 days was 600 rads (4200–3600). The extra dose required in a constant overall time when the fraction number was increased from 5 to 21 was 1400 rads (5600–4200). From Fowler *et al.* (1963).

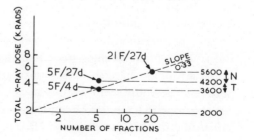

If the clinical data (Fig. 12) are plotted logarithmically against overall time using "daily" fractions, a straight-line relationship is observed. The slope of this line is approximately 0.33, corresponding to the rough cube-root law that has been used for many years, for five or six "daily" doses per week:

$$\text{total dose} = \text{constant} \times (\text{overall time})^{0.33}$$

In 1944, Strandqvist found a slope of 0.22 (i.e., a less marked time dependence) for both skin reactions and for cure of squamous cell carcinoma. Because other data indicated 0.33, Strandqvist's skin reaction slope has been discarded, but Ellis (1969) used his value for tumors to estimate the effect of fraction number only, on the assumption that compensatory proliferation played no part in the response of the carcinomas.

In this way, using the $T^{0.33}$ for normal tissues, which should proliferate to compensate for damage, and subtracting $T^{0.22}$ for tumors, Ellis was able to devise a formula which takes both time and fraction number into account:

$$\text{total dose} = \text{constant} \times (\text{time})^{0.11} \times (\text{fraction number})^{0.24}$$

(The 0.24 is derived from 0.22 in changing from six to five fractions per week.) The constant in this equation is the NSD. It gives the extrapolation of the straight log–log line to the one-fraction axis of the graph, although it does not represent a real single dose that could be used in practice. Values of NSD are given in rets.

This formula is now widely used and seems to give a reasonable fit to a large volume of experimental and clinical data, between four and 30 fractions and with the important exceptions described in the next section. A slide rule is available to calculate doses using this formula, or they can be read from the tables published by Orton and Ellis (1973). In particular, these tables are useful for determining doses for two different parts of a fractionated course of therapy (i.e., for adding "partial tolerance" dose equivalents).

A different formula has been proposed by Kirk *et al.* (1971): the CRE or cumulative radiation effect concept. This formula uses the same exponent of 0.24 for fraction number, but assumes an exponential decay of radiation injury with time, instead of following the (time)$^{0.11}$ term exactly. In practice, the differences are small, with the Kirk CRE formula suggesting more loss of damage early on, so that larger added doses would be calculated for short gaps in treatment.

6.1.1. Comparison of Dose–Time Formulas and Observations

Turesson and Notter (1975) have recently shown that CRE is a useful formula for predicting tolerance doses for skin erythema and pigmentation in patients when the fractionation schemes were markedly altered, although they have not yet tested it for late changes. Most clinical information, however, cannot distinguish between these different empirical formulas, and so long as the therapist is concerned with a modest change in overall time or fraction number, it makes no practical difference whether the NSD or the CRE formula is used.

Berry *et al.* (1974) have found experimentally that the Ellis NSD was able to predict accurately the tolerance doses for late skin necrosis in pigs, but predicted poorly the doses for early reactions and for late fibrosis and contraction. In these cases, the measured tolerance doses were higher for early reactions and lower for fibrosis and contraction than predicted by the NSD formula. For vascular damage, measured by the ability of a skin flap to survive from an irradiated pedicle, the prediction was good (Wiernik *et al.*, 1974). For kidney tolerance in the pig, the fraction number component of 0.24 was an underestimate (Hopewell and Berry, 1975).

In treating skin cancer with small fields, Young *et al.* (1976) found that the (fraction number)$^{0.24}$ term fitted both early and late (atrophy and fibrosis) effects but that the time factor should be smaller than the (time)$^{0.11}$ term suggests.

Other recent animal experiments have indicated, however, that the effect of fraction number—i.e., the capacity for repair of sublethal injury—is larger than the 0.24 power of N for lung damage and for spinal cord injury. The exponent of N appears to be about 0.4 both for LD_{50} lung experiments in mice (Wara *et al.*, 1973; Field *et al.*, 1976) and for spinal cord injury leading to paraplegia (Van der Kogel and Barendsen, 1974; Wara *et al.*, 1975; Van der Kogel *et al.*, 1976). This means a larger change of tolerance dose with fraction number for those organs than is predicted by NSD or CRE. The evidence from kidney function injury in animals is contradictory, but the same trend has been reported in some of the experiments (Caldwell, 1974; Hopewell and Berry, 1975; Glatstein *et al.*, 1975). Gauwerky *et al.* (1972) have also reported an exponent of about 0.4 for late subcutaneous fibrosis in ^{60}Co-irradiated patients.

The time exponent in the formulas is rather small: for example, any doubling of the overall time requires only an 8% increase of total dose, according to the term $T^{0.11}$. The effect of time has been found to be even smaller than $T^{0.11}$ for lung damage in mice, being about 0.07 (Phillips and Fu, 1974; Field *et al.*, 1976). The same trend was observed for human skin reactions in small fields, as mentioned above (Young *et al.*, 1976).

While there are few such instances of data sufficiently precise to enable significant differences from the exponents $N^{0.24}$ and $T^{0.11}$ to be established, it is wise to consider that such an approximate formula should at best have only a general form $N^x T^y$ and that the exponents x and y will, in principle, differ for different tissues and different types of injury. They are in any case no more than convenient ways of quantitating different factors which may not even be completely independent.

It is remarkable that the Ellis NSD formula $N^{0.24} T^{0.11}$ works as well as it does for certain types of injury, but not including the vital organs in the trunk; the formula was derived from skin and subcutaneous connective tissue effects. Its success is probably due to the avoidance of extreme changes in fraction number or overall time. Increasing the overall time to 90 days, for example, leads to less acute skin reactions than the NSD or CRE formulas would predict, although late fibrosis is not avoided (Sambrook, personal communication; Notter and Turreson, personal communication).

In order to make with confidence any major change away from conventional fractionation schemes, a more basic understanding of the biological processes behind these two exponents is necessary. This can be obtained only from animal experiments.

6.1.2. Repair during Fractionated Radiotherapy

All the tissues so far reported clinically and tested in experimental animals show exponents for fraction number between about $N^{0.24}$ and $N^{0.44}$, except for one clinical report of $N^{0.75}$ (Phillips and Bushke, 1969). This implies that repair of sublethal injury is large for all these tissues after irradiation with X- or γ-rays.

The dose recovered between successive small fractions often amounts to 60–80% of the administered dose; the reasons for this are the subject of much recent research and discussion (e.g., Alper, 1974). It appears that for the small doses used in each clinical fraction the cell-killing processes are less effective, per rad, than the higher doses used in many radiobiological experiments. This is supported by the observation that the reparable fraction is high for very low doses and falls as the dose per fraction increases (Fig. 14). If the curves were exactly horizontal at the lower doses in Fig. 14, this could be explained in terms of a "two-component" cell survival curve, with an inefficient single-hit killing process operating at low doses, and with about two-thirds of the dose being absorbed as sublethal reparable damage.* This model was proposed by Dutreix et al. (1973) to explain their data on human skin and on mouse intestine. Dutreix's model, however, leads to a clinical formula which, for fraction numbers greater than 20, suggests no further increase in total dose for additional numbers of fractions (Fig. 15). This lack of further increase is contradicted by other observations. The data of Dutreix et al. suffer from the fact that a low level of cell killing was being studied (i.e., modest erythema), so that their conclusions do not remain valid for more extensive cell killing corresponding to a full tolerance level of injury. They would underestimate repair, as illustrated by the lowest curves in Fig. 14.

---

* $S = e^{-D/D_1}[1-(1-e^{-D/D_0})^m]$, where S is the surviving proportion of cells, D is the radiation dose (in one fraction), D_1 is the average dose required to inactivate a cell by the one-hit process, and D_0 is the average dose to inactivate each of m identical targets.

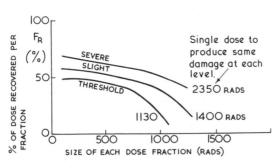

FIGURE 14. Variation in the percentage of dose repaired per fraction with the size of each dose fraction and also with the level of damage that is being studied. The percentage of each dose fraction repaired is $F_R = [(D_n - D_1)/(n-1)]/D_n/n \times 100\%$, where D_n is the total dose, n is the number of equal fractions, and D_1 is the single dose which produces the same reaction. If the total dose, and hence the level of damage, is smaller, the proportion of dose repaired is lower, as shown for three levels of skin reaction.

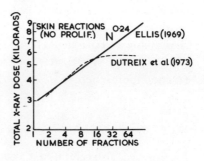

FIGURE 15. Total X-ray dose vs. number of fractions (log-scale) as predicted by the NSD formula (Ellis, 1969) and as measured in patients by Dutreix *et al.* (1973). The latter workers, however, used a modest degree of erythema only, so they found less repair than in higher doses (see Fig. 14). These two curves are significantly different only for more than 16 fractions.

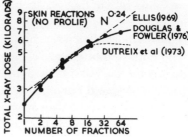

FIGURE 16. As Fig. 15, with the data of Douglas and Fowler (1976) for mouse skin reactions added. These results were for an overall time of 8 days or less, so proliferation did not contribute significantly.

Similar multifraction experiments extending to 32 fractions were performed by Field *et al.* (1975) on mouse skin, and higher doses were required for 32 than for 16 fractions, in accordance with the NSD formula.

When the fraction number was extended to 64 fractions, given in 8 days overall time in order to avoid repopulation, the curve shown in Fig. 16 was obtained (Douglas and Fowler, 1976). A significantly larger dose was required than for Dutreix's formula, but less than that predicted by NSD. There was a clear decrease in the dose increments required as the fraction number increased, as shown by the curvature of the line in Fig. 17. This set of data has been shown to provide a good fit to a cell survival formula containing a dose term and a dose-squared term:

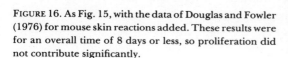

$$S = e^{-(\alpha D + \beta D^2)}$$

where S is the surviving proportion of cells, D is the radiation dose (in one fraction), α is the rate of single-hit killing per rad ($= 1/D_1$ in previous formula), and β is the rate of two-hit killing per rad. This formula has a sounder biophysical basis than the two-component model just described above. Douglas and Fowler (1975) also showed that a plot of reciprocal total dose against fraction size was linear.

The meaning of such dose–response formulas, both for clinical application and for an understanding of the basic mechanism of radiation-induced cell death, was the subject of several conferences, and obviously cannot be adequately covered in this chapter. The reader is referred to proceedings of the Sixth L. H. Gray Conference (Alper, 1974), the Carmel Conference (1969), and the Madison Time–Dose Conference (Caldwell and Tolbert, 1974). In summary, however, a large amount of extra dose is needed if the fraction number is increased, because of the repair of low-dose sublethal radiation damage. This dose increment can be reasonably well predicted by several formulas over the range of 4–30 fractions for skin and for other tissues, but care must be taken in adopting widely differing fractionation schemes.

6.1.3. Repopulation during Fractionated Radiotherapy

Extra dose is also tolerated if a course of fractionated radiotherapy is given over an extended period of time. This is obviously likely to result from proliferation of surviving cells in tissues capable of proliferation (e.g., skin, gut), but in nondividing or slowly dividing tissues a slow repair process has recently been reported that requires more than a few hours for completion.

The Ellis exponent of $T^{0.11}$ corresponds to an increase of only 8% in tolerated dose if the overall time is doubled. The dose increments predicted by $T^{0.11}$ are large initially and fall off with successive weeks, as is illustrated in Table 6. Some workers have assumed an approximate average value of 25–30 rads per day (e.g., Cohen, 1968), and this has been consistent with animal data averaged over 2–4 weeks. Liversage (1971), however, thought that a value of 30 rads per day applied only up to 20 days overall time, but 20 rads per day was more appropriate for longer overall times. Such a decreasing value of dose per day over extending periods of time is more consistent with a repair process that is exponentially decreasing and has a long halving time. Just such a slow repair has been reported by Field *et al.* (1976) for lung damage (a slowly proliferating tissue) and by Van den

TABLE 6

Weekly Dose Increments Calculated from the NSD Formula When Only Overall Time T is Varied and the Fraction Number N is Constant or Ignored, i.e., Total Dose = $1800 \times T^{0.11}$

Overall time T (days)	Total dose (rets)	Dose increment per week (rets)
1	1800	430
7	2230	175
14	2405	110
21	2515	80
28	2595	65
35	2660	55
42	2715	45
49	2760	

^a From Withers (1974, Table 2, p. 37). As explained in the text, the steady decrease of the increments is not consistent with the compensatory proliferation which begins in skin 2 or 3 weeks after starting daily treatment.

TABLE 7

Compensatory Proliferation in Mouse Skin after Fractionated X-Irradiation

	Population doubling time	
	From split-dose experiments[a] (hr)	From continuous-labeling studies[b] (hr)
Control before irradiation	—	84[c]–129[d]
4 × 300 rads	No measurable proliferation	74[c]–131[d]
9 × 300 rads	48–60	49[c]–119[d]
14 × 300 rads	15–21	<26[c]–<32[d]

[a] From Denekamp (1973).
[b] From Denekamp *et al.* (1976).
[c] For sole of foot.
[d] For upper surface of foot.

Brenk *et al.*, (1974) and Reinhold and Buisman (1975) for capillary damage (again, a slowly dividing system).

In skin, however, or any other rapidly dividing normal tissue, compensatory proliferation will be evoked when the radiation-induced cell depletion is recognized. This means that after an initial lag period (in which no extra dose will be tolerated) proliferation will accelerate and more dose will then be tolerated as the compensation becomes effective. This is not consistent with the Ellis NSD, the Kirk CRE, or the Liversage exponentially decreasing repair models, but is supported by some experimental work in rodents.

In order to determine the importance of repopulation at various stages during a course of fractionated radiotherapy, daily doses of 300 rads were administered for either 1, 2, or 3 weeks. At the end of these periods, repopulation was tested in two ways: one was by determining the extra dose to produce the desired "tolerance level"; the other was to label repeatedly with tritiated thymidine and to score in autoradiographs the fraction of cells progressing through DNA synthesis. These two experiments agreed in showing that repopulation was not important after 1 week of therapy; it was worth 60 rads/day after 2 weeks, i.e., the cell doubling time had been halved; and it was worth 130 rads/day after 3 weeks, i.e., a reduction by a factor of 4–6 in cell doubling time (Denekamp, 1973). See Table 7.

This shows either that the biological process resulting in the Ellis NSD or the Kirk CRE time factors is not repopulation or that the form of their time factors is not correct. Since the important clinical end point is subcutaneous or connective tissue damage, which concerns slowly dividing tissue, rather than acute desquamation arising from depletion of rapidly proliferating epithelial cells, it may be that the time factor in radiotherapy is due to slow repair, not repopulation (Fig. 17). This topic has been poorly researched so far, and is discussed in the preceding chapter (Denekamp and Fowler, this volume).

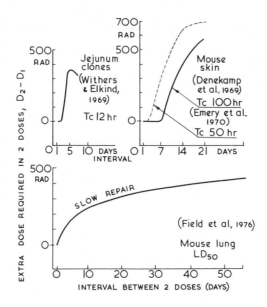

FIGURE 17. Additional dose required to counteract proliferation (upper diagrams) or "slow repair" (lower diagram) as measured by two-dose experiments using the stated intervals. T_C is the cell-cycle time before irradiation.

6.1.4. Dose-Rate Effects

Apart from the overall time of fractionated treatments, another consideration is the effect of dose rate within individual treatments. Most clinical radiotherapy is delivered at a dose rate of 50–300 rads/min, as in much of the radiobiological work. However, interstitial treatments using radium or radioisotopic sources are delivered at much lower dose rates (0.1–1 rad/min) and the processes of rapid repair of sublethal injury can then occur within the treatment time, which usually extends over several days. Dose-rate effects have been studied in experimental systems, and repair has certainly been shown to occur within the treatment period if the treatment time is extended to hours instead of minutes, as would be expected on the basis of the shapes of the cell survival curves (Hall, 1972). For interstitial therapy, this can be taken into account by formulae published by Liversage (1969).

If the treatment is given in seconds rather than minutes, no repair differences have been observed except in the small intestine, when significant repair can occur during a 10-min overall irradiation period (Hornsey and Alper, 1966). No other tissue has been shown to have such rapid repair. A completely different effect of high dose rate which might protect normal tissues, has sometimes been thought to be a possible way of dealing with hypoxic cells in tumors; however, it does not now seem feasible. At very high dose rates, such as can be obtained with electron beams from linear accelerators (kilorads delivered in milliseconds), the oxygen which is in the tissue will be radiochemically depleted and an anoxic tissue response (i.e., more radioresistant) may result. This has been demonstrated with single doses for skin reactions by Field and Bewley (1974) at dose rates in excess of 6000 rads/min and for 4-day death of mice by Hornsey and Bewley (1971). However, much larger doses per fraction are necessary (1 or 2 krads) than are used in radiotherapy.

6.2. Hypoxia and Radiation Modifiers

169

RADIATION
EFFECTS ON
NORMAL
TISSUES

Hypoxic cells exist in tumors, and these are more resistant to conventional radiation by a dose factor of 2.5–3. Thus the radiotherapist starts at a disadvantage since the normal, well-oxygenated tissues which he wants to protect are radiosensitive and the tumor tissue, which he wants to destroy, is resistant. Some of the new approaches to radical radiotherapy are aimed at overcoming this disadvantage. They include the following (Fig. 18).

1. Deliberate anoxia: Normal tissues can be made equally resistant by cutting off their blood supply with a tourniquet (Baker *et al.*, 1966; Suit, 1965). This can be painful, has not proved to be very effective, and is limited to limbs.

2. Hyperbaric oxygen: When a patient breathes oxygen at normal pressure or at a raised pressure of 3 atm before and during irradiation, the oxygen concentration is increased in the blood, and hence in the tumor cells (Thomlinson and Gray, 1955; Du Sault, 1963). This appears to yield only modest gains in a few types of tumor (including larynx carcinoma and squamous carcinoma of the cervix stage III) because the body responds physiologically to excessive oxygen, which can be toxic, by peripheral vasoconstriction (Lambertsen, 1966). Thus, although the blood carries more oxygen, less blood perfuses the tumor.

3. High-LET* radiation: More densely ionizing radiation kills cells in a way that is less dependent on the oxygen concentration than when X-rays are used. Thus

---

* "Linear energy transfer" is a term describing the density of ionization in the tracks of charged particles which traverse tissue during irradiation. X-rays, γ-rays, and electrons are "low-LET" radiations.

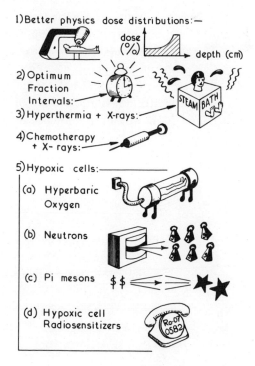

FIGURE 18. Some of the current growing points in radiotherapy: methods by which enhanced effects on tumors may be achieved.

hypoxic cells are only 1.6 times more resistant to neutrons, and no more resistant to very heavy accelerated nuclei, in contrast to being 2.5–3 times more resistant to X-rays. Fast neutrons produced by small cyclotrons (up to 50 MeV) or even more expensive π-mesons produced by 500 MeV proton synchrotrons are prime candidates (Barendsen et al., 1971; Fowler, 1976).

4. Electron-affinic drugs: The increased radiosensitivity in the presence of oxygen is believed to be due to oxygen's affinity for electrons produced by the ionization of biological molecules, thus preventing chemical repair by the electron returning to the molecule from which it was released and helping to "fix" the damage. This electron affinity can be supplied by molecules other than oxygen, in particular by certain compounds which are not metabolized by respiration and therefore can diffuse from capillaries to distant hypoxic cells and cause radiosensitization (Adams et al., 1976). The nitroaromatic drugs are currently of great biological interest and have recently been introduced clinically (Dische et al., 1976).

Any of these approaches depends on the assumption that it is *only* the tumor cells that are hypoxic, and that there will be no corresponding increase in damage to the normal tissues. Since normal tissues have adequate vascular beds, with the exception of cartilage, this assumption seems to be a reasonable one for most if not all tissues. It was found in the early studies with hyperbaric oxygen that a slight sensitization of skin may occur (equivalent to increasing the X-ray dose by 10%) if the same dose is given in oxygen as in air (Van den Brenk, 1965), but that much more severe cartilage necrosis was observed after hyperbaric oxygen (Van den Brenk, 1968).

The only other normal tissues which are suspected of containing hypoxic cells under normal conditions are the testis and perhaps the esophagus. Experiments using fast neutrons to determine relative biological effectiveness (RBE) for various tissues have shown the esophagus to be particularly sensitive to neutrons (high RBE). This could be a result of different repair capacities, but a study using the electron-affinic drug Ro-07-0582 (Field and Hornsey, personal communication) suggests rather that it is due to normal tissue hypoxia in the anesthetized mice.

Normal tissue studies in animals can identify hypoxic tissues and thus help to avoid unexpected increases in sensitivities in particular organs when the new form of therapy is tried.

6.3. High-LET Radiation

In addition to the reduced oxygen effect with high-LET radiation, there may be an advantage from the geometry at the depth-dose distribution or from the difference in the accumulation and repair of sublethal injury.

The physical distribution advantage results from the fact that high-energy charged particles (π^- mesons and accelerated nuclear particles) do not deposit energy uniformly along their track. They initially have a low linear energy transfer, but as they slow down, more energy is imparted per micrometer of track (higher keV/μm, i.e., higher LET), and the locally absorbed dose increases. This can result in a Bragg peak which varies in depth from one particle beam to another, but can be very narrow if it comes from a beam of monoenergetic particles passing through a uniform medium. This is used, for example, in treating pituitary lesions with helium ions. It requires a very precise knowledge of the location and extent of the tumor, but it can certainly be used as a means of sparing normal tissue that must inevitably be included in the beam. This localization advantage is not present with beams of uncharged particles, including neutrons and X- or γ-rays.

Because of the increased density of ionizations with high-LET radiation, cells are less likely to receive a sublethal dose of irradiation (i.e., a hit is more likely to be lethal). Thus the initial part of the survival curves is steeper for cells *in vitro*, i.e., the repair capacity represented by the width of the shoulder is smaller for beams of neutrons and heavy particles than for X-rays. Similarly, for tissues *in vivo* the fraction number exponent is much less important for neutrons than for other tissues. For skin, for example, it is reduced from $N^{0.24}$ to $N^{0.07}$, while the time component is unchanged (Field, 1972). This reduced ability in inflict sublethal damage means that the RBE, for any cell line or tissue, decreases with increasing size of dose per fraction administered. This was shown for a range of normal tissues by Field and Hornsey (1971, 1974) and Hornsey and Field (1974) (Fig. 19). The exact biological reason for the different RBE values of different tissues at any one dose per fraction is not known, but it may relate to oxygenation status, as well as to the proportions of single hit/multihit damage, i.e., to the ratios of α and β in the $\alpha D + \beta D^2$ model. These in turn depend on the small distances in the cell within which two damaged molecules can interact with each other. An understanding of these processes for different normal tissues is obviously required for a confident application of high-LET radiation to any particular tumor site.

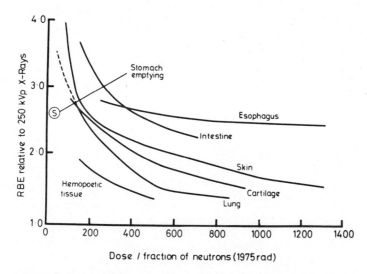

FIGURE 19. Relative biological effectiveness of fast neutrons vs. size of neutron dose per fraction for several normal tissues. From Field (1976).

J. F. FOWLER
AND
J. DENEKAMP

6.4. Modification of Injury by Drugs and Other Factors

It is well known that certain cancer chemotherapuetic agents will markedly enhance radiation injury when given either before, during, or after irradiation, and that this interaction can cause severe morbidity (see *Committee for Radiation Oncology Studies*, 1976). The best-known example of this is the enhancement of skin and lung reactions when actinomycin D is used. Other newer agents, including Adriamycin, appear to cause enhanced radiation damage as well. Some of the DNA base analogs, such as BUdR, also enhance normal tissue reactions. However, the electron-affinic radiosensitizers of hypoxic cells do not change the response of well-oxygenated tissues so they are not expected to sensitize normal tissues except mature cartilage and possibly, as mentioned above, esophageal epithelium.

A number of sulfur-containing radioprotective compounds have been shown to reduce injury in normal tissues which are accessible to the drug, especially bone marrow, by X-ray dose-modifying factors varying from 1 (no protection) to about 3, when administered in large amounts before irradiation. However, the variability of the protective effect in certain tissues, especially gut, the toxicity of the compounds, and the lack of knowledge about differentially less protection in tumors have prevented their application to radiotherapy. A practical disadvantage is that higher radiation doses would have to be given, and this presents an ethical problem to the radiotherapist unless he can be much more certain than at present that full protection is guaranteed in all normal tissues.

Hormone compounds such as thyroid or adrenal steroid hormones may modify radiation damage if given before irradiation or during the appearance of radiation damage. Certain treatments given after irradiation may modify the degree of injury. For example, they may delay the expression of injury or alter its amplification by fibrosis. Such treatments include fluoride to prevent caries, pilocarpine treatment to stimulate salivation, and adrenal steroid treatment of radiation pneumonitis.

It is clear that the type of tissue, the age of the subject, the proliferative state of the tissue in relation to growth and development, the presence of other illnesses such as diabetes and hypertension, or the presence of metastases (e.g., in the spine at the time of cord irradiation) may modify the dose tolerated by a given critical organ. Each of these is recognized as important, and radiotherapists often make allowances for them, but their interrelationship requires further work. Beyond all this, occasional patients demonstrate a general but unexplained radiosensitivity of both tumor and normal tissues that is 10–25% greater than the average. Some of these cases might be explained by the repair deficiency in cells of patients with xeroderma pigmentosum or ataxia telangiectasia (Taylor *et al.*, 1975).

6.5. Hyperthermia and X-rays

The application of high temperatures in the range of 40–45°C as a method of cancer treatment, with or without ionizing radiation added, is under intensive study both clinically and in laboratories. The basis for this approach depends on observations that partial regressions of established human tumors took place after febrile episodes during infectious diseases or artificially induced fever (Cavaliere *et al.*, 1967). Laboratory work provides a more scientific basis which is not yet complete (Westra and Dewey, 1971).

There is agreement that a single exposure of 1 hr to a temperature of 42°C will halve the tolerance dose of X-rays for skin desquamation, if a single dose of X-rays is given at the same time (Stewart and Denekamp, 1977). This amount of heat alone would produce a minimal effect on the skin. There is a large amount of repair of "sublethal" injury due to heat alone, although it requires 8 hr or more for completion as compared with 3–5 hr for repair of sublethal X-ray injury (Henle and Leeper, 1975; Kal *et al.*, 1975). Hyperthermia with simultaneous irradiation is always more effective than when the two treatments are given separately. Normal tissue damage appeared to be greater when hyperthermia preceded irradiation than when it followed irradiation (Thrall *et al.*, 1973), although a rather high temperature of 44.1°C was applied for 15 min. More data on the relationships between heat and radiation injury will gradually become available.

One of the interesting aspects of hyperthermia is that it can be used to enhance the known effects of cytotoxic drugs (including the hypoxic cell radiosensitizer Ro-07-0582; Stratford and Adams, 1977). This provides a warning, therefore, that the combined effects of radiation and cytotoxic drugs on normal tissues may be enhanced if hyperthermia is also used.

7. Prophylactic Irradiation

It is becoming increasingly common to irradiate prophylactically areas of the body which are not symptomatically involved but which have a high probability of developing metastases. These areas include the draining lymph nodes in Hodgkin's lymphoma, the lung for osteosarcoma, the brain and spinal cord for leukemia, and the lymph nodes in the neck and in the axilla for breast tumors (Fletcher, 1973). Such prophylactic irradiations are performed in the knowledge that much lower doses than are needed to eradicate large primary tumors of 10^{10} cells will be adequate to sterilize small subclinical or "pinhead" tumor deposits of about 10^6 cells. Radiobiological data from *in vitro* cell survival curves would suggest that little more than two-thirds of the dose would be required to sterilize 10^6 instead of 10^9 cells. The doses used prophylactically can therefore be kept well below the tolerance doses used for the volume enclosing the primary tumor. Such prophylactic irradiations have resulted in a reduced incidence of metastases in certain patients (Rosenberg and Kaplan, 1966) and are still being evaluated in other clinical trials. However, there are three risks attendant upon this treatment: (1) the inability to treat again to full normal tissue tolerance if cancer should arise in the previously irradiated field, (2) the risk of additional seeding from tumor cells borne into an irradiated area, and (3) the risk of inducing new tumors by misrepair of DNA damage inflicted on sublethally irradiated cells.

7.1. Normal Tissue Tolerance to Prophylactic Irradiation

Total-body irradiation is now being used together with intensive chemotherapy in the treatment of certain leukemic patients. Because of the success of this treatment in controlling the leukemic proliferation, these patients are surviving long enough to develop late normal tissue injury, particularly to the CNS. Prophylactic irradiation of the brain is often combined with intrathecal methotrexate, and the tolerance to the radiation is affected by the concurrent chemotherapy. Van der Kogel *et al.* (1976) have recently evaluated the risk of severe CNS damage in these circumstances. The tolerance level of 7000 rads in 7 weeks for a small portion of the brain (Kramer *et al.*, 1972) is reduced by 20% for a child relative to an adult, and the methotrexate is thought to be worth another 20% in terms of radiation dose. Thus the estimated normal tissue tolerance for a child's brain is thought to be about 4050 rads in 7 weeks instead of 7000 rads, when used in combination with methotrexate. The large factor of 0.4 for the N exponent, when corrected for CNS from the Ellis formula, makes it critical just how many fractions are given, although the overall time (T exponent) does not seem to be very important. Van der Kogel *et al.* (1976) have emphasized that, although the factors they have used are rough approximations, the prophylactic doses in current use for children may in practice be close to the normal tissue tolerance for whole brain under those conditions. Therefore, some late CNS damage might possibly occur if 4000 rads in 7 weeks or 2500 rads in $2\frac{1}{2}$ weeks is used. However, in an evaluation of 22 children surviving 28–36 months after 2400 rads to the brain in $2\frac{1}{2}$ weeks, together with five doses of intrathecal methotrexate and prolonged chemotherapy, no prohibitive toxicity was evident (Verzosa *et al.*, 1976). No leukemic deposits were evident in the CNS, so the main purpose of the prophylactic irradiation appeared to be achieved at this level of dose.

7.2. Metastases in Irradiated Normal Tissues

An enhancing effect on the development of metastases in certain tissues which had been locally irradiated to high dosage has been reported, especially for lungs (Withers and Milas, 1973; Van den Brenk *et al.*, 1976; Peters, 1975). The mechanism is unknown but is believed to relate to changes in the ease with which malignant cells in the bloodstream are trapped in the tissue which has been damaged by irradiation. This may be due to swelling of the capillary endothelium, more rigidity in the capillary bed, or reduced surfactant production and therefore less elasticity of the lungs. The production of fibrin as irradiated cells die may also be a means of enmeshing some microfoci of tumor cells (Peters and Hewitt, 1974). Other stimuli can also alter the incidence of lung metastases in experimental

animals after intravenous administration of tumor cells, including topical and
systemic stress from cytotoxic drugs or even from constant activity in a tumbling box (Van den Brenk *et al.*, 1976).

The risk of increasing subsequent entrapment of tumor cells in a capillary bed is therefore not just restricted to irradiation. It raises questions about the desirability of such prophylactic treatments, and undoubtedly points to the general principle that radical treatment of a primary tumor that could release cells into the bloodstream should be completed *before* any prophylactic therapy.

7.3. Carcinogenesis

Radiation-induced cancers are not unknown in long-term survivors of radiotherapy, but their occurrence is in practice a much lower risk than that of recurrence of the original tumor. There appear to be two types of tissues, one in which there may be a continuous increase in cancer incidence as the radiation rises from zero dose (leukemia, thyroid carcinoma, breast cancer), and one in which there may be a threshold with negligible cancer induction below a certain dose (skin, bone). The effect of high-dose delivery to limited volumes of tissue is not clear with respect to leukemia, but a general trend to an increased tumor incidence up to equivalent single doses of about 1000 rads, followed by a decrease in the incidence at higher doses, has been reported by a number of authors. The decrease at these higher doses may occur because the proportion of cells killed by the radiation will include a higher proportion of the potentially carcinogenic cells. The main quantitative evidence comes from cases of ankylosing spondylitis treated with 200–250 kV X-rays in the United Kingdom in the 1930s, from children in the United States treated for benign conditions of the neck in the period 1930–1955 (Coleman, personal communication), and from survivors of the atomic bomb explosions in Japan. The hazards from internally deposited radioisotopes are shown by cases of bone cancer developed by some of the radium dial painters and patients given radium injections for assorted benign conditions in Germany in the 1940s and 1950s. Malignancies may appear between 4 and 30 years after irradiation. The risk of radiation carcinogenesis depends on age, being greater for children because of their longer life expectancy. The overall risk of cancer induction has been assessed as 10^{-6} per rad per individual exposed per year of lifetime remaining. This is probably a somewhat pessimistic estimate in order to be on the safe side, and is derived from evidence where the whole body or large parts of it were exposed. It does not take into account localized irradiation, as in most radiotherapy, nor the decrease in cancer risk as the dose approaches the tolerance limit for normal tissue complications, as discussed above. Certainly the incidence of new cancers arising in the irradiated volume after successful radiotherapy is not as high as 10%. Thus recurrence of the existing cancer is a much more important risk for the patient than induction of a new tumor. Although benign conditions are no longer treated by radiotherapy, there is no case for refraining from the treatment of malignant disease for this reason.

ACKNOWLEDGMENTS

We have pleasure in thanking the following colleagues for permission to quote unpublished data: Dr. G. E. Adams, Dr. I. J. Stratford, and Dr. J. Moulder. For permission to reproduce published figures and tables, we thank Dr. T. Alper, Dr. G. W. Casarett, Dr. B. G. Douglas, Dr. E. W. Emery, Dr. S. B. Field, Dr. S. Hornsey, Dr. R. Morrison, Dr. P. Rubin, and Dr. H. R. Withers.

We are grateful to many other colleagues, too, for discussions, especially Dr. Frank Ellis, Dr. Raul Urtasun and Dr. Bill Liversage, although any deficiencies in our chapter are, of course, our own responsibility.

8. References

ADAMS, G. E., DENEKAMP, J., AND FOWLER, J. F., 1976, Biological basis of radiosensitization by hypoxic-cell radiosensitizers, in *Proceedings of the 9th International Congress of Chemotherapy* (London, July 1975) (K. HELLMAN, ed.), Plenum Press, New York.

ALPER, T., 1973, Relevance of experimental radiobiology to radiotherapy, *Br. Med. Bull.* **29**:3.

ALPER, T., 1974, *Cell Survival after Low Doses of Irradiation, Proceedings of the Sixth L. H. Gray Conference* (T. ALPER, ed.), Institute of Physics and Wiley, London.

BACLESSE, F., 1958, Clinical experience with ultra-fractionated radiotherapy, in: *Progress in Radiation Therapy*, p. 128, Grune and Stratton, New York.

BAKER, D. J., LINDPOP, P. J., MORGAN, B. W. G., SKEGGS, D. B. L., WHITTLE, R. J. M., AND WILLIAMS, I. G., 1966, Monitored regional hypoxia in radiotherapy, *Br. J. Radiol.* **39**:908.

BARENDSEN, G. W., BROERSE, J. J., AND VAN PUTTEN, L. M. (eds.), 1971, Fundamental and practical aspects of the application of fast neutrons in clinical radiotherapy, Proc. Rijswijk meeting (1970), *Eur. J. Cancer* **7**:97; see also Proc. 2nd Rijswijk meeting (1973), *Eur. J. Cancer* **10**:199.

BATES, T., 1975, A prospective clinical trial of post-operative radiotherapy delivered in 3 fractions per week versus 2 fractions per week in breast carcinoma, *Clin. Radiol.* **26**:297.

BERGONIE, J., AND TRIBONDEAU, L., 1906, Interprétation de quelques resultats de la radiotherapie et assai de fixation d'une technique rationale, *C. R. Acad. Sci.* **143**:983. See English translation by G. Fletcher, 1959, *Radiat. Res.* **11**:587.

BERRY, R. J., 1969, Radiotherapy plus chemotherapy—Have we gained anything by combining them in the treatment of human cancer? in: *Frontiers of Radiation Therapy and Oncology*, Vol. 4 (G. VAETH, ed.), pp. 1–16, Karger, Basel.

BERRY, R. J., WIERNIK, G., AND PATTERSON, T. J. S., 1974, Skin tolerance to fractionated X-irradiation in the pig—How good a predictor is the N.S.D. formula? *Br. J. Radiol.* **47**:185; see also *Br. J. Radiol.* **47**:277.

BROWN, J. M., AND PROBERT, J., 1973, Long-term recovery of connective tissue after irradiation, *Radiology* **108**:205.

BROWN, J. M., AND PROBERT, J. C., 1975, Early and late radiation changes following a second course of irradiation, *Radiology* **115**:711.

CALDWELL, W. L., 1974, Tolerance of skin and kidneys to conventional or split course fractionation, in: *Proceedings of the Madison Conference on the Time–Dose Relationships in Clinical Therapy* (W. L. CALDWELL AND D. D. TOLBERT, eds.), pp. 38–42, University of Wisconsin, Madison.

Carmel Conference on Time and Dose Relationships in Radiation Biology as Applied to Radiotherapy, 1969, BNL 50203 (C-57), Clearinghouse for Federal Scientific and Technical Information, NBS, Springfield, Va.

CALDWELL, W. L., AND TOLBERT, D. D. (eds.), 1974, *Proceedings of the Madison Conference on the Time–Dose Relationships in Clinical Therapy*, University of Wisconsin, Madison.

CAVALIERE, R., CIOCATTO, E. C., GIOVANELLA, B. C., HEIDELBERGER, C., JOHNSON, R. O., MARGOTTINI, M., MANDOVI, B., MORRICA, G., AND ROSSI-FANELLI, A., 1967, Selective heat sensitivity of cancer cells, *Cancer* **20**:1351.

CHEN, K. Y., AND WITHERS, H. R., 1972, Survival characteristics of stem cells of gastric mucosa in C3H mice exposed to local gamma irradiation, *Int. J. Radiat. Biol.* **21**:521.

COHEN, L., 1968, A cell population kinetic model for fractionated radiation therapy, *Br. J. Radiol.* **41**:522.

COHEN, L., AND KERRICK, J. E., 1951, Estimation of biological dosage factors in clinical radiation therapy, *Br. J. Cancer* **5**:180.

COMMITTEE FOR RADIATION ONCOLOGY STUDIES, 1975, Research Plan for Radiation Therapy, *Cancer Suppl.* **37**:2031.

COUTARD, H., 1932, Roentgen therapy of epitheliomas of tonsillar regions, hypopharynx and larynx from 1920 to 1926, *Am. J. Roentgenol.* **28**:313.

DENEKAMP, J., 1973, Changes in the rate of repopulation during multifraction irradiation of mouse skin, *Br. J. Radiol.* **46**:381.

DENEKAMP, J., 1975, Residual radiation damage in mouse skin 5 to 8 months after irradiation, *Radiology* **115**:191.

DENEKAMP, J., BALL, M. M., AND FOWLER, J. F., 1969, Recovery and repopulation in mouse skin as a function of time after irradiation, *Radiat. Res.* **37**:361.

DISCHE, S., GRAY, A. J., ADAMS, G. E., FLOCKHART, I. R., FOSTER, J. L., ZANELLI, G. D., THOMLINSON, R. H., AND ERRINGTON, L. M., 1976, Clinical testing of the radiosensitizer Ro-07-0582 (4 papers), *Clin. Radiol.* **27**:151.

DOUGLAS, B. G., AND FOWLER, J. F., 1975, Fractionation schedules and a quadratic dose–effect relationship, *Br. J. Radiol.* **48**:502.

DOUGLAS, B. G., AND FOWLER, J. F., 1976, The effect of multiple small doses of X-rays on skin reactions in the mouse and a basic interpretation, *Radiat. Res.* **66**:401.

DU SAULT, L. A., 1963, The effect of oxygen on the response of spontaneous tumours in mice to radiotherapy, *Br. J. Radiol.* **36**:749.

DUTREIX, J., 1975, Clinical trials on fractionation, in: *Proceedings of the XI International Cancer Congress* (Florence 1974), Vol. 5, (P. BUCALOSSI, U. VERONESI, AND N. CASCINELLI, eds.), Excerpta Medica, Amsterdam.

DUTREIX, J., WAMBERSIE, A., AND BOUNIK, C., 1973, Cellular recovery in human skin reactions: Application to dose fraction number overall time relationship in radiotherapy, *Eur. J. Cancer* **9**:159.

ELKIND, M. M., SWAIN, R. W., ALESCIO, T., SUTTON, H., AND MOSES, W. B., 1965, Oxygen, nitrogen, recovery and radiation therapy, in: *Cellular Radiation Biology*, pp. 442–468, Williams and Wilkins, Baltimore.

ELLIS, F., 1969, Dose, time and fractionation: A clinical hypothesis, *Clin. Radiol.* **20**:1.

ELLIS, F., 1974, The NSD concept and the treatment of resistant tumours, in: *Proceedings of the Conference on the Time–Dose Relationships in Clinical Therapy* (W. CALDWELL AND D. D. TOLBERT, eds.), pp. 74–81, 188–189, 208–209, University of Wisconsin, Madison.

EMERY, E. W., DENEKAMP, J., BALL, M. M., AND FIELD, S. B., 1970, Survival of mouse skin epithelial cells following single and divided doses of X-rays, *Radiat. Res.* **41**:450.

FIELD, S. B., 1969, Early and late reactions in skin of rats following irradiation with X-rays or fast neutrons, *Radiology* **92**:381.

FIELD, S. B., 1972, The Ellis formula for X-rays and fast neutrons, *Br. J. Radiol.* **45**:315.

FIELD, S. B., 1976, An historical survey of radiobiology and radiotherapy with fast neutrons, *Curr. Top. Radiat. Res. Q.* **11**:1.

FIELD, S. B., AND BEWLEY, D. K., 1974, Effects of dose rate on the radiation response of rat skin, *Int. J. Rad. Biol.* **26**:259.

FIELD, S. B., AND HORNSEY, S., 1971, RBE values for cyclotron neutrons for effects on normal tissues and tumours as a function of doses and dose fractionations, *Eur. J. Cancer* **7**:161.

FIELD, S. B., AND HORNSEY, S., 1974, The link between animal experiments and clinical practice, in: *Biomedical, Chemical, and Physical Perspectives* (O. F. NYGAARD, H. I. ADLER, AND W. K. SINCLAIR, eds.), pp. 1125–1135, Academic Press, New York.

FIELD, S. B., MORRIS, C., DENEKAMP, J., AND FOWLER, J. F., 1975, The response of mouse skin to fractionated X-rays, *Eur. J. Cancer* **11**:291.

FIELD, S. B., HORNSEY, S., AND KUTSUTANI, Y., 1976, Effects of fractionated irradiation on mouse lung and a phenomenon of slow repair, *Br. J. Radiol.* **49**:700.

FLETCHER, G. H., 1966, *Textbook of Radiotherapy*, Lea and Febiger, Philadelphia.

FLETCHER, G. H., 1973, Clinical dose–response curves of human malignant epithelial tumours, *Br. J. Radiol.* **46**:1.

FOWLER, J. F., 1976, The relationship between pion therapy and other new modalities: Neutrons, hypoxic-cell radiosensitizers and non-standard fractionation, *Atomkernenergie* **27**:161.

FOWLER, J. F., AND DENEKAMP, J., 1976, Regulation of epidermal stem cells, in: *Proceedings of the Leblond Symposium on Stem Cells* (Montreal, October 1975), (A. B. CAIRNIE, ed.), p. 117, Academic Press, New York.

FOWLER, J. F., AND STERN, B. E., 1963, Dose–time relationships in radiotherapy and the validity of cell survival curve models, *Br. J. Radiol.* **36**:163.

FOWLER, J. F., MORGAN, R. L. SILVESTER, J. A., BEWLEY, D. K., AND TURNER, B. A., 1963, Experiments with fractionated X-ray treatment of the skin of pigs. I. Fractionation up to 28 days, *Br. J. Radiol.* **36**:188.

GAUWERKY, F., LANGHEIM, F., AND TEEBKEN, F., 1972, Ein Zeitfaktoruntersuchung zur Strahlenfibrose der Unterhaut nach Telekobaltbestrahlung, *Beiheft der Fortschr. a. d. Gebiete Röntgenstr. u. d. Nuklearmedizin*, p. 15, Thieme, Stuttgart.

GLATSTEIN, E. J., 1973, Alterations in rubidium-86 extraction in normal mouse tissues after irradiation. An estimate of long-term blood flow changes in kidney, lung, liver, skin and muscle, *Pediat. Res.* **53**:88.

GLATSTEIN, E. J., BROWN, R. C., ZANELLI, G. D., AND FOWLER, J. F., 1975, The uptake of Rb-86 in mouse kidneys irradiated with fractionated doses of X-rays, *Radiat. Res.* **61**:417.

HALL, E. J., 1972, Radiation dose-rate: A factor of importance in radiobiology and radiotherapy, *Br. J. Radiol.* **45**:81.

HENLE, K. J., AND LEEPER, D. B., 1975, The interaction of hyperthermia and radiation in CHO cells: Recovery kinetics of sublethal damage. *Radiat. Res.* **65**:591 (abst.).

HOCKLY, J. D. L., AND SEALY, R., 1977, The treatment of carcinoma of the cervix using 2 or 5 fractions per week in air and in hyperbaric oxygen, *S. Afr. Med. J.* (in press).

HOPEWELL, J. W., AND BERRY, R. J., 1975, Radiation tolerance of the pig kidney: A model for determining overall time and fraction factors for preserving renal function, *Int. J. Radiat. Oncol. Biol. Physics* **1**:61.

HORNSEY, S., AND ALPER, T., 1966, Unexpected dose-rate effect in the killing of mice by irradiation, *Nature (London)* **210**:212.

HORNSEY, S., AND BEWLEY, D. K., 1971, Hypoxia in mouse intestine induced by electron irradiation at high dose-rates, *Int. J. Radiat. Biol.* **19**:479.

HORNSEY, S., AND FIELD, S. B., 1974, The RBE of cyclotron neutrons for effects on normal tissues, *Eur. J. Cancer* **10**:231.

HORNSEY, S., AND VATISTAS, S., 1963, Some characteristics of the survival curves of crypt cells of the small intestine characteristics of the survival curves of crypt cells of the small intestine of the mouse deduced after whole body X-irradiation, *Br. J. Radiol.* **36**:795.

JARDINE, J. H., HUSSEY, D. H., BOYD, D. D., RAULSTON, G. L., AND DAVIDSON, T. J., 1975, Acute and late effects of 16 and 50 MeVd on Be neutrons (and cobalt-60 radiation) on the oral mucosa of rhesus monkeys, *Radiology* **117**:185.

KAL, H. B., JANSE, H. C., AND GAISER, F. J., 1975, Repair of radiation and hyperthermic induced lesions in rat rhabdomyosarcoma cells *in vitro*, *REP Annual Report 1975* pp. 30–32, TNO Radiobiological Institute, Rijswijk, the Netherlands.

KIRK, J., GRAY, W. M., AND WATSON, E. R., 1971, Cumulative radiation effect. Part I: Fractionated treatment regimes, *Clin. Radiol.* **22**:145.

KRAMER, S., SOUTHARD, M. E., AND MANSFIELD, C. M., 1972, Radiation effect and tolerance of the CNS, in: *Frontiers of Radiation Therapy and Oncology*, Vol. 6 (G. M. VAETH, ed.), p. 332, Karger, Basel.

KRÖNIG, B., AND FRIEDRICH, W., 1918, *Physikalische und biologische Grundlagen der Strahlentherapie*, Urban and Schwarzenberg, Berlin.

LAMBERTSEN, C. J., 1966, Physiological effects of oxygen inhalation at high partial pressures, in: *Fundamentals of Hyperbaric Medicine*, p. 17, Publication No. 1298, National Academy of Sciences, Washington, D.C.

LIVERSAGE, W. E., 1969, A general formula for equating protracted and acute regimes of radiation, *Br. J. Radiol.* **42**:432.

LIVERSAGE, W. E., 1971, A critical look at the ret, *Br. J. Radiol.* **44**:91.

MCNALLY, N. J., 1972, A low O.E.R. for tumour cell survival as compared with that for tumour growth delay, *Int. J. Radiat. Biol.* **22**:407.

MCNALLY, N. J., 1975, The effect of an hypoxic cell sensitizer on tumour growth delay and cell survival: Implications for cell survival *in situ* and *in vitro*, *Br. J. Cancer* **32**:610.

MENDELSOHN, M. L., 1969, The biology of dose-limiting tissues, in: *Time and Dose Relationships in Radiation Biology as Applied to Radiotherapy*, BNL 50203, p. 154.

MONTAGUE, E. D., 1968, Experience with altered fractionation in radiation therapy of breast cancer, *Radiology* 90:962.

MORRISON, R., 1975, The results of treatment of cancer of the bladder—A clinical contribution to radiobiology, *Clin. Radiol.* 26:67.

MOSS, W. T., BRAND, W. N., AND BATTIFORA, H., 1973, *Radiation Oncology: Rationale, Technique, Results*, C. V. Mosby Co., St. Louis.

ORTON, C. G., AND ELLIS, F., 1973, A simplification in the use of the NSD concept in practical radiotherapy, *Br. J. Radiol.* 46:529.

PATERSON, R., 1948, *The Treatment of Malignant Disease by Radiotherapy*, Edwin Arnold Co., London.

PETERS, L. J., 1975, Enhancement of syngeneic murine tumour transplantability by whole-body irradiation: A non-immunogenic phenomenon, *Br. J. Cancer* 31:293.

PETERS, L. J., AND HEWITT, H. B., 1974, The influence of fibrin formation on the transplantability of murine tumour cells: Implications for the mechanism of the Révész effect, *Br. J. Cancer* 29:279.

PHILLIPS, T. L., AND BUSHKE, F., 1969, Radiation tolerance of the thoracic spinal cord, *Am. J. Roentgenol.* 105:659.

PHILLIPS, T. L., AND FU, K., 1974, Derivation of time–dose factors for normal tissues using experimental end-points in the mouse, in: *Proceedings of the Conference on the Time–Dose Relationships in Clinical Therapy* (W. L. CALDWELL AND D. D. TOLBERT, eds.), pp. 42–47, University of Wisconsin, Madison.

PHILLIPS, T. L., AND MARGOLIS, L. W., 1972, Radiation pathology and clinical response of lung and esophagus, in: *Frontiers of Radiation Therapy and Oncology*, Vol. 6 (J. M. VAETH, ed.), pp. 254–273, Karger, Basel.

REGAUD, C., AND FERROUX, R., 1937, Discordance des effets des rayons X, d'une part dan la peau, d'autre part dans le testicule par le fractionnement de la dose, diminution d'efficacité dans la peau, maintien de l'efficacité dans le testicule, *C. R. Soc. Biol.* 97:431.

REINHOLD, H. S., AND BUISMAN, G. H., 1975, Repair of radiation damage to capillary endothelium, *Br. J. Radiol.* 48:727.

ROSENBERG, S. A., AND KAPLAN, H. A. S., 1966, Evidence for an orderly progression in the spread of Hodgkin's disease, *Cancer Res.* 26:1225.

RUBIN, P., AND CASARETT, G. W., 1968, *Clinical Radiation Pathology*, Vols. I and II, p. 1057, Saunders, Philadelphia.

RUBIN, P., AND CASARETT, G. W., 1972, A direction for clinical radiation pathology: The tolerance dose, in: *Frontiers of Radiation Therapy and Oncology*, Vol. 6 (J. M. VAETH, ed.), pp. 1–16, Karger, Basel.

SEITZ, L., AND WINTZ, W., 1920, *Unsere Methode der Röntgentherapie*, Berlin.

SHUKOVSKY, L. J., 1970, Dose, time, volume relationships in squamous cell carcinoma of the supraglottic larynx, *Am. J. Roentgenol.* 108:27.

SHUKOVSKY, L. J., 1974, Clinical applications of time–dose data to tumour control, in *Proceedings of the Madison Conference on the Time–Dose Relationships in Clinical Therapy* (W. L. CALDWELL and D. D. TOLBERT, eds.), pp. 118–130, University of Wisconsin, Madison.

SHUKOVSKY, L. J., AND FLETCHER, G. H., 1973, Time–dose and tumour volume relationships in squamous cell carcinoma of the tonsillar fossa, *Radiology* 107:621.

STEWART, F. A., AND DENEKAMP, J., 1977, Sensitization of mouse skin to X-irradiation by moderate heating, *Radiology* 123:195.

STEWART, J. G., AND JACKSON, A. W., 1975, The steepness of the dose response curve both for tumour cure and normal tissue injury, *Laryngoscope* 85:1107.

STRATFORD, I. J., AND ADAMS, G. E., 1977, Effect of hyperthermia on differential cytotoxicity of a hypoxic cell radiosensitizer, Ro-07-0582, on mammalian cells *in vitro*, *Br. J. Cancer* 35:307.

SUIT, H. D., 1965, Radiation therapy given under conditions of local hypoxia for bone and soft tissue sarcoma, in: *Tumours of Bone and Soft Tissue*, pp. 143–163, Year Book Medical Publishers, Chicago.

TAYLOR, A. M. R., HARNDEN, D. G., ARLETT, C. F., HARCOURT, S. A., LEHMANN, A. R., STEVENS, S., AND BRIDGES, B. A., 1975, Ataxia telangiectasia: A human mutation with abnormal radiation sensitivity, *Nature (London)* 258:427.

THOMLINSON, R. H., AND GRAY, L. H., 1955, The histological structure of some human lung cancers and the possible implications for radiotherapy, *Br. J. Cancer* 9:539.

180

J. F. FOWLER
AND
J. DENEKAMP

THRALL, D. E., GILLETTE, E. L., AND BAUMAN, C. L., 1973, Effect of heat on the C3H mouse mammary adenocarcinoma evaluated in terms of tumour growth, *Eur. J. Cancer* **9**:871.

TILL, J. E., AND MCCULLOCH, E. A., 1961, A direct measurement of the radiation sensitivity of normal mouse bone marrow cells, *Radiat. Res.* **14**:213.

TILL, J. E., AND MCCULLOCH, E. A., 1963, Early repair processes in marrow cells irradiated and proliferating *in vivo*, *Radiat. Res.* **18**:96.

TURESSON, I., AND NOTTER, G., 1975, Skin reactions after different fractionation schedules giving the same cumulative radiation effect, *Acta Radiol. Ther. Phys. Biol.* **14**:475.

VAETH, J. M., 1972, *Frontiers of Radiation Therapy and Oncology*, Vol. 6, Karger, Basel.

VAN DEN BRENK, H. A. S., 1965, Enhancement of radiosensitivity of skin of patients by high pressure oxygen, *Br. J. Radiol.* **38**:857.

VAN DEN BRENK, H. A. S., 1968, Hyperbaric oxygen in radiation therapy, *Am. J. Roentgenol.* **52**:8.

VAN DEN BRENK, H. A. S., 1971, Radiation effects on the pulmonary system, in: *Pathology of Irradiation* (C. G. BERDJIS, ed.), p. 569, Williams and Wilkins, Baltimore.

VAN DEN BRENK, H. A. S., BURCH, W. M., ORTON, C., AND SHARPINGTON, C., 1973, Stimulation of clonogenic growth of tumour cells and metastases in the lungs by local X-radiation, *Br. J. Cancer* **27**:291.

VAN DEN BRENK, H. A. S., SHARPINGTON, C., OORTON, C., AND STONE, M., 1974, Effects of X-radiation on growth and function of the repair blastema (granulation tissue). II. Measurements of angiogenesis in the Selye pouch in the rat, *Int. J. Radiat. Biol.* **25**:277.

VAN DEN BRENK, H. A. S., STONE, M. G., KELLY, H., AND SHARPINGTON, C., 1976. Lowering of innate resistance of the lungs to the growth of blood-borne cancer cells in states of topical and systemic stress, *Br. J. Cancer* **33**:60.

VAN DER KOGEL, A. J., AND BARENDSEN, G. W., 1974, Late effects of spinal cord irradiation with 300 kV X-rays and 15 MeV neutrons, *Br. J. Radiol.* **47**:393.

VAN DER KOGEL, A. J., AND SISSINGH, H. A., 1975, Dose–latent-period relationships for radiation induced damage of the rat spinal cord, *REP Annual Report*, pp. 19–21, TNO Radiobiological Institute, Rijswijk, the Netherlands.

VAN DER KOGEL, A. J., VAN BEKKUM, D. W., AND BARENDSEN, G. W., 1976, Tolerance of CNS to total body irradiation combined with chemotherapy applied for the treatment of leukaemia, *Eur. J. Cancer* **12**:675.

VERZOSA, M. S., AUR, R. J. A., SIMONE, J. V., HUSTER, H. O., AND PINKEL, D. P., 1976, Five years after CNS irradiation of children with leukaemia, *Int. J. Radiat. Oncol. Biol. Phys.* **1**:209.

WARA, W. M., PHILLIPS, T. L., MARGOLIS, L. W., AND SMITH, V., 1973, Radiation pneumonitis: A new approach to the derivation of time–dose factors, *Cancer* **32**:547.

WARA, W. M., PHILLIPS, T. L., SHELINE, G. E. AND SCHWADE, J. G., 1975, Radiation tolerance of the spinal cord, *Cancer* **35**:1558.

WESTRA, A., AND DEWEY, W. C., 1971, Varition in sensitivity to heat shock during the cell cycle of Chinese hamster cells *in vitro*, *Int. J. Radiat. Biol.* **19**:467.

WIERNIK, G., PATTERSON, T. J. S., AND BERRY, R. J., 1974, The effect of fractionated dose-patterns of X-radiation on the survival of experimental skin flabs in the pig, *Brit. J. Radiol.* **47**:343.

WITHERS, H. R., 1967, The dose–survival relationships for irradiation of epithelial cells of mouse skin, *Br. J. Radiol.* **40**:187.

WITHERS, H. R., 1971, Regeneration of intestinal mucosa after irradiation, *Cancer* **28**:75.

WITHERS, H. R., 1974, Iso-effect curves for various proliferative tissues in experimental animals, in: *Proceedings of the Conference on the Time–Dose Relationships in Clinical Therapy* (W. L. CALDWELL AND D. D. TOLBERT, eds.), pp. 30–38, University of Wisconsin, Madison.

WITHERS, H. R., AND ELKIND, M. M., 1969, Radiosensitivity and fractionation response of crypt cells of mouse jejunum, *Radiat. Res.* **38**:598.

WITHERS, H. R., AND ELKIND, M. M., 1970, Microcolony survival assay for cells of mouse intestinal mucosa exposed to radiation, *Int. J. Radiat. Biol.* **17**:261.

WITHERS, H. R., AND MILAS, L., 1973, The influence of pre-irradiation of lung on development of artificial pulmonary metastases of fibrosarcoma in mice, *Cancer Res.* **33**:1931.

WITHERS, H. R., HUNTER, N., BARKLEY, H. T., AND REID, B. O., 1974, Radiation survival and regeneration characteristics of spermatogenic stem cells of mouse testis, *Radiat. Res.* **57**:58.

YOUNG, C. M. A., BRENNAN, D., DURRANT, K., HOPEWELL, J. W., AND WIERNIK, G., 1976, The effects of varied numbers of dose fractions and overall treatment time on the radiation response of normal human skin, *Br. J. Radiol.* **49**:558.

6

Hypoxic Cell Sensitizers for Radiotherapy

G. E. ADAMS

1. Introduction

1.1. Adjunctive Agents, Potentiating Agents, and Radiation Sensitizers

In the treatment of malignant disease with combinations of chemotherapy and radiotherapy, it is important to draw distinctions between adjunctive agents, so-called potentiating agents, and true radiation sensitizers (Bleehen, 1973). This is illustrated by Fig. 1. For the truly adjunctive agent, the overall effect results from the separate but additive effects of both modalities, althought there is little or no gain in overall therapeutic ratio. Potentiation arises (Fig. 1b) when the combined effect of both modalities is greater than the sum of the effects of each of the separate treatments. True potentiation is, however, difficult to characterize since, depending on the criteria of measurement, the complex nature of dose–response curves can sometimes indicate apparent potentiation when, in reality, the drug and radiation treatments are giving a purely additive affect in terms of cell killing.

True sensitization arises when the drug alone has little or no cytocidal action without radiation, but significantly increases the efficiency of radiation-induced cell killing when present during irradiation (Fig. 1c). For any radiation sensitizer to be of value in the radiation treatment of cancer, it is essential that the drug enhance the radiation effect on the tumor more than any increased effect on normal tissue. At the present time, about 50% of all cancer patients receive

G. E. ADAMS • Gray Laboratory, Cancer Research Campaign, Mount Vernon Hospital, Northwood, Middlesex HA6 2RN, England. Present address: Division of Physics as Applied to Medicine, Institute of Cancer Research, Sutton, Surrey SM2 5PX, England.

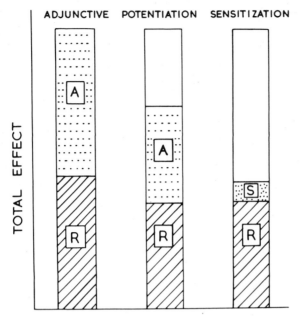

FIGURE 1. Adjunctive agents, potentiating agents, and radiation sensitizers. From Bleehen (1976).

radiotherapy, and many are cured. Nevertheless, failures in local control do occur, and even a modest improvement in the radiosensitivity of tumors relative to that of normal tissue would result in a substantial improvement in control of local disease. It is for this reason that there is a rapidly developing interest in the application of radiosensitizing drugs in radiotherapy.

This chapter describes the current status of one particular class of drug, the hypoxic cell sensitizer. However, before discussion of this promising current approach, it would be useful to comment on the classification of radiation sensitizers generally.

1.2. Classification of Radiation Sensitizers

1.2.1. Sulfhydryl-Binding Agents

One of the earliest suggested mechanisms for radiation sensitization arose from the observation that the compound N-ethylmaleimide (NEM) greatly sensitized the radiation-induced inactivation of bacteria (Bridges, 1960). While subsequent investigations have shown that some sensitization may occur in the presence of oxygen, it is generally found that the sensitization is usually much greater for hypoxic bacteria. The rationale behind these early studies was that NEM, a recognized antoxidant used in the rubber industry, might oxidize intracellular SH-containing compounds. It was reasoned that, if natural cellular radiosensitivity is conditioned to some extent by the level of SH compounds which are present in cells and which act as endogenous radioprotectors, then their removal by oxidation by NEM might increase the radiosensitivity.

It is true that NEM does react efficiently with SH compounds, and there is convincing evidence from studies with synchronized mammalian cells *in vitro* (Sinclair, 1975) that this process contributes to sensitization. Nevertheless, studies of the radiosensitization of hypoxic bacteria by NEM using a rapid-mixing technique (Adams *et al.*, 1968) have shown that sensitization can still occur even though the irradiation is carried out only a few milliseconds after the cells are brought into contact with the sensitizer. Since the contact time is almost certainly too short for the occurrence of any chemical reaction between NEM and endogenous SH compounds, it was concluded that the main mechanism of NEM sensitization involves the participation of fast radiation chemical free-radical processes.

More recently, sensitization of hypoxic mammalian cells by the reagent Diamide has been demostrated (Harris and Powers, 1973). This compound reacts more rapidly than NEM with SH compounds, and there is good evidence that SH suppression contributes to the overall sensitization. However, rapid-mix evidence indicates that another mechanism involving fast free-radical processes is involved, possibly to a major extent (Watts *et al.*, 1975).

1.2.2. Radiation-Induced Cytotoxicity

There are a few compounds that exhibit an apparent sensitizing effect due to cytotoxic substances formed as a result of radiation action on the original compound. One example of this type of sensitizer is iodoacetamide, which undergoes radiolytic breakdown to form several products, including iodine. The sensitizing action of iodoacetamide in bacterial systems is probably attributable to iodine production. Other iodine-containing compounds, including some radiobiological contrast media, e.g., iothalamic acid, also exhibit sensitizing action (Quintiliani, 1974), although here the mechanism of action remains unclear.

Of particular interest mechanistically is the sensitizing action of some copper compounds. Cupric ion (Cu^{2+}) is a very effective sensitizer for hypoxic bacteria, but has no effect on oxic cells (Cramp, 1967). The effect is due entirely to the highly toxic cuprous ion (Cu^+) formed by radiation-induced reduction of cupric ion, which itself is relatively nontoxic. The absence of sensitization in oxic bacteria is due to the rapid conversion of the cuprous ion back to the cupric ion by direct chemical reaction with molecular oxygen.

1.2.3. Structural Incorporation of DNA Analogues

Analogues of DNA precursors such as bromodeoxyuridine (BUdR) can be incorporated into the DNA of metabolizing cells. It is now well established that cells containing BUdR are more radiosensitive than normal cells (Szybalski, 1962). The incorporation of BUdR at the expense of thymine occurs because the van den Waals radius of the bromine atom in the 5-position of the uridine ring is similar to that of the 5-methyl group in thymine. Incorporation can occur, therefore, with little distortion of the three-dimensional structure of DNA.

The sensitization effect is not due to any increase in the amount of energy absorption by the DNA which may occur with some types of radiation, nor is it due to weakening of the hydrogen bonds in the DNA. Interference with repair processes has been implicated, but it is most likely that the effect is due to an increase in the number of discrete radiation-chemical lesions, each of which may give rise to irreversible biological damage (Kaplan, 1970). A mechanism involving long-range intramolecular electron migration has been proposed (see Adams, 1972), and fast-luminescence studies with DNA containing incorporated BUdR have shown that energy in some form can certainly migrate considerable distances along the DNA chain (Fielden and Lillicrap, 1970).

Studies with this type of sensitizer have been valuable in mechanistic studies in radiobiology, but there has been only limited success in radiotherapy using this approach. Major obstacles are that the incorporation occurs in both normal and malignant dividing cells, and that sensitization occurs in oxygenated cells but not in cells that were hypoxic at the time of exposure to the drug. Some success has been achieved, however, using local infusion techniques (see Bleehen, 1973).

1.2.4. Modification of Cellular Processes

Various agents or treatments that modify endogenous protective or repair mechanisms provide valuable knowledge concerning the mechanisms of cellular radiation resistance and sensitivity. Sensitization arising from the prevention of fast radiation-chemical repair by SH binding, as discussed above, is a specific example of this general class of sensitization. There is clear evidence that sensitization can result from the inhibition of slow repair mechanisms. This can occur either by rendering inactive the enzyme system responsible for the repair or by modification of the initial lesion in such a way as to prevent its subsequent repair. The relationship between radiation sensitivity and repair generally is better understood in bacterial systems. However, there is good evidence that some sensitizing agents for mammalian cells act by repair inhibition, e.g., actinomycin D (Elkind et al., 1968).

An interesting and promising new development involves radiation modification studies on the melanin-producing systems. Radiation resistance can be substantially decreased in a variety of pigmented tissues including melanotic tumor cells irradiated in vitro and in vivo. These investigations have led to a pilot clinical study in patients with melanoma (Lukiewicz, 1976).

1.2.5. Hypoxic Cell Sensitizers

The generality of the oxygen effect in radiobiology has for many years encouraged the search for other chemical agents that might act by a similar mechanism. During the last 20 years, many different types of chemical compounds have been found which have the ability to increase the radiation sensitivity of hypoxic cells without affecting the sensitivity of oxic cells.

A subgroup of this class of sensitizer is the nitroxyl stable free radical, of which there are now numerous examples (Emmerson, 1972). Nitroxyl sensitizers developed out of earlier studies on the radiation-sensitizing properties of nitric oxide itself. Some of these agents are very efficient sensitizers for mammalian cells *in vitro* (Emmerson, 1972; Cooke *et al.*, 1976) and as such have proved to be useful for mechanistic studies in radiation biology. Their drawback, however, is that as free radicals they are highly reactive and have very short lifetimes *in vivo*. At the present time, the problem of instability is restricting sensitization studies to *in vitro* systems.

Recently, some drugs in the general class of anesthetics, analgesics, and tranquilizers have been shown to sensitize hypoxic bacteria and hypoxic mammalian cells to radiation. There appears to be some differential action in favor of hypoxic cells, but the mechanism of their action is unknown, although membrane interaction is suggested to be involved (Shenoy *et al.*, 1976).

The largest groups in the hypoxic cell sensitizer class are the "electron-affinic" agents, so called because of the relationship between their efficiencies and the electron affinities of the compounds. Much of the remainder of this chapter is devoted to a discussion of the status of the radiobiological and clinical investigations with these drugs.

2. Methods of Overcoming the Hypoxia Problem

For any sensitizing drug to be of value in the radiotherapy of cancer, it must increase radiation damage to malignant tissue more than any increased effect on normal tissue which falls within the irradiated area. Interest in drugs which specifically radiosensitize hypoxic cells rests on the beliefs (1) that hypoxic cells occur in a significant proportion of human tumors and (2) that they are a major obstacle to improvement in local control by radiotherapy.

Oxygen status is the largest single factor affecting the radiosensitivity of the mammalian cell. Hypoxic cells, that is, cells where the oxygen concentration is $< 10^{-6}$ moles, are approximately 3 times more radioresistant than oxic cells. The blood supply to most normal tissues is sufficient to maintain an intracellular oxygen concentration of at least 30 μM, which is more than enough to maintain high radiosensitivity. However, in tumors, the disorganized process of growth is such that tumor cells proliferate more rapidly than the microvasculature of the tumor. Histological examinations of tumor sections show that areas of necrosis often occur at distances greater than about 150–200 μm from a microcapillary (Thomlinson and Gray, 1955). According to these authors, the necrosis arises as a result of oxygen depletion caused by oxygen metabolism occurring in the cells in the intervening region. Therefore, some cells near the limit of oxygen diffusion will have an oxygen content low enough for the cells to be radiobiologically resistant. In many rodent tumors, the proportion of hypoxic cells lies between 10% and 20%, and in some cases may be even higher. Because of their relative radioresistance, these cells will survive a radiation dose that is sufficient to completely sterilize all the oxygenated cells. Subsequent to the radiation, these dead cells will be absorbed, the tumor may shrink, the previously hypoxic cells will become reoxygenated, and the tumor will regrow.

Since regions of extensive necrosis are often present in human tumors, it is reasonable to conclude that hypoxic cells will be present, also.

2.1. Optimum Fractionation

It is general experience that better results are obtained in radiotherapy when the radiation is given in multiple small fractions rather than in a large single dose. One reason for this is that reoxygenation of hypoxic cells can occur between successive fractions. While some optimum fractionation schedules have already evolved empirically following many years of experience, the search continues for new schedules which may maximize the benefit to be gained from reoxygenation.

2.2. High-LET Radiation

There is much current interest in radiotherapy with densely ionizing radiation such as neutrons, protons, π^- mesons, and other particles of high LET. Linear energy transfer (LET) is a parameter describing the rate of energy loss of a fast particle passing through a medium and is usually expressed in units of keV/μm. Part of the rationale behind this approach is that the magnitude of the oxygen effect decreases as the LET of the radiation increases. Thus the radioresistance of hypoxic tumor cells relative to that of well-oxygenated normal tissue is decreased, with a consequent gain in overall therapeutic ratio. For π^- mesons, the LET is extremely high, and cells irradiated with such beams show only a small oxygen effect. There are additional advantages with this type of radiation associated with the penetration and energy deposition characteristics in tissue. However, the high cost of future treatments will be a disadvantage.

For high-energy neutrons such as those used in current clinical trials, the oxygen effect is about 1.7, i.e., considerably lower than with conventional X- or γ-radiation.

2.3. Hyperbaric Oxygen

It is now over 20 years since Churchill-Davidson and his colleagues reported on their clinical findings using the hyperbaric oxygen technique (Churchill-Davidson et al., 1955). This attempt at overcoming the problem of the hypoxic cell rested on laboratory observations that the radiosensitivity of some animal tumors increased if the animals were treated while breathing oxygen at greater than 1 atm pressure. The rationale was that administration of hyperbaric oxygen should provide a substantial increase in the concentration of dissolved oxygen in the blood supply to the tumor. It was argued that the extent to which oxygen would diffuse from the tumor capillaries would increase and, it was hoped, oxygen would reach the distant hypoxic cells at a concentration sufficient to oxygenate these cells and thus lower their radioresistance. Since that time, numerous controlled clinical trials have been carried out, with benefit reported in some but not in others. Overall, the results have been disappointing, and this has caused much speculation that hypoxic cell radioresistance is not so important a factor in local control as was anticipated. However, there have been suggestions (e.g., Milne *et al.*, 1973) that the failure to observe a large degree of benefit is attributable to HBO-induced arteriolar constriction leading to a reduction in the blood-flow through the capillaries. Alternatively, the question has been raised whether or not the increased oxygen supply with HBO would be sufficient to oxygenate *all* the hypoxic cells in the tumor because of the rapid rate of oxygen metabolism during diffusion through the intervening tumor tissue. It is worth examining this question is some detail using the following model.

Let us consider the hypothetical single-dose radiation response of a tumor containing 10^{10} viable cells, of which 10% are hypoxic. For reasons of simplicity, the dose–response relationships of both the oxic and the hypoxic cell populations, expressed as cell survival, are assumed to be entirely exponential. The values of D_{10}, i.e., the dose required to reduce the surviving population by a factor of 10, are, respectively, 300 rads for the oxic and 900 rads for the hypoxic cells. The theoretical survival "curve" for this model cell population is shown by the heavy line in Fig. 2. The survival curve is biphasic in that, at low doses, cell survival decreases rapidly due to radiation killing of the more sensitive oxic cells (90% of the total population). At higher does, i.e., beyond the "break point," survival is governed almost entirely by the response of the hypoxic fraction. Thus "curative dose" (the dose required to reduce the overall population by a factor of more than 10^{-10}) will be > 8100 rads according to this simple model. Let us imagine the effect on the sensitivity if the hypoxic cell population is decreased by an order of magnitude (for example, by oxygenation in HBO). Under these conditions, the limiting dose necessary to reduce the cell population by 10^{-10} is now 7200 rads rather than 8100 rads. Thus the "gain factor" is the ratio of these doses, i.e., 1.12. The remaining biphasic survival curves in Fig. 2 have been constructed on the basis of reduction of the initial hypoxic cell population by 2, 3, 4, etc., orders of magnitude. The corresponding gain factors calculated from the respective doses required to reduce the overall population to one cell or less are plotted in Fig. 3 as a function of the proportion of the initial hypoxic cell population sensitized by oxygenation.

The striking feature of this plot is that the gain factor is relatively small even when 99% of the original hypoxic cells have been sensitized. Indeed, the gain factors become large when the remaining hypoxic cell fraction becomes vanishingly small in that the maximum gain of 2.7 is achieved only when the hypoxic cell fraction is reduced to less than 0.0001% of the original hypoxic population.

A plausible, indeed, a likely explanation, therefore, of the failure of HBO to produce a large degree of benefit is that, notwithstanding the large increase in the oxygen supply to the tumor, some of the more distant of the hypoxic cells fail to oxygenate. Clearly, even if such cells were relatively few in number, their radioresistance would still govern the overall radiation response of the tumor.

G. E. ADAMS

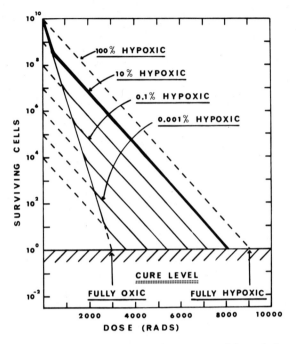

FIGURE 2. Theoretical single-dose exponential survival curves for a population of 10^{10} cells containing various proportions of hypoxic cells (see text).

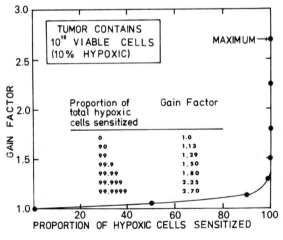

FIGURE 3. Theoretical single-dose gain for "tumor cure" as a function of the proportion of initial hypoxic cells sensitized (see text).

2.4. Electron–Affinic Sensitizers

Electron-affinic sensitizers for hypoxic cells, so called because the efficiencies of such drugs are related directly to the electron affinities of the compounds, represent a promising alternative approach to the hypoxia problem. The rationale for their use is that they diffuse out of the tumor blood supply and are absorbed by, and thus sensitize, distant hypoxic cells. In principle, these drugs mimic the sensitizing effect of oxygen and therefore do not increase the radiation response of well-oxygenated cells in surrounding normal tissue irradiated during radiotherapy.

Many experiments *in vitro* have shown that hypoxic cell sensitizers of this type vary enormously in their efficiencies defined in terms of the concentrations required to produce a given degree of sensitization. Invariably, these efficiencies are less than that of oxygen itself. However, a fundamental difference is that, unlike oxygen, some of these sensitizers have extremely long metabolic lifetimes *in vivo*. This provides the time necessary for their diffusion from the tumor blood supply to the distant hypoxic cells. Therefore, despite the lower *efficiency* of the chemical sensitizer with respect to oxygen, they are more *effective* because of this property of relative metabolic stability. This is illustrated by the diagram in Fig. 4.

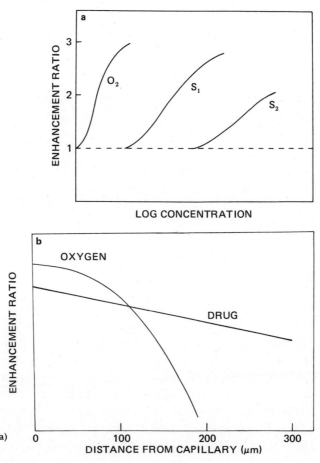

FIGURE 4. Sensitizer *efficiency* (a) and sensitizer *effectiveness* (b).

The upper panel in Fig. 1 shows a hypothetical relationship between the enhancement ratios (ER) for oxygen and two hypoxic cell sensitizers, S_1 and S_2. The concentration of oxygen required for a given enhancement ratio is much less than that for S_1. In turn, the required concentration of S_1 is much less than that for S_2. The order of efficiency is, therefore, $O_2 > S_1 > S_2$. However, the lower figure illustrates how oxygen can be less *effective* with respect to sensitization of hypoxic cells situated some distance from a capillary in a tumor. The lower panel shows hypothetically the relationship between enhancement ratios and this distance. Even if initially the enhancement ratio for O_2 is greater than that of the sensitizer (the latter may be smaller, for example, because toxicity *in vivo* limits the drug dose to a value less than that required to give the maximum possible degree of sensitization), the OER rapidly falls off. In contrast, the sensitizer can diffuse much farther because of its greater metabolic stability and thus reach all hypoxic cells. The large sensitization gain factors observed for many different animal tumors treated with radiation and electron-affinic sensitizers must be attributable to their ability to reach *all* and not 90%, or even 99%, of hypoxic cells in tumors.

3. Development of Electron-Affinic Sensitizers

More than 20 years ago, Mitchell and colleagues (see Mitchell, 1960) carried out many clinical and laboratory studies on radiosensitization with the compound Synkavit ®. This substance, a synthetic analogue of vitamin K, has the chemical structure I:

I. Synkavit   II. Menadione

Interest in the application of this drug subsided partly because many workers failed to demonstrate significant sensitization either *in vitro* or *in vivo*. The mechanism by which it was believed to act was never unequivocably established, and, indeed, hypoxic cell sensitization was not believed to be involved. However, from a historical viewpoint, the compound is interesting because of its relationship to another compound, 2-methylnaphthaquinone (menadione) II. This substance was one of a group of highly electron-affinic compounds studied as bacterial radiosensitizers (Adams and Cooke, 1969) in the early stages of the development of these agents. It was found to be extremely effective in bacteria, although toxicity and solubility problems prevented much further study in mammalian systems. Dephosphorylation of synkavit leads to the formation of the corresponding hydroquinone. Since menadione is the oxidation product of this substance, it is possible that early reports of tumor sensitization by synkavit were due to the physiological production of menadione.

3.1. The Electron-Affinic Relationship

Before the 1960s, few chemical sensitizers were known, and most of these were believed to act by the SH suppression mechanism (Section 1). Studies were generally carried out with bacteria since there was little scope for investigation with mammalian cells, due to the lack of test systems available.

The electron-affinity hypothesis arose partly out of basic pulse radiolysis studies concerned with the general phenomena of electron attachment to organic molecules. Combined radiation-chemical and bacterial studies led to the proposal that the efficiency of hypoxic cell sensitizers was related directly to the electron affinities of the compounds (Adams and Dewey, 1963). Subsequent work with bacterial cells (Adams and Cooke, 1969; Ashwood-Smith *et al.*, 1970) and bacterial spores (Tallentire *et al.*, 1968) showed that many organic compounds of diverse chemical structure could act as radiation sensitizers. These early compounds included conjugate diketones, aromatic ketones, quinones, unsaturated diesters, and various other conjugate structures.

At first, the electron-affinic relationship was simply a qualitative correlation between sensitizer efficiencies on the one hand and radiation-chemical estimates of relative electron capture efficiencies on the other. The correlation was supported by many pulse studies on one-electron transfer reactions between known sensitizers. Later, a more quantitative correlation was established (Raleigh *et al.*, 1973) following demonstrations of sensitization of irradiated hypoxic mammalian cells by the nitrobenzene compound paranitroacetophenone (PNAP) (Chapman *et al.*, 1971; Adams *et al.*, 1971). Raleigh and co-workers showed that the sensitizing efficiencies of a range of substituted nitrobenzenes closely correlate with the Hammett σ coefficients of the various substituents. Their data are shown in Fig. 5.

The σ constants for substituents in benzenoid compounds are a measure of the electron-withdrawing properties of the substituents and reflect differences in the

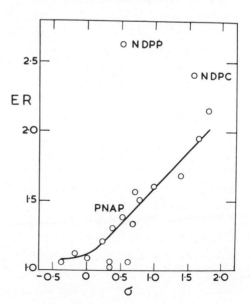

FIGURE 5. Relationship between sensitizing efficiencies of some substituted nitrobenzenes and the Hammett σ coefficients for the substituents. From Raleigh *et al.* (1973).

overall oxidizing abilities, i.e., the electron affinities, of the compounds. Although some deviation from the plot was noted, overall the correlation was good and represented the first quantitative expression of the electron-affinic relationship. This method had much value in the search for new sensitizers.

A more direct approach is to compare sensitization efficiencies with a property more fundamentally related to electron affinity. Such a property is the one-electron reduction potential, which is a direct expression of the standard free-energy change associated with electron attachment to the sensitizer.

Simic and Powers (1974), using anoxic bacterial spores, observed a trend between the sensitization efficiencies of various compounds and their reduction potentials taken from the literature. Although it is now known that some of these potentials are not true one-electron potentials, the errors involved were probably small compared to the very wide range of potentials of the compounds studied.

Accurate one-electron reduction potentials can now be determined by an accurate pulse radiolysis method based on the measurement of one-electron transfer equilibria between a given compound and a reference solute of known potential (Arai and Dorfman, 1968; Patel and Wilson, 1973; Meisel and Czapski, 1975; Meisel and Neta, 1975; Wardman and Clarke, 1976). This method is currently being used in the systematic study of structure–activity relationships of mammalian cell sensitizers, and its application to the development of new sensitizers is discussed later in this chapter.

3.2. The Search for Mammalian Cell Sensitizers

In the 1960s, almost all reports of hypoxic cell sensitization were confined to studies with anoxic suspensions of vegetative bacteria or bacterial spores (Tallentire et al., 1968). During this time, mammalian cell sensitization by the stable nitroxyl free radicals had been reported (Parker et al., 1969), but usually sensitization occurred only with concentrations near the toxic limits. Studies on the sensitization of ascites tumor cells by indanetrione (Scott and Sturrock, 1967), on hypoxic mouse gut (Hornsey et al., 1968), also by indane trione, and on hypoxic Chinese hamster cells by phenylglyoxal (Ashwood-Smith et al., 1970) showed some sensitization.

3.2.1. Paranitroacetophenone

Paranitroacetophenone (PNAP) was the first example of the purely electron-affinic type of sensitizer to show appreciable radiosensitization of hypoxic mammalian cells in vitro.(Chapman et al., 1971; Adams et al., 1971).

$$CH_3CO \langle\!\!\!\bigcirc\!\!\!\rangle NO_2$$

PNAP

In Chinese hamster V79 cells, sensitization occurs at low concentrations, the enhancement ratio attaining a maximum value of 1.6–1.7 at about 0.4 mM. Sensitization by PNAP showed several encouraging features. Apart from its activity in several mammalian cell lines, the sensitization of V79 cells is not significantly affected when the cells are irradiated in contact with full growth medium. Further, in these cells, PNAP sensitizes almost equally at all phases of the cell cycle (Chapman *et al.*, 1971).

These promising results led to studies aimed at demonstrating hypoxic cell sensitization *in vivo*. However, solubility problems prevented appropriate experiments from being carried out and attempts were made to synthesize related water-soluble derivatives.

3.2.2. NDPP (4'-Nitro-3-dimethylamino-propiophenone hydrochloride)

NDPP is a Mannich base of paranitroacetophenone and is considerably more water soluble than the parent compound. In both radioresistant and radiosensitive hypoxic bacteria, sensitization occurs up to the level of the full oxygen effect. In Chinese hamster cells, marked sensitization is sometimes evident at extremely low concentrations (Adams *et al.*, 1972). However, detailed studies have shown that this sensitizer operates by more than one mechanism. Whitmore *et al.* (1975) have shown that the extent of sensitization is very dependent on the preirradiation contact time and the pH of the medium. While it is clear that electron-affinic sensitization is involved, there is evidence that suppression of the endogenous sulfhydryl groups contributes to the sensitization and that protein binding is an additional factor affecting the overall sensitization efficiency.

This compound was used in one of the earlier demonstrations of hypoxic cell sensitization *in vitro*. Denekamp and Michael (1972) used the skin clone technique developed by Withers (1967) to show sensitization of hypoxic mouse epithelial cells.

Test areas on the back of mice were plucked about 1 day before irradiation from a pulsed electron beam. The mice were made anoxic by breathing nitrogen for 35 sec before and during rapid irradiation, and after introperitoneal administration of the sensitizer. Mice breathing oxygen during irradiation showed a rapid fall in cell survival over the dose range 1550–1850 rads, whereas in nitrogen the corresponding effect occurred at 3800–4800 rads. The oxygen enhancement ratio calculated from the data is 2.5–2.7, indicating that administration of nitrogen for 35 sec suffices to produce radiobiological hypoxia in the skin.

Mice receiving the sensitizer before hypoxic irradiation were appreciably more sensitive to radiation-induced skin damage, but, significantly, there was no additional sensitization in air-breathing animals. The enhancement ratio for NDPP increased with drug dose and, near the toxic limit of about 5 mg/30 g mouse, reached a value of 1.5.

Sensitization with this compound was also observed with P388 leukemia cells irradiated as mouse ascites tumors (Berry and Asquith, 1974), and slight sensitization has been reported with a solid mouse tumor (Sheldon and Smith, 1975).

3.2.3. Nitrofurans

Following the demonstration of sensitizing ability in the nitrobenzenes, Chapman and co-workers searched for sensitization with other nitro-containing aromatic compounds. These authors found the nitrofurans of general formula

were potent hypoxic cell sensitizers *in vitro* and were generally more active than the nitrobenzenes (Chapman *et al.*, 1973*b*) because of their greater electron-affinities. These findings were of considerable interest at the time because several nitrofurans were already in clinical use as antibacterials: therefore, there was considerable information available on their toxicology and pharmacology. However, since then, *in vivo* studies with the nitrofurans have been generally disappointing, often because of their metabolic instability and toxicity at the high doses necessary for sensitization.

It was while the studies with the nitrofurans were in progress that reports appeared of hypoxic cell sensitization with another class of nitro-heterocyclic compounds, the nitroimidazoles, sensitizers which have now proved to be by far the most promising. The nitroimidazoles are relatively less toxic than other nitro sensitizers and possess a high degree of metabolic stability. It is these properties which are responsible for the high sensitization factors now observed routinely in numerous mouse tumor systems. The remainder of the chapter is devoted to discussion of the present research status with this class of sensitizer and with a summary of the encouraging but as yet preliminary results from studies at the clinical level.

4. The Nitroimidazoles

4.1. Basic Structure

The nitroimidazoles of the most current interest as clinical radiation sensitizers are the derivatives of the 5-nitro- and the 2-nitro-substituted structures

On theoretical grounds, it would be expected that the 2-nitro compounds should have electron affinities greater than those of the 5-nitro compounds. Electron-spin resonance studies of the radical anions derived from those structures have shown that this is generally true (Whillans *et al.*, 1975; Greenstock *et al.*, 1976). In accord with the electron-affinic relationship, the 2-nitroimidazoles are more efficient hypoxic cell sensitizers than the 5-substituted analogues.

While many nitroimidazoles have been shown to be active sensitizers *in vitro*, the two which have been most studied are metronidazole, or Flagyl (a 5-nitroimidazole), and the experimental 2-nitroimidazole drug Ro-07-0582. Both compounds have been shown to sensitize a wide range of experimental solid tumors in mice and both are under current clinical investigation.

$$CH_2CH_2OH \qquad\qquad CH_2CH(OH)CH_2OCH_3$$

$$O_2N-\underset{N}{\overset{N}{\bigcirc}}-CH_3 \qquad\qquad \underset{N}{\overset{N}{\bigcirc}}-NO_2$$

Metronidazole Ro-07-0582

4.2. Metronidazole

In 1973, both Foster and Willson and Chapman and colleagues reported that hypoxic Chinese hamster cells were radiation sensitized by the antiflagellant metronidazole, or Flagyl. Figure 6 shows survival data for hypoxic cells irradiated in the presence of 8 mM drug. Sensitization is appreciable, although less than the full oxygen effect. However, the enhancement ratio is unaffected by the presence of full growth medium and, as with PNAP and the nitrofurans, shows little change with the position of the cells in the mitotic cycle. Although metronidazole is only moderately active on a concentration basis, interest was aroused by the relatively long metabolic half-life of the drug in experimental animals, and evidence soon followed of its sensitizing activity *in vivo*.

Denekamp *et al.* (1974) used the artificially hypoxic mouse skin system (see Section 3.2.2) and demonstrated enhancement ratios of up to 1.6 with 2 mg/mouse of the drug (see Fig. 10). No sensitization was found when the mice

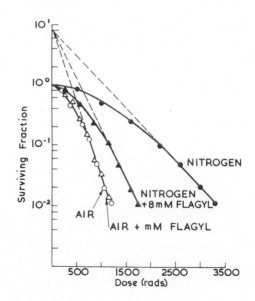

FIGURE 6. Survival data for hypoxic Chinese hamster V79-GL1 cells irradiated *in vitro* with X-rays in the presence of 1 and 10 mM metronidazole. Data from Asquith *et al.* (1974).

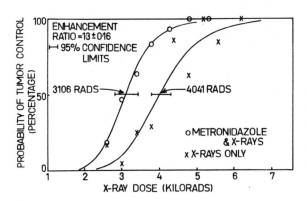

FIGURE 7. Proportion of C3H mice with transplanted mammary tumors cured as a fraction of X-ray dose. Right curve, X-rays only; left curve, X-rays given 30 min after intraperitoneal administration of 1 mg/g metronidazole. From Begg *et al.* (1974).

were breathing air or when the drug was administered 5 min after irradiation under hypoxia.

Studies were extended to include solid mouse tumors. Sensitization was demonstrated in several systems in which various endpoints were used, including local control, tumor-regrowth delay, and assay of surviving cell fraction. Figure 7 shows an example of improvement of local cure in a transplantable C3H mouse mammary tumor irradiated with single doses of radiation after administration of 2.5 mg/g of metronidazole 30 min before irradiation. The reduction in the TCD_{50}, i.e., the dose required to cure 50% of the tumors, represents an enhancement ratio of 1.3 (Begg *et al.*, 1974). The sensitization generally observed in a range of mouse tumors led to preliminary clinical evaluation of the drug; the current status of these studies is discussed later in this chapter. However, the very large doses of drug required to produce sensitization *in vivo* prompted a search for more active nitroimidazoles. Theoretical consideration led to investigation *in vitro* of the 2-nitroimidazoles, and several of these compounds were found to be more active than metronidazole (Asquith *et al.*, 1974b). One of these was the Roche compound Ro-07-0582, synthesized originally as a prototype antiflagellant.

4.3. The 2-Nitroimidazole Ro-07-0582

4.3.1. In Vitro

Figure 8 illustrates the sensitization of cultured Chinese hamster V79 cells irradiated *in vitro* in the presence of 1 and 10 mM 0582 (data from Adams *et al.*, 1976). These and other data (Asquith *et al.*, 1974b; Hall and Roizin-Towle, 1975) show that the sensitization efficiency of 0582 is considerably greater than that of metronidazole (about 5–10 on a concentration basis). Further, the enhancement ratio for 10 mM 0582 approaches that of the full oxygen effect. Like metronidazole, sensitization is unaffected by the presence of serum protein in the irradiation medium, is absent in aerated cells, and is virtually independent of the position of the cells in the mitotic cycle (Asquith *et al.*, 1974b).

While, in general, the sensitization of mammalian cells by the electron-affinic sensitizers, including 0582, appears to mimic the sensitizing effect of oxygen,

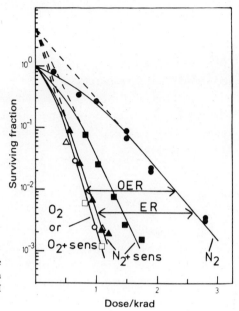

FIGURE 8. Survival data for hypoxic Chinese hamster V79-379A cells irradiated *in vitro* with X-rays in the presence of 1 mM (■) and 10 mM (▲) Ro-07-0582. Data from Adams *et al.* (1976).

there are some differences. One of the most striking of these relates to the phenomenon of repair of sublethal damage. Hall and Roizin-Towle investigated the effect of 0582 on the survival of hypoxic V79 cells irradiated with split doses of ^{60}Co γ-irradiation. Oxic cells were irradiated in oxygen with either 1200 rads in a single dose or two separate 600-rad doses separated by 1, 2, 3, or 4 hrs. The cells irradiated in two fractions showed the expected high survival consistent with repair of sublethal damage occurring between fractions. Figure 9 shows the recovery factor as a function of the time interval between the two fractions. Under oxic conditions, repair occurs efficiently in that two doses of 600 rads separated by 4 hr result in a surviving fraction 3 times as large as that following a single dose of 1200 rads. In air, the recovery factor is unaffected by the presence of 1 mM 0582.

In hypoxia, where the cells are irradiated with a single dose of 4000 rads, the survival is the same as that found when the radiation dose is split into two fractions

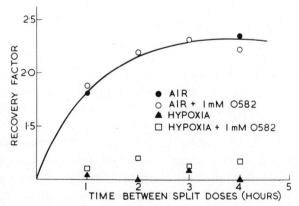

FIGURE 9. Recovery factor for V79 cells irradiated under aerobic and hypoxic conditions in the presence of 1.0 mM Ro-07-0582. Aerobic: single dose of 1200 rads compared with two single doses of 600 rads separated by various intervals. Hypoxic: single dose of 4000 rads compared with two fractions. From Hall *et al.* (1975).

of 2000 rads, confirming that repair of sublethal damage does not occur under hypoxic conditions. Similar experiments were carried out in hypoxia with 0582 present. Within the limits of experimental error, the surviving fraction following irradiation with two fractions of 2000 rads was the same as that found for a single 4000-rad dose irrespective of the time interval between fractions. Thus, at a concentration of 1 mM 0582, repair of sublethal damage is almost completely inhibited, i.e., at a concentration sufficient to mimic about 60% of the oxygen effect on cell killing. Thus 0582 does *not* mimic oxygen with respect to the repair of sublethal damage.

4.3.2. Sensitization in Vivo

4.3.2a. Hypoxic Mouse Skin. Figure 10 shows data of Denekamp *et al.* (1974) on the comparative sensitizing efficiencies of 0582 and metronidazole in the hypoxic mouse skin system (see Section 3.2.2). Over the dose range of 0.1–1.25 mg/g body weight for 0582, the enhancement ratio rises from 1.4 to 2.2. Over a comparable dose range for metronidazole, the enhancement ratio would be only 1.2–1.3. The greater sensitizing efficiency of 0582 confirms the findings in the *in vitro* systems. As with metronidazole, no sensitization was found when 0582 was given to O_2-breathing mice before irradiation or when the drug was administered a short time after irradiation under hypoxia.

4.3.2b. Solid Mouse Tumors. The *in vivo* mouse tumor systems used to investigate radiosensitization by 0582 have covered a wide range of histological type, growth rate, and proportion of hypoxic cells. Several methods of assessing tumor response have been used, including regrowth delay, local control (i.e., cure), resection of the tumor for cell dilution assays, and loss of activity from tumors containing cells labeled with [125]IUdR. Sensitization experiments are usually designed to determine the ratio of two X-ray doses, one given with the sensitizer present, the other without, which produce the same biological effect on the tumor. This ratio is often called the enhancement ratio of gain factor, but it is strictly a dose-reduction factor for a given degree of tumor response.

As was discussed in Section 2.2, tumor response to radiation has two components because the tumor contains both sensitive oxygenated cells and resistant hypoxic cells. At low single doses of X-rays, tumor response is mainly that of the oxic fraction, but at higher doses when most of the oxic cells have been killed, the tumor becomes more resistant as the hypoxic cells predominate.

It is convenient to review the current status of hypoxic cell sensitization by 0582 *in vivo* according to the method of assay of tumor response.

Tumor Growth Delay: Figure 11 shows some typical results for the sensitizing effect of 0582 on the mouse transplantable carcinoma NT (Denekamp and Harris, 1975). Growth of the tumor is delayed for about 20 days following a single-dose X-irradiation of 2000 rads. When 0582 (or metronidazole) is given before irradiation, the delay is increased. For 1 mg/g 0582, the delay is 35 days. Similar

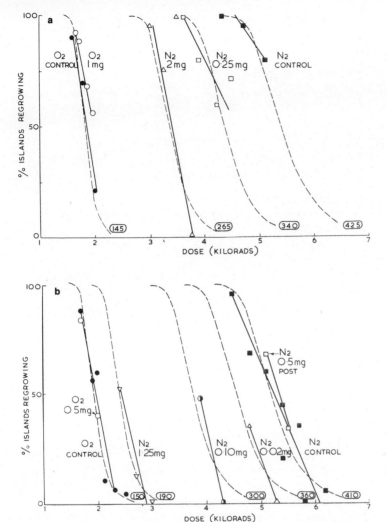

FIGURE 10. Response of mouse epidermal cells to radiation (Denekamp *et al.* 1974). Skin irradiated in mice breathing nitrogen for 35 sec before and during irradiation is 2.5 times less sensitive compared to that in oxygen-breathing mice. Sensitivity is partly restored if (a) metronidazole or (b) Ro-07-0582 is administered before hypoxic irradiation. No effect in oxygen.

regrowth curves were obtained for a range of X-ray doses given after different doses of 0582 to batches of mice. Figure 12 shows the plots of delay as a function of X-ray dose for 1 mg/g 0582 given before irradiation. The figure shows the response of "normal" tumors in mice, and also tumors where the blood supply was clamped off before and during irradiation in order to make them uniformly hypoxic. In the clamped tumors, the observed enhancement ratio is 2.1 for all levels of damage. For the unclamped tumors, the enhancement ratio is low for doses below 1200 rads, since under these conditions the aerobic cells are dominating the response. At higher radiation doses, the ratio reaches 2.1, i.e., the same

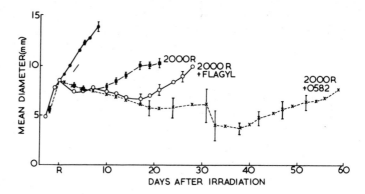

FIGURE 11. Regrowth curves for mouse carcinoma NT irradiated with single doses of X-rays. Drug dose 1 mg/g. From Denekamp and Harris (1975).

level as for the clamped tumors. These results show that the sensitizer is just as effective on the naturally occurring hypoxic cells in the tumor as it is on the previously aerobic tumor cells rendered temporarily hypoxic by clamping. These cells probably lie close to capillaries. The smooth curves for the sensitized tumors (above 1200 rads) indicate that the sensitizer reaches *all* the hypoxic tumor cells

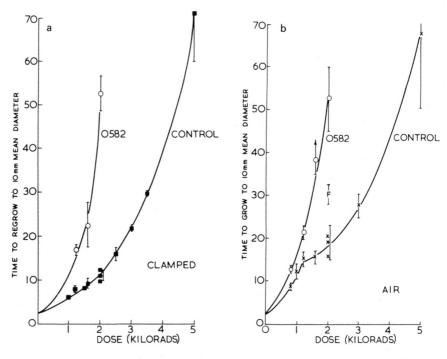

FIGURE 12. Dose-response curves for regrowth delay in irradiated mouse carcinoma NT in the presence of 1 mg/g Ro-07-0582. (a) Tumors clamped off before irradiation to make all cells hypoxic. (b) Tumors in air-breathing mice. From Denekamp and Harris (1975).

since the presence of unsensitized cells would be revealed by "break points" in the curves.

Cell Assay Methods: All cell assay methods involve irradiation of a mouse tumor *in vivo*, subsequent excision of the tumor, preparation of serially diluted cell suspensions, and assay of the surviving fraction of the cell population by various methods. One method developed by Hewitt and Wilson (1959) is to inject serially diluted cells into mice of the same line and assay the frequency of tumor takes: a cell survival curve can be constructed from the results. This method was used (Hewitt and Blake, 1970) to investigate sensitization by the nitroxyl free radical tri-acetoneamine-*N*-oxyl (TAN) on anoxic leukemia cells irradiated *in situ* in the infiltrated livers of leukemic mice. No sensitization was observed in spite of the favorable conditions provided by this system for the detection and measurement of sensitization. However, when 0582 was used (0.44 mg/g), Hewitt and Blake (1974) obtained an enhancement ratio of 1.7 with this system. The very short lifetime of the nitroxyls *in vivo* (Hill *et al.*, 1975) is probably responsible for the negative results found for this type of sensitizer (Hewitt and Blake, 1970; Olive *et al.*, 1972).

The surviving cell population of an irradiated tumor can sometimes be assessed by *in vitro* culture of serially diluted suspensions prepared from the excised tumor. This method has been used by several workers to measure sensitization by 0582, particularly in the mouse tumor system EMT6.

Figure 13 shows survival data for the tumor X-irradiated 30 min after intraperitoneal administration of 1 mg/g 0582 (Bleehen, 1976). Comparison of the survival curve for air-breathing mice (open circles) with that obtained when

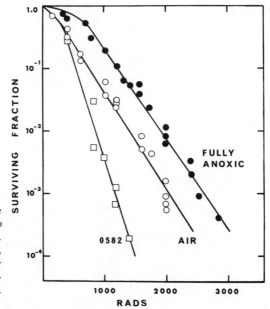

FIGURE 13. Radiation dose-response curve for EMT6 mouse tumor irradiated *in vivo* and assayed *in vitro* for surviving fraction. ●, Mice killed and irradiated in nitrogen; ○, mice breathing air; □, mice breathing air and given 1 mg/g Ro-07-0582, intra-peritoneally 30 min before irradiation. From Bleehen (1976).

the tumor-bearing mice are killed before irradiation (i.e., all tumor cells are rendered hypoxic) shows that the tumor normally contains about 20% hypoxic cells. When 1 mg/g 0582 is administered before irradiation (open squares), the survival curve is much steeper. The enhancement ratio calculated from the ratio of the linear portion of the survival curve is about 2.2.

Brown (1975) used the same tumor system to measure sensitization by both metronidazole and 0582. The enhancement ratios expressed again as the ratios of the linear portion of the survival curves are dependent on both drug dose and, significantly, the timing between administration of the drugs and irradiation (see Section 5). For 1 mg/g metronidazole given 30 min before the start of the irradiations, the ER is 1.84, one of the highest values obtained with this drug. The ratio falls to 1.61 when the contact time is reduced to 10 min. Sensitization with 0582 is again greater than with metronidazole. Overall enhancement ratios range

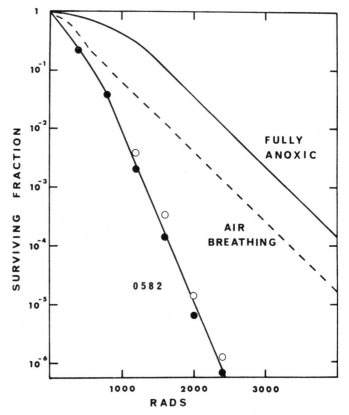

FIGURE 14. Sensitization of hypoxic cells in irradiated KHT mouse tumors. Survival assayed by the lung colony technique. – – –, Survival curve for tumors in air-breathing mice; ———, survival curve for fully hypoxic tumors; ○, ●, duplicate survival data for tumors in air-breathing mice irradiated 1 hr after administration of 1.5 mg/g Ro-07-0582. Data from Rauth and Kaufman (1975 and private communication).

from 1.17 for the very low dose of 0.025 mg/g up to 2.4–3.1 for doses between 0.1 and 1.2 mg/g.

McNally (1975) used a similar cell dilution assay system to study sensitization by 0582 of a transplantable mouse sarcoma. Sensitization is obtained for all levels of cell survival below 10^{-1}, and the effect increases with drug concentration. For 0.2 and 1.0 mg/g doses of 0582, the enhancement ratios are about 1.3 and 2.2, respectively.

One of the most sensitive cell-assay systems for measurement of tumor response *in vivo* was that developed by Hill and Bush (1969). In this method, the serially diluted cell suspensions prepared from the excised tumor are injected into recipient mice and the cell survival is measured by the number of tumor nodules which appear in the lungs. Figure 14 shows sensitization data obtained by Rauth and co-workers (Rauth and Kaufman, 1975; Rauth *et al.*, 1975) using this system. The dotted line in the figure is the normal survival curve applicable to tumors in air-breathing mice. The upper solid line is that obtained for fully hypoxic tumors obtained when the mice are killed shortly before irradiation. The lateral displacement of the curve indicates a normal hypoxic cell fraction in the tumor of about 10%. In the live mice, Milne *et al.* (1973) found that administration of excess oxygen produced little or no sensitization. Rauth's data are in sharp contrast. Administration of 1 mg/g 0582 at 1 hr before irradiation causes considerable sensitization, with an enhancement ratio of over 2. Significantly, down to the limit of the considerable sensitivity of the system (about 10^{-6} surviving fraction), there is no evidence whatsoever of a break point in the survival curve. If present, such a break point would indicate that not all of the hypoxic cells were sensitized. This result emphasizes the great advantage of this type of sensitizer over that of administered oxygen. The rate of metabolism is sufficiently slow to permit diffusion of the sensitizer to *all* hypoxic cells.

4.3.2c. Assay of Tumor Cure. Measurement of tumor response by local control is, in some respects, the most realistic method from the viewpoint of present and future applications of sensitizers in the clinic. Figure 15 shows some data of Sheldon *et al.* (1974) on sensitization by 0582 of first-generation transplants of spontaneous mammary tumors in C3H mice. These results can be compared with those obtained using metronidazole in the same tumor system. The tumors were irradiated with single doses of X-rays while at a diameter of 6.5 ± 1 mm, with the drug given 30 min before the start of the irradiation. The ordinate gives the proportion of tumors locally controlled, i.e., tumors which did not recur within 150 days. The ratio of the doses required to cure 50% of the tumors (TCD_{50}) indicates an enhancement ratio of 1.8 under these conditions. This means that the use of the drug can increase the cure rate, for example, at a dose of 3200 rads, from 10% to about 90%. Further, the dose–response curve for X-rays with 0582 is considerably steeper than the control curve, almost in the ratio of 1.8, suggesting that also in these experiments the drug reached and sensitized all the hypoxic cells in the tumors.

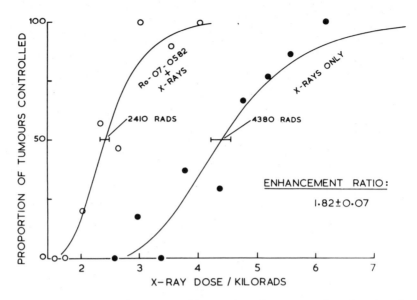

FIGURE 15. Proportion of C3H mice with transplanted tumors cured as a function of X-ray dose. Dose of Ro-07-0582 1 mg/g. From Sheldon *et al.* (1974).

Similar data have been obtained for a radiation-resistant transplantable anaplastic tumor MT in WHT/Ht mice (Sheldon and Hill, 1976). It was found that single-dose irradiation after drug doses of 0.1, 0.3, and 1.0 mg/g body weight gave enhancement ratios of 1.4, 1.7, and 2.0, respectively.

Brown (1975) measured single-dose enhancement ratios by local control for sensitization of 0582 of the mouse tumor MDAH/MCa4. In the absence of 0582, the TCD_{50} of the tumor is about 7100 rads. When 0.3 mg/g of 0582 was administered 30 min before irradiation, the TCD_{50} dropped to < 4000 rads, indicating an enhancement ratio of > 1.78. For a high drug dose of 1.0 mg/g, the enhancement ratio was 2.30. Enhancement ratios of up to 2.4 have also been reported by Stone and Withers (1975) for local control of this tumor irradiated in the presence of 1 mg/g 0582.

In summary, these large enhancement ratios now found routinely in a large number of different tumor systems (see Table 1 for summary) represent the most effective enhancements of treatment achievable by any agent used in combination with radiation for treatment of cancer in experimental animals. A drug dose of 1 mg/g is outside the range acceptable in man, so it would be expected that sensitization factors achievable in man would be somewhat less. Further, when the radiation is given in a fractionated course of treatment, sensitization might be further reduced. However, based on animal data, quite modest enhancement ratios could lead to a large improvement in the local control of human tumors. Some of the more important criteria that have to be satisfied before sensitizers can be generally applied clinically are discussed in the next section in the light of the laboratory data so far accumulated.

TABLE 1

Sensitization by Ro-07-0582 of Solid Tumors in Mice Irradiated with Single Doses

Assay method	Tumor	Doubling time	Hypoxic fraction	X-ray dose 0.2–0.3 mg/g	Enhancement 1.0 mg/g	References
Cell survival	EMT6	—	20	—	2.2	Bleehen (1976)
	EMT6	—	—	—	2.4–2.9 (for 1.2 mg/g)	Brown(1975)
	WHT MT (anap)	1	50	—	1.6	McNally and Sheldon (1976)
	WHT sq ca D	1	18	—	1.0 (0.4 mg/g +0.4 mg/g)	Hewitt and Blake (1974)
	CBA sarc F	1	10	1.3	2.2	McNally (1975)
	C3H KHT	2	6	—	2.0 (1.5 mg/g)	Rauth and Kaufman (1975)
Regrowth delay	CBA sarc F	1	10	1.0	1.5	Begg (1976)[a]
	CBA ca NT	3	6	—	2.1	Denekamp and Harris (1975)
	Osteosa. C22LR	—	—	—	large (1.2 mg/g)	van Putten and Smink (1976)
Tumor cure	WHT sq ca D	1	18	—	2.0	Hill and Fowler (1976)
	WHT sq ca D (intradermal)	1	0.3	1.9	2.1	Peters (1976)
	WHT MT (anap)	1	50	1.7	2.1	Sheldon and Hill (1976)
	C3H mamm ca	6	10	1.7	1.8	Sheldon et al. (1974)
	C3H mamm ca	—	—	>1.8	2.3	Brown (1975)
	C3H mamm ca	—	—	—	2.4	Stone and Withers (1975)

[a] Also measured by release of ^{127}I from $^{127}IudR$ incorporation.

5. Criteria for the Application of Sensitizers in Radiotherapy

5.1. Differential Sensitization with Respect to Normal Tissue

The basis for the therapeutic value of the nitroimidazoles or other electron-affinic sensitizers is that sensitization is confined to tumor tissue. Since most normal tissues probably do not contain a significant number of hypoxic cells, this criterion would appear to be satisfied.

There is evidence from clinical trials of hyperbaric oxygen indicating a small but significant increase in normal tissue morbidity relative to air. There are sound reasons why this should not occur with hypoxic cell sensitizers. Figure 16 shows a theoretical curve for relating the oxygen enhancement ratio (OER) in irradiated

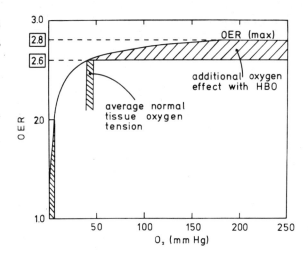

FIGURE 16. Theoretical curve relating OER for irradiated mammalian cells to concentration of oxygen (see text).

mammalian cells to the concentration of oxygen in the tissue. This curve (Howard-Flanders and Alper, 1957) agrees very well with *in vitro* measurements of the OER measured as a function of oxygen concentration in the medium. If this curve applies *in vivo*, then at the average concentration of oxygen in venous blood, i.e., 40 mm Hg, the equivalent OER is about 2.6. Administration of HBO will greatly increase the free oxygen dissolved in the blood, and this should be sufficient to raise the OER of normal tissue cells to the maximum level, i.e., about 2.8. There will, therefore, be an effective increase in radiation sensitivity of about 10%.

Consider the effect on normal tissue radiation sensitivity of a clinical sensitizer present at a concentration sufficient to give rise to an enhancement ratio of 2.0 with respect to anoxic cells. From Fig. 16, sensitization by the drug will be equivalent to that produced by about 10 mm Hg pressure of oxygen. In normal tissue *already* containing 40 mm Hg oxygen, this additional sensitizing capacity will be equivalent to an oxygen tension of about 50 mm Hg (indicated by the double hatched area). The increase in OER will therefore be negligible and no additional sensitization should be apparent. Evidence from the laboratory and the clinic supports this conclusion.

In studies using the clone method of assessing radiation damage in mouse skin, neither 0582 nor metronidazole caused any additional sensitization when administered before irradiation of O_2 breathing mice (Denekamp *et al.*, 1974). Further radiation-induced pigmentation of human skin appears to be unaffected by prior administration of 0582 (Dische *et al.*, 1976) and general clinical experience with both metronidazole and 0582 has so far revealed no sensitization of normal tissue in any site within the irradiated field (Dische, Urtasun, private communications).

5.2. Wide Distribution in Tissues

For a sensitizer to have the greatest value in radiotherapy, it is necessary that the distribution of the drug be in no way limited by tissue specificity. This would enable the sensitizer to be used for the radiation treatment of tumors irrespective of the site of occurrence. In man, information on tissue distribution of either 0582 or metronidazole is not yet available, although it is known that the levels in human plasma show a roughly one-to-one correlation with the average tissue concentration calculated on the basis of body weight dose (Gray *et al.*, 1976).

More information is available from mouse studies. Both 0582 and its reduction products are found to be generally distributed throughout various organs, including skin, brain, liver, and spleen, as well as tumor (Flockhart *et al.*, 1976; Varghese *et al.*, 1976). The question of levels likely to be attainable in human tumors is discussed below.

5.3. Stability with Respect to Tumor Penetration

During the development of hypoxic cell sensitizers suitable for clinical use, it was recognized that an appreciable time might be required for the sensitizer to diffuse out of the tumor blood vessels to the distant hypoxic cells. This requires, therefore, that the sensitizer must not only be capable of wide distribution through different tissues but also be sufficiently stable to metabolic breakdown and have a fairly long clearance time.

Metabolic instability has been the main reason behind the lack of effect *in vivo* of many of the earlier sensitizers, but this is not so for the nitroimidazoles. Clearance of both metronidazole and 0582 from mouse plasma occurs with a half-life of about 1.0–1.5 hr. In man, both drugs are metabolized much more slowly, and overall clearance has a half-life of about 12 hr (Urtasun *et al.*, 1975; Gray *et al.*, 1976). The relative stability of these two drugs is undoubtedly one of the main factors influencing the large sensitization ratios seen in numerous experimental mouse tumors.

However, it is clear from these studies that the doses of drug required to produce a given amount of sensitization in mouse tumors are larger than those predicted from sensitization data *in vitro*, usually by a factor of about 2–4. Further, the degree of sensitization is sometimes critically dependent on the time interval between administration of the drug and radiation treatment of the tumor. In C3H mouse mammary tumors, Brown (1975) and Stone and Withers (1975) observed a greater sensitizing efficiency of 0582 when it was administered 30 min before irradiation compared with that for shorter times. Similarly, Sheldon and Hill (1976) found that the tumor control probability for WHT MT mouse tumors irradiated with a single 5000-rad dose of X-rays at various times following intraperitoneal administration of 0.2 mg/g 0582 rose from about 35% for a 15-min interval up to >90% when this was increased to 45–60 min. For longer intervals, the cure probability then decreased.

A likely reason for these results is that the maximum concentration of 0582 achieved in mouse tumors rarely exceeds about 30–40% of peak plasma levels (Flockhart, private communication). This is probably due to the lifetime in plasma being too short to permit full buildup of the drug in the tumor. If so, then the much longer lifetimes of both metronidazole and 0582 in man (Urtasun *et al.*, 1975; Gray *et al.*, 1976) should enable concentration in tumors to approach that in plasma. For both drugs, biopsy of human tumors shows drug levels in most cases comparable to those in plasma (Urtasun *et al.*, 1975; Dische *et al.*, 1976).

5.4. Acceptable Toxicology

Large-animal toxicological studies have been carried out in dogs and primates using various nitroimidazoles including metronidazole, 0582, and other related 2-nitroimidazoles. Schärer (1972) investigated neurotoxicity in dogs and found that administration of large daily doses of these drugs (50–200 mg/kg) produced ataxia and convulsions and could lead to death. If, however, the drug was stopped at the onset of symptoms, recovery occurred. Histological changes were found indicating degeneration of the Purkinje cells of the cerebellum. However, these changes were not found in mice, rats, guinea pigs, or rabbits given large doses of 400–1000 mg/kg.

Baboons given daily doses of 100 and 200 mg/kg for 28 days tolerated 0582 (Parkes, personal communication). However, 500 mg/kg doses resulted in severe muscular incoordination and incipient convulsions by day 11. There was no evidence of cerebellar lesions, but other brain lesions were found with all three doses. Similarly, Johnson *et al.* (1976) found that doses of 800 mg/kg caused intermittent convulsions and death within 3 days of administration of the drug. In both studies, lower doses were found to be safe and, if applicable in man, were believed to be sufficient to give appreciable sensitization (see Section 6).

Possible carcinogenicity of metronidazole has been investigated in mice and implicated for high doses given throughout life. Rustia and Shubik (1972) administered 100, 250, 500, and 830 mg/kg daily to Swiss albino mice and observed slight increase in the normal incidence of lung tumors, which were predominantly adenomas. At the two highest dose levels, the incidence of lymphomas was approximately doubled in female but not in male mice. This strain has a very high natural incidence of lymphomas. In contrast, Cohen *et al.* (1973) found no carcinogenicity in rats administered 0.14% of diet weight from birth to 66 weeks. More long-term studies with both metronidazole and 0582 would be desirable, although, on the combined evidence, carcinogenicity would not be envisaged to be a serious hazard in the administration of a limited number of doses to patients already suffering from cancer.

5.5. Effectiveness of Sensitization and Position in the Cell Cycle

Little is known so far about the detailed biochemical characteristics of hypoxic cells in mouse or human tumors, although it is reasonable to believe that such cells are in a presynthetic resting phase. It is relevant, therefore, to know how the sensitization efficiencies of electron-affinic sensitizers vary with the position of the cell in the mitotic cycle. Clearly, a sensitizer whose activity is restricted to cells well advanced in the cycle would have little practical value.

The results of *in vitro* studies of sensitization of synchronized cells were discussed earlier (Sections 3.2 and 4.3). While there is evidence that some cycle-dependence can occur in sensitization by compounds other than the strictly electron-affinic type, sensitization by the nitroimidazoles, nitrofurans, and paranitroacetophenone shows very little variation with position in the cycle.

5.6. Sensitization with Fractionated Radiation

In clinical radiotherapy, radiation is given in multiple fractions since the overall therapeutic gain is greater. One reason for this is that some hypoxic cells become reoxygenated between fractions and if the fractionation is such that reoxygenation is optimized in a particular tumor, the hypoxic cells may be eliminated by the X-rays alone without the necessity of using sensitizers. Many of the experimental data for mouse tumors have been obtained using single doses of radiation. It is, therefore, of paramount importance to ascertain in the laboratory whether or not worthwhile gains will still be obtained with sensitizers administered with multi-fraction radiation. Results of mouse tumor studies of sensitization using multif-raction radiation are generally encouraging. Fowler and colleagues have used a C3H mouse mammary tumor to study sensitization by 0582. Figure 17 shows tumor cure data as a function of overall treatment time for one, three, and five fractions of X-rays (Sheldon *et al.*, 1976). For each treatment, the X-ray doses were such that a constant level of skin reaction was produced. Thus the greater the local control probability for the constant amount of normal tissue damage, the greater is the therapeutic ratio. In two of the schedules, i.e., five fractions in 4 or 9 days, the results for X-rays alone were mediocre ($\sim 20\%$ local control). This is probably due to inadequate reoxygenation of hypoxic cells between fractions.

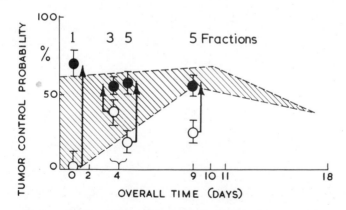

FIGURE 17. Tumor control probability for skin reactions of 1.5 vs. time in days. ●, Ro-07-0582 with X-rays; ○, tumor response without drug present. Vertical arrows show the improvements in tumor control with Ro-07-0582. Shaded area shows range of tumor control probabilities previously obtained with these and other fractionated X-ray schedules for skin reactions of 1.5. Data from Fowler *et al.* (1976).

The vertical arrows show improvement in local control when 0.67 mg/g 0582 was given 30 min before the start of each radiation. For all schedules including the single-dose treatment where, for X-rays alone, no local cures were found, administration of 0582 brings the tumor rate up to about 50–60%. This improvement is similar to that found for similar fractionated treatment with neutrons compared with X-rays alone (Fowler *et al.*, 1976), suggesting that, like neutrons, 0582 can take some of the criticality out of the choice of a fractionation schedule. In the clinic, if the fractionation schedule is such as to optimize reoxygenation for a particular type of tumor, the sensitizer will be less effective. If, however, reoxygenation is inadequate, the remaining hypoxic cells will be sensitized and should lead to a better clinical response.

In other systems, sensitization has been observed with fractionated radiation. Brown (unpublished observations) compared the effect of ten fractions of X-rays given over 9 days with and without 0.3 mg/g 0582 administered 30 min before irradiation. The TCD_{50} values changed from ~ 9700 rads to ~ 7000 rads, indicating a sensitization factor of ~ 1.4.

Denekamp and colleagues measured the effect of 0582 on regrowth delay of irradiated carcinoma NT irradiated with fractionated X-rays (Denekamp and Harris, 1976) or cyclotron neutrons (Denekamp *et al.*, 1976). For a constant level of skin damage (erythema and moist desquamation), about 16 days' delay in tumor growth was observed for a single X-ray dose (Fig. 18). This was increased to 40 days with five fractions over 9 days. More delay still was found when the X-rays were given after administration of 0–67 mg/g 0582 with each fraction. A similar beneficial effect was found for neutron irradiation alone. Significantly, tumors irradiated with a single dose of neutrons following 0582 administration gave a response equivalent to that of multifraction neutrons alone, or multifraction X-rays with 0582. Recently, further gain has been demonstrated for two and five fractions of neutrons given with 0582 (Denekamp, Morris, and Field, unpublished).

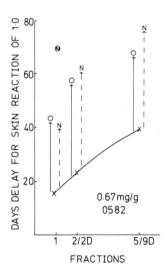

FIGURE 18. Regrowth delay for CBA carcinoma NT for a constant skin reaction irradiated with X: 1, 2, and 5 fractions of X-rays; O: 1, 2, and 5 fractions of X-rays and Ro-07-0582; N: 1, 2, and 5 fractions of neutrons; Ⓝ: single-dose neutrons with Ro-07-0582. From Denekamp and Harris (1976).

Van Putten and Smink (1976) used the poorly reoxygenating mouse osteosarcoma C22LR to investigate by regrowth delay sensitization by 0582 with fractionated X-rays. Single doses of 1000 rads gave an improved response with 1.2 mg/g 0582 1 hr before irradiation. Similarly, 0582 given daily with five fractions of 300 rads gave considerable sensitization, as did a schedule employing 6×800 rad X-rays with 0582, given twice weekly over 3 weeks. Appreciable sensitization was also found for the latter schedule when 0582 was given with the first three X-ray fractions only. However, no overall sensitization was found when the drug was given with daily 300-rad fractions over 3 weeks.

In conclusion, the experimental mouse tumor data available indicate that sensitization occurs with multifraction radiation, although the enhancement ratios are smaller than for single-dose irradiation. With the limited amount of either experimental or clinical data available, there is little point in speculating about fractionation regimes which will optimize hypoxic cell sensitization in radiotherapy, although there are some grounds for anticipating that unconventional regimes utilizing relatively few large-dose fractionations may prove to be the most valuable.

6. Clinical Studies

6.1. Metronidazole

Some preliminary phase 1 studies using single doses of metronidazole in conjunction with radiation were started in 1974 in two centers, Mount Vernon Hospital, Northwood, Middlesex, England (Deutsch *et al.*, 1975), and The Cross Cancer Institute, Edmonton, Canada (Urtasun *et al.*, 1974, 1975, 1976). The early studies were designed primarily to establish minimum safe drug doses and showed that patients could tolerate up to about 300 mg/g (10–15 g) administered orally in a single dose. The upper limit was set by nausea and vomiting.

The peak concentration in the plasma was found to be proportional to dose over the range 80–300 mg/kg and was reached about 1–2 hr after administration provided that the patient had no food during the previous 3 hr. If food had been taken, the peak level was lower and occurred later: the half-life was about 12 hr. Blood count and liver function were normal.

With multiple doses, Urtasun *et al.* (1975) found that patients could usually tolerate 2.5 g/m^2 (about 4 g) daily for 2–4 weeks and somewhat higher doses, 6 g/m^2, administered two or three times weekly for 3 weeks. However, nausea was a problem in some patients. Bush (private communication) has also given 3 g of metronidazole daily to several patients, including one for 24 days and another for 36 days.

Urtasun has extended his studies to include a phase II randomized clinical trial using ^{60}Co γ-radiation and multiple doses of metronidazole to treat supratentorial glioblastoma (Urtasum *et al.*, 1976). The main purpose of this study was to evaluate the effectiveness of metronidazole as a sensitizer, using survival times as the endpoint. Glioblastoma was chosen because of the very high failure rate.

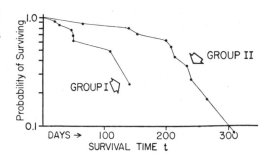

FIGURE 19. Kaplan–Meier survival plots for trial of human glioblastomas treated with metronidazole and radiation. From Urtasun *et al.* (1976).

A total of 36 patients were entered into the trial and five were subsequently withdrawn. Of the remainder, 15 received radiation alone and 16 radiation with metronidazole. Patients were treated with 3000 rads in nine fractions in an overall time of 18 days (1288 rets). Metronidazole (6 g/m²) was given 4 hr before each radiation treatment, and no food was permitted for 7 hours prior to drug administration. The peak plasma levels at 4 hr were 180–200 μg/ml, i.e., > 1 mM.

The difference in survival between the two groups is shown in Fig. 19 as actuarial plots of the probability of surviving to time t as a function of t. The curves for the two groups are significantly different at the $P = 0.02$ level, with the metronidazole group giving the longer survival time by about 4.5 months.

In this study, the unconventional fractionation regime gave a somewhat shorter survival for the radiation-alone group than has been achieved with some other treatment schedules. However, the significant improvement in survival time in the metronidazole group is convincing evidence that the radiation response of the tumor is affected by the presence of radiation-resistant hypoxic cells. It is to be hoped that the improvement will be maintained when metronidazole is used with other radiation treatment schedules (Urtasun, work in progress).

6.2. Ro-07-0582: Single-Dose Studies

6.2.1. Tolerance

In preliminary work at Mount Vernon Hospital, up to 4 g of Ro-07-0582 was given to normal volunteers. Plasma levels as high as 63 μg/ml (about 0.32 mM) were achieved, and the volunteers showed few side effects (Foster *et al.*, 1975). This was followed by the administration of between 4 and 10 g of the drug to eight patients who each received radiotherapy about 4 hr thereafter (Gray *et al.*, 1976). Peak plasma levels in excess of 100 μg/ml were obtained in all patients; in five patients, levels were equal to or greater than 200 μg/ml. Levels of this order in hypoxic cells in tumors give very large enhancement ratios. The clearance rate indicated an average half-life of approximately 12 hr, i.e., similar to that observed with metronidazole. Again, like metronidazole, the plasma levels at 4 hr showed an approximately linear relationship with body-weight dose except that for the patient given the highest dose. Here, the plasma level was unusually high

($\sim$400 μg/g) (Gray *et al.*, 1976). The drug concentrations in the tumors were measured following biopsy in five patients and gave values relative to plasma of 92%, 70%, 64%, 14%, and 12%. The last two samples were very sclerotic, which made it difficult to extract and measure accurately the drug concentration.

The immediate symptoms limiting drug dose were anorexia, nausea, and vomiting. At this point, it was felt that a dose of about 120 mg/kg would be a practical dose.

6.2.2. Sensitization

Seven of the patients with measurable multiple metastases were assessed for evidence of sensitization (Thomlinson *et al.*, 1976). The delay imposed on the growth of tumor was compared to that of tumor in the same patient treated with radiation alone. Two patients died before any response could be assessed, but qualitative evidence from a further three patients suggested some enhancement of radiation response in two, but not in the third. In one, a patient with multiple pulmonary metastases from carcinoma of the breast, no enhancement was seen.

The most striking result came from a patient with multiple subcutaneous metastases from a carcinoma of the cervix. Measurement of two groups of seven nodules showed a significant difference ($P = 0.05$) in the time of regrowth after single doses of 960 rads and 1120 rads, giving a measure of the discriminatory sensitivity of the system. In a third group of seven nodules treated with 800 rads combined with a 4-g dose of 0582, the regrowth was similar to that after 960 rads alone, indicating a dose enhancement factor of 1.2. In another patient, there was evidence of enhancement, although this did not reach significance in the period of survival of the patient.

An enhancement ratio of 1.2 represents a large degree of sensitization of the hypoxic cells since, for a single dose of only 800 rads, much of the radiation would be spent in sterilizing the oxic cellular component.

6.2.3. Human Skin Studies

To determine whether 0582 would sensitize hypoxic cells in man, Dische *et al.* (1976) used a radiostrontium plaque to irradiate with single doses of 800–1100 rads small test areas in the skin of some patients already receiving the drug with radiotherapy. It was found that the degree of late pigmentation was closely related to dose. When the limb was rendered temporarily hypoxic by tourniquet, about 2000 rads were required to produce the same degree of pigmentation as that following 1000 rads in oxic skin. Ro-07-0582 greatly increased radiation response in the temporarily hypoxic skin, but did not significantly affect that under oxic conditions. The effectiveness of the drug in restoring the sensitivity of the hypoxic skin relative to that of oxic skin can be expressed as a percentage of the oxygen effect measured in the same limb. In the six patients given a variable dose of 0582, the values ranged from 27 to 71%; in three patients given metronidazole, the values were 11–14%.

6.2.4. Multiple Doses of Ro-07-0582

In a recent study (Dische *et al.*, 1977), multiple doses of 0582 were given with radiotherapy to 16 patients with advanced disease. They each received a total dose of from 15 to 51 g in 3–20 doses. Immediate tolerance was good, and consistently satisfactory plasma levels of the drug were obtained. However, neurotoxicity was troublesome. The first patient was given 120 mg/kg repeated six times over 3 weeks, with a six-fraction regime, but at the end of treatment he developed a severe neurotoxicity. Fifteen further patients received lower doses (15–32.5 g total) in from 3–20 doses. However, about 75% of these patients developed a peripheral neuropathy of varying degrees of severity. Some patients received daily doses for 20 days; other received 4–6 doses over 3 weeks. The neurotoxicity appeared to be critically dependent on total dose, and, at the present time, a maximum safe dose in the region of 300 mg/kg or 12 g/m² is indicated.

Analysis of drug concentration in tumor specimens were obtained from two patients 2, 4, and 6 hr after administration of 0582. In one patient, biopsies were performed after five separate treatments in a six-fraction schedule. Drug levels in most instances were close to plasma levels (see Fig. 20).

Figure 21 shows the relationship between enhancement ratios and 0582 concentration for X-irradiation of Chinese hamster cells *in vitro*. On the basis that this curve is applicable to hypoxic cells in human tumors, Dische *et al.* (1977) estimated the enhancement ratios that might be attainable clinically with safe drug dosages. These ratios are ∼1.65 for twice-weekly administration over 3 weeks. For single doses or for a few doses given with longer periods in between, the ratios would be higher.

If these estimates are correct, then the degree of overall benefit should be considerable even allowing for reduction in the overall enhancement ratio due to reoxygenation between fractions.

7. Future Developments

7.1. Differential Toxicity to Hypoxic Cells

Electron-affinic sensitizers are considerably more toxic to hypoxic cells than to normal mammalian cells. This property, first reported for metronidazole by Sutherland (1974) using the multicellular spheroid system, has considerable implications for selective cancer chemotherapy on noncycling cells. This effect is also found in hypoxic single cells *in vitro* (Mohindra and Rauth, 1976) and in mouse tumors containing hypoxic cells (Begg *et al.*, 1974; Inch *et al.*, 1976; Foster *et al.*, 1976; Brown, 1976). Some other electron-affinic sensitizers show this differential toxicity *in vitro*, including 0582 (Hall and Roizin-Towle, 1975; Moore *et al.*, 1976; Stratford and Adams, 1977) and a nitrofuran (Nifurazone) (Mohindra and Rauth, 1976). Further, for 0582, there is a particularly marked effect of temperature on the differential toxicity (Stratford and Adams, 1977; Hall and Biaglow, 1976) i.e., at 41°C the slope of the survival vs. contact time plot with 1 mM

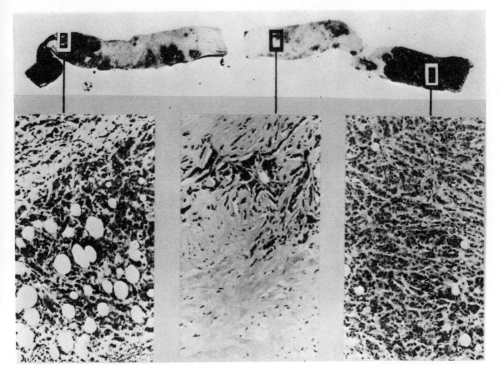

FIGURE 20. Histological study of biopsy specimen (36 mm) from human breast tumor 6 hr after administration of Ro-07-0582. The specimen was divided into three sections. The two outer sections are magnified ×6 (above); selected areas are magnified ×120. (Reduced 18% for reproduction.) At the margins, the tumor is densely cellular without evidence of necrosis. Near center, tumor cells appear to be surviving only around blood vessels, and much of the material consists of fibrous tissue. Center section showed a mean concentration of 79 μg/g, which was 99% of the plasma level at that time. From Dische *et al.* (1977).

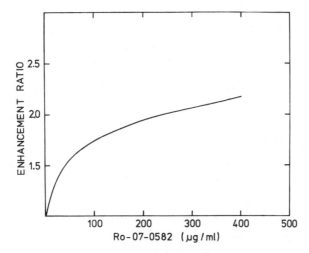

FIGURE 21. Sensitization of hypoxic Chinese hamster cells: enhancement ratio vs. concentration for Ro-07-0582. Data for V79 cells irradiated *in vitro*. From Adams *et al.* (1976).

0582 increases twofold relative to that at 37°C. This enhancement of hypoxic cell toxicity with hyperthermia has also been observed in solid tumors in mice given 1 mg/g 0582 (Bleehen *et al.*, 1976; George *et al.*, 1977).

Also related to the effect of metronidazole on hypoxic cells is the finding of Biaglow and colleagues (Durand and Biaglow, 1976; Nygaard and Biaglow, 1975; Biaglow and Durand, 1976) that sensitizers, depending on their electron affinity, can either inhibit or accelerate oxygen respiration. For compounds of relatively low electron affinity, i.e., metronidazole, respiration is considerably inhibited, and it is concluded that this contributes to the overall effect of metronidazole in eliminating hypoxic cells in small multicellular spheroids by extending the diffusion distance of oxygen. Implications of this interesting observation to the use of metronidazole or other sensitizers in combination cancer therapy are obvious, particularly in view of the finding that very small tumors in mice have been shown to contain hypoxic cells (Suith and Maeda, 1967; Shipley *et al.*, 1976).

7.2. Combination of Sensitizers and High-LET Radiation

Since the relative radioresistance of hypoxic cells is reduced with radiations of high LET due to the decrease in OER, it might be expected that sensitization by the oxygen-mimetic sensitizers could also increase. Hall *et al.* (1975) showed that the OER for hypoxic V79 cells irradiated with ~ 15 MeV neutrons falls from 1.5 to 1.25 in the presence of 10 mM metronidazole. This corresponds to a reduction in the sensitizer enhancement ratio for hypoxic cells from ~ 1.7 to 1.2. Consistent with these results, McNally (1976) found that the ER for 5 mM 0582 was reduced from 2.3 for X-irradiated V79 cells to 1.6 when the cells were irradiated with neutrons from a 2 MeV Van de Graaff generator.

Similar effects have been found in other sensitization experiments using radiation beams of various LET values. Raju *et al.* (1976) irradiated mammalian cells in the presence of 0.4 mM 0582 with 250 kVp X-rays and with a mixed dose of 15% α-particles from a ^{258}Pu source and 85% X-rays. For the latter radiation quality, the OER was 1.6, and in both cell lines the hypoxic cells were sensitized by 0582, giving a further reduction in the OER.

Sensitization of V79 cells by metronidazole, 0582, and a related 2-nitroimidazole, Ro-07-0741, has been studied with a wide range of high-LET beams from the high-energy installations at Berkeley (Chapman *et al.*, 1976). The radiations used were (1) X-rays (250 kV), (2) He ions (230 MeV/n), (3) C ions (400 MeV/n), (4) Ne ions (400 MeV/n), and (5) Ar ions (500 MeV/n). The associated OERs measured at the 10% survival level were, respectively, 2.8, 2.3, 1.7, 1.6, and 1.4. Sensitization of hypoxic cells was observed for all three compounds, and, argon ions excepted, the enhancement ratios when expressed as a percentage reduction of the appropriate value of the OER appeared to be fairly independent of radiation quality.

Since toxicity at present limits the doses of sensitizer that can be used clinically to levels that decrease but do not entirely remove the full oxygen effect, these results hold promise that sensitizers should give an even greater therapeutic benefit when used in conjunction with high-LET radiation.

7.3. Shoulder Effects

In vitro studies appear to show that most electron-affinic sensitizers are dose modifying in behavior. However, in a detailed series of investigations, including studies with 0582 (Révèscz and Littbrand, 1976), Révèscz and colleagues have given evidence that for *severely* hypoxic cells there is little if any shoulder on the radiation survival curve. This implies that, for low doses, the oxygen effect is very small. A similar lack of sensitization was found for 0582 under these conditions. If such extreme hypoxia occurs in solid tumors, it would follow from these results that little sensitization would occur with multifraction schedules using very small doses per fraction. However, Hall and Roizin-Towle (1975) found no shoulder loss for cells irradiated with 0582 when severe hypoxia was induced by oxygen respiration.

Whitmore and Wong (private communication) have obtained evidence suggesting that low dose-per-pulse fractionation might be advantageous. Cells incubated with 0582 for several hours before irradiation in hypoxia showed a survival curve with a reduced shoulder. The shoulder for oxic cells with 0582 remained unchanged. If this were to apply for hypoxic cells in human tumors, then the use of many small fractions could result in even greater sensitization. A differential effect on the shoulder of the hypoxic survival curve has also been observed for diamide (Harris and Power, 1973) and for a nitroxyl sensitizer (Cooke *et al.*, 1976). This general area is one of some priority in mechanistic studies with sensitizers.

7.4. Mechanisms and the Search for New Drugs

There is little doubt that electron-affinic sensitizers act, at least in part, by very fast free-radical processes. The oxygen effect itself is free radical in nature, and studies with bacterial spores (Powers and Tallentire, 1968), and mammalian cells (Shenoy *et al.*, 1975) indicate that more than one process is involved. Many radiation-chemical studies, usually by pulse radiolysis, have shown that sensitizers can undergo both addition and oxidation reactions with "target" free radicals produced in vital molecules within the cell, either by direct radiation action or via the mediation of radiolysis of intracellular water (Adams, 1968; Wilson and Emmerson, 1970; Greenstock *et al.*, 1970, 1973; Chapman *et al.*, 1973a, 1974; Willson *et al.*, 1974). There is no point, because of space limitations, in attempting to review the many and often conflicting lines of evidence regarding the precise molecular, radiation-chemical, or biochemical mechanism or mechanisms involved in hypoxic cell sensitization. However, it is clear from all these basic molecular studies that electron affinity is by far the dominant property affecting sensitization efficiency in mammalian cells *in vitro*. Naturally, the relationship has been of great value in studying structure-activity relationships in a broad range of chemical

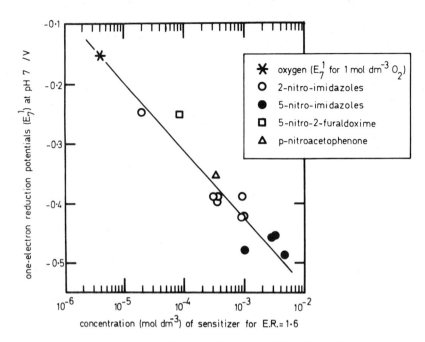

FIGURE 22. Dependence of sensitization efficiency for V79 cells irradiated *in vitro* on electron affinity expressed as one-electron reduction potentials. From Adams *et al.* (1976).

compounds. As discussed earlier, one-electron redox potentials are a fairly accurate measure of the electron affinities of chemical radiosensitizers.

Figure 22 shows the sensitizing efficiencies of various sensitizers, including nitroimidazoles, for hypoxic Chinese hamster V79 cells plotted as a function of their one-electron redox potentials (Adams *et al.*, 1976). The efficiencies are arbitrarily expressed as the concentration of sensitizer required to give a common enhancement ratio of 1.6. The plot includes data for oxygen, a nitrofuran, paranitroacetophenone, and both 2- and 5-nitroimidazoles. The implications of the correlation, which holds over about a 2000-fold range of efficiencies, are considerable. Sensitizing efficiencies *in vitro* should be reasonably predictable provided that no other factors are involved in the sensitization phenomenon.

The octanol/water partition coefficients for the compounds in Fig. 22 vary by a factor of about 300, suggesting that lipophilicity may not be an important factor affecting sensitization *in vitro*. However, *in vivo*, it may be very important, both for the rate at which sensitizers penetrate to the distant hypoxic cells in tumors and for the pharmacokinetics of the drugs. In particular, lipophilicity may be a factor influencing the neurotoxicity of these drugs.

Much remains to be done. However, the existence of a theoretical basis for relating structure and redox properties with sensitizing efficiencies provides at least one foundation for the search for sensitizers with even greater therapeutic ratios.

ADAMS, G. E., 1968, Pulse radiolysis in radiobiology: Some recent studies on model systems, in: *Radiation Chemistry of Aqueous systems* (G. STEIN, ed.), pp. 289–308, Weizman New Science Press with Interscience, New York.

ADAMS, G. E., 1972, Radiation chemical mechanisms in radiation biology, in: *Advances in Radiation Chemistry*, Vol. 3 (M. BURTON AND J. L. MAGEE, eds.), pp. 125–207, Wiley, New York.

ADAMS, G. E., COOKE, M. S., AND MICHAEL, B. D., 1968, Rapid-mixing in radiobiology, *Nature* **219:**1368.

ADAMS, G. E., AND COOKE, M. S., 1969, Electron-affinic sensitization. I. A structural basis for chemical radiosensitizers in bacteria, *Int. J. Radiat. Biol.* **15:**457.

ADAMS, G. E., AND DEWEY, D. L., 1963, Hydrated electrons and radiobiological sensitization, *Biochem. Biophys. Res. Commun.* **12:**473.

ADAMS, G. E., ASQUITH, J. C., DEWEY, D. L., FOSTER, J. L., MICHAEL, B. D., AND WILLSON, R. L., 1971, Electron-affinic sensitization. II. Paranitroacetophenone, a radiosensitizer for anoxic bacterial and mammalian cells, *Int. J. Radiat. Biol.* **19:**575.

ADAMS, G. E., ASQUITH, J. C., WATTS, M. E., AND SMITHEN, C. E., 1972, Radiosensitization of hypoxic cells *in vitro*, a water-soluble derivative of *p*-nitroacetophenone, *Nature (London) New Biol.* **239:**23.

ADAMS, G. E., FLOCKHART, I. R., SMITHEN, C. E., STRATFORD, I. J., WARDMAN, P., AND WATTS, M. E., 1976, Electron-affinic sensitization. VII. A correlation between structures, one-electron reduction potentials and efficiencies of some nitroimidazoles as hypoxic cell radiosensitizers, *Radiat. Res.* **67:**9.

ARAI, S., AND DORFMAN, L. M., 1968, Rate constants and equilibrium constants for electron transfer reactions of aromatic molecules in solution, *Adv. Chem. Ser.* **82:**378.

ASHWOOD-SMITH, M. J., BARNES, J., HUCKLE, J., AND BRIDGES, B. A., 1970, Radiosensitization of bacterial and mammalian cells with carbonyl compounds and ketoaldehydes with special reference to the properties of phenylglyoxal, in: *Radiation Protection and Sensitization* (H. L. MOROSON AND M. QUINTILIANI, eds.), pp. 183–188, Taylor and Francis, London.

ASQUITH, J. C., FOSTER, J. L., WILLSON, R. L., INGS, R., AND McFADZEAN, J. A., 1974a, Metronidazole ("Flagyl"), a radiosensitizer of hypoxic cells, *Br. J. Radiol.* **47:**474.

ASQUITH, J. C., WATTS, M. E., PATEL, K. B., SMITHEN, C. E., AND ADAMS, G. E., 1974b, Electron-affinic sensitization. V. Radiosensitization of hypoxic bacterial and mammalian cells *in vitro* by some nitroimidazoles and nitropyrazoles, *Radiat. Res.* **60:**108.

BEGG, A. C., 1976, The use of ^{125}IUdR to measure hypoxic cell radiosensitization by Ro-07-0582 in a solid murine tumour, *Radiat. Res.* (in press).

BEGG, A. C., SHELDON, P. W., AND FOSTER J. L., 1974, Demonstration of radiosensitization of hypoxic cells in solid tumors by metronidazole, *Br. J. Radiol.* **47:**399.

BERRY, R. J., AND ASQUITH, J. C., 1974, Cell cycle-dependent and hypoxic radiosensitizers, in: *Advances in Chemical Radiosensitization*, pp. 25–36, International Atomic Energy Agency, Vienna.

BIAGLOW, J. E., AND DURAND, R. E., 1976, The effects of nitrobenzene derivatives on oxygen utilization and radiation response of an *in vitro* tumour model, *Radiat. Res.* **65:**529.

BLEEHEN, N. M., 1973, Combination therapy with drugs and radiation, in: *Biological Basis of Radiotherapy, Br. Med. Bull.* **29:**54.

BLEEHEN, N. M., 1976, A radiotherapist's view of radiosensitizers, in: *Modification of Radiosensitivity of Biological Systems*, International Atomic Energy Agency, Vienna.

BLEEHEN, N. M., HONESS, D., AND MORGAN, J., 1977, The interaction of hyperthermia and the hypoxic cell sensitizer Ro-07-0582 on the EMT 6 mouse tumour, *Br. J. Cancer* **35:**299.

BRIDGES, B. A., 1960, Sensitization of *Escherichia coli* to gamma-radiation by *N*-ethylmaleimide, *Nature (London)* **188:**415.

BROWN, J. M., 1975, Selective radiosensitization of the hypoxic cells of mouse tumours with the nitroimidazoles, metronidazole and Ro-07-0582, *Radiat. Res.* **64:**633.

BROWN, J. M., 1977 Cytotoxic effects of the hypoxic cell radiosensitizer Ro-07-0582 to tumour cells *in vivo, Radiat. Res.* (in press).

CHAPMAN, J. D., WEBB, R. G., AND BORSA, J., 1971, Radiosensitization of mammalian cells by *p*-nitroacetophenone. I. Characterization in asynchronous and synchronous populations, *Int. J. Radiat. Biol.* **19:**561.

CHAPMAN, J. D., REUVERS, A. P., BORSA, J., PETKAU, A., AND McCALLA, D. R., 1972, Nitrofurans as radiosenitizers of hypoxic mammalian cells, *Cancer Res.* **32:**2630.

CHAPMAN, J. D., GREENSTOCK, C. L., REUVERS, A. P., McDONALD E., AND DUNLOP, I., 1973a, Radiation chemical studies with nitrofurazone as related to its mechanism of radiosensitization, *Radiat. Res.* **53**:190.

CHAPMAN, J. D., REUVERS, A. P., AND BORSA, J., 1973b, Effectiveness of nitrofuran derivatives in sensitizing hypoxic mammalian cells to X-rays, *Br. J. Radiol.* **46**:623.

CHAPMAN, J. D., REUVERS, A. P., BORSA, J., HENDERSON, J. S., AND MIGLIORE, R. D., 1974, Nitro-heterocyclic drugs as selective radiosensitizers of hypoxic mammalian cells, *Cancer Chemother. Rep. Part 1* **58(4)**:559.

CHAPMAN, J. D., BLAKELY, E. A., SMITH, K. C., AND URTASUN, R. C., 1976, Radiobiological characterization of the inactivating events produced in mammalian cells by helium and heavy ions, in: *Proceedings of the International Conference on High LET Radiation*, Berkeley.

CHURCHILL-DAVIDSON, I., SANGER, C., AND THOMLINSON, R. H., 1955, High pressure oxygen and radiotherapy, *Lancet* 1091.

COHEN, S. M., ETURK, E., VON ESCH, A. M., CROVEHI, A. J., AND BRYAN, S. T., 1973, Carcinogenicity of 5-nitrofurans, 5-nitroimidazole, 4-nitrobenzenes and related compounds, *J. Natl. Cancer Inst.* **51**:403.

COOKE, B. C., FIELDEN, E. M., AND JOHNSON, M., 1976, Polyfunctional radiosensitizers: Effects of a nitroxyl biradical on the survival of mammalian cells *in vitro*, *Radiat. Res.* **65**:152.

CRAMP, W. A., 1967, The toxic action on bacteria of irradiated solutions of copper compounds, *Radiat. Res.* **30**:221.

DENEKAMP, J., AND HARRIS, S. R., 1975, Tests of two electron-affinic radiosensitizers *in vivo* using regrowth of an experimental carcinoma, *Radiat. Res.* **61**:191.

DENEKAMP, J., AND HARRIS, S. R., 1976, The response of a transplantable tumour to fractionated irradiation. Part I. X-rays and the hypoxic cell sensitizer Ro-07-0582, *Radiat. Res.* **66**:66.

DENEKAMP, J., AND MICHAEL, B. D., 1972, Preferential sensitization of hypoxic cells to radiation *in vivo*, *Nature (London) New Biol.* **239**:21.

DENEKAMP, J., MICHAEL, B. D., AND HARRIS, S. R., 1974, Hypoxic cell radiosensitizers. Comparative tests of some electron-affinic compounds using epidermal cell survival *in vivo*, *Radiat. Res.* **60**:119.

DENEKAMP, J., HARRIS, S. R., MORRIS, C., AND FIELD, S. B., 1976, The response of a transplantable tumour to fractionated irradiation. Part II. Fast neutrons, *Radiat. Res.* **68**:93–103.

DEUTSCH, G., FOSTER, J. L., McFADZEAN, J. A., AND PARNELL, M., 1975, Studies with "high dose" metronidazole: A non-toxic radiosensitizer of hypoxic cells, *Br. J. Cancer* **31**:75.

DISCHE, S., GRAY, A. J., AND ZANELLI, G. D., 1976, Clinical testing of the radiosensitizer Ro-07-0582. II. Radiosensitization of normal and hypoxic skin, *Clin. Radiol.* **27**:159–166.

DISCHE, S., SAUNDERS, M. I., LEE, M. E., ADAMS, G. E., AND FLOCKHART, I. F., 1977, Clinical testing of the radiosensitizer Ro-07-0582: Experience with multiple doses, *Br. J. Cancer* (in press).

DURAND, R. E., AND BIAGLOW, J. E., 1976, Modification of the radiation response of an *in vitro* tumour model by control of cellular respiration, *Int. J. Radiat. Biol.* **26**:597.

ELKIND, M. M., SAKAMOTO, K., AND KAMPER, C., 1968, Age-dependent toxic properties of actinomycin D and X-rays in cultured Chinese hamster cells, *Cell Tissue Kinet.* **1**:209.

EMMERSON, P. T., 1972, X-ray damage to DNA and loss of biological function: Effects of sensitizing aspects, in: *Advances in Radiation Chemistry*, Vol. 3, (M. BURTON AND J. L. MAGEE, eds.), pp. 209–282, Wiley, New York.

FIELDEN, E. M., AND LILLICRAP, S. C., 1970, The effect of 5-bromouracil on energy transfer in irradiated DNA, in: *Radiation Protection and Sensitization* (H. L. MOROSON AND M. QUINTILIANI, eds.), pp. 81–86, Taylor Francis, London.

FLOCKHART, I. R., LARGE, P., MALCOLM, S. L., MARTEN, T. R., AND TROUP, D., 1976, Studies on the metabolism of the hypoxic cell radiosensitizer, Ro-07-0582 in man and other mammals, *Zenobiotica* (submitted).

FOSTER, J. L., AND WILLSON, R. L., 1973, Radiosensitization of anoxic cells by metronidazole, *Br. J. Radiol.* **6**:234.

FOSTER, J. L., FLOCKHART, I. R., DISCHE, S., GRAY, A., LENOX-SMITH, I., AND SMITHEN, C. E., 1975, Serum concentration measurements in man of the radiosensitizer Ro-07-0582. Some preliminary results, *Br. J. Cancer* **31**:679.

FOSTER, J. L., CONROY, P. J., SEARLE, A. J., AND WILLSON, R. L., 1976, Metronidazole ("Flagyl"): Characterization as a cytotoxic drug specific for hypoxic tumour cells, *Br. J. Cancer* **33**:485.

FOWLER, J. F., SHELDON, P. W., DENEKAMP, J., AND FIELD, S. B., 1976, Optimum fractionation of the C₃H mouse mammary tumour using X-rays, the hypoxic cell sensitizer Ro-07-0582 or fast neutrons, *Int. J. Radiat. Oncol. Biol. Phys.* **1**:579.

GEORGE, K. C., HIRST, D. G., AND McNALLY, N. J., 1977, The effect of hyperthermia on the cytotoxicity of the radiosensitizer Ro-07-0582 on a solid mouse tumour, *Br. J. Cancer* **35**:372.

GRAY, A. J., DISCHE, S., ADAMS, G. E., FLOCKHART, I. R., AND FOSTER, J. L., 1976, Clinical testing of the radiosensitizer Ro-07-0582. I. Dose, tolerance, serum and tumour concentration, *Clin. Radiol.* **27**:151.

GREENSTOCK, C. L., ADAMS, G. E., AND WILLSON, R. L., 1970, Electron transfer studies of nucleic acid derivatives in solution containing radiosensitizers, in: *Radiation Protection and Sensitization* (H. L. MOROSON AND M. QUINTILIANI, eds.), pp. 65–71, Taylor and Francis, London.

GREENSTOCK, C. L., RALEIGH, J., McDONALD, E., AND WHITEHOUSE, R., 1973, Nucleotide radical oxidation and addition reactions with cellular radiation sensitizers, *Biochem. Biophys. Res. Commun.* **52**:276.

GREENSTOCK, C. L., RUDDICK, G. W., AND NETA, P., 1976, Pulse radiolysis and ESR studies of the electron-affinic properties of nitroheterocyclic radiosensitizers, *Radiat. Res.* **66**:472.

HALL, E. J., AND BIAGLOW, J. E., 1977, Ro-07-0582 as a radiosensitizer and cytotoxic agent, *Int. J. Radiat. Oncol. Biol. Phys.* (in press).

HALL, E. J., AND ROIZIN-TOWLE, L., 1975, Hypoxic sensitizers: Radiobiological studies at the cellular level, *Radiology* **117**:453.

HALL, E. J., ROIZIN-TOWLE, L., THEUS, R. B., AND AUGUST, L. S., 1975, Radiobiological properties of high energy cyclotron produced neutrons used for radiotherapy, *Radiology* **117**:173.

HARRIS, J. W., AND POWER, J. A., 1973, Diamide: A new radiosensitizer for anoxic cells, *Radiat. Res.* **56**:97.

HEWITT, H. B., AND BLAKE, E. R., 1970, Studies of the toxicity and radio-sensitizing ability of triacetone-*N*-oxyl in mice, *Br. J. Radiol.* **43**:91.

HEWITT, H. B., AND BLAKE, E. R., 1974, *In vivo* studies of a radiosensitizer (Ro-07-0582) using murine leukaemia and squamous carcinoma, *Annu. Rep. Gray Lab. Cancer Res. Campaign, U.K.,* p. 20.

HEWITT, H. B., AND WILSON, C. W., 1959, A survival curve for mammalian leukaemia cells irradiated *in vivo*: Implications for the treatment of mouse leukaemia by whole body irradiation, *Br. J. Cancer,* **13**:69.

HILL, R. P., AND BUSH, R. S., 1969, A lung-colony assay to determine the radiosensitivity of the cells of a solid tumour, *Int. J. Radiat. Biol.* **15**:435.

HILL, S., AND FOWLER, J. F., 1976, Radiosensitizing and cytocidal effects on hypoxic cells of Ro-07-0582 and repair of X-ray injury in an experimental carcinoma, *Br. J. Cancer* (in press).

HILL, R. P., FIELDEN, E. M., LILLICRAP, S. C., AND STANLEY, J. A., 1975, Studies on the radiosensitizing action *in vivo* of 2,2,6,6 tetramethyl-4-piperidonl-*N*-oxyl (TMPN), *Int. J. Radiat. Biol.* **27**:499.

HORNSEY, S., HEDGES, M. J., AND BRYANT, P. E., 1968, The sensitization of the hypoxic gastrointestinal tract *in vivo* to radiation damage by indane trione, *Int. J. Radiat. Biol.* **13**:581.

HOWARD-FLANDERS, P., AND ALPER, T., 1957, The sensitivity of micro-organisms to irradiation under controlled gas conditions, *Radiat. Res.* **7**:518.

INCH, W. R., McCREDIE, J. A., SUTHERLAND, R. M., AND HAYNES, M. J., 1977, Effect of metronidazole on C_3H/HeJ mice and growth of the C_3H BA adenocarcinoma, *Growth* (in press).

JOHNSON, R., GOMER, C., AMBRUS, J., PEARA, J., AND BOYLE, D., 1976, An investigation of the pharmacological and radiosensitizing effects of the 2-nitroimidazole Ro-07-0582 in primates, *Br. J. Radiol.* **49**:294.

KAPLAN, H. S., 1970, Radiosensitization by the halogenated pyrimidine analogues: Laboratory and clinical investigations, in: *Radiation Protection and Sensitization* (H. L. MOROSON AND M. QUINTILIANI, eds.), pp. 35–42, Taylor and Francis, London.

LUKIEWICZ, S., 1976, Interference with endogenous radioprotectors as a method of sensitization, in: *Modification of Radiosensitivity of Biological Systems*, pp. 61–76, International Energy Atomic Agency, Vienna.

McNALLY, N. J., 1975, The effect of a hypoxic cell sensitizer on tumour growth delay and cell survival, *Br. J. Cancer* **32**:610.

McNALLY, N. J., 1976, The effect of a change in radiation quality on the ability of electron-affinic sensitizers to sensitive hypoxic cells, *Int. J. Radiat. Biol.* **29**:191.

McNALLY, N. J., AND SHELDON, P. W., 1977, The effect of radiation on tumour growth delay, cell survival and cure of the animal using one tumour system, *Br. J. Radiol.* **50**:321.

MEISEL, D., AND CZAPSKI, G., 1975, One-electron transfer equilibria and redox potentials of radicals studied by pulse radiolysis, *J. Phys. Chem.* **79**:1503.

MEISEL, D., AND NETA, P., 1975, One-electron reduction potential of riboflavine studied by pulse radiolysis, *J. Phys. Chem.* **79:**2459.

MILNE, N., HILL, R. P., AND BUSH, R. S., 1973, Factors affecting hypoxic KHT tumour cells in mice breathing O_2, O_2 and CO_2, or hyperbaric oxygen with or without anaesthetic, *Radiology* **106:**663.

MITCHELL, J. S., 1960, *Studies in Radiotherapeutics*, Blackwell, Oxford.

MOHINDRA, J. K., AND RAUTH, A. M., 1976, Increased cell killing by metronidazole and nitrofurazone of hypoxic compared to aerobic mammalian cells, *Cancer Res.* **36:**930.

MOORE, B. A., PALCIC, B., AND SKARSGARD, L. D., 1976, Radiosensitizing and toxic effects of the 2-nitroimidazole Ro-07-0582 in hypoxic mammalian cells, *Radiat. Res.* **67:**459.

NYGAARD, O. F., AND BIAGLOW, J. E., 1975, Metabolic limitations in the use of anoxic radiosensitizers, *Radiat. Res.* **59:**159.

OLIVE, P. L., INCH, W. R., AND SUTHERLAND, R. M., 1972, The effect of triacetoneamine-*N*-oxyl on oxygenation and radiocurability of a mouse mammary carcinoma, *Radiat. Res.* **52:**618.

PARKER, L., SKARSGARD, L. D., AND EMMERSON, P. T., 1969, Sensitization of anoxic mammalian cells to X-rays by triacetoneamine-*N*-oxyl, *Radiat. Res.* **38:**493.

PATEL, K. B., AND WILLSON, R. L., 1976, Semiquinone free radicals and oxygen. Pulse radiolysis study of one-electron transfer equilibria, *J. Chem. Soc. Faraday Trans. 1* **69:**814.

PETERS, L. J., 1976, Modification of the radiocurability of a syngeneic murine squamous carcinoma by its site of growth, by electron-affinic drugs and by ICRF 159, *Br. J. Radiol.* **49:**708.

POWERS, E. L., 1972, The hydrated electron, the hydroxyl radical and hydrogen peroxide in radiation damage in cells, *Isr. J. Chem.* **10:**1199.

POWERS, E. L., AND TALLENTIRE, A., 1968, The roles of water in the cellular effects of ionizing radiation, in: *Action Chimiques et biologiques des radiations*, Vol. 12 (M. HAISSINSKY, ed.), pp. 3–67, Masson et Cie, Paris.

QUINTILIANI, M., 1974, Molecular mechanism of radiosensitization by iodine-containing compounds, in: *Advances in Chemical radiosensitization*, pp. 87–103, International Atomic Energy Agency, Vienna.

RAJU, M. R., FRANK, J. P., TRUJILLO, T. T., AND BAIN, E., 1976, A high LET and hypoxic cell radiosensitizer, private communication.

RALEIGH, J. A., CHAPMAN, J. D., BORSA, J., KREMER, S. W., AND REUVERS, A. P., 1973, Radiosensitization by *p*-nitroacetophenone. III. Effectiveness of nitrobenzene analogues, *Int. J. Radiat. Biol.* **23:**377.

RAUTH, A. M., AND KAUFMAN, K., 1975, *In vivo* testing of hypoxic radiosensitizers using the KHT mouse tumour assayed by the lung colony technique, *Br. J. Radiol.* **48:**209.

RAUTH, A. M., KAUFMAN, K., AND THOMSON, J. E., 1975, *In vivo* testing of hypoxic cell radiosensitizers, in: *Radiation Research Biomedical, Chemical and Physical Perspectives* (O. F. NYGAARD, H. I. ADLER, AND W. K. SINCLAIR, eds.), pp. 761–772, Academic Press, New York.

RÉVÈSCZ, L., AND LITTBRAND, B., 1976, Radiation dose dependence of sensitization by electron-affinic compounds, in: *Modification of Radiosensitivity of Biological Systems*, pp. 155–162, International Atomic Energy Agency, Vienna.

RUSTIA, M., AND SHUBIK, P., 1972, Induction of lung tumours and malignant lymphomas in mice by metronidazole, *J. Natl. Cancer Inst.* **48:**721.

SCHÄRER, K., 1972, Selective injury to Purkinje cells in the dog after oral administration of high doses of nitroimidazole derivatives, *Vetl. Deutsch. Ges. Pathol.* **56:**407.

SCOTT, O. C. A., AND STURROCK, J. E., 1967, Search for radiosensitization of ascites tumour cells by indanetrione, *Int. J. Radiat. Biol.* **13:**573.

SHELDON, P. W., AND HILL, S. A., 1977, unpublished results.

SHELDON, P. W., AND SMITH, A. M., 1975, Modest radiosensitization of solid tumours in C_3H mice by NDPP, *Br. J. Cancer* **31:**81.

SHELDON, P. W., FOSTER, J. L., AND FOWLER, J. F., 1974, Radiosensitization of C_3H mouse mammary tumours by a 2-nitroimidazole drug, *Br. J. Cancer* **30:**560.

SHELDON, P. W., FOSTER, J. L., HILL, S. A., AND FOWLER, J. F., 1976, Radiosensitization of C_3H mouse mammary tumours using fractionated doses of X-rays with the drug Ro-07-0582, *Br. J. Radiol.* **49:**76.

SHENOY, M. A., ASQUITH, J. C., ADAMS, G. E., MICHAEL, B. D., AND WATTS, M. E., 1975, Time-resolved oxygen effects in irradiated bacteria and mammalian cells: a rapid-mix study, *Radiat. Res.* **62:**498.

SHENOY, M. A., GEORGE, K. C., SRINIVASAN, V. T., SINGH, B. B., AND SUNDARAM, K., 1976, Radiation sensitization by membrane-specific drugs, in: *Modification of Radiosensitivity of Biological Systems*, pp. 131–140, International Atomic Energy Agency, Vienna.

SHIPLEY, W. V., STANLEY, J. A., AND STEEL, G. G., 1976, Enhanced tumour cell radiosensitivity in artificial pulmonary metastases of the Lewis lung carcinoma, *Int. J. Radiat. Oncol. Biol. Phys.* **1**:261.

SIMIC, M., AND POWERS, E. L., 1974, Correlation of the efficiencies of some radiation sensitizers and their redox potentials, *Int. J. Radiat. Biol.* **26**:87.

SINCLAIR, W. K., 1975, Mammalian cell sensitization repair and the cell cycle, in: *Radiation Research, Biomedical, Chemical and Physical Perspectives* (O. F. NYGAARD, H. I. ADLER, AND W. K. SINCLAIR, eds.), pp. 742–751, Academic Press, New York.

STONE, H. B., AND WITHERS, H. R., 1975, Enhancement by the radioresponse of a murine tumour by a nitroimidazole, *Br. J. Radiol.* **48**:411.

STRATFORD, I. J., AND ADAMS, G. E., 1977, The effect of hyperthermia on the differential cytotoxicity of a hypoxic cell radiosensitizer, the 2-nitroimidazole Ro-07-0582, on mammalian cells *in vitro*, *Br. J. Cancer* **35**:307.

SUIT, H. D., AND MAEDA, M. M., 1967, Hyperbaric oxygen and radiobiology of a C_3H mouse mammary carcinoma, *J. Natl. Cancer Inst.* **39**:639.

SUTHERLAND, R. M., 1974, Selective chemotherapy of noncycling cells in an *in vitro* tumour model, *Cancer Res.* **34**:3501.

SZYBALSKI, W., 1962, Properties and applications of halogenated deoxyribonucleic acids, in: *The Molecular Basis of Neoplasia*, pp. 147–171, University of Texas Press, Austin.

TALLENTIRE, A., SCHILLER, N. L., AND POWERS, E. L., 1968, 2.3 Butadiene, an electron stabilising compound as a modifier of *Bacillus megaterium* spores to X-rays, *Int. J. Radiat. Biol.* **14**:397.

THOMLINSON, R. H., AND GRAY, L. H., 1955, The histological structure of some human lung cancers and the possible implication for radiotherapy, *Br. J. Cancer* **9**:539.

THOMLINSON, R. H., DISCHE, S., GRAY, A. J., AND ERRINGTON, L. M., 1976, Clinical testing of the radiosensitizer Ro-07-0582. III. Response of tumours, *Clin. Radiol.* **27**:167.

URTASUN, R. C., STURMWIND, J., RABIN, H., BAND, P. R., AND CHAPMAN, J. D., 1974, High dose metronidazole: A preliminary pharmacological study prior to its investigational use in clinical radiotherapy trials, *Br. J. Radiol.* **47**:297.

URTASUN, R. C., CHAPMAN, J. D., BAND, P., RABIN, H., FRIER, C., AND STURMWIND, J., 1975, Phase 1 study of high dose Metronidazole, an "*in vivo*" and "*in vitro*" specific radiosensitizer of hypoxic cells, *Radiology* **117**:129.

URTASUN, R. C., BAND, P., CHAPMAN, J. D., FELDSTEIN, M. C., MIELKE, B., AND FRYER, C., 1976, Radiation and high dose metronidazole ("Flagyl^R") in supratentorial glioblastomas, *N. Engl. J. Med.* **294**:1364.

VAN PUTTEN, L. M., AND SMINK, T., 1976, Effect of Ro-07-0582 and radiation on a poorly reoxygenating mouse osteosarcoma, in: *Modification of Radiosensitivity of Biological systems*, pp. 179–190, International Atomic Energy Agency, Vienna.

VARGHESE, A. J., GULYAS, S., AND MOHINDRA, J. K., 1976, Hypoxia dependent reduction of 1-(2-nitro-1-imidazolyl)-3-methoxy-2-propanol by Chinese hamster cells *in vitro* and *in vivo*, *Cancer res.* **36**:3761.

WARDMAN, P., AND CLARKE, E., 1976, One-electron reduction potentials of substituted nitroimidazoles measured by pulse radiolysis, *J. Chem. Soc. Faraday Trans. 1*, **72**:1377.

WATTS, M. E., WHILLANS, D. W., AND ADAMS, G. E., 1975, Studies of the mechanisms of radiosensitization of bacteria and mammalian cells by diamide, *Int. J. Radiat. Biol.* **27**:259.

WHILLANS, D. W., ADAMS, G. E., AND NETA, P., 1975, Electron-affinic sensitization. VI. A pulse radiolysis and esr comparison of some 2- and 5-nitroimidazoles, *Radiat. Res.* **62**:407.

WHITMORE, G. F., GULYAS, S., AND VARGHESE, A. J., 1975, Studies on the radiosensitizing action of NDPP, a sensitizer of hypoxic cells, *Radiat. Res.* **61**:325.

WILLSON, R. L., AND EMMERSON, P. T., 1970, Reaction of triacetoneamine-*N*-oxyl with radiation-induced radicals from DNA and deoxyribonucleotides in aqueous solution, in: *Radiation Protection and Sensitization* (H. L. MOROSON AND M. QUINTILIANI, eds.), pp. 73–79, Taylor and Francis, London.

WILLSON, R. L., CRAMP, W. A., AND INGS, R. M. J., 1974, Metronidazole ("Flagyl"): Mechanisms of radiosensitization, *Int. J. Radiat. Biol.* **26**:557.

WITHERS, H. R., 1967, The dose–survival relationship for irradiation of epithelial cells of mouse skins, *Br. J. Radiol.* **40**:187.

7

Effects of Radiation on Animal Tumor Models

ROBERT F. KALLMAN and SARA ROCKWELL

1. Introduction

Irradiation of a malignant tumor in a patient or in an experimental animal produces a variety of changes in the physiology, growth, and behavior of the neoplasm. Many of these changes are of significance in the therapy of human cancer, because they alter the sensitivity of the tumor to subsequent treatments with radiation or with other therapeutic modalities. A better understanding of the effects of radiation on tumors is therefore necessary in order that improved regimens may be developed in which therapy with radiation or radiation combined with other agents is delivered in a more optimum fashion. However, it is difficult to examine a subject of this complexity in the clinic, because severe technical problems and ethical considerations limit the observations that can be made and the phenomena that can be studied quantitatively. As a result, most of the available data defining the effects of radiation on tumors have been obtained from experiments with tumors in experimental animals or with experimental tumor models *in vitro*.

In this chapter, we will attempt to provide an overview of the effects of radiation on experimental animal tumors. In the discussion, we will consider in detail the experimental tumor systems, the techniques used to analyze their therapeutic responses, and the advantages and limitations of the different experimental systems as models for human cancer. We will also discuss the basic phenomena

ROBERT F. KALLMAN ● Department of Radiology, Stanford University School of Medicine, Stanford, California 94305.   SARA ROCKWELL ● Department of Therapeutic Radiology, Yale University School of Medicine, New Haven, Connecticut 06510.

226

ROBERT F.
KALLMAN
AND
SARA
ROCKWELL

and problems of current interest, and give a brief, up-to-date summary of the experimental data relating to these subjects. Although we will be concerned primarily with radiation, the discussions of the experimental tumor models, the criteria of experimental design, the concepts, and even many of the findings can be extrapolated to treatment with other therapeutic modalities, especially chemotherapy. We hope that this approach will provide an appreciation for the use, potential, and limitations of the available experimental models for human cancer which will be of use to those who are beginning work in experimental therapeutics and to those who are extrapolating data obtained with these models to the clinical situation.

It would be impossible to include in this chapter detailed discussions of all of the aspects of tumor radiobiology. Many of the topics that we will consider only briefly are discussed in detail in other chapters in these volumes. Others are well reviewed in other publications, including "Methods for the Study of Radiation Effects on Cancer Cells," by R. F. Kallman (1968); "Radiobiology's Contribution to Radiotherapy: Promise or Mirage? Failla Memorial Lecture," by H. S. Kaplan (1970); the symposium proceedings, *Time–Dose Relationships in Radiation Biology as Applied to Radiotherapy* (1970); the Proceedings of the 13th Annual Hanford Biology Symposium, *The Cell Cycle in Malignancy and Immunity* (1975); the Proceedings of the Sixth L. H. Gray Conference, *Cell Survival after Low Doses of Radiation: Theoretical and Clinical Applications* (T. Alper, ed., 1975); and "The Four R's of Radiotherapy," by H. R. Withers (1975).

2. Kinds of Tumors and Experimental Systems

2.1. Experimental Animal Tumors

2.1.1. "Spontaneous" Tumors

The experimental model system which is closest to the tumor/patient population encountered clinically is the heterogeneous population of tumors of all types arising in a natural or experimental animal population. These may be found arising essentially at random in experimental rat or mouse breeding colonies, or they may be found by veterinarians in zoos or in private practice as individual animal patients are brought in with tumors. Many practical considerations limit the usefulness of such tumors in experimental cancer therapy. Ideally, the experimental oncologist would like to accumulate a large number of uniform tumors in similar hosts for each experiment. The great variability of the spontaneous tumors in histology, natural history, stage at presentation, immunogenicity, etc., and the variability of the hosts in age, sex, health, and possibly breed, presents the same problems of selection and randomization to the experimental oncologist that the variability of clinical material presents to the clinician planning or performing a clinical trial. In using tumors discovered in veterinary practice, ethical considerations also arise which may limit experimental procedures to those that are both potentially curative and of minimal morbidity. Because of such limitations, the size of the population of uniform tumors which may be accumulated for an experiment is very small and the types of experiments which can be performed are limited. However, spontaneous tumors in pets or zoo animals are practically the only available experimental tumor material in animals larger than the rodents that are customarily used in the laboratory. They are therefore invaluable as models for experiments in which the size of the host, the biology of the therapy-limiting normal tissues, or the cell proliferation kinetics of the host and/or tumor should be similar to those in man. Examples of the use of such tumor systems include the study of cell population kinetics in dog tumors (Owen and Steel, 1969) and preclinical evaluations of neutrons (Banks, 1974).

2.1.2. Autochthonous or Autogenous Tumors

The autochthonous, or autogenous, tumor is a tumor studied in its host of origin. The *spontaneous* tumors discussed above are of unknown etiology; i.e., they occur without the involvement of a known virus or chemical carcinogen, and are found in strains or breeds of animals generally regarded as low-tumor (see Hewitt *et al.*, 1976). Tumors induced by viruses or carcinogens and studied in the host in which they arose are autochthonous tumors. Many of the strain-specific tumors characteristic of specific inbred mouse and rat lines are also in this category. Mammary tumors arising in female C3H mice, which are caused by the interaction of mammary tumor virus, sex hormones, and mammary gland cells of a susceptible genotype, constitute a prime example (see Moore, Vol. 2, this series). Similarly, this category would include AKR lymphoma, which results from endogenous virus(es) acting on the cells of genetically susceptible hosts, and the radiation-induced leukemia produced in C57Bl mice (Kaplan, 1964) by the combination of a virus, genetic susceptibility, and irradiation. Several technical problems limit the experiments that are possible with autochthonous tumors, such as those harvested from a "high-tumor" mouse colony (Kallman and Tapley, 1964; Kallman, 1968). First, it is difficult to obtain sufficient numbers of tumors. Because the latent period for the development of many of the tumors is long and because not all animals develop tumors, it is generally necessary to maintain a large population of animals at risk. Second, there is heterogeneity in the tumor population. Even under the best of circumstances, tumors will arise at different sites, at different times, in animals of different ages, and will show a wider variability in growth rate, histology, and response to treatments than will transplanted tumors. Third, multiple tumors per animal may arise both simultaneously and sequentially. These may seriously complicate the experiments and the interpretation of experimental results. A similar problem in the AKR lymphoma system is that the hosts used in curative experiments may develop a second primary tumor, which may be difficult to distinguish from a late recurrence of a treated first primary and which may make interpretation of curative experiments difficult. Fourth, the quantitative measurements that can be used with these tumors are very limited and usually

228

ROBERT F.
KALLMAN
AND
SARA
ROCKWELL

confined to gross tumor responses. Therefore, the kind and number of experiments which can be performed with autochthonous tumors are limited by the number of tumors of a uniform size, biology, and host which can be collected and by the few types of experimental assays which can be performed unambiguously.

On the other hand, such tumors provide superior models for the human disease. First, most are relatively slow growing. In this respect, their cell proliferation kinetics resemble those of primary human tumors more closely than do the kinetics of typical transplanted tumor lines. Second, their antigenicity is that of a natural tumor growing in its host of origin; such tumors are free of the incompatibilities which can arise during the course of the frequent serial passaging associated with the propagation of transplantable tumors. Third, an animal in which a carcinogenic event has occurred and a slow-growing primary tumor has developed may differ substantially from an animal into which a rapidly growing transplantable tumor has been implanted—in its immune response to the tumor, its hormonal status, and many other features of its physiology. Therefore, autochthonous tumors may be the systems of choice for experiments in which host factors are critical.

2.1.3. Transplanted Tumors

Transplanted tumor lines have been started from both spontaneous tumors and carcinogen- or virus-induced tumors. Traditionally, a tumor line is propagated continuously by serial passage in the animal species, and preferably the inbred strain, of origin. More recently, it has become common practice to store an early transplantation passage in the frozen state (in liquid nitrogen) and to thaw samples as needed to inoculate large numbers of tumors in appropriate, syngeneic recipient animals for experiments (Suit et al., 1965). The latter procedure is most likely to ensure a uniform stock of tumor material which closely approximates the primary tumor. The former method greatly favors selection for rapid growth and against the original cell proliferation kinetics and state of partial differentiation of the primary. Also, with long-continued serial passage, many tumors acquire the ability to grow in allogeneic hosts and, perhaps paradoxically, take on increased immunological incompatibility with the host of origin.

2.1.4. Animal Species

On the bases of their similarities to man in physiology, pharmacology, and cell or tissue proliferation patterns, large animals (dogs, monkeys, pigs, etc.) are preferable for many oncological experiments. In addition, larger size is convenient or essential for certain kinds of studies, e.g., accurate localization for irradiation, surgery, tests of diagnostic techniques. Such animals have proved extremely useful in studying the radiation responses of the normal tissues which may limit therapy (Probert and Hughes, 1975). However, the cost, life span, heterogeneity, and variability of spontaneous tumors in these species make planned experimentation with tumors in large animals difficult, and the lack of inbred lines or strains precludes experiments using transplanted tumors (Brown, 1975).

Small animals are therefore the models of choice for most of experimental oncology. The vast majority of the experimental literature deals with tumors of the mouse and rat, although studies with the hamster, rabbit, and guinea pig are also to be found. Experiments with nonmammalian species such as fowl or frogs are almost always concerned with the process of carcinogenesis rather than tumor therapy.

The utility of small rodent species, especially the mouse, is directly attributable to the availability of inbred strains (Kallman, 1975). A suitably propagated inbred strain ensures the availability of large numbers of genetically identical animals, in which one can transplant normal tissues (skin, bone marrow, endocrine glands, etc.) from one animal to another without immunological recognition and destruction of the graft by the recipient animal. Tumors also obey the laws of transplantation and may be transplanted freely into syngeneic recipients. Although this minimizes immunological differences between tumor and host, it may not eliminate them entirely: a tumor may express antigens which were not expressed either in the normal tissues of the original host or in normal animals of the same inbred strain (Klein *et al.*, 1960). Because of this, every tumor–host system must be analyzed for the presence and strength of tumor antigenicity, i.e., incompatibility between the host and tumor (Scott, 1961; Kallman, 1968). Because of the expected enhancement of therapeutic effects by immunological rejection, tumors of easily demonstrable antigenicity generally are poor models for use in sensitive or sophisticated studies of cancer therapy.

2.2. Human Tumors Grown in Animals

Tumors from man may be transplanted xenogeneically (i.e., into other species), but either the recipient animals must be immunologically deficient or the graft must be placed in an immunologically privileged site, such as the hamster cheek pouch (Toolan, 1953) or the anterior chamber of the eye (Gimbrone *et al.*, 1974). Laboratory rodents may be immunosuppressed sufficiently to permit the growth of xenogeneic transplants by any one of several means: thymectomy followed by whole-body X-irradiation (Cobb and Mitchley, 1974), cortisone (Toolan, 1953), or antilymphocyte serum (ALS) and/or antithymocyte serum (ATS) (Stanbridge *et al.*, 1975). A related approach is to utilize as an immunologically incompetent host the athymic nude mouse (Rygaard and Povlsen, 1969). Mice homozygous for the recessive gene *nu* (nude) are born with a severely defective thymus and are extremely deficient in T-cell production. Because these animals are severely deficient in cell-mediated immunity, they will accept nonsyngeneic transplants with minimal immunological reactivity. Although tumors of a variety of types and origins may be grown successfully in immunologically deficient hosts, xenografted tumors do not provide an unambiguous model system. Because host immune responses are never completely or permanently absent, but only impaired, some host immune responses to the tumor will occur and may alter the behavior of the tumor from that seen in the original host. Because the tumor stroma is of host

230

ROBERT F.
KALLMAN
AND
SARA
ROCKWELL

(animal) origin, those tumor characteristics which are dependent upon the stroma or the interactions of the stroma with the malignant parenchymal cells will reflect the host rather than the species of origin of the tumor. In addition, some tumors developing after transplantation of human tumors into animals have proved to be induced in the animal by a virus or by the transplantation process or to be derived from hybrid cells that resulted from the fusion of a malignant human cell and a normal host cell (Goldenberg *et al.*, 1971). Nevertheless, one should not underestimate the potential of these methods for studying the biology or therapeutic responses of human tumor cells as solid tumors and for performing experiments which cannot ethically be performed on a human patient.

2.3. In Vitro Models

Short-term cultures of tissue fragments or of malignant cells explanted from human or animal tumors have been used to examine a variety of features of tumor physiology, including the cell proliferation patterns, the hormone dependence, and the biochemical activities of the malignant cells, and also the interactions between the tumor cells and the host immune system. In addition, short-term cell and tissue cultures have been used to examine the responses of tumors to treatment with radiation or chemotherapeutic agents. Short-term cultures from human tumors are also useful as a diagnostic tool and may eventually provide a rapid and reliable means of screening individual tumors for drug sensitivity. The techniques and clinical applications of short-term cultures from human tumors have recently been reviewed (Dendy, 1976).

Established cell lines (cell lines capable of indefinite or prolonged propagation under proper culture conditions) from a variety of origins have been used to study the effects of radiation, chemotherapeutic agents, hyperthermia, and immunological strategies as therapeutic modalities. Cell lines which have proved valuable include not only cells of malignant origin, both human (e.g., HeLa) and animal (L1210, Ehrlich ascites, EMT6), but also cells of normal origin (L cells from the mouse; ovarian cells from the Chinese hamster; WI-38, Chang liver, and T1 kidney cells from man) and their transformed counterparts. The use of established cell lines to study the effects of therapeutic agents offers many advantages, including precise control of growth and culture conditions; optimum control over treatment conditions (radiation distribution and dose, drug doses and exposure times, etc.); the capability of preparing and treating special subpopulations (e.g., synchronous cells); and the availability of easy, reliable, and precise assays for measuring effects on cell populations (e.g., growth of colonies from surviving cells).

Most experiments with cultured mammalian cells are performed during the period of exponential growth, in which the cells are actively proliferating in a nutrient medium. Another valuable model for experimental therapeutics is the plateau-phase culture (Hahn and Little, 1972), which is composed of cells that have been planted at relatively low cell densities and allowed to grow in the same culture vessels until the cell number has ceased to increase. The cells in plateau-phase cultures are deprived of nutrients and coexist in cell densities that are

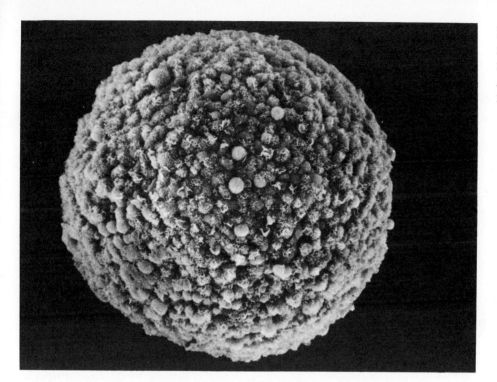

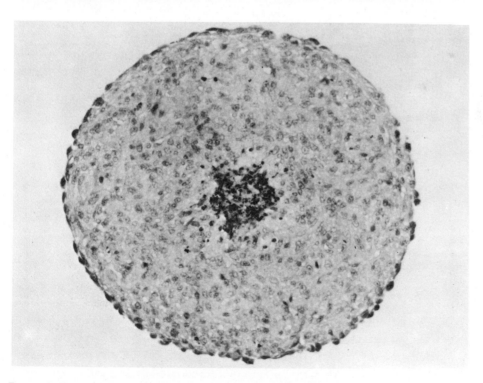

FIGURE 1. Top panel: Scanning electron microscope picture of a spheroid of EMT6 cells. This spheroid is 500–600 μm in diameter. Bottom panel: Cross-section of an EMT6 cell spheroid the same size as the spheroid shown in the top panel. The exterior portion of the spheroid is composed of tightly packed, viable cells. A small region of necrosis is present in the center of the spheroid. Courtesy of Dr. Robert M. Sutherland.

232

ROBERT F.
KALLMAN
AND
SARA
ROCKWELL

sufficiently high to alter the pattern of proliferation from the exponential growth generally seen in less crowded cultures. The exact pattern of the cell proliferation in plateau-phase cultures varies with the cell line. In some lines, the cell-cycle time lengthens greatly and most cells continue to cycle, although at an abnormally slow rate. In other lines, cells are inhibited from progressing through the G_1 phase, and the majority of the cells accumulate in a resting, G_1-like state while only a few of the cells progress through the cycle. In both of these cases, the cultures more closely resemble the cell populations in tumors than do exponentially growing cultures, and studies of their drug sensitivity, repair processes, and the like may prove extremely useful in the analysis of the effects of therapeutic agents on tumors *in vivo*.

Another type of *in vitro* model is the three-dimensional cultured tumor model, which is exemplified by the spheroids introduced by Sutherland *et al.* (1971). Some cells placed in suspension culture under proper conditions will stick together and form small rounded masses of packed cells. As the cells in this "spheroid" proliferate, the spheroid grows larger. When the radius of the spheroid becomes large enough that oxygen and nutrients cannot diffuse to the cells in its center, the central cells die and the spheroid develops a characteristic morphology: a rind of intact cells with a central zone of necrosis. This is shown in Fig. 1. Cells near the surface of the spheroid are fully oxygenated and have adequate nutrient levels, cells in the central necrotic zone are dead, and cells on the edge of the necrotic zone are radiobiologically hypoxic and are noncycling, probably as a result of nutrient deficiencies (Sutherland and Durand, 1973). The spheroid system therefore constitutes an *in vitro* model for many of the effects of vascular insufficiency in tumors *in vivo*, including oxygen and nutrient deficiencies and proliferative changes. Other three-dimensional models that have been developed but not yet extensively applied to therapy include systems in which cells grow to high densities inside of capillary tubes that are constantly perfused with nutrient medium (Knazek *et al.*, 1972) and models in which cells grow on the interior surfaces of a three-dimensional matrix of solid supportive materials (Leighton, 1968).

3. Measurement of Therapeutic Effect

3.1. Tumor Control or Tumor Cure

The measurement of tumor cure is perhaps the most clinically relevant end point for assessing therapeutic effects, and is the ultimate test of any therapeutic agent. Speaking strictly, a tumor is cured if it disappears completely after treatment and does not recur either at the primary site or as metastases while the host lives out its complete, normal life span. Because these criteria can seldom be met experimentally, the term "tumor control" is preferable; this implies that the tumor disappears completely and does not recur locally during an adequate period of observation.

Therapeutic effectiveness is best measured by determining the treatment necessary to cure 50% of the tumors, the *tumor control dose 50* (TCD_{50}) or *curative dose 50* (CD_{50}) (Suit and Shalek, 1963; Kallman and Tapley, 1964; Reinhold and DeBree, 1968). For this, a large number of tumor-bearing animals are randomized into several groups, each of which receives a different graded treatment, e.g., a different dose of radiation. Doses are chosen so that the smallest treatments are expected to cure none of the tumors while the largest treatments are expected to cure all of them. The number of treatment doses and the spacing of the doses will depend on the precision desired in the TCD_{50}. As a useful rule of thumb, there should be at least three points between 0 and 100% effect on the curve of cure vs. dose. The number of animals used per point will depend on the desired confidence limits, but generally there should be no fewer than six animals per group. The animals must be carefully matched at the time of treatment, both for the characteristics of the host (age, sex, health, size, etc.) and for the characteristics of the tumor (size, growth rate, site, etc.).

After treatment, each animal must be observed periodically until essentially all recurrences have been noted. This may require a follow-up period of only 2 or 3 months for some rapidly growing transplantable tumors, but may require 6 months or longer for some slowly growing transplantable tumors and for many autochthonous tumors. It is essential to determine the necessary posttreatment observation period for every tumor system to be used for TCD_{50} experiments. Starting shortly after the completion of treatment, the TCD_{50} will increase as the time of observation increases. The rate of increase in the TCD_{50} will slow as the majority of the recurrences are accumulated. The tumors should be observed until the TCD_{50} ceases to rise appreciably, and the period of observation should be specified with the TCD_{50}. The necessity for long follow-up periods makes it difficult, and frequently impossible, to do rigorous TCD_{50} analyses on tumors which metastasize early in their natural history, simply because the hosts generally die from metastases before even the earliest recurrences develop. A long follow-up time may also result in animals dying with no outward evidence of the malignancy, but still at risk of recurrence. Such animals should be necropsied, if possible, for evidence of residual tumor, metastases, and cause of death. Extreme caution must be exercised in deciding on criteria for including or excluding these animals from the TCD_{50} analysis. For example, suppose it is known from past experiments that a particular mouse tumor must be observed for at least 3 months after treatment to detect essentially all of the recurrences. In an experiment with this tumor line, every tumor in a group of ten mice disappears completely within a few weeks after irradiation, recurrent tumors are observed at 47, 53, 55, 60, and 67 days, and one animal dies at 79 days of intercurent disease without evidence of a recurrent tumor. In calculating the TCD_{50} at 3 months after treatment, it would be incorrect to score the response of the group as 50% (i.e., 5/10) controlled. The correct value would be 44% (i.e., 4/9) controlled, because the animal that died was still at risk and must be eliminated.

The TCD_{50} and its error limits must be calculated from a complete set of data relating the dose and the proportion of tumors cured. This is usually performed

234

ROBERT F.
KALLMAN
AND
SARA
ROCKWELL

by fitting a least-squares curve to a probit or a logit transformation of the tumor control rates as a function of either the dose or the logarithm of the dose (Suit *et al.*, 1965; Finney, 1964) and calculating the TCD_{50} and its error limits on the basis of this curve.

The measurement of tumor cure has the additional advantage of being usable with autochthonous, primary tumors, but this assay also has several limitations. Because intensive treatments are necessary to cure a tumor, the assay can be used only with effective treatment agents in high doses. Large numbers of animals must be followed for long periods of time, which is tedious and usually expensive. The assay provides little information about the response of individual tumor cells to the treatment, but instead reflects the overall effect of the therapy on the tumor–host system. Because of these limitations, it is desirable to use other assays, which are less clinically relevant, but which give more or different information about the effects of the agents.

3.2. Tumor Growth and Regrowth

It is perhaps simplest to measure therapeutic effects by analyzing the changes induced in the tumor growth patterns by the treatment. Generally, tumors are implanted or selected and their growth is followed until they reach a certain, predetermined size. The tumors are then randomized into different treatment groups and treated. After treatment, the size of each tumor is measured frequently until the tumor reaches a predetermined size, usually in the range of 2–4 times the size at the time of treatment. The growth pattern, growth rate, and the times for treated groups and untreated control groups to reach this larger predetermined size may be compared.

The techniques for measuring tumor growth and regrowth are relatively simple. For ascites tumors, it is possible to remove the tumor cells from the peritoneal cavity quantitatively by repeated washings of the cavity. A simple count of the resulting cell suspension gives a direct measurement of the number of tumor cells in the peritoneal cavity. For solid tumors, repeated measurements of the same tumor are usually limited to external measurements of the tumor. These are generally caliper measurements of the tumor dimensions, although other techniques of measurement have been used (e.g., displacement of liquid by the tumors or measurement of the dimensions of nonpalpable nodules from radiographs). While it is most desirable to measure the length, breadth, and depth of the tumor so that tumor volume may be calculated, some tumors may be followed more conveniently by determining the area, which is based only on length and breadth of the nodule. The volume of the tumor is related to the number of malignant cells in the tumor, but this relationship is not always straightforward. Such factors as the ratio of parenchyma to stroma, the proportion of necrosis, the volume of the tumor cells, and the amount of extracellular fluid in the tissue may vary during the natural history of the tumor and frequently change dramatically after treatment.

Growth/regrowth alterations are useful in comparing the therapeutic effectiveness of different agents, modes of treatment administration, sequencing of treatments, etc. Because a wide range of responses can be measured, from no change in tumor growth to the cure of the tumors, the technique is especially applicable to the analysis of treatments of unknown efficacy, which are difficult to analyze by many other methods. Growth/regrowth assays can be performed with autochthonous tumors, and are therefore useful when the experiment requires the special features of these tumors. Growth/regrowth assays are performed on tumors remaining *in situ* after treatment; this is advantageous in situations where cell counting and/or suspension of tumor cells is undesirable or impossible, e.g., in clinical trials or in tests of agents which result in rapid lysis of the killed cells.

However, several disadvantages must be recognized. First, changes in the tumor volume need not necessarily reflect changes in the tumor cell number or the tumor-cell viability. Thus growth/regrowth assays cannot always distinguish between cytotoxic agents (agents which kill the tumor cells) and cytostatic agents (those which inhibit proliferation in the tumor cells but do not kill them), as either would result in a delay in the growth of the tumor. Second, the growth of a treated tumor reflects the effects of the treatment on the normal stromal elements as well as the effects on the tumor-cell parenchyma. For example, localized irradiation of the subcutaneous tissues changes the function and structure of the vasculature and alters the ability of the tissue to support the growth of tumors injected weeks or months later (Hewitt and Blake, 1968; Jirtle and Clifton, 1973; Takahashi and Kallman, 1977). The regrowth of an irradiated tumor may likewise reflect this damage to the tumor bed (Thomlinson and Craddock, 1967). As another example, treatments which are immunosuppressive to the host are likely to affect tumor-directed immunity, and this in turn may alter the behavior of the treated tumor. Such effects are frequently of interest and importance in themselves; however, failure to recognize them and control for them appropriately in tumor growth/regrowth analyses may lead to erroneous conclusions about the cytocidal properties of the tested modalities. Perhaps the most serious disadvantage of regrowth measurements is the strictly empirical nature of this kind of data.

It is the pattern of tumor growth, rather than the pattern or rate of tumor shrinkage, which should be evaluated after treatment. The time when shrinkage of a tumor begins and the rate and extent of tumor shrinkage are more closely related to the structure of the tumor stroma, the kinetics of cell death after treatment, and the ability of a host to remove and dispose of dead or dying cells than they are to the viability of the surviving malignant cells *per se*. For example, some tumors do not shrink immediately after treatment; the relatively rigid stromal elements of these tumors maintain the treated tumor volume, and the density of the tumor cells decreases within this volume. Therefore, in evaluating the tumor response, it is the growth of the recurrent tumor, i.e., the regrowth, that must be observed and analyzed.

In some systems, it is possible to relate more or less quantitatively the growth of the treated tumor to the survival of the cells after treatment (Suit and Shalek, 1963; Van Peperzeel, 1972; Hermens, 1973). Such analyses require a thorough

236

ROBERT F.
KALLMAN
AND
SARA
ROCKWELL

previous knowledge of both the tumor system and the likely mode(s) of action of the treatment agent. In addition, one must have a thorough knowledge of the patterns of cell proliferation in the treated tumors. This is difficult to achieve. As will be discussed later in this chapter, the proliferative changes induced by treatment of a tumor may include delays in cell progression, shortening of the cell cycle, and changes in the proportion of proliferating cells. These changes will be dose dependent, and the proliferative patterns may be quite different at different times after treatment. In addition, the pattern and kinetics of cell death and the rate of the removal of dead cells from the treated tumor must be known for both the malignant and stromal elements. The changes in cell density (cells/volume) must also be known, because changes in the noncellular matrix (e.g., swelling caused by edema) may alter the volume of the tumor without changing the total number of cells in the tumor. Finally, it must be emphasized that for growth delay to be related quantitatively to the number of surviving proliferating tumor cells, the slope of the regrowth curve should be identical with that of the growth curve, i.e., the curve of growth before treatment. Although this may be achieved in tumors in experimental animals, painstakingly careful measurements of human tumors have established that posttreatment growth rates are rarely if ever identical with those determined prior to treatment (R. H. Thomlinson, personal communication; Thomlinson *et al.*, 1976). Because all such essential data are seldom available, quantitative analyses relating tumor-cell survival to tumor growth and regrowth data must be based on numerous assumptions about cell proliferation and cell death in the tumor. Estimates of tumor-cell survival derived from tumor growth/regrowth data must therefore be regarded as, at best, very approximate.

Even though information gained from growth/regrowth experiments must be considered as empirical, it may nonetheless be of great value in comparing different treatments or treatment modalities. An example of a carefully designed study using this assay is an experiment in which Brown *et al.* (1971) examined the radiosensitizing properties of some pyrimidine analogues. Figure 2 shows the regrowth patterns of a well-characterized solid tumor, the KHT sarcoma in C3H mice, after a fractionated course of X-irradiation. Plotting the delay in the time necessary for irradiated tumors to increase from the size at treatment to double that size, as a function of total radiation dose, yields a conveniently linear relationship (Fig. 3, open circles) which is not altered by infusing the animals with either saline (closed circles) or FUdR (open squares). No growth delay was seen in tumors infused with BCdR but not irradiated. Tumors infused with BCdR before irradiation were sensitized to the effects of the irradiation, as shown by the increased slope of the dose–response curve (closed squares).

3.3. Prolongation of Host Survival

Prolongation of host survival is frequently used as a measure of therapeutic effectiveness, especially in screening experiments with new chemotherapeutic agents or combinations. The general protocol for this type of analysis is to inject the host animal with a known number of malignant cells, wait some fixed time (a

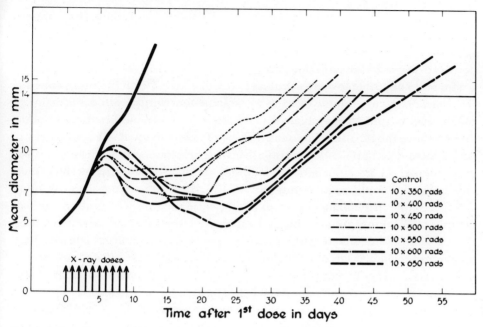

FIGURE 2. Growth curves of KHT sarcomas after fractionated courses of daily irradiation. Each curve was obtained by plotting as a function of time the mean of the diameters of a group of six tumors. From Brown *et al.* (1971).

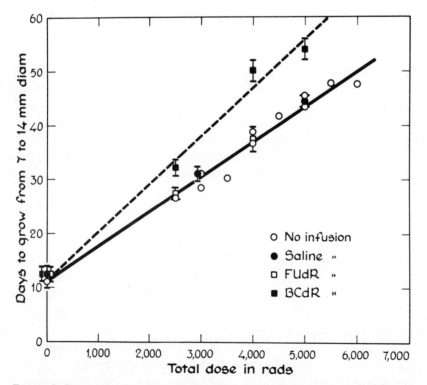

FIGURE 3. Dose–response curves for growth delay in KHT sarcomas treated with fractionated irradiation alone (noninfused mice, saline-infused controls) or in combination with infused FUdR or BCdR. From Brown *et al.* (1971).

238
ROBERT F.
KALLMAN
AND
SARA
ROCKWELL

few minutes to a few days), treat the tumor, and observe and compare the time of death in treated and control animals. In essence, this is a variation of the tumor growth/regrowth method: death occurs when the tumor size, cell number, or body burden reaches some maximum level. In general, this endpoint is most useful and applicable to ascites tumors and leukemias. Death of animals bearing these tumors occurs rapidly (days to weeks), the time until death is a function of the number of tumor cells inoculated, and this end point is sufficiently reproducible to ensure the reliability and sensitivity of the assay method. The popularity of such systems as L1210 leukemia and S180 ascites rests upon these properties. For solid tumors, the growth/regrowth method described above is generally preferable to the time-until-death end point, because these tumors usually grow more slowly than the disseminated diseases and because the causes of death in animals bearing solid tumors are multiple and variable—secondary infection, metastases, hemorrhage, or invasion of vital structures. As a result, the time until death is both longer and far more variable for solid tumors than for disseminated tumors.

The relative rapidity and simplicity of the survival-time method are probably the main factors responsible for its wide use in the rapid screening of new agents or combinations. Unfortunately, while the method is sound, it frequently has been used with a number of unsuitable tumor–host combinations. The response to systemic therapy of allogeneic tumors, e.g., Ehrlich ascites carcinoma, may be influenced disproportionately by effects of the treatment on the host immune system, which are not easily distinguished from direct effects on the tumor. Thus the validity of such a system as a model for the treatment of human tumors is highly questionable. This method also suffers from the same difficulties noted above, i.e., distinguishing between cytostatic and cytotoxic effects and relating changes in host survival to changes in tumor-cell survival after treatment. When testing ascites tumors, there is an additional problem, namely, that the pharmacokinetics of a drug injected into the peritoneal cavity and acting upon an intraperitoneal tumor-cell suspension is very different from the pharmacokinetics of the same drug acting on the cells of a solid tumor after entering the bloodstream. For these reasons, the applicability of this technique to realistic, quantitative studies of modalities under consideration for the therapy of solid human tumors is limited, although its utility in screening novel agents for activity is extensive.

3.4. Assays of Cell Survival

During the past 20 years, a variety of techniques have been developed which allow measurement of the viability of malignant cells suspended from animal tumors. These can be divided into three general types: end-point dilution assays, assays based on colony formation *in vivo*, and assays based on colony formation *in vitro*. All of these require the removal of tumor cells from the original animal, dispersal into single-cell suspension, enumeration of the cells, and a test of the growth potential of the cells, either in new hosts or in cell culture.

3.4.1. Preparation of Tumor-Cell Suspensions

239

EFFECTS OF
RADIATION ON
ANIMAL TUMOR
MODELS

Some tumors (e.g., ascites tumors, lymphomas, and leukemias), occur naturally as single-cell suspensions and need only be harvested from the animals in which they have grown. For solid tumors, however, the cells must be suspended; i.e., they must be released from the stromal elements and separated from one another. Single-cell suspensions may be prepared from solid tumors by mechanical means, by enzymatic digestion, or by a combination of both. Tumors with loose stroma frequently may be disrupted satisfactorily by mincing the tumor with sharp scissors or razor blades. Forcing crude suspensions through a fine sieve or back and forth through a needle may aid in mechanical disruption. Such techniques have been used with solid lymphomas or with tumor-involved lymph nodes. Although mechanical tissue homogenizers have been used occasionally, most of the commercially available models are designed for the disruption of tissues for biochemistry, and produce suspensions containing very few intact, viable cells.

Tumors may also be suspended by treating the solid tumor pieces with enzymes that break down the intercellular matrix of proteins and glycoproteins. Trypsin, collagenase, and pronase have all been effective in certain situations. Trypsin is probably the most widely used enzyme, primarily because of its relatively low cost and ready availability. Enzymatic disruption of the tumor cannot proceed indefinitely, because the proteolytic enzymes will attack and destroy the cell membranes. Enzymatic activity must therefore be stopped before the cells are killed or seriously injured. This can be done conveniently by centrifuging the cells from the enzyme-containing medium, by chilling the suspension, or, in the case of trypsin, by adding serum, which inhibits the activity of the enzyme.

Enumeration of the suspended tumor cells requires differentiation of the malignant cells from the blood and stromal elements present in the same suspension. In many cases, this is a major problem, because the classification of some of the cells is almost inevitably arbitrary. It is also desirable, if not essential, to identify cells which have been killed during the suspension process or which were physiologically dead prior to suspension and withstood complete digestion by the enzymes. This is commonly done by applying a dye exclusion test to the cells in a hemacytometer chamber. Several supravital dyes, such as trypan blue and erythrosin B, selectively stain dead cells, i.e., cells which have damaged cellular membranes and compromised active transport systems. While these are usually cells which have had their membranes damaged during suspension, some may also be cells in the final stages of dying from experimental treatments or natural causes. Although it is widely agreed that cells stained in this manner are dead, dying, or incapable of proliferation, it is not true that all unstained cells are either physiologically "viable" or potentially clonogenic. Nonetheless, dye exclusion methods are useful in differentiating definitely dead from possibly viable cells, especially when observation is made with phase contrast optics.

Automatic counting equipment and flow microfluorometry (FMF) systems are now widely used to enumerate suspensions of cultured cells. However, it is not yet practicable to use these systems to enumerate viable tumor cells in suspensions

240

ROBERT F.
KALLMAN
AND
SARA
ROCKWELL

prepared from solid tumors. The available FMF systems, which can discriminate between trypan blue stained and unstained cells, are often unable to distinguish the malignant and stromal cell populations on the basis of size and morphology, and the complicated staining procedures necessary for more sophisticated analyses of cellular contents or biochemistry are still too long and complex to allow real-time application of the techniques to routine differential counts of cell suspensions for cell survival analyses. It is to be hoped that the next few years will bring sufficient progress in instrument design and in the formulation of sufficiently comprehensive algorithms for cell recognition so that superior cell-enumeration systems will become available for this task and the present dependence on tedious, and frequently subjective, microscopic counts can be eliminated.

Most suspension and enumeration procedures in common use involve a combination of mechanical and enzymatic disruption (Reinhold, 1965; Kallman *et al.*, 1967). A typical suspension procedure, used for suspending cells from EMT6 tumors, is illustrated in Fig. 4. The tumors are removed aseptically, freed from the overlying skin, fat, and other extraneous normal tissues, and placed in a watch glass containing a few drops of Hanks' balanced salt solution supplemented with 0.05% trypsin. After a group of tumors (generally three to eight tumors, depending on the number of cells required) have been pooled in the same watch glass, they are minced with a small curved surgical scissors, forming a fine brei. This is transferred to a fluted trypsinizing flask with 200 ml of a solution of 0.05% trypsin in Ca^{2+}, Mg^{2+}-free Hanks' balanced salt solution at 37°C. The brei is then trypsinized for 15 min with agitation, and the resulting suspension is filtered through a fine wire mesh to remove any intact tumor fragments. The filtrate is centrifuged at 1000 rpm for 10 min at 4°C and the pellet of cells is resuspended in cell culture medium (Waymouth's 752/1) containing 15% serum to inhibit any residual trypsin. An aliquot is then removed, diluted, and mixed with trypan blue. A differential count is performed with a hemacytometer using phase contrast microscope optics. Serial dilutions are then prepared and plated in petri dishes so that survival may be determined from colony counts after 13–14 days of growth *in vitro*.

One potential problem associated with all suspension procedures is the danger of selecting a subpopulation not typical of the entire tumor cell population. If, for example, a tumor were to contain abundant necrotic regions from which the cells would be released quickly, incomplete trypsinization would yield a suspension enriched in cells from these necrotic regions. Conversely, too vigorous a trypsinization might result in the complete destruction of these cells and yield a suspension consisting only of the last cells to be released, which would probably be those from the most solid, nonnecrotic regions of the tumor. In many tumor models, however, the viable, suspended cells have been shown to be suitably representative of the initial tumor cell population (Reinhold and DeBree, 1968; Barendsen *et al.*, 1973; Rockwell *et al.*, 1976). It must also be borne in mind that any suspension prepared from a solid tumor is no more than a sample of the total tumor cell population, and that it is virtually impossible to suspend quantitatively all of the

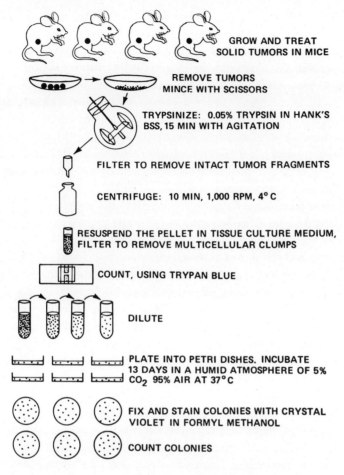

GROW AND TREAT
SOLID TUMORS IN MICE

REMOVE TUMORS
MINCE WITH SCISSORS

TRYPSINIZE: 0.05% TRYPSIN IN HANK'S
BSS, 15 MIN WITH AGITATION

FILTER TO REMOVE INTACT TUMOR FRAGMENTS

CENTRIFUGE: 10 MIN, 1,000 RPM, 4° C

RESUSPEND THE PELLET IN TISSUE CULTURE MEDIUM,
FILTER TO REMOVE MULTICELLULAR CLUMPS

COUNT, USING TRYPAN BLUE

DILUTE

PLATE INTO PETRI DISHES. INCUBATE
13 DAYS IN A HUMID ATMOSPHERE OF 5%
CO_2 95% AIR AT 37° C

FIX AND STAIN COLONIES WITH CRYSTAL
VIOLET IN FORMYL METHANOL

COUNT COLONIES

FIGURE 4. Schematic representation of the techniques used for the *in vitro* measurement of the survival of cells from solid EMT6 tumors. A complete discussion of these techniques is found in the text.

relevant parenchymal cells from any solid tumor. Furthermore, it is difficult, if not impossible, to ensure that any suspension technique will yield a constant percentage of the tumor cells, especially in treated tumors. For a therapeutic modality such as radiation, which produces a lesion that is not immediately lethal but causes the cells to die hours or days after treatment, samples of tumor cells suspended soon after treatment can provide valuable and unambiguous information. If, on the other hand, one is considering an agent, such as hyperthermia, which damages cells in such a way that they die and lyse during or very soon after the treatment, the dying cells may be lost from the tumor before they can be suspended in intact, recognizable form. In this case, subsequent measurements of cell survival would be artificially high, and should not be performed. One would then be constrained to employ more empirical methods, such as TCD_{50} or growth/regrowth assays, which do not involve suspension and enumeration of the tumor cells.

ROBERT F.
KALLMAN
AND
SARA
ROCKWELL

3.4.2. Clonogenic Assays

All of the tumor-cell survival assay methods discussed in this section measure the ability of malignant cells to proliferate essentially indefinitely, i.e., the capacity for clonogenicity. This criterion of cell survival is necessary and especially appropriate in radiation oncology for several reasons. First, a single clonogenic cell can, under appropriate conditions, cause the growth or regrowth of a tumor and the death of the host. Therefore, it is the definition of cell death as the loss of clonogenic capacity which is clinically important. Second, cells killed by irradiation continue to metabolize and proliferate quasi-normally for considerable periods of time after irradiation. For example, Elkind *et al.* (1963) showed that virtually all of the V79 Chinese hamster cells in a cell population irradiated with 200 rads (a commonly used dose in fractionated radiotherapy regimens) proliferated relatively normally for several cell cycles, i.e., for days. However, only about half the cells of the irradiated cell population retained the capacity to proliferate indefinitely and to produce a macroscopic colony. Therefore, measuring cell survival by the use of metabolic indicators of cell function such as [^{3}H]TdR uptake, the presence of mitoses, trypan blue exclusion, or indicators of differentiated function shortly after irradiation can be dangerously misleading. By the time metabolic death begins to occur, repopulation and other processes in the tumor would make measurement with these assays of cell death essentially meaningless as measurements of cell survival. In the absence of direct evidence to the contrary, cytotoxic agents other than radiation, e.g., chemotherapeutic agents or hyperthermia, should be assumed to kill cells slowly rather than instantaneously, and should be similarly evaluated in terms of their effects on the clonogenic potential of target cells.

Additional problems with cell survival assays may result from the fact that the suspended cells are tested for clonogenicity by removing them from the original tumor and testing them for growth in new hosts or *in vitro*. If only a small fraction (5% or less) of the cells from untreated tumors are capable of forming colonies under the assay conditions, it is overwhelmingly likely that the cells examined by the assay are but a small subpopulation of the cells that would be clonogenic if left *in situ*. The behavior and therapeutic responses of this subpopulation of cells may not be representative of the responses of the entire clonogenic tumor cell population. Because of this, it is desirable to use cell lines and assay systems in which the proportion of clonogenic cells is high (i.e., where the plating efficiency is greater than approximately 20% or the TD$_{50}$ is less than approximately 50 cells). In all cases, the system must be examined critically to ensure that the tested population is representative of the total population.

The results of cell-survival analyses are not sufficient to predict or interpret therapeutic responses of tumors *in situ*, simply because cells suspended and tested in cell culture or in untreated animals have a very different environment than cells remaining *in situ* after treatment. Environmental factors can be critical in determining the ability of the cells to recover from damage produced by the treatment. As discussed below, noncycling cells remaining in a tumor treated with radiation or drugs may exhibit recovery from potentially lethal damage, while the same cells explanted into a more favorable environment immediately after treatment would not have the opportunity to recover (Little *et al.*, 1973; Hahn *et al.*, 1974). Similarly, cells remaining in the hypoxic regions of irradiated tumors may repair sublethal damage less well than the same cells which have been suspended and therefore well oxygenated after treatment (Koch and Kruuv, 1971). Such factors do not invalidate results obtained with clonogenic assays. In fact, clonogenic assay methods have allowed the identification of such phenomena and the examination of their biological bases, their importance, and their implications for the treatment of human cancer. However, such phenomena do influence the survival of tumor cells remaining *in situ* after treatment and must be considered whenever data from cell-survival assays are used to interpret, analyze, or model the survival and behavior of cells in treated tumors *in vivo*.

3.4.3. The End-Point Dilution Method

End-point dilution was the first quantitative method used for the *in vivo* analysis of tumor-cell survival (Hewitt, 1953; Hewitt and Wilson, 1959a). The method basically consists of the preparation of serial dilutions of a counted tumor-cell suspension, the placement of replicate inocula of each dilution into a given site in appropriate normal recipients, the scoring of tumor takes, and calculation of the TD_{50} (the number of cells necessary to give tumors in 50% of the inoculation sites). The number of dilutions tested, the number of cells/dilution, and the difference in cell count from dilution to dilution are all determined by the degree of precision required in the TD_{50} and the accuracy with which the TD_{50} may be predicted from other data. TD_{50}'s measured for unperturbed, i.e., control, tumors may range from one cell to 5×10^5 cells. Ideally, the recipient animals should be syngeneic with the tumor to be tested (Hewitt *et al.*, 1976), but if this cannot be assured, immunosuppressed or immunologically incompetent (e.g., neonatal) recipients may be used (Silini and Hornsey, 1961). The choice of the inoculation site depends on the kind of tumor and its compatibility with the recipient. Cell suspensions prepared from solid tumors syngeneic with the recipients are conveniently inoculated subcutaneously or intradermally, while immunologically privileged sites may be preferable with immunogenic tumors. Dilutions of leukemia cells or ascites tumors are conveniently inoculated intraperitoneally. The use of multiple inocula per recipient, although convenient and economical, introduces other difficulties. If the tumor cells are recognized as foreign, there is likely to be significant interaction between multiple sites in the same recipient. Even independent inocula may interact operationally if there should be a take at one site with subsequent rapid growth, culminating in death of the animal before the end of the observation period. In this case, the fate of other inocula in the same animal cannot be determined, and appropriate and troublesome corrections must be performed during the statistical data analysis. There is no universally applicable observation period; this must be determined separately for every tumor. While 100 days is frequently satisfactory, either longer or shorter times may be

244

ROBERT F.
KALLMAN
AND
SARA
ROCKWELL

required or adequate. Once the final tally of tumor takes as a function of inoculum size has been completed, the TD_{50} may be computed by routine statistical analysis (Finney, 1964; Kallman *et al.*, 1967).

Because it has been determined that the TD_{50} can be changed greatly by the admixture in the inocula of large numbers of heavily irradiated (HR) cells (Révész, 1958; Hewitt *et al.*, 1973), it is necessary to determine experimentally for every tumor to be used with this kind of assay whether such a "Révész" effect occurs. The mechanism for this effect remains elusive, despite several notable attempts to explain it. It does not appear to be a simple feeder-layer effect, although the dying HR cells do release macromolecules, macromolecular fragments, and small molecules which are incorporated by the viable tumor cells (Yatvin *et al.*, 1970). Hewitt and his collaborators have suggested that the thromboplastic effects of the dying HR cells result in increased fibrin formation at the inoculation site and therefore increase entrapment or survival of the viable cells (Hewitt *et al.*, 1973; Peters and Hewitt, 1974). For demonstrably immunogenic tumors, the phenomenon is complicated by immunological effects, and HR cells may either stimulate or inhibit tumor development (Révész, 1958). However, the Révész effect also occurs in tumors without demonstrable immunogenicity and immunological factors do not appear to be solely responsible for the Révész effect.

3.4.4. Colony Formation in Vivo

Several techniques are now available for studying tumor cell survival by measuring the ability of individual malignant cells to form colonies, i.e., small tumors, in specific organs of a mouse. Generally, the tumor cells are injected into the bloodstream as a single-cell suspension and the tumors are observed in the tissue which provides a suitable bed for their entrapment and proliferation. This type of assay is operationally and theoretically similar to the method of Till and McCulloch (1961), in which hematopoietic stem cells form macroscopically distinct colonies in the spleen after intravenous inoculation into a lethally irradiated mouse. A modification of the Till and McCulloch method was used by Bush and Bruce (1964) to study the survival of lymphoma cells by their ability to form spleen colonies, and has been used by these authors and others for the analysis of therapeutic responses in this type of tumor.

Single-cell suspensions prepared from certain solid tumors and injected intravenously will be trapped in the lungs of the recipients and grow into discrete colonies, which may be counted 2–3 weeks later (Hill and Bush, 1969). The colony-forming efficiency, analogous to the plating efficiency in cell culture, is low (one colony per 10^4–10^5 cells inoculated), but this may be increased markedly either by admixing synthetic microspheres or radiation-sterilized tumor cells with the viable cell suspension or by irradiating the lungs (i.e., bilateral thorax) of the recipients before inoculation (Hill and Bush, 1969; Brown, 1973; Withers and Milas, 1973). Enhancement by either of these methods is related to the formation of emboli in the pulmonary microcirculation, which favors the lodgement of colony-forming tumor cells, rather than to any immunological mechanism.

3.4.5. Colony Formation in Vitro

245

EFFECTS OF
RADIATION ON
ANIMAL TUMOR
MODELS

Unfortunately, most tumors cannot be grown or cloned *in vitro* after direct passage from animals, and it is necessary to employ methods such as TCD_{50}, growth/regrowth, or TD_{50} to study their sensitivity to therapy. Recently, however, a few tumor systems have been developed which permit the *in vitro* analysis of the survival of cells from tumors treated *in vivo*. Development of a tumor-cell line which will grow well both *in vitro* and *in vivo* may require selection and/or adaptation of the tumor-cell population. A cell suspension prepared from an autochthonous tumor may be very heterogeneous and contain many subpopulations of parenchymal tumor cells having a wide range of cell proliferation patterns, metastic potentials, degrees of differentiation, and abilities to proliferate *in vitro*. With repeated passage *in vivo* or *in vitro*, more uniform subpopulations may be selected and these may progressively predominate, resulting in the emergence of a relatively homogeneous and stable subline. To develop a tumor-cell line capable of proliferating either *in vivo* or *in vitro*, a serially transplanted animal tumor is chosen which has desirable experimental properties as a transplantable tumor line. Cells are put into cell culture and passaged for several weeks or months until a subline that grows well *in vitro* has evolved. There is great variability in the adaptability of tumor lines to cell culture. Some grow well from the earliest passages; others have never been successfully adapted to *in vitro* growth in spite of intensive effort. The cell line is often cloned, so that a population derived from a single cell may be studied and propagated. The line is then examined for its ability to produce tumors in suitable, preferably syngeneic, host animals with a "plating efficiency" that is high, i.e., with a low TD_{50}, and with a reasonably low antigenicity. Cells then may be passaged alternately in animals and cell culture to avoid selection for growth in one growth mode, or they may be stored in liquid nitrogen. Ideally, an *in vivo/in vitro* system should have a low TD_{50} when either cells from tumors or cells from culture are inoculated into animals and a high plating efficiency when either cells from culture or cells from tumors are plated in cell culture. Because of the selection processes, *in vivo/in vitro* systems tend to be rapidly growing, relatively uniform, anaplastic tumors. They therefore have limitations as models for all of the biological properties of tumors seen in patients, which are always more slowly growing and usually more differentiated. They also may differ appreciably from the animal tumor lines from which they were derived. *In vivo/in vitro* systems are nonetheless invaluable for the investigation of fundamental questions in experimental therapeutics, because of the rapid, precise, and quantitative data which they afford. Current *in vivo/in vitro* systems include the R-1 rhabdomyosarcoma grown in the WAG/Rij rat (Barendsen and Broerse, 1969), the EMT6 mammary tumor grown in the BALB/c mouse (Rockwell *et al.*, 1972), the NCTC 2472 fibrosarcoma grown in the C3H mouse (Frindel *et al.*, 1972), the RIB5C fibrosarcoma grown in the Wistar rat (McNally, 1972), a brain tumor grown in the Fischer 340 rat (Leith *et al.*, 1975; Rosenblum *et al.*, 1975), and the HLAC lung adenocarcinomas grown in the Syrian hamster (Terzaghi and Little, 1975). Although all of these systems are relatively new,

246

ROBERT F.
KALLMAN
AND
SARA
ROCKWELL

several of them have already become widely used, and are being applied to the study of a variety of treatment modalities including radiation, a variety of chemotherapeutic agents, and hyperthermia, as well as to basic studies of the immunology, metastasis, and biology of tumors *in vivo* and tumor cells *in vitro*.

The inability to develop *in vivo/in vitro* lines from some animal tumors probably arises because many of the standard tissue culture conditions, including the existing nutrient media, buffers, and growth surfaces, are suboptimal for supporting the growth and viability of cells with exacting nutritional or environmental requirements. Because cells in mass culture alter their environment by "conditioning" the nutrient medium and growth surfaces, such factors become exceedingly critical when cells are grown at the low densities necessary for colony formation. Progress in understanding the environmental requirements of cells *in vitro* should result in the improvement of nutrient media, buffers, two- and three-dimensional growth matrices, and other components of cell culture as well as the development of techniques for better cell culture. It is to be hoped that this will enable other, less hardy tumor cells to be grown in culture and will permit the development of additional *in vivo/in vitro* systems that resemble more closely the primary tumors from which they were derived.

The use of *in vivo/in vitro* systems has two major advantages. First, these systems allow cells from the same cell line to be studied both as tumors *in vivo*, where the complicated tumor architecture, host–tumor interactions, and complex tumor-cell population structure interact to yield the observed tumor responses, and *in vitro*, where cell populations with simpler population structures and environments may be studied in isolation. Second, they allow rapid and precise measurement of the survival of cells from tumors treated *in vivo*. The type of technique used for the *in vitro* measurement of the viability of cells from solid tumors is shown in Fig. 4, which illustrates the manner in which the authors work with cells from EMT6 tumors. The suspension technique, which was described earlier in this chapter, is similar to those used with *in vivo* assays such as the TD_{50} or lung colony assays, but greater care is necessary to ensure the sterility of the final cell suspension. Briefly, the suspended, counted, diluted tumor cells are plated into petri dishes containing a rich nutrient medium (Waymouth's 752/1) supplemented with antibiotics and serum, which has been equilibrated to the proper temperature and pH in a CO_2 incubator. The cells are plated at low concentrations, so that approximately 100 colonies may be expected to develop in each petri dish. Dishes are incubated in a 95% air/5% CO_2 atmosphere for approximately 13 days without feeding or disturbing the cells, to allow the clonogenic cells to develop into macroscopic colonies. These are then fixed and stained with formyl methanol containing crystal violet, and are counted. The cell culture techniques used with *in vivo/in vitro* tumor systems for plating cells from solid tumors are similar to those used with established cell lines *in vitro*. However, the *in vivo/in vitro* lines are frequently less hardy than lines such as HeLa or CHO, and require gentler handling and more favorable cell culture conditions, including richer growth media, more and better serum, and better-controlled pH. For some lines (the R-1, the NCTC 2472, the brain tumor), feeder-layers of radiation-sterilized cells, or medium conditioned by the growth of cells, or both have proved necessary for clonal growth with high and reproducible plating efficiencies.

In addition to the *in vivo/in vitro* tumors, which can be cloned *in vivo* using standard conditions, there are other tumor lines which do not grow or clone well under standard culture conditions but which can be assayed for cell survival *in vitro* by cloning the cells in suspension in a semisolid gel. In these assays, single-cell suspensions are prepared from the tumors as described above and the cells are counted and adjusted to the desired concentration. The cells are then mixed into a semisolid growth medium composed of tissue culture medium supplemented with serum and gelled with either agar or methylcelluose. The cells grow into three-dimensional colonies suspended in the gel. Because culture in this mode frequently offers a more permissive and favorable environment for the growth of malignant cells, this type of assay sometimes permits the clonal growth of cells from tumors which cannot be cloned in liquid medium on petri dishes. After incubation for colony formation, the clones are counted, generally without staining or fixation, using a low-power microscope. This approach has been used to study the effects of treatment on the L5178Y leukemia (Chu and Fischer, 1968), the KHT sarcoma (Thomson and Rauth, 1974), and the Lewis lung carcinoma (Shipley *et al.*, 1975; Courtenay, 1976).

4. Experimental Findings Relating to Further Understanding of Tumor Therapy

The effects of radiation treatments on animal tumor models can be summarized most simply by a consideration of the phenomena which have been widely referred to as the four R's of tumor radiobiology (Withers, 1975): repair, repopulation, redistribution, and reoxygenation. The first three of these occur in varying degrees in normal tissues as well as in tumors. Only the last appears to be unique to tumors. Other phenomena which are related to the four R's, not only mnemonically but also mechanistically, include recruitment and immunological rejection.

4.1. Reoxygenation

"Reoxygenation" is the term used to denote the reacquisition of radiosensitivity by cells which have survived a radiation treatment because they were hypoxic at the time of irradiation. It was originally inferred, and subsequently shown experimentally, that the hypoxic cells surviving in a tumor do become better oxygenated after irradiation, so that the term has proved to be entirely appropriate.

It has been known for about 55 years that irradiation given in the presence of oxygen produces more damage than irradiation given under hypoxic conditions (Holthusen, 1921). To act as a radiation sensitizer, oxygen must be present during

248

ROBERT F.
KALLMAN
AND
SARA
ROCKWELL

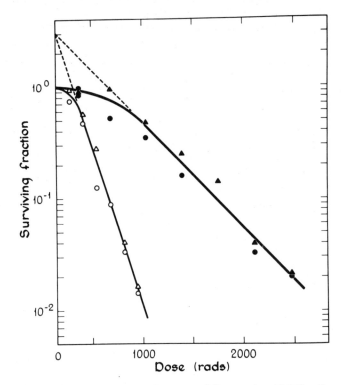

FIGURE 5. Survival curves of exponentially growing EMT6 cells irradiated *in vitro* under conditions of normal aeration (○, △) and severe hypoxia (●, ▲). From Rockwell and Kallman (1973).

the irradiation process. The concentration of oxygen required to produce complete radiation sensitization is low: essentially complete sensitization of mammalian cells is obtained at intracellular oxygen concentrations of approximately 70 μM (corresponding to a partial pressure of 40 mm Hg); lower oxygen concentrations produce less sensitization (Gray, 1961). The effect of oxygen on the survival of irradiated mammalian cells is illustrated in Fig. 5, which shows survival curves for exponentially growing EMT6 cells irradiated *in vitro* in the presence of oxygen and under acute, artificial hypoxia. Under the conditions of this experiment, oxygen acts as a dose-modifying factor, decreasing the D_0 of the survival curve from the value of 475 rads obtained in severe hypoxia to 155 rads, without changing the extrapolation number significantly.* The oxygen enhancement ratio (OER), calculated as the ratio of the anoxic and oxic D_0's, is 3.0, a value typical of the OERs found for mammalian cells *in vitro*.

Because many tumors have either a limited or a grossly inadequate blood supply, it has long been suspected that certain radioresistant tumors contain clonogenic cells that are not killed by the usual therapeutic radiation regimens

---

* The D_0 is the dose necessary to reduce survival by a factor of $1/e$ along the exponential portion of a survival curve. The extrapolation number, $\tilde{n}$, is the number obtained when the exponential portion of the survival curve is extrapolated back to 0 dose. For a complete discussion of these terms, see Elkind and Whitmore (1967).

simply because they are hypoxic and therefore radioresistant (Mottram, 1936). A firm histological basis for the presence of hypoxic cells in human tumors was established by Thomlinson and Gray (1955), who described in sections of human bronchogenic carcinoma, cords of healthy-looking tumor cells surrounding necrotic tumor cells. The stroma at the periphery of each cord was well supplied with capillaries, while the parenchymal tumor-cell and necrotic regions were avascular. Their calculations showed that the distance which oxygen could diffuse from a capillary through respiring tissue was similar to the radii of the viable tumor cords, and that viable cells on the periphery of the necrotic zone were probably hypoxic. Subsequently, similar patterns have been described in other human and murine tumors (Tannock, 1968, 1972; Tannock and Steel, 1970). The corded pattern with capillaries disposed along the outer peripheries of individual cords is not universal. Other tumors with corded morphology have capillaries located axially along the centers of their cords, while many other tumors completely lack characteristic corded patterns. In all instances where tumor cells are in cords or nests, the architectural dimensions are consistent with the expectation that there would be hypoxic zones containing viable tumor cells beyond the oxygen diffusion radius of 90–200 μm from the capillary walls (Tannock, 1972).

Because they are resistant to the cytocidal effects of ionizing radiation, the hypoxic cells in tumors are critical in determining the response of tumors to single treatments with large doses of radiation. Survival curves for a variety of solid tumors *in vivo* have now been obtained. Many of them have the characteristic shape first described by Powers and Tolmach (1963): a biphasic pattern with an initial portion similar to survival curves of well-oxygenated cells *in vitro* and a resistant tail with a slope similar to those of hypoxic cells *in vitro* or cells in tumors made hypoxic *in vivo*. This is illustrated in Fig. 6, which shows the survival curve for cells of solid EMT6 mouse mammary tumors *in vivo* irradiated under normal oxygenation (in air-breathing mice) and in hypoxia (in nitrogen-asphyxiated mice). The shape of the survival curve for the cells in a solid tumor reflects the proportion of hypoxic cells in the tumor as well as the intrinsic radiosensitivity of the tumor cells, and the proportion of hypoxic cells in the tumor can be estimated from the survival curve using the model of Hewitt and Wilson (1959b). Progress in the quantitative determination of tumor oxygenation and reoxygenation has been limited by the inability to measure local oxygen tensions within tumor or tissue beds reliably and directly. Consequently, virtually all data available on this subject stem from indirect measurements, such as analyses of tumor-cell survival curves or TCD_{50}'s, and are confined to tumors in experimental animals. In most experimental animal tumors, the proportion of the clonogenic cells which have survival curves that are characteristic of hypoxic cells, i.e., the "hypoxic fraction", is between 0.12 and 0.35 (see review by Kallman, 1972).

Immediately after a single, large dose of irradiation, the hypoxic fraction of the surviving, clonogenic tumor cells has been found to approach 1.0, reflecting the fact that the well-oxygenated cells of the tumor have been killed selectively by the radiation. After irradiation, reoxygenation occurs. At least four different patterns of reoxygenation occur in experimental tumors, as shown in Fig. 7. The different

250

ROBERT F.
KALLMAN
AND
SARA
ROCKWELL

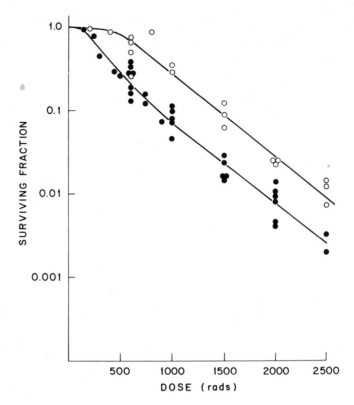

FIGURE 6. Survival curves for cells of solid EMT6 tumors irradiated *in situ* under normal oxygenation in air-breathing mice (●) and under artificial hypoxia in nitrogen-asphyxiated mice (○).

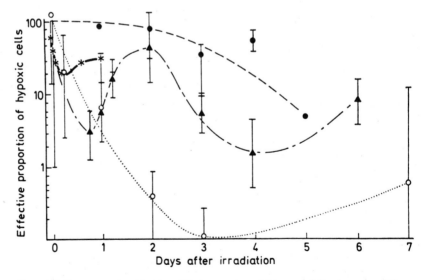

FIGURE 7. Reoxygenation kinetics of four experimental tumors following a conditioning irradiation (1000 or 1500 rads) at 0 time. The data are as follows: ▲, Thomlinson (1970); ○, Howes (1969); ●, van Putten (1968); *, Kallman (1974). From Kallman (1975).

kinetic patterns shown in Fig. 7 may be related to the different methods used in tracing reoxygenation, but it is more likely that the differences are characteristic of different kinds of tumors. With the exception of the osteosarcoma (van Putten, 1968), reoxygenation is prompt and rapid: the effective proportion of hypoxic cells begins to decrease immediately after irradiation. In addition, Fig. 7 shows that the proportion of hypoxic cells does not simply decrease to its preirradiation value, to stay there indefinitely or until some further insult is added. In some tumors, there is a suggestion of a second rise in the hypoxic fraction, possibly resulting from the expression of radiation damage to the vasculature (cf. Thomlinson, 1970). Also, in some tumors the hypoxic fraction eventually falls to values far lower than those of unirradiated tumors, possibly as a result of extensive shrinkage or improved microcirculation (cf. Howes, 1969).

Table 1 illustrates the rapidity of reoxygenation in three mouse tumors which were studied by the same technique in the same laboratory (Kallman, 1974). These tabulated data illustrate another potentially important fact, namely, that the kinetics of reoxygenation in a tumor is a function of its radiation history. Thus, in contrast to the pattern of prompt reoxygenation seen after a single dose of 1000 rads, reoxygenation does not start until about 12 hr after 2000 rads. Although this is a provocative finding, it may not be directly applicable to human tumors undergoing fractionated radiotherapy by the customary daily irradiation regimens, because a single dose of 2000 rads cannot be equated with a fractionated course reaching the same or even higher total dose. In fact, earlier evidence (van Putten and Kallman, 1968) suggests that reoxygenation is not noticeably inhibited in tumors exposed to large total doses by daily treatment with, for example, 200 rads.

In attempting to conceptualize models which account for radiobiological findings and which, in turn, would correctly predict radiation and drug effects, it is necessary to understand the mechanism responsible for reoxygenation. Unfortunately, it is not possible to implicate decisively any single mechanism as the cause of

TABLE 1

Hypoxic Fractions in Three Mouse Tumors at Different Times after Conditioning Doses of 1000 or 2000 rads[a]

Time after conditioning irradiation (hr)	KHT sarcoma (1000 rads)	KHJJ carcinoma (1000 rads)	EMT6 sarcoma	
			1000 rads	2000 rads
0	1.00	0.67	0.61	0.86
1	0.24	0.34	0.44	0.79
3	0.18	0.32	0.29	0.81
6	0.29	0.21	0.35	0.79
12	0.23	0.31	0.24	0.87
24	0.32	0.34	0.46	0.29
Unirradiated tumors	0.16	0.19	0.35	0.35

[a] Modified from Kallman (1975).

252

ROBERT F.
KALLMAN
AND
SARA
ROCKWELL

all reoxygenation. Four possibilities have been suggested (Kallman, 1972): first, radiation-sterilized cells may be assumed to consume less oxygen, thus advancing the limit of diffusion of the available oxygen without changes in the patency of the tumor vasculature. Second, if the capillaries were to become more patent without a concomitant decrease in intravascular pressure, the diffusion distance of oxygen would be increased, thereby improving tumor-cell oxygenation; in other words, the capillaries would be capable of carrying more blood per unit length and therefore of releasing more oxygen per capillary cross-section. Third, if killed cells were to die promptly and were to be scavenged equally promptly, shrinkage of the tumor mass should occur and capillaries unchanged in their blood- and oxygen-carrying capacity would be able to supply oxygen to a greater proportion of the tumor cells. Fourth, surviving hypoxic cells might be capable of migration to more favorable environments in positions within the effective diffusion radius of oxygen-carrying capillaries. The finding that reoxygenation is inhibited by giving large single radiation doses (described above) casts doubt on the first hypothesis— the assumption of reduced oxygen consumption by irradiated cells. Although tumor shrinkage is probably involved in the later phases of reoxygenation, the death of radiation-sterilized cells and the concomitant changes in cell density and tumor volume occur too late to explain rapid reoxygenation. Although several recent studies demonstrate significant changes in tumor microcirculation (Reinhold, 1971; Kallman et al., 1972; Song *et al.*, 1972; Hilmas and Gillette, 1974), most of these observed changes occur too long after irradiation to account for prompt reoxygenation. Thus, while such microcirculatory changes are of great importance in the physiology of treated tumors, they do not satisfactorily explain the process of prompt reoxygenation. Therefore, the mechanism, or combination of mechanisms, responsible for reoxygenation remains to be established.

Hypoxic cells limit the effectiveness of single doses of radiation in eradicating the cells of solid tumors in animals and probably in people as well. The greater therapeutic effectiveness of fractionated radiotherapy, relative to large single radiation treatments, probably results largely from reoxygenation, as the reoxygenation induced by each radiation treatment tends to ensure that more, formerly hypoxic, cells would be treated in an oxic environment in subsequent fractions, and therefore would be sterilized. However, not all fractionation schedules are equally successful in eliminating hypoxic cells in experimental rat and mouse tumors. In certain experimental tumors, after treatment the proportion of hypoxic cells falls slowly or falls rapidly, only to rise again (Table 1), and hypoxic cells could continue to be a problem during many fractionation regimens. For some experimental tumors, the efficacy of many fractionation schemes has been compared. The therapeutic ratios of the different fraction regimens vary significantly as a result of differences in reoxygenation and repopulation between fractions (Fowler *et al.*, 1974; Moulder *et al.*, 1976). Similarly, there is evidence that the problem of hypoxic cells is not completely eliminated for all human tumors by reoxygenation occurring during the conventional courses of fractionated radiotherapy, and that residual, chronically hypoxic cells may limit the curability of certain human tumors by present therapeutic regimens (Bush and Hill, 1975).

Several different approaches have been tried or are currently being examined to enhance the killing of hypoxic cells during radiotherapy. The most obvious approach is to tailor the fractionation regimens for a specific tumor type to achieve the maximum therapeutic ratio for that tumor. For some tumors, this may necessitate such approaches as the use of prolonged fractionation schemes, doses larger or smaller than the conventional doses per fraction, multiple small fractions per day, fractions of varying size, split courses of radiotherapy, or the use of low-dose-rate irradiation (e.g., implants) to obtain the optimal scheduling of the radiation treatments. Another approach is to treat tumors with radiations of high linear energy transfer (LET), which produce tracks of dense ionization in the irradiated volume. In the regions of dense ionization, oxygen becomes far less important in the radiochemistry leading to the production of cytocidal damage than it is for the sparsely ionizing, low-LET radiation generally used for radiotherapy. As a result, the oxygen enhancement ratio (OER) is reduced from the value of about 3 found for such low-LET radiations as X- or γ-rays to values of 1.5–2.0 (e.g., for neutrons or many fast charged particles) or even 1 at very high LETs (e.g., 2.5 MeV α particles).

A third means of reducing the problem of hypoxic cells is to improve the net tumor oxygenation. Because hemoglobin is saturated with oxygen under normal physiological circumstances, one approach which has been used clinically is to attempt to increase the oxygen carried in solution by the blood, by having the patient breath 100% oxygen, a 95% oxygen/5% CO_2 mixture, or 95% oxygen under increased barometric pressures (3–4 atm). Although such techniques have been shown to increase the radiosensitivity of animal tumors and some improvement in therapeutic results have been claimed, the clinical results as a whole have proved to be equivocal. As a result, such procedures have not been widely applied (see review by Duncan, 1973). Another approach, which is very appealing theoretically and is currently in vogue, is to use as an adjuvant to radiotherapy a chemical agent which will selectively sensitize the hypoxic cells in a tumor to radiation. One interesting type of hypoxic cell sensitizer is the class of electron-affinic compounds which have radiochemical effects similar to those of oxygen but which are not metabolized and therefore diffuse farther from the blood vessels than oxygen and are able to reach the hypoxic cells. These electron-affinic radiosensitizers, especially the nitroimidazoles, have been shown to be very promising, both in the laboratory and in the clinic. These compounds are described and discussed by Adams (this volume). Another approach which has recently begun to receive extensive investigation is to combine radiotherapy with treatments using a second modality that is selectively toxic to hypoxic cells. Possible agents presently being investigated include hyperthermia (Hahn, 1974; Gerner *et al.*, 1975), the nitroimidazoles (Hall and Roizin-Towle, 1975), and bioreductive alkylating agents, which are reduced to an active alkylating form at intracellular pH's lower than those generally found in well-oxygenated tissues (Lin *et al.*, 1974).

ROBERT F.
KALLMAN
AND
SARA
ROCKWELL

4.2. Repair

"Repair" may be defined as the return or recovery of a biological system, in this case a cell, to the preirradiation state after it has been injured by exposure to radiation or other therapeutic modalities. As this is the subject of another chapter (Elkind, this volume), it will not be discussed at length here. However, it is relevant to mention that there are two broad classes of repair phenomena of proven or potential importance in tumor radiobiology: sublethal damage (SLD) repair and potentially lethal damage (PLD) repair. As originally reported by Elkind and Sutton (1959), radiation may inflict injury which is insufficient to kill the cell and which may be repaired in a matter of hours if no further insult is received. This is known as sublethal damage. So long as this damage is not completely repaired, additional injury may sum with it to kill the cell. Consequently, a given dose of X-rays is less effective delivered in several fractions than delivered in a single exposure, because sublethal damage is repaired during the intervals between the treatments. Sublethal damage is detected only by comparing the survival of cells exposed to single treatments with the survival of cells exposed to two or more radiation treatments.

If cells are damaged by radiation, some of the injury that they experience may become lethal under certain conditions of growth or metabolism, but may be repaired, and therefore not lethal, under other conditions. This constitutes potentially lethal damage, and it requires manipulation of the postirradiation environment, rather than a second radiation exposure, for its detection. Both of these kinds of damage and repair have been extensively studied in cells grown and held *in vitro* (Elkind *et al.*, 1961; Phillips and Tolmach, 1966; Hahn *et al.*, 1973*a*) and have also been demonstrated *in vivo* both in tumors (Little *et al.*, 1973; Hahn et al., 1974; Shipley *et al.*, 1975) and in normal tissues (Withers, 1967; Withers and Mason, 1974). Both SLD and PLD repair have been demonstrated to occur after exposure to chemotherapeutic agents, as well as after treatment with irradiation (Hahn *et al.*, 1973*b*; Mauro and Elkind, 1968).

As discussed above, tumors *in vivo* contain cells in various states of oxygenation, and it is the proportion and radiosensitivity of the hypoxic cells which governs the response of many tumors to single radiation treatments. For radiation treatments, both the changes in the oxygenation of the tumor cells and the capacity of the tumor cells to repair radiation damage become important, and it is critical to determine whether all of the cells in a tumor share equally the capacities for the repair of SLD and PLD, regardless of their proliferative state, their state of oxygenation, and the characteristics of their nutritional and chemical environment.

Contrary to the opinion which was popular several years ago, that all tumors are made up of wildly proliferating cells, it is now generally acknowledged that appreciable numbers of tumor cells are not actively proliferating. Mendelsohn (1962) demonstrated that experimental tumors contain large numbers of viable, normal-looking cells which are either temporarily or permanently nonproliferating. The actively proliferating cells comprise the *growth fraction* of the tumor, and it is not at all uncommon for the growth fraction to include fewer than half of the

tumor cells. It is intuitively obvious that cells in the growth fraction must be regarded as potentially clonogenic, although some tumors do contain cycling, but nonclonogenic cells. For example, certain well-differentiated tumors, including human and animal leukemias as well as solid tumors, contain cells which are cycling but partially differentiated and capable of only limited proliferation before terminal differentiation to a noncycling end cell. In addition, tumors treated with radiation may contain large numbers of cells which are proliferating but doomed to die and therefore nonclonogenic. It is less clear whether noncycling tumor cells are generally clonogenic. In many experimental tumors, there is now ample evidence that noncycling cells are potentially clonogenic, and may return to proliferation under the proper stimulus. This is discussed in detail later in this chapter.

A conservative attitude to the therapy of tumors, therefore, is to regard all tumor cells as potentially clonogenic, whether or not they are actively proliferating. It is probable that many of the chronically hypoxic tumor cells are in the noncycling population. Severe, chronic hypoxia applied to exponentially growing cells *in vitro* causes a decrease in the proportion of cells engaged in DNA synthesis, a significant prolongation of the S phase, a significant and still greater prolongation of the G_1 phase, an accumulation of cells in a G_1-like state, a prolongation and increased variability in the cell-cycle time, and a gradual cessation of cell division (Bedford and Mitchell, 1974; Koch *et al.*, 1973; Born *et al.*, 1976). Nutrient deficiencies and/or acid environments, both of which would be correlated with hypoxia *in vivo*, likewise inhibit the proliferation of cells in culture (Fodge and Rubin, 1975). Therefore, cell culture data suggest a variety of mechanisms by which hypoxic cells *in vivo* might be inhibited from proliferation. An examination of cell proliferation patterns in a variety of solid tumors has shown that cell proliferation is depressed in regions of vascular insufficiency (Tannock, 1968; Rockwell *et al.*, 1972). In corded tumors, the depression of cell proliferation is accentuated as the distance from the blood vessel increases (Tannock, 1968). Therefore, it seems probable that many of the chronically hypoxic cells *in vivo* are nonproliferating. However, not all of the quiescent tumor cells are hypoxic; the hypoxic fraction in many experimental tumors is approximately 15%, while the fraction of nonproliferating cells in the same tumors is usually about 50%. In view of this appreciable discrepancy, the noncycling tumor cells must include both hypoxic and well-oxygenated cells.

Experimental tumors, and presumably the clinical tumors for which they are models, therefore contain proliferating and nonproliferating cells in a variety of states of nutrition and oxygenation, and one must ask whether the capacities of cells in these different states to repair radiation damage are similar. This problem can best be approached by examining data on cultured mammalian cells. As discussed above, exponentially growing cultures of mammalian cells provide a laboratory model for actively proliferating tumor cells *in vivo*, while plateau-phase cultures of mammalian cells provide a model for quiescent tumor cells *in vivo*.

256

ROBERT F.
KALLMAN
AND
SARA
ROCKWELL

Exponentially growing mammalian cells *in vitro* generally display a radiation survival curve characterized by a shoulder region of progressively increasing negative slope, followed by a more rapid decrease in survival which is essentially exponential, or a straight line if the log of survival is plotted as a function of dose. The capacity of cells to accumulate sublethal damage is related to the shoulder of this survival curve; a cell exhibiting this type of survival curve is capable of accumulating SLD and usually capable of its repair. For exponentially growing cells, the quantity of SLD which may be accumulated and the rate and extent of the repair vary with the cell line, the cellular environment, and the conditions of irradiation. The effect of hypoxia on the accumulation and repair of sublethal damage is not yet firmly established. At moderate levels of hypoxia, both accumulation and repair of sublethal damage occur, and only the slope of the survival curve is changed. Littbrand and Révész (1969) reported that cells irradiated under extreme hypoxia had a reduced extrapolation number (i.e., a diminished shoulder), which was reduced to a value of 1 in anoxia (<2 ppm O_2). No increase in survival was observed if this dose was fractionated, even when the cells were aerated between treatments. They concluded that severely hypoxic cells had a reduced capacity to accumulate SLD and that anoxic cells could not accumulate SLD. Other investigations contradicted this finding (Koch and Kruuv, 1971; Elkind *et al.*, 1965). The effect of extreme hypoxia on the repair of SLD is also open to debate. Some investigations have shown that cells irradiated in extreme hypoxia are able to accumulate SLD, but are either partially or totally unable to repair SLD if held in extreme hypoxia between radiation treatments (Koch and Kruuv, 1971; Hall, 1972). Others have reported normal SLD repair in extremely hypoxic cells (Elkind *et al.*, 1965). Whether these discrepancies are attributable to differences in the degree of intracellular hypoxia (extreme hypoxia vs. complete anoxia, i.e., the complete absence of oxygen) or to other factors (different cells, experimental methods, etc.) is still unresolved. Should the severely hypoxic cells in tumors have a reduced or abolished capacity for SLD repair, this would constitute an advantage for the therapist, because the well-oxygenated normal tissues would repair SLD during fractionated radiotherapy, while the severely hypxic tumor cells could not.

In general, cells growing exponentially under optimum conditions do not exhibit repair of PLD. It is only when conditions are made suboptimal, e.g., by reducing the quality of the growth medium or by inhibiting cell proliferation with drugs, that PLD repair is detectable (Phillips and Tolmach, 1966; Hahn *et al*, 1973*a*). We are unaware of data on the reparability of PLD in exponentially growing cultures irradiated under hypoxia or maintained in hypoxia after irradiation.

Cells in plateau phase under oxygenated conditions are variably capable of SLD repair. The ability to sustain and repair SLD is related to the single-dose response of the cells and is found only in cells whose survival curves have shoulders. For many cell lines, survival curves obtained during the plateau phase have smaller shoulders than those obtained during exponential growth; for some cell lines, the plateau-phase survival curves are exponential, with no shoulder and an extrapolation number of 1. Concomitantly, plateau-phase cells have been found to have a reduced or abolished capacity to sustain and repair SLD (Hahn and Little, 1972). In contrast, plateau-phase cells have a greater capacity for the repair of potentially lethal damage than do exponentially growing cells under the same environmental conditions. Unlike SLD repair, PLD repair involves a change in the slope of the survival curve and is essentially independent of the shoulder. Several experimental observations *in vitro* suggest that noncycling cells in solid tumors should be especially capable of PLD repair: (1) Intercellular contact appears to increase the capacity for PLD recovery; cells in dense monolayers exhibit 2–5 times as much PLD repair as the same cells irradiated after exposure in suspension. (2) Repair of PLD is enhanced when the irradiated cells are held in a nonoptimum nutrient medium which supports proliferation only poorly, and is greater still in a medium which does not support proliferation at all (Little, 1969; Hahn *et al.*, 1973a). (3) Cultured plateau-phase cells are capable of extensive PLD repair under conditions of moderate hypoxia (Hahn *et al.*, 1973a).

For the purposes of understanding—and, it is to be hoped, controlling—tumor-cell killing by irradiation and by other modalities, it is important to determine the molecular basis for SLD and PLD. On the one hand, Elkind *et al.* (1967) have examined the interaction of actinomycin D and irradiation and have concluded that sublethal and lethal damage are equivalent in kind, with respect to both the forward process of damage registration and the reverse process of damage repair. Winans *et al.* (1972) reached a similar conclusion after determining that the rates of repair of PLD and SLD were similar and that the same treatment (hypertonic medium) of irradiated S-phase cells blocked both types of repair, and after considering the correlations between chromosomal damage and cell killing. They suggest that potentially lethal lesions result from the interaction of sublethal lesions in chromatin structures. On the other hand, Hahn and Little (1972) have pointed out that stronger evidence indicates that the two types of repair are different: repair of SLD is dose independent over a wide range of doses, while repair of PLD is not; the two kinds of repair are additive; and PLD repair can occur under conditions where cells can neither sustain nor repair SLD (i.e., in some fed plateau-phase cultures).

To summarize, it is apparent that repair processes are of great importance in cancer therapy, in both the choice of the treatment modality(s) and the scheduling of treatments. As pointed out by Hahn and Little (1972), in predicting the response of cells to fractionated irradiation, one must consider the change in the effective D_0 due to the repair of PLD as well as the return of the shoulder due to the repair of SLD. One must also consider the many different subpopulations within the tumor, and the differing capacities of cells in these subpopulations for the repair of PLD and SLD.

4.3. Redistribution

"Redistribution," or "reassortment," refers to changes in the distribution of the cells surviving a treatment among the phases of the generation cycle. Populations

258

ROBERT F.
KALLMAN
AND
SARA
ROCKWELL

which are in active growth are composed of individual cells at different stages of the cell cycle. In addition to those cells which are actively traversing the cell cycle, designated for convenience as "P cells," significant numbers of cells may be nonproliferating, i.e., resting in a G_1-like, or occasionally a G_2-like, state out of the cell cycle; these are designated as "Q cells." Treatment with radiation or other therapeutic modalities will change the viability and proliferation pattern of the cells, and the surviving cells will be redistributed among the phases of the cell cycle. The redistribution of Q cells into the proliferating compartment may be regarded as a special case of redistribution and deserving of a specific term, namely "recruitment."

Changes in the P-cell compartment were both understood and expected following the classical reports by Terasima and Tolmach (1963) and later by Sinclair and Morton (1965) that cellular radiosensitivity undergoes pronounced and regular changes as cells progress through the generation cycle. This variation of the radiation response of the cell as a function of the "age," or position in the cell cycle, has been termed the "age–response function" (Elkind and Whitmore, 1967). It is not the purpose of this chapter to review the extensive literature on age–response functions; this can be summarized by stating that most cells are sensitive to X-rays during mitosis and near the beginning of DNA synthesis (in late G_1 and early S) and that resistance is characteristic of the mid-G_1 phase (provided that the G_1 phase is sufficiently long) and, increasingly, toward the end of S and into G_2. In addition to their well-known findings defining the sensitivity of cells to killing by X-rays as a function of age, Terasima and Tolmach (1963) reported another phenomenon which is frequently overlooked: irradiated cells experience delay before entering their next mitotic division and the duration of this division delay depends not only on the radiation dose but also on the cell age. There is extensive evidence that division delay is manifested by a block in the G_2 phase (Whitmore *et al.*, 1961) and that the closer a cell is to this point of blockage at the time of irradiation the longer the division delay per unit dose (Terasima and Tolmach, 1963).

It was suggested (Kallman, 1963) that the surviving clonogenic cells in an exponentially growing asynchronous cell population will undergo redistribution upon irradiation, roughly as follows: Cells in the more sensitive phases of the cycle will be killed preferentially, leaving survivors from the more resistant phases, e.g., late S and mid-G_1. As the surviving cells progress, they will tend to accumulate in G_2, at the "X-ray transition point" (Leeper *et al.*, 1972, 1973), the point of blockage that accounts for much of the division delay. Older cells, i.e., cells closer to the transition point in G_2, will remain blocked longer than younger cells. At the end of the block, the cells will tend to progress beyond the transition point as a synchronous cohort. Delay in cell division is seen as an effect of radiation in virtually all proliferating mammalian cells. The nature of the lesion responsible for division delay has been investigated extensively by Dewey and his collaborators (Dewey and Highfield, 1976).

The expected redistribution following irradiation of an asynchronous cell population *in vitro* was shown by the experiments of Elkind (1967), in which the

survival of Chinese hamster cells was examined as a function of the time between
two doses of X-rays. The survival probability of cells held at 37°C between
treatments was found to increase rapidly as a result of SLD repair and to reach a
maximum with approximately 2 hr between doses. With increasing times between
treatments, the surviving fractions fell, and then rose in a manner which could be
explained by partial growth synchrony in the surviving, clonogenic cells. Another
group of cells was held between treatments at 24°C, a temperature which
effectively inhibits progression of the cells through the cell cycle. SLD repair
proceeded normally at 24°C, and the rapid increase in the survival probability
during the first 2 hr was similar to that observed at 37°C. However, cells held at
24°C between treatments had very similar survival probabilities when irradiated
with a second dose between 2 and 10 hr after the first treatment; the fall and rise in
cell survival observed at 37°C did not occur. This is because the cells did not
progress at the lower temperature and therefore could not assume the different
states of radiosensitivity which normally would follow their initial redistribution.

It may be seen that redistribution as postulated here leads to a state of partial
proliferative synchrony among surviving cycling cells, that this state might be
expected to appear shortly after irradiation or comparable perturbation, and that
it should be evidenced by changes in net cellular radiosensitivity as the surviving
cohort continues to progress through the cell cycle. Owing to the heterogeneous
nature of cell populations and the possibly stochastic nature of the control of
growth and of the transition from one phase of the cycle to the next, synchrony
would not be expected to persist more than approximately one average cycle time
for the cells in question. Relatively early evidence that these expectations are
borne out experimentally has been summarized (Kallman *et al.*, 1967), and more
recent experiments from the same laboratory (Rockwell and Kallman, 1974) both
substantiate and extend the earlier findings. In Fig. 8, data are shown for the
surviving fractions of tumor cells taken from EMT6 mouse tumors which had
been irradiated *in situ* with a conditioning, or first, dose of 300 rads, and at 2-hr
intervals thereafter with a second, test dose of 600 rads. To avoid complications
arising from reoxygenation, the latter dose was always given to tumors which had
been rendered maximally hypoxic, i.e., 5 min after nitrogen asphyxiation of the
host animals. The surviving fraction changed cyclically, or periodically, as a
function of the interval between the two dose fractions. On the average, survival
varied over a two- or three-fold range. Time series analysis of these data
established that the periodicity was statistically significant and that the period
averaged 10–12 hr. Additional experiments showed that EMT6 cells had two
periods of radiosensitivity and two periods of radioresistance during each cell
cycle and that the mean cell-cycle time of the tumor cells was 20–22 hr. Separate
control experiments were carefully performed to investigate whether the radiation sensitivity of these tumor cells displayed any diurnal variations; none was
found.

Clearly, redistribution and the ensuing variations in radiosensitivity are confined to actively cycling cells, i.e., cells in active growth. The phenomenon is to be
expected in all kinds of cells, not just tumor cells. Evidence for it has been

260

ROBERT F.
KALLMAN
AND
SARA
ROCKWELL

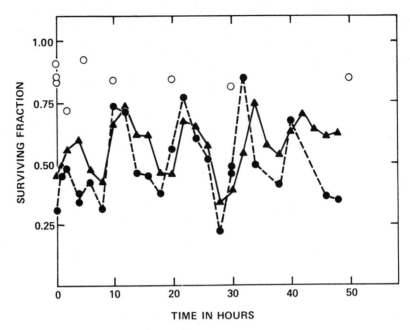

FIGURE 8. Survival of cells in solid EMT6 tumors after two doses of radiation. All tumors were irradiated locally with 300 rads of X-rays at time 0. At the specified times after this first treatment, tumors received a second treatment with 600 rads delivered in hypoxia. ●, ▲, Two independent experiments; ○, △ survivals of cells irradiated only with the first dose of irradiation and explanted at different times after treatment to test for PLD repair.

presented for bone marrow stem cells (Kallman *et al.*, 1966), skin (Denekamp *et al.*, 1969), and spermatogenic stem cells of the testis (Withers *et al.*, 1974). It is therefore apparent that the deliberate induction of redistribution by radiation or by drugs (Madoc-Jones and Mauro, 1970) is not a simple strategy to which one might turn in order to increase the effectiveness of therapy. The intriguing possibility remains that the therapist who can capitalize upon induced redistribution should be able to increase the therapeutic ratio appreciably. This would be a monumental task, however, as it would necessitate that cell-cycle progression be monitored continuously and closely in the clonogenic, surviving cells of both the treated tumor and the dose-limiting normal tissues. It should be emphasized that it is the redistribution of the *surviving* cells which is critical in determining the response of the population to fractionated therapy. This may be difficult to monitor experimentally, because the dying cells in a population treated with radiation will still be present and indistinguishable from the surviving cells, and these doomed-to-die cells will even proliferate for one or several cell-cycle times before dying and lysing. This makes it necessary to use assays of clonogenic cell proliferation to monitor the reassortment (Vassort *et al.*, 1973; Rockwell *et al.*, 1976) rather than assays of cell proliferation such as the labeling index or mitotic index. These latter assays measure proliferation in the total cell population (surviving and doomed-to-die) and may underestimate or incorrectly predict the proliferation of the redistributed, surviving cells (Rockwell *et al.*, 1976). There are

no methods currently available for monitoring the proliferation of the clonogenic
cells in tumors and normal tissues in the clinical situation, nor can any be foreseen
in the near future.

Nonetheless, an appreciation of the importance of redistribution and of the
differential effect that can be generated in proliferating, as contrasted with
nonproliferating, cell populations is provided by the hypothetical situation
sketched by Withers (1972) and shown in Fig. 9. As he has pointed out, if

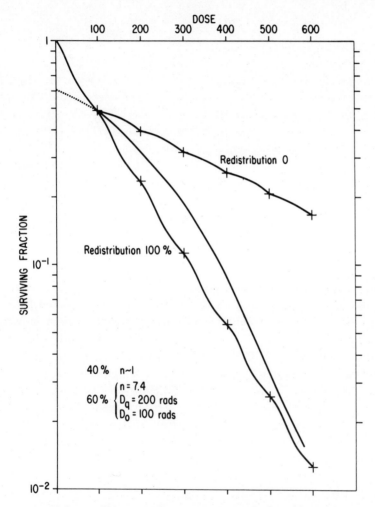

FIGURE 9. Hypothetical survival curves for a mixture of cells in two phases
of the cell cycle with different radiosensitivities. The sensitive phase is
assumed to have no capacity for the repair of sublethal injury ($n = 1$, $D_0 =$
100 rads). The resistant phase is assumed to have a large capacity for SLD
repair ($n = 7.4$, $D_q = 200$ rads, $D_0 = 100$ rads). The middle curve represents the single-dose–response curve for this population. The top curve
illustrates the multifraction response with no proliferation between doses
(i.e., no redistribution). The bottom curve represents the multifraction
response of the cells if proliferation results in complete redistribution of
the cells between treatments. From Withers (1972).

262

ROBERT F.
KALLMAN
AND
SARA
ROCKWELL

redistribution were complete between successive doses of 100 rads, the tissue response would be governed largely by the more sensitive cells and cell survival would be defined by the bottom curve in Fig. 9. If there were no redistribution (nonproliferating tissues), the response would soon become that of the more resistant cells and those cells would dominate the response to the second and all succeeding doses. Thus, in the case of an actively proliferating tumor being treated simultaneously with nonproliferating normal tissue cells, redistribution should provide a significant advantage to the therapist.

4.4. Recruitment

Earlier in this chapter it was pointed out that tumors are comprised of both cycling, or proliferating (P), cells and noncycling, or quiescent (Q), cells. Quiescent tumor cells are frequently referred to as "G_0 cells." However, this usage is not strictly correct. The term "G_0" was originally introduced (Lajtha, 1963), and is still used, to designate cells in certain normal tissues, such as the liver, intestinal crypts, and bone marrow, which are noncycling, which contain the amount of DNA characteristic of pre-DNA-synthetic cells, and which can be induced to begin proliferating upon appropriate specific stimulation. Thus G_0 cells in normal tissues may be either quiescent stem cells or functioning differentiated cells subject to specific regulatory processes that control their proliferation. Although some noncycling cells in well-differentiated tumors may be held from proliferation because they have not escaped completely from the homeostatic control mechanisms regulating the tissue of origin, most noncycling cells in experimental tumors, which are generally very anaplastic, have probably ceased proliferation because nonspecific environmental deficiencies prevent them from expressing their capacity for proliferation. In this sense, they may be regarded as analogous to plateau-phase cells *in vitro*. Cells such as those in plateau phase might react very differently to therapy and/or to subsequent environmental alterations than would G_0 cells in normal tissues.

Several models have been developed to describe tumor-cell proliferation kinetics in terms of two compartments and the transit of cells between these two compartments (Steel, 1972; Burns, 1975; Mendelsohn, 1975). However, until very recently, noncycling tumor cells had not been shown to possess the capacity for unlimited or extensive proliferation under any circumstances; i.e., they had not been shown conclusively to be clonogenic.

The clonogenic potential of Q cells was demonstrated convincingly by Bardensen *et al.* (1973) and later by Kallman (1976) in experiments of similar design. As the findings of the latter author are as of yet largely unpublished, they will be presented in slightly greater detail here. In these experiments, Q cells were defined operationally as cells determined to be noncycling on the basis of their inability to incorporate tritiated thymidine ([^{3}H]TdR) upon continuous or semicontinuous exposure to this DNA precursor for a period of at least 1 standard deviation longer than the mean cell-cycle time of the cells which are easily assignable to the P compartment on the basis of PLM analyses. In both sets of experiments, solid tumor systems have been used which are capable of alternate growth *in vivo* and *in vitro* as discussed earlier in this chapter; this capability is an absolute requirement of this experimental approach. Solid tumors (the R-1 rhabdomyosarcoma by Barendsen and colleagues and the EMT6 tumor by Kallman and his associates) were grown in syngeneic animals (rats and mice, respectively) and were exposed to [^{3}H]TdR semicontinuously, by repeated intraperitoneal injection, or continuously, by intravenous infusion, for 16 and 24 hr, respectively. The tumors were then excised and dispersed into single-cell suspensions, which were counted, diluted, plated in culture vessels, and incubated to permit the growth of colonies. Autoradiographs of the cultures were prepared, and the distribution of the [^{3}H]TdR in the colonies was examined and analyzed. Because the radioactive label would be excessively diluted by the 15–20 doublings necessary for the formation of macrocolonies, it is virtually impossible to distinguish labeled and unlabeled cells in traditional macroscopic colonies and small colonies must be used in the analyses. This procedure is illustrated in Fig. 10.

With this technique, it is possible to determine whether a given colony arose from a P or a Q cell, i.e., whether the progenitor cell had participated in at least one round of DNA replication during the period of exposure to [^{2}H]TdR. An unlabeled colony must have descended from a Q cell. Although it is to be expected that there would be some P cells with cell cycles only slightly longer than the period of [^{3}HT]TdR infusion, these would be rare. In the case of the microcolonies from R-1 tumor cells labeled *in vivo* for 16 hr as just described, the colony-labeling indices were 0.45 at 72 hr and 0.42 at 96 hr of colony growth. For the EMT6 tumor, the labeling index for all the colonies (containing 2–22 cells) scored at 72 hr was 0.80. Therefore, approximately 55% of the R-1 colonies and 20% of the EMT6 colonies arose from unlabeled or Q cells. These data provide conclusive proof that cells defined by the experimental conditions as nonproliferating have retained their clonogenic capacity. Of course, in these experiments, clonogenic capacity is expressed *in vitro*. While it is reasonable to assume that these cells would have the same capacity for clonogenicity *in situ*, i.e., within the tumors from which they were suspended, concrete proof for this is not yet available. Interestingly, the labeling indices obtained by scoring labeled and unlabeled microcolonies in the experiments described for the R-1 and EMT6 tumors are higher than the growth fractions derived from analysis of PLM data. This discrepancy probably results from two sources: (1) There is probably a steady flow of cells from P to Q. Therefore, some of the Q cells present at the end of the 24-hr infusion would have been derived from P cells which incorporated [^{3}H]TdR and divided earlier during the infusion period. That is, the tumor would contain some new, labeled Q cells. (2) P cells which had incorporated label near the beginning of the 24-hr labeling period would have divided at least once, so that the proportion of cells containing [^{3}H]TdR (i.e., the proportion of labeled cells) in the suspension would be greater than the proportion of cells incorporating [^{3}H]TdR during the incubation. Even though the grain counts of these cells would have been halved by division, they would still contain sufficient ^{3}H to be labeled autoradiographically.

264

ROBERT F.
KALLMAN
AND
SARA
ROCKWELL

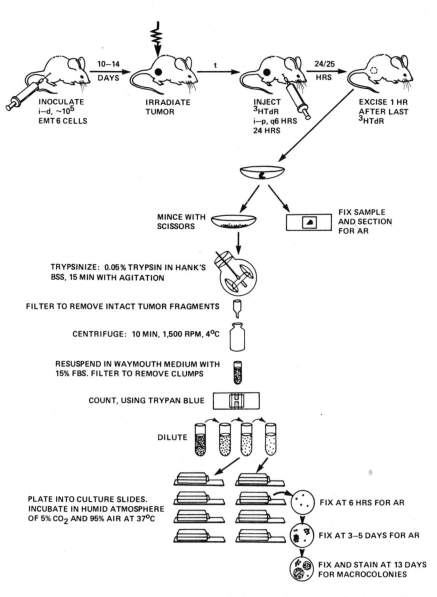

FIGURE 10. Schematic representation of the techniques used to analyze the clonogenicity of P and Q cells in solid EMT6 tumors. The techniques are discussed in detail in the text.

Having established that Q cells are potentially clonogenic, it is essential to obtain a better understanding of the factors that can cause the conversion of Q cells to P cells *in vivo*, i.e., the factors which cause recruitment. In designing optimum therapeutic schedules, it is important to know whether treatment with each of the possible therapeutic modalities causes recruitment. If recruitment does occur, one must ask when it occurs and how the magnitude and timing of the recruitment are related to the dose. Answers to such key questions are currently unavailable. The beginnings of informative answers, however, are emerging from experiments in which EMT6 tumors have been irradiated with either 300 or 600 rads

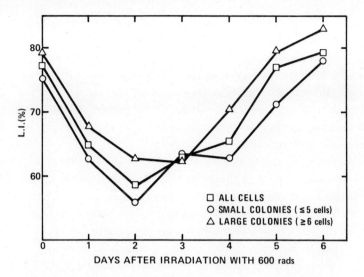

FIGURE 11. Changes in the labeling index of colonies derived from cells suspended from EMT6 tumors which were X-irradiated and then labeled *in situ.* The times relative to irradiation (abscissa) are times at the end of a 24-hr period of [³H]TdR administration. As discussed in the text, these changes reflect changes in the proportions of clonogenic P cells and clonogenic Q cells in the irradiated tumors. From Kallman (1976).

and then, at increasing times after irradiation, have been labeled with [³H]TdR for a standard 24-hr period. Analyses of labeled and unlabeled microcolonies derived from cells of these tumors reveal that Q cells were changed back into the P state, i.e., they were recruited in cycle, especially for the higher dose tested. This is shown in Fig. 11: tumors that were irradiated and labeled with [³H]TdR for the 24-hr period 5 days later contained more P cells than did unirradiated tumors. The rise of the curve, which starts at 2 days, suggests that recruitment began at this time and that, for approximately 3–4 days, recruited Q cells were replacing the P cells which had disappeared because of their greater radiosensitivity at the time of radiation exposure (Kallman, 1976).

4.5. Repopulation

The term "repopulation" refers to the replacement of cells which have been destroyed by treatment and is synonymous with the older term "regeneration." As this chapter is concerned primarily with tumors, only brief mention will be made of the fact that repopulation has been studied and characterized in a number of irradiated normal tissues, including intestinal mucosa, hematopoietic tissues, skin, and oropharyngeal mucosa (Chen and Withers, 1972; Vos, 1968; Withers, 1967; Withers and Mason, 1974; Lesher and Bauman, 1969; Moulder and Fischer, 1976). It is difficult to study repopulation in tumors because the lack of appropriate, direct methods necessitates the use of indirect approaches. Nevertheless, it

266

ROBERT F.
KALLMAN
AND
SARA
ROCKWELL

is essential to understand the kinetics of repopulation in tumors, because effective radiotherapy utilizes multifraction regimens, with daily or near-daily irradiation given over a period of several weeks; and repopulation occurring in the tumor between doses may be critical in determining the responses of the tumors to multifraction therapy with certain treatment schedules. In contrast, the exact pattern of repopulation after a large single dose, or even after two relatively large doses with the spacing used in most split-dose experiments, is largely of academic interest, and has little practical significance.

The importance of repopulation in radiotherapy is well illustrated by the findings of Suit *et al.* (1977), as shown in Fig. 12. In these experiments, third- and fourth-generation isotransplants of a tumor originally derived from a spontaneous mammary carcinoma in C3H/He mice were implanted in the leg and irradiated locally after they had reached a mean diameter of 8 mm. Tumors were irradiated either in hypoxia (with the blood supply to the tumor occluded by application of a heavy clamp across the proximal portion of the thigh), or with the mice breathing air, or in conditions where the mice were breathing oxygen at a pressure of 30 psi. TCD_{50}'s were calculated based on the presence or absence of tumor at 120 days following completion of irradiation. Tumors were irradiated with ν equal fraction, where $\nu = 1, 2, 5, 10,$ or 20. The maximum overall treatment time for these fractionated regimens was 30 days, and the interfraction interval ranged from $\frac{1}{3}$ day to 4 days. Figure 12 shows that for tumors irradiated under clamped conditions, which rules out any complicating effects of reoxygenation, the TCD_{50} for a specified ν appears to be independent of the time between treatments until some critical time is reached, beyond which the TCD_{50} increases

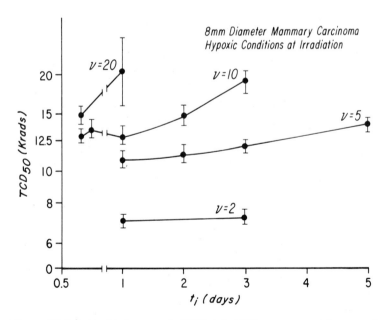

FIGURE 12. Relationship between the TCD_{50} of a C3H mammary carcinoma and the intertreatment interval (t_i). The tumors were irradiated with 2, 5, 10, or 20 equal fractions delivered in hypoxia. From Suit *et al.* (1977).

rapidly. For example, the TCD_{50}'s for ten fractions delivered 3 times per day, 2 times per day, or every 24 hr (i.e., in total times of 3, 5, or 9 days), were all approximately 13,000 rads. However, when the ten fractions were given with 2 days between fractions i.e., in a total time of 18 days, the TCD_{50} rose to 14,910 rads, and when the interfraction interval was 3 days the TCD_{50} rose to 18,980 rads. The *critical time*, when the tumor control dose starts to increase with increasing intertreatment time, becomes smaller as ν is increased and as the dose per fraction is decreased. The increasing steepness of the slope of the curve of TCD_{50} vs. overall treatment time suggests that repopulation becomes relatively more and more important (compared with repair) in determining the TCD_{50} as the treatment time increases. This is most likely the result of a stimulated, rapid rate of repopulation by the surviving tumor cells, an effect that has also been observed in normal tissues.

In contrast, studies by Moulder *et al.* (1976) with the BA1112 rhabdomyosarcoma did not reveal any significant effect of repopulation on the TCD_{50} of that tumor when irradiation was given 3 times per week in total treatment times of 1–49 days (1–22 fractions). However, the therapeutic ratio obtained by comparing tumor cure and skin damage under the same fractionation schedule became more favorable at the longest treatment times, because repopulation in the skin between treatments increased the tolerance of that normal tissue. This illustrates the fact that the effects of repopulation are not the same for all tumors and that repopulation in both the tumor and the dose-limiting normal tissue needs to be considered in optimizing therapeutic regimens.

Clinically, it is popular to use formulations such as that of Ellis (1968) for estimating the modification of total dose which should be made when the total treatment time or fractionation is altered, so that a specified and tolerable normal tissue response may be obtained. Although these formulations are reliable under certain limited circumstances (see Fowler and Denekamp, this volume), it is obvious that they cannot be applied with any confidence in situations such as those described above, in which cell proliferation occurs between fractional treatments, at times and rates dependent on the treatments and the tissue.

It is impossible to dissociate repopulation from redistribution and recruitment, as both of the latter processes are part of repopulation. Data of the kind described above suggest some different mechanisms that must be considered in defining the basis of repopulation in treated tumors. The finding that repopulation after irradiation may be more rapid than the increase in cell number in unperturbed tumors raises the question of whether this rapidity of repopulation is due to the recruitment of more cells into cycle (i.e., an elevated growth fraction) or to a shortening of the cycle time in cells that were proliferating prior to irradiation, or both.

In a recent series of experiments designed to examine the postirradiation proliferation kinetics of cells from the R-1 rhabdomysarcoma, Hermens and Barendsen (1976) present evidence that newly recruited Q cells cycle more rapidly than cells that were proliferating at the time of treatment. These authors speculate that the recruitment of such clonogenic Q cells into proliferation may provide an

268
ROBERT F.
KALLMAN
AND
SARA
ROCKWELL

important contribution to the repopulation of a tumor after treatment with noncurative doses of radiation. Interestingly, they also report that rapid repopulation in R-1 tumors is brought about by cells which were severely hypoxic at the time of irradiation.

Table 2 summarizes the effects of irradiation on cell proliferation in several experimental animal tumors. It should be noted that all of these results were obtained using the percent labeled mitosis (PLM) technique. This method suffers from some severe deficiencies when applied to treated tumors, because the analytical techniques are not strictly applicable to perturbed or partially synchronous cell populations. In addition, it is impossible to distinguish morphologically between the surviving cells and doomed-to-die cells, and the autoradiographic data, the tumor growth data, and therefore the cell-cycle time and growth fraction derived from them reflect the proliferation and disappearance of the dying cells as well as the proliferation of the surviving cells. Because of these technical limitations, the values shown in Table 2 must be regarded as tenuous and approximate.

As a brief examination of Table 2 will show, it is presently impossible to formulate any general rule about the effect of irradiation on tumor-cell proliferation. The cell-cycle time has been reported to lengthen, to shorten, and to remain constant. The growth fraction has been reported to increase, to decrease, and to remain constant. When cell proliferation has been examined as a function of time after irradiation, different tumors have shown different changes with time. Some of these differences may reflect the limitations of the techniques. Others may result from the variations in doses and times examined in the investigations. Still others may reflect real differences in the response of the different tumor systems to irradiation. It is to be hoped that future experiments will clarify this problem and provide additional data which will lead to a better understanding of the proliferative changes and repopulation processes in treated tumors.

4.6. Rejection and Other Host Phenomena

The behavior of a tumor *in situ* is influenced by the interactions between the tumor and the host as well as by the behavior and characteristics of the malignant cells. Therefore, a treatment which affects the normal tissues of the host in any way that alters their interactions with the malignant cells may indirectly produce changes in the characteristics of the tumor. Such phenomena would not, in general, influence the survival curves obtained by explanting the malignant cells immediately after treatment and cloning them in new hosts or in cell culture. They might be detectable by pretreating the host animal before implanting untreated tumor cells. The phenomena would occur, and might be studied in, tumors which remain *in situ* after the treatment and are examined for their growth rate, cure, metastatic capability, or response to fractionated treatment.

Many experimental tumors are influenced by the activities of the host's immune system. The viability and behavior of malignant cells and the growth, metastatic potential, invasiveness, and therapeutic responses of tumors have been shown to be affected by such nonspecific factors as activated macrophages as well as by such specific immunological factors as antibodies and cytoxic lymphocytes. The effects of immune attacks on a tumor are seen most clearly for allogeneically transplanted tumors. In this case, genetic differences between the tumor and host are extensive, and tumors transplanted into normal adult animals are very frequently rejected. Such tumors were used extensively in experimental oncology before the availability of inbred strains of mice and rats. Several allogeneically transplanted tumor lines, such as the Ehrlich ascites carcinoma, are still widely studied. However, the immune response to allogeneically transplanted tumors actually represents a strong homgraft rejection rather than the more specific and subtle tumor-directed immune response observed in experimental syngeneic tumor–host systems or in human tumors. Allogeneic tumor–host systems are therefore poor systems for modeling the immunobiology of human cancer. Neoantigens, antigens found on the cells of a tumor but not on the cells of the syngeneic host, may be easily demonstrable in tumors of viral origin (which may express virus-specific antigens), in tumors induced by many chemical carcinogens, and in tumors which have been passaged repeatedly in animals or in cell culture. These neoantigens are generally immunogenic in the syngeneic tumor-bearing host and may influence the development and growth of the tumor.

Spontaneous tumors in inbred rats and mice are less immunogenic, and it is unclear whether tumor-directed immune responses influence the behavior of these neoplasms significantly. Hewitt *et al.* (1976) examined the effects of immune perturbations on the TD_{50}, growth, and behavior of 27 spontaneous tumors arising in the low-tumor strains of their animal colony. They failed to detect any immune rejection responses to these tumors in either autochthonous hosts or hosts of the first few transplant generations of the tumors in syngeneic mice. Baldwin and Price (1976) have demonstrated that spontaneous tumors in Wistar rats are generally less immunogenic than tumors induced by viruses or most chemical carcinogens, and that many spontaneous tumors do not induce rejection responses in syngeneic hosts. However, these investigators also have demonstrated that even tumors which normally do not elicit effective rejection responses in syngeneic hosts do exhibit neoantigens (generally embryonic antigens) when examined with appropriate tests *in vitro*, and have suggested that these antigens may be able to elicit rejection responses under certain, limited conditions.

The experimental tumor–host systems which have been studied by various investigators range from those in which tumor-directed immune responses are either absent or negligible to those with sufficient immunological incompatibility that the host must be immunosuppressed to allow growth of the tumor without rejection. In using animal tumors as models for the immunobiology of human cancer, it is therefore necessary to ensure that the immunological incompatibilities between the tumor and host being studied are similar to those which might reasonably be expected to occur in the human tumors being modeled.

The presence and strength of immune attacks on the malignant cells of a tumor *in vivo* will influence the curability of the tumor, because the immune attacks will

270

ROBERT F.
KALLMAN
AND
SARA
ROCKWELL

TABLE 2

Cell-Cycle Time and Growth Fraction of Several Experimental Tumors Before and After Irradiation

Tumor	Dose (rads)	Time between treatment and measurement	Before irradiation		After irradiation		References
			Cell-cycle time (hr)	Growth fraction	Cell-cycle time (hr)	Growth fraction	
R-1 rhabdomyosarcoma	2000	4 days	21	0.32	11	0.26	Hermens (1973)
		8 days			12	0.28	
		10 days			12	0.22	
		14 days			13	0.20	
Adenocarcinoma 282	600	1 day	14	0.25	18	—	Szczepanski and Trott (1975)
		2 days			16	"Unchanged"	
		3 days			15	"Increased"	
		4 days			17	"Increased"	
	1200	4 days			12	"Increased"	
		6 days			12	"Increased"	
		8 days			20	"Unchanged"	
NCTC 2472 fibrosarcoma (ascites)[a]	250	20 hr	17	0.74–0.86	30	0.83	Frindel et al. (1970)
		48 hr			28	0.71	

RIB5 fibrosarcoma	1500	7 days	13	0.45	13	0.57	Denekamp and Thomlinson (1971)
SSO fibrosarcoma	1000	10 days	21	0.48	21	0.55	
SSB1 fibrosarcoma	1000	28 days	39	0.60	39	0.43	
C3H mammary carcinoma	1500	14 days	15	0.37	15	0.40	
Ehrlich ascites carcinoma (diploid)	500 r	1 hr	23	—[b]	45	—	Adler et al. (1972)
Ehrlich ascites carcinoma (hypertetraploid)	500 r	1 hr	41	—	50	—	
EMT6 mammary tumor	300	24 hr	20	—	18	—	Rockwell and Kallman (1974)
DMBA-induced carcinoma	500	24 hr	12	0.31	13	—	Brown (1970)
	1000	3 days	11	0.31	13	—	
Adenocarcinoma, M8013	210	45 hr	15	0.87	12	1.0	Van Peperzeel (1972)

[a] In the solid NCTC 2472 fibrosarcoma, the cell-cycle time is reported to be unchanged 48 hr after 600 rads delivered in hypoxia, but quantitative data are not reported (Tubiana et al., 1968).
[b] Not reported.

272

ROBERT F.
KALLMAN
AND
SARA
ROCKWELL

kill malignant cells, and therefore decrease the number of cells which must be killed directly by the treatment agent to cure the malignancy (Powers *et al.*, 1967; Suit and Kastelan, 1970). Current studies of immunotherapy, described in other chapters of this volume, are aimed at maximizing this effect and using the immune response to destroy the malignant cells remaining after treatment with other modalities.

The effects of radiation on the immune response to an established tumor are complex, because the immune response to an established tumor includes a variety of facets, both specific and nonspecific, both cellular and humoral, which may have very different radiation responses. The type of treatment, the dose, and the prior immune status of the host will obviously affect the changes in the immune response (Suit and Kastelan, 1970; Rockwell and Hahn, 1974). For localized, fractionated irradiation, the size and location of the treated field, the recovery and repopulation occurring within the treated volume, the seeding of the treated region by stem cells from untreated sites, and compensatory proliferative processes throughout the hematopoietic system all influence the changes in the immune response (Croizat *et al.*, 1970; LeFrancois *et al.*, 1974; Vaage *et al.*, 1974). The changes in the immune response following therapy with radiation, chemotherapy, or surgery may be significant, and may either stimulate or inhibit the growth and survival of malignant cells in the treated site or elsewhere in the host (LeFrancois *et al.*, 1974; Vaage *et al.*, 1974). Unfortunately, data on this important subject are still so limited and contradictory that generalizations and extrapolations to human tumors are not yet possible.

Radiation may alter the ability of the normal tissues of the host to support the growth of a recurrent, metastatic, or second primary tumor in the treated site, and therefore alter the natural history of the malignancy from that which would be observed in an untreated site. For example, irradiation of the subcutaneous tissues alters the ability of the vascular endothelium to form new vessels, and this may inhibit the growth of either newly implanted or recurrent tumors in irradiated sites (Thomlinson and Craddock, 1967; Hewitt and Blake, 1968; Jirtle and Clifton, 1973). In contrast, irradiation of the lungs increases the entrapment of circulating tumor cells in the lungs, and increases both the number of tumor nodules developing subsequent to intravenous injection of tumor cells and the number of metastases developing from tumor lines which metastasize to the lung (Brown, 1973; Van der Brenk *et al.*, 1973; Withers and Milas, 1973). In addition, it should be noted that tumor growth, behavior, and response to treatment are sensitive to modification by a variety of other physiological factors, including alimentation, in terms of both specific nutrients such as vitamin B_6 or A (Ferrer and Mihich, 1967; Tannock *et al.*, 1972) and general nutrient intake (Steiger *et al.*, 1975), the presence of anemia (Hewitt and Blake, 1971), stress (DeChambre and Goss, 1973), hormonal factors, and so on. Therefore, any significant physiological changes occurring in the host as a result of treatment must be considered as potentially capable of altering the behavior of a tumor developing in that host, whether this malignancy is the uncured treated primary, a metastasis, or a newly arising second neoplasm. Such processes have not yet been extensively investigated using animal tumor models, but they should, and undoubtedly will, receive

increasing attention in the future because of their implications for the late effects of cancer therapy and for the therapy of recurrent, metastic, or second primary neoplasms in man.

ACKNOWLEDGMENTS

The authors' research is supported by Grants CA-03353 and CA-10372 (R.F.K.) and Grant CA-06519 (S.R.) from the National Cancer Institute. We offer our sincere thanks to Marion Mangino for her assistance with the preparation of the manuscript.

5. *References*

ADLER, D., BLANKENSTEIN, U., AND LENNARTZ, K.-J., 1972, Der Einfluss von Röntgenbestrahlung (500 R OD) unter *in vivo*-Bedingungen auf die Anderung der Wachstumskinetik von Ehrlich-Aszites-Tumoren Unterschiedlicher Ploidie, *Strahlenterapie* **144**:491.

ALPER, T. (ed.), 1975, *Cell Survival after Low Doses of Radiation: Theoretical and Clinical Implications*, Proceedings of the Sixth L. H. Gray Conference, Sept. 16–21, 1974, Institute of Physics and Wiley, London.

BALDWIN, R. W., AND PRICE, M. R., 1976, Immunobiology of rat neoplasia, *Ann. N. Y. Acad. Sci.* **276**:3.

BANKS, W. C., 1974, Radiation therapy of animals using gamma rays and neutrons, *J. Am. Vet. Radiol. Soc.* **15**:104.

BARENDSEN, G. W., AND BROERSE, J. J., 1969, Experimental radiotherapy of a rat rhabdomyosarcoma with 15 MeV neutrons and 300 kV X-rays. I. Effects of single exposures, *Eur. J. Cancer* **5**:373.

BARENDSEN, G. W., ROELSE, H., HERMENS, A. F., MADHUIZEN, H. T., VAN PEPERZEEL, H. A., AND RUTGERS, D. H., 1973, Clonogenic capacity of proliferating and non-proliferating cells of a transplantable rat rhabdomyosarcoma in relation to its radiosensitivity, *J. Natl. Cancer Inst.* **51**:1521.

BEDFORD, J. S., AND MITCHELL, J. B., 1974, The effect of hypoxia on the growth and radiation response of mammalian cells in culture, *Br. J. Radiol.* **47**:687.

BORN, R., HUG, O., AND TROTT, K.-R., 1976, The effect of prolonged hypoxia on growth and viability of Chinese hamster cells, *Int. J. Radiat. Oncol. Biol. Phys.* **1**:687.

BROWN, J. M., 1970, The effect of acute X-irradiation on the cell proliferation kinetics of induced carcinomas and their normal counterpart, *Radiat. Res.* **43**:627.

BROWN, J. M., 1973, The effect of lung irradiation on the incidence of pulmonary metastases in mice, *Br. J. Radiol.* **46**:613.

BROWN, J. M., 1975, Animal experiments in radiotherapy. III. Large versus small animals, *J. Can. Assoc. Radiol.* **26**:35.

BROWN, J. M., GOFFINET, D. R., CLEAVER, J. E., AND KALLMAN, R. F., 1971, Preferential radiosensitization of mouse sarcoma relative to normal skin by chronic intra-arterial infusion of halogenated pyrimidine analogs, *J. Natl. Cancer Inst.* **47**:75.

BURNS, F. J., 1975, Theoretical aspects of growth fraction in a G_0 model, in: *The Cell Cycle in Malignancy and Immunity*, pp. 315–322, Proceedings of the 13th Annual Hanford Biology Symposium, Richland, Wash., October 1–3, 1973, CONF-731005, ERDA Symposium Series.

BUSH, R. S., AND BRUCE, W. R., 1964, The radiation sensitivity of transplanted lymphoma cells as determined by the spleen colony method, *Radiat. Res.* **21**:612.

BUSH, R. S., AND HILL, R. P., 1975, Biologic discussions augmenting radiation effects and model systems, *Laryngoscope* **85**:1119.

The Cell Cycle in Malignancy and Immunity, 1975, Proceedings of the 13th Annual Hanford Biology Symposium, Richland, Wash., October 1–3, 1973, CONF-731005, Technical Information Center,

274
ROBERT F.
KALLMAN
AND
SARA
ROCKWELL

Office of Public Affairs, U.S. ERDA National Technical Information Service, Department of Commerce, Springfield, Va.

CHEN, K. Y., AND WITHERS, H. R., 1972, Survival characteristics of stem cells of gastric mucosa in C3H mice subjected to localized gamma irradiation, *Int. J. Radiat. Biol.* **21**:521.

CHU, M. Y., AND FISCHER, G. A., 1968, The incorporation of ^{3}H cytosine arabinoside and its effect on murine leukemic cells (L5178Y), *Biochem. Pharmacol.* **17**:753.

COBB, L. M., AND MITCHLEY, B. C. V., 1974, The growth of human tumors in immune deprived mice, *Eur. J. Cancer* **10**:473.

COURTENAY, V. D., 1976, A soft agar colony assay for Lewis lung tumour and B16 melanoma taken directly from the mouse, *Br. J. Cancer* **34**:39.

CROIZAT, H., FRINDEL, E., AND TUBIANA, M., 1970, Proliferative activity of the stem cells in the bone-marrow of mice after single and multiple irradiations (total- or partial-body exposure), *Int. J. Radiat. Biol.* **18**:347.

DECHAMBRE, R. P., AND GOSS, C., 1973, Individual versus group caging of mice with grafted tumors, *Cancer Res.* **33**:140.

DENDY, P. P. (ed.), 1976, *Human Tumours in Short Term Culture: Techniques and Clinical Applications,* Academic Press, New York.

DENEKAMP, J., AND THOMLINSON, R. H., 1971, The cell proliferation kinetics of four experimental tumors after acute X-irradiation, *Cancer Res.* **31**:1279.

DENEKAMP, J., BALL, M. M., AND FOWLER, J. F., 1969, Recovery and repopulation in mouse skin as a function of time after X-irradiation, *Radiat. Res.* **37**:361.

DEWEY, W. C., AND HIGHFIELD, D. P., 1976, G_2 block in Chinese hamster cells induced by X-irradiation, hyperthermia, cycloheximide, or actinomycin D, *Radiat. Res.* **65**:511.

DUNCAN, W., 1973, Exploitation of the oxygen enhancement ratio in clinical practice, *Br. Med. Bull.* **29**:33.

ELKIND, M. M., 1967, Sublethal X-ray damage and its repair in mammalian cells, in: *Radiation Research* (G. SILINI, ed.), pp. 558–586, North-Holland, Amsterdam.

ELKIND, M. M., AND SUTTON, H., 1959, X-ray damage and recovery in mammalian cells in culture, *Nature (London)* **184**:1293.

ELKIND, M. M., AND WHITMORE, G. F., 1967, *The Radiobiology of Cultured Mammalian Cells,* Gordon and Breach, New York.

ELKIND, M. M., SUTTON, H., AND MOSES, W. B., 1961, Postirradiation survival kinetics of mammalian cells grown in culture, *J. Cell. Comp. Physiol.* **58**:113 (Suppl. 1).

ELKIND, M. M., HAN, A., AND VOLZ, K. W., 1963, Radiation response of mammalian cells grown in culture. IV. Dose dependence of division delay and postirradiation growth of surviving and nonsurviving Chinese hamster cells, *J. Natl. Cancer Inst.* **30**:705.

ELKIND, M. M., SWAIN, R. W., ALESCIO, T., SUTTON, H., AND MOSES, W. B., 1965, Oxygen, nitrogen, recovery, and radiation therapy, in: *Cellular Radiation Biology,* pp. 442–461, Williams and Wilkins, Baltimore.

ELKIND, M. M., SUTTON-GILBERT, H., MOSES, W. B., AND KAMPER, C., 1967, Sublethal and lethal radiation damage, *Nature (London)* **214**:1088.

ELLIS, F., 1968, The relationship of biological effect to dose–time–fractionation factors in radiotherapy, *Current Topics Radiat. Res.* **4**:357.

EVANS, R. G., BAGSHAW, M. A., GORDON, L. F., KURKJIAN, S. D., AND HAHN, G. M., 1974, Modification of recovery from potentially lethal X-ray damage in plateau phase Chinese hamster cells, *Radiat. Res.* **59**:597.

FERRER, J. F., AND MIHICH, E., 1967, Dependence of the regression of sarcoma 180 in vitamin B_6-deficient mice upon the immunologic competence of the host, *Cancer Res.* **27**:456.

FINNEY, D. J., 1964, *Statistical Method in Biological Assay,* 2nd ed., Griffin and Company, London.

FODGE, D. W., AND RUBIN, H., 1975, Glucose utilization, pH reduction, and density inhibition in cultures of chick embryo fibroblasts, *J. Cell. Physiol.* **85**:635.

FOWLER, J. F., DENEKAMP, J., SHELDON, P. W., SMITH, A. M., BEGG, A. C., HARRIS, S. R., AND PAGE, A. L., 1974, Optimum fractionation in the X-ray treatment of C3H mouse mammary tumors, *Br. J. Radiol.* **47**:781.

FRINDEL, E., VASSORT, F., AND TUBIANA, M., 1970, Effects of irradiation on the cell cycle of an experimental ascites tumour of the mouse, *Int. J. Radiat. Biol.* **17**:329.

FRINDEL, E., HAHN, G. M., ROBAGLIA, D., AND TUBIANA, M., 1972, Responses of bone marrow and tumor cells to acute and protracted irradiation, *Cancer Res.* **32**:2096.

GERNER, E. W., CONNOR, W. G., BOONE, M. W., DOSS, J. D., MAYER, E. G., AND MILLER, R. C., 1975, The potential of localized heating as an adjuvant to radiation therapy, *Radiology* **116**:433.

GIMBRONE, M. A., JR., COTRAN, R. S., LEAPMAN, S. B., AND FOLKMAN, J., 1974, Tumor growth and neovascularization: An experimental model using rabbit cornea, *J. Natl. Cancer Inst.* **52**:413.

GOLDENBERG, D. M., BHAN, R. D., AND PAVIA, R. A., 1971, *In vivo* human–hamster somatic cell fusion indicated by glucose-6-phosphate dehydrogenase and lactic dehydrogenase profiles, *Cancer Res.* **31**:1148.

GRAY, L. H., 1961, Radiobiologic basis of oxygen as a modifying factor in radiation therapy, *Am. J. Roentgenol.* **85**:803.

HAHN, G. M., 1974, Metabolic aspects of the role of hyperthermia in mammalian cell inactivation and their possible relevance to cancer treatment, *Cancer Res.* **34**:3117.

HAHN, G. M., AND LITTLE, J. B., 1972, Plateau phase cultures of mammalian cells: An *in vitro* model for human cancer, *Current Topics Radiat. Res.* **8**:39.

HAHN, G. M., BAGSHAW, M. A., EVANS, R. G., AND GORDON, L. F., 1973*a*, Repair of potentially lethal lesions in X-irradiated, density-inhibited Chinese hamster cells: Metabolic effects and hypoxia, *Radiat. Res.* **55**:280.

HAHN, G. M., RAY, G. R., GORDON, L. F., AND KALLMAN, R. F., 1973*b*, Response of solid tumor cells exposed to chemotherapeutic agents *in vivo*: Cell survival after 2- and 24-hour exposure, *J. Natl. Cancer Inst.* **50**:529.

HAHN, G. M., ROCKWELL, S., KALLMAN, R. F., GORDON, L. F., AND FRINDEL, E., 1974, Repair of potentially lethal damage *in vivo* in solid tumor cells after X-irradiation, *Cancer Res.* **34**:351.

HALL, E. J., 1972, The effect of hypoxia on the repair of sublethal radiation damage in cultured mammalian cells, *Radiat. Res.* **49**:405.

HALL, E. J., AND ROIZIN-TOWLE, L., 1975, Hypoxic sensitizers: Radiobiological studies at the cellular level, *Radiology* **117**:453.

HERMENS, A. F., 1973, Variations in the cell kinetics and the growth rate in an experimental tumour during natural growth and after irradiation, Publ. No. 835, Radiobiological Institute TNO, Rijswijk (ZH), the Netherlands.

HERMENS, A. F., AND BARENDSEN, G. W., 1976, Effects of ionizing radiation on the growth kinetics of tumors, in: *Growth Kinetics and Biochemical Regulation of Normal and Malignant Cells*, Proceedings of the 29th Annual M. D. Anderson Symposium, March 10–12, 1976, Houston, Texas.

HEWITT, H. B., 1953, Studies of the quantitative transplantation of mouse sarcoma, *Br. J. Cancer* **7**:367.

HEWITT, H. B., AND BLAKE, E. R., 1968, The growth of transplanted murine tumors in pre-irradiated sites, *Br. J. Cancer* **22**:808.

HEWITT, H. B., AND BLAKE, E. R., 1971, Effect of induced host anaemia on the viability and radiosensitivity of murine malignant cells *in vivo*, *Br. J. Cancer* **25**:323.

HEWITT, H. B., AND WILSON, C. W., 1959*a*, A survival curve for mammalian leukaemia cells: Irradiated *in vivo* (implications for the treatment of mouse leukaemia by whole-body irradiation), *Br. J. Cancer* **13**:69.

HEWITT, H. B., AND WILSON, C. W., 1959*b*, The effect of tissue oxygen tension on the radiosensitivity of leukaemia cells irradiated *in situ* in the livers of leukaemic mice, *Br. J. Cancer* **13**:675.

HEWITT, H. B., BLAKE, E., AND PORTER, E. H., 1973, The effect of lethally irradiated cells on the transplantability of murine tumors, *Br. J. Cancer* **28**:123.

HEWITT, H. B., BLAKE, E. R., AND WALDER, A. S., 1976, A critique of the evidence for active host defence against cancer, based on personal studies of 27 murine tumours of spontaneous origin, *Br. J. Cancer* **33**:241.

HILL, R. P., AND BUSH, R. S., 1969, A lung colony assay to determine the radiosensitivity of the cells of a solid tumour, *Int. J. Radiat. Biol.* **15**:435.

HILMAS, D. E., AND GILLETTE, E. L., 1974, Morphometric analysis of the microvasculature of tumors during growth and after X-irradiation, *Cancer* **33**:103.

HOLTHUSEN, H., 1921, Beiträge zur Biologie der Strahlenwirkung: Untersuchungen an Askarideneirn, *Pfluegers Arch.* **187**:1.

HOWES, A. E., 1969, An estimation of changes in the proportions and absolute numbers of hypoxic cells after irradiation of transplanted C3H mouse mammary tumours, *Br. J. Radiol.* **42**:441.

JIRTLE, R., AND CLIFTON, K. H., 1973, Effect of preirradiation of the tumor bed on the relative vascular space of the mouse gastric adenocarcinoma 328 and mammary adenocarcinoma CA755, *Cancer Res.* **33**:764.

276

ROBERT F.
KALLMAN
AND
SARA
ROCKWELL

KALLMAN, R. F., 1963, Recovery from radiation injury: A proposed mechanism, *Nature (London)* **197**:557.

KALLMAN, R. F., 1968, Methods for the study of radiation effects on cancer cells, in: *Methods in Cancer Research*, Vol. IV (H. BUSCH, ed.), pp. 309–354, Academic Press, New York.

KALLMAN, R. F., 1972, The phenomenon of reoxygenation and its implications for fractionated radiotherapy, *Radiology* **105**: 135.

KALLMAN, R. F., 1974, The oxygen effect and reoxygenation, in: *Excerpta Medica International Congress Series No. 353*, Vol. 5: *Surgery, Radiotherapy, and Chemotherapy of Cancer*, pp. 136–140, Proceedings of the XI International Cancer Congress, Florence, 1974.

KALLMAN, R. F., 1975, Animal experiments in radiotherapy. I. Small animals, *J. Can. Assoc. Radiol.* **26**:15.

KALLMAN, R. F., 1976, On the recruitment of non-cycling tumor cells by irradiation, in: *Growth Kinetics and Biochemical Regulation of Normal and Malignant Cells*, Proceedings of the 29th Annual M. D. Anderson Symposium, Houston, Texas, March 10–12, 1976.

KALLMAN, R. F., AND TAPLEY, N. DUV., 1964, Radiation sensitivity and recovery patterns of spontaneous and isologously transplanted mouse tumors, *Acta Unio Int. Contra Cancrum* **20**:1216.

KALLMAN, R. F., SILINI, G., AND TAYLOR, H. M., III, 1966, Recuperation from lethal injury by whole-body irradiation. II. Kinetic aspects in radiosensitive BALB/c mice, and cyclic fine structure during the four days after conditioning irradiation, *Radiat. Res.* **29**:362.

KALLMAN, R. F., SILINI, G., AND VAN PUTTEN, L. M., 1967, Factors influencing the quantitative estimation of the *in vivo* survival of cells from solid tumors, *J. Natl. Cancer Inst.* **39**:539.

KALLMAN, R. F., DeNARDO, G. L., AND STASCH, M. J., 1972, Blood flow in irradiated mouse sarcoma as determined by the clearance of xenon-133, *Cancer Res.* **32**:483.

KAPLAN, H. S., 1964, The role of radiation in experimental leukemogenesis, *Nat. Cancer Inst. Monogr.* **14**:207.

KAPLAN, H. S., 1970, Radiobiology's contribution to radiotherapy: Promise or mirage? Failla Memorial Lecture, *Radiat. Res.* **43**:460.

KLEIN, G., SJÖGREN, H. O., KLEIN, E., AND HELLSTRÖM, K. E., 1960, Demonstration of resistance against methylcholanthrene-induced sarcomas in the primary autochthonous host, *Cancer Res.* **20**:1561.

KNAZEK, R. A., GULLINO, P. M., KOHLER, P. O., AND DEDRICK, R. L., 1972, Cell culture on artificial capillaries: An approach to tissue growth *in vitro*, *Science* **178**:65.

KOCH, C. J., AND KRUUV, J., 1971, The effect of extreme hypoxia on recovery after radiation by synchronized mammalian cells, *Radiat. Res.* **48**:74.

KOCH, C. J., KRUUV, J., FREY, H. E., AND SNYDER, R. A., 1973, Plateau phase in growth induced by hypoxia, *Int. J. Radiat. Biol.* **23**:67.

LAJTHA, L. G., 1963, On the concept of the cell cycle, *J. Cell. Comp. Physiol.* **62**:143 (Suppl. 1).

LEEPER, D. B., SCHNEIDERMAN, M. H., AND DEWEY, W. C., 1972, Radiation-induced division delay in synchronized Chinese hamster ovary cells in monlayer culture, *Radiat. Res.* **50**:401.

LEEPER, D. B., SCHNEIDERMAN, M. H., AND DEWEY, W. C., 1973, Radiation-induced cycle delay in synchronized Chinese hamster cells: Comparison between DNA synthesis and division, *Radiat. Res.* **53**:326.

LeFRANCOIS, D., TROISE, G. D., CHAVAUDRA, N., MALAISE, E. P., AND BARSKI, G., 1974, Comparative effect of local radiotherapy and surgery on cell-mediated immunity against a mouse transplantable mammary tumor, *Int. J. Cancer* **13**:629.

LEIGHTON, J., 1968, Invasive growth and metastasis in tissue culture systems, in: *Methods in Cancer Research*, Vol. 4 (H. BUSCH, ed.), p. 85, Academic Press, New York.

LEITH, J. T., SCHILLINGS, W. A., AND WHEELER, K. T., 1975, Cellular radiosensitivity of a rat brain tumor, *Cancer* **35**:1545.

LESHER, S., AND BAUMAN, J., 1969, Cell kinetic studies of the intestinal epithelium: Maintenance of the intestinal epithelium in normal and irradiated animals, *Natl. Cancer Inst. Monogr.* **30**:185.

LIN, A. J., SHANSKY, C. W., AND SARTORELLI, A. C., 1974, Potential bioreductive alkylating agents. 3. Synthesis and antineoplastic activity of acetomethyl and corresponding ethyl carbonate derivatives of benzoquinones, *J. Med. Chem.* **17**:558.

LITTBRAND, B., AND RÉVÉSZ, L., 1969, The effect of oxygen on cellular survival and recovery after radiation, *Br. J. Radiol.* **42**:914.

LITTLE, J. B., 1969, Repair of sub-lethal and potentially lethal radiation damage in plateau phase cultures of human cells, *Nature (London)* **224**:804.

LITTLE, J. B., AND HAHN, G. M., 1973, Life-cycle dependence of repair of potentially-lethal radiation damage, *Int. J. Radiat. Biol.* **23**:401.

LITTLE, J. B., HAHN, G. M., FRINDEL, E., AND TUBIANA, M., 1973, Repair of potentially lethal radiation damage *in vitro* and *in vivo*, *Radiology* **106**:689.

MADOC-JONES, H., AND MAURO, F., 1970, Age responses to X-rays, *Vinca* alkaloids, and hydroxyurea of murine lymphoma cells synchronized *in vivo*, *J. Natl. Cancer Inst.* **45**:1131.

MAURO, F., AND ELKIND, M. M., 1968, Comparison of repair of sublethal damage in cultured Chinese hamster cells exposed to sulfur mustard and X-rays, *Cancer Res.* **28**:1156.

MCNALLY, N. J., 1972, A low oxygen-enhancement ratio for tumour-cell survival as compared with that for tumour-growth delay, *Int. J. Radiat. Biol.* **22**:407.

MENDELSOHN, M. L., 1962, Autoradiographic analysis of cell proliferation in spontaneous breast cancer of the C3H mouse. III. The growth fraction, *J. Natl. Cancer Inst.* **28**:1015.

MENDELSOHN, M. L., 1975, The cell cycle in malignant and normal tissues, in: *The Cell Cycle in Malignancy and Immunity*, pp. 293–314, Proceedings of the 13th Annual Hanford Biology Symposium, Richland, Wash., Oct. 1–3, 1973, CONF-731005 ERDA Symposium Series.

MOORE, D. H., 1975, Mammary tumor virus, in: *Cancer: A Comprehensive Treatise*, Vol. 2 (F. F. BECKER, ed.), pp. 131–167, Plenum, New York.

MOTTRAM, J. C., 1936, A factor of importance in the radiosensitivity of tumors, *Br. J. Radiol.* **9**:606.

MOULDER, J. E., AND FISCHER, J. J., 1976, Radiation reaction of rat skin: The role of the number of fractions and the overall treatment time, *Cancer* **37**:2762.

MOULDER, J. E., FISCHER, J. J., AND MILARDO, R., 1976, Time–dose relationships for the cure of an experimental rat tumor with fractionated radiation, *Int. J. Radiat. Oncol. Biol. Phys.* **1**:431.

OWEN, L. N., AND STEEL, G. G., 1969, The growth and cell population kinetics of spontaneous tumours in domestic animals, *Br. J. Cancer* **23**:493.

PETERS, L. J., AND HEWITT, H. B., 1974, The influence of fibrin formation on the transplantability of murine tumour cells: Implications for the mechanisms of the Révész effect, *Br. J. Cancer* **29**:279.

PHILLIPS, R. A., AND TOLMACH, L. J., 1966, Repair of potentially lethal damage in X-irradiated HeLa cells, *Radiat. Res.* **29**:413.

POWERS, W. E., AND TOLMACH, L. J., 1963, A multicomponent X-ray survival curve for mouse lymphosarcoma cells irradiated in *in vivo*, *Nature (London)* **197**:710.

POWERS, W. E., PALMER, L. A., AND TOLMACH, L. J., 1967, Cellular radiosensitivity and tumor curability, *J. Natl. Cancer Inst. Monogr.* **24**:169.

PROBERT, J. C., AND HUGHES, D. B., 1975, Animal experiments in radiotherapy. II. Large animals, *J. Can. Assoc. Radiol.* **26**:25.

REINHOLD, H. S., 1965, A cell dispersion technique for use in quantitative transplantation studies with solid tumours, *Eur. J. Cancer* **1**:67.

REINHOLD, H. S., 1971, Improved microcirculation in irradiated tumours, *Eur. J. Cancer* **7**:273.

REINHOLD, H. S., AND DEBREE, C., 1968, Tumour cure rate and cell survival of a transplantable rat rhabdomyosarcoma following X-irradiation, *Eur. J. Cancer* **4**:367.

RÉVÉSZ, L., 1958, Effect of lethally damaged tumour cells upon the development of admixed viable cells, *J. Natl. Cancer Inst.* **20**:1157.

ROCKWELL, S., 1971, Cellular radiosensitivity, cell population kinetics, and tumor radiation response in two related mouse mammary carcinomas, Ph.D. thesis, Stanford University.

ROCKWELL, S., AND HAHN, G. M., 1974, An assay permitting quantitative comparison of tumor-directed immunity and tumor cell survival, *J. Natl. Cancer Inst.* **53**:1379.

ROCKWELL, S., AND KALLMAN, R. F., 1973, Cellular radiosensitivity and tumor radiation response in the EMT6 tumor cell system, *Radiat. Res.* **53**:281.

ROCKWELL, S., AND KALLMAN, R. F., 1974, Cyclic radiation-induced variations in cellular radiosensitivity in a mouse mammary tumor, *Radiat. Res.* **57**:132.

ROCKWELL, S. C., KALLMAN, R. F., AND FAJARDO, L. F., 1972, Characteristics of a serially transplanted mouse mammary tumor and its tissue-culture-adapted derivative, *J. Natl. Cancer Inst.* **49**:735.

ROCKWELL, S., FRINDEL, E., AND TUBIANA, M., 1976, A technique for determining the proportion of the clonogenic cells in S phase in EMT6 cell cultures and tumors, *Cell Tissue Kinet.* **9**:313.

ROSENBLUM, M., KNEBAL, K. D., WHEELER, K. T., BARKER, M., AND WILSON, C., 1975, Development of an *in vitro* colony formation assay for the evaluation of *in vivo* chemotherapy of a rat brain tumor, *In Vitro* **11**:264.

RYGAARD, J., AND POVLSEN, C. O., 1969, Heterotransplantation of a human malignant tumor into "nude" mice, *Acta Pathol. Microbiol. Scand.* **77**:758.

278

ROBERT F.
KALLMAN
AND
SARA
ROCKWELL

SCOTT, O. C. A., 1961, Some observations on the use of transplanted tumors in radiobiological research, *Radiat. Res.* **14**:643.

SHIPLEY, W. U., STANLEY, J. A., COURTENAY, V. D., AND FIELD, S. B., 1975, Repair of radiation damage in Lewis lung carcinoma cells following *in situ* treatment with fast neutrons and γ-rays, *Cancer Res.* **35**:932.

SILINI, G., AND HORNSEY, S., 1961, Studies on cell-survival of irradiated Ehrlich ascites tumor. I. The effect of the host's age and the presence of non-viable cells on tumour takes, *Int. J. Radiat. Biol.* **4**:127.

SINCLAIR, W. K., AND MORTON, R. A., 1965, X-ray and ultraviolet sensitivity of synchronized Chinese hamster cells at various stages of the cell cycle, *Biophys. J.* **5**:1.

SONG, C. W., PAYNE, J. T., AND LEVITT, S. H., 1972, Vascularity and blood flow in X-irradiated Walker carcinoma 256 of rats, *Radiology* **104**:693.

STANBRIDGE, E. J., BOULGER, L. R., FRANKS, C. R., GARRETT, J. A., REESON, D. E., BISHOP, D., AND PERKINS, F. T., 1975, Optimal conditions for the growth of malignant human and animal cell populations in immunosuppressed mice, *Cancer Res.* **35**:2203.

STEEL, G. G., 1972, The cell cycle in tumours: An examination of data gained by the technique of labelled mitoses, *Cell Tissue Kinet.* **5**:87.

STEIGER, E., ORAM-SMITH, J., MILLER, E., KUO, L., AND VARS, H., 1975, Effect of nutrition on tumor growth and tolerance to chemotherapy, *J. Surg. Res.* **18**:455.

SUIT, H. D., AND KASTELAN, A., 1970, Immunologic status of host and response of a methylcholanthrene-induced sarcoma to local X irradiation, *Cancer* **26**:232.

SUIT, H. D., AND SHALEK, R. J., 1963, The response of anoxic C3H mouse mammary carcinoma isotransplants ($1-25 \text{ mm}^3$) to X-irradiation, *J. Natl. Cancer Inst.* **31**:479.

SUIT, H. D., SHALEK, R. J., AND WETTE, R., 1965, Radiation response of C3H mouse mammary carcinoma evaluated in terms of cellular radiation sensitivity, in: *Cellular Radiation Biology*, pp. 514–530, Williams and Wilkins, Baltimore.

SUIT, H. D., HOWES, A. E., AND HUNTER, N., 1977, Dependence of response of a C3H mammary carcinoma to fractionated irradiation on fractionation number and intertreatment interval, *Radiat. Res.* (in press).

SUTHERLAND, R. M., AND DURAND, R. E., 1973, Hypoxic cells in an *in vitro* tumor model, *Int. J. Radiat. Biol.* **23**:235.

SUTHERLAND, R. M., MCCREDIE, J. A., AND INCH, W. R., 1971, Growth of multicell spheroids in tissue culture as a model of nodular carcinomas, *J. Natl. Cancer Inst.* **46**:113.

SZCZEPANSKI, L., AND TROTT, K. R., 1975, Post-irradiation proliferation kinetics of a serially transplanted murine adenocarinoma, *Br. J. Radiol.* **48**:200.

TAKAHASHI, M., AND KALLMAN, R. F., 1977, Quantitative estimation of histological changes in subcutaneous vasculature of the mouse after X-irradiation. *Int. J. Radiat. Oncol. Biol. Phys.* **2**:61.

TANNOCK, I. F., 1968, The relation between cell proliferation and the vascular systems in a transplanted mouse mammary tumour, *Br. J. Cancer* **22**:258.

TANNOCK, I. F., 1972, Oxygen diffusion and the distribution of cellular radiosensitivity in tumours, *Br. J. Radiol.* **45**:515.

TANNOCK, I. F., AND STEEL, G. G., 1970, Tumor growth and cell kinetics in chronically hypoxic animals, *J. Natl. Cancer Inst.* **45**:123.

TANNOCK, I. F., SUIT, H. D., AND MARSHALL, N., 1972, Vitamin A and the radiation response of experimental tumors: An immune-mediated effect, *J. Nat. Cancer Inst.* **48**:731.

TERASIMA, T., AND TOLMACH, L. J., 1963, Variation in several responses of HeLa cells to X-irradiaton during the division cycle, *Biophys. J.* **3**:11.

TERZAGHI, M., AND LITTLE, J. B., 1975, Establishment and characteristics of a hamster lung adenocarinoma *in vivo* and *in vitro*, *J. Natl. Cancer Inst.* **55**:865.

THOMLINSON, R. H., 1970, Reoxygenation as a function of tumor size and histopathologic type, in: *Conference in Time and Dose Relationships in Radiobiology as Applied to Radiotherapy*, pp. 242–247, BNL50230 (C-57), Clearinghouse for Federal Scientific and Technical Information, Springfield, Va.

THOMLINSON, R. H., AND CRADDOCK, E. A., 1967, The gross response of an experimental tumour to single doses of X-rays, *Br. J. Cancer* **21**:108.

THOMLINSON, R. H., AND GRAY, L. H., 1955, The histological structure of some human lung cancers and the possible implications for radiotherapy, *Br. J. Cancer* **9**:539.

THOMLINSON, R. H., DISCHE, S., GRAY, A. J., AND ERRINGTON, L. M., 1976, Clinical testing of the radiosensitiser Ro-07-0582. III. Response of tumours, *Clin. Radiol.* **27**:167.

THOMSON, J. E., AND RAUTH, A. M., 1974, An *in vitro* assay to measure the viability of KHT tumor cells not previously exposed to culture conditions, *Radiat. Res.* **58**:262.

TILL, J. E., AND MCCULLOCH, E. A., 1961, A direct measurement of the radiation sensitivity normal mouse bone marrow cells, *Radiat. Res.* **14**:213.

Time–Dose Relationships in Radiaton Biology as Applied to Radiotherapy, 1970, BNL 50203(C-57) (Biology and Medicine-TID-4500), Proceedings of the Conference at Carmel, Calif., Sept. 15–18, 1969, Clearinghouse for Federal Scientific and Technical Information, NBS, Department of Commerce, Springfield, Va.

TOOLAN, H. W., 1953, Growth of human tumors in cortisone-treated laboratory animals: The possibility of obtaining permanently transplantable human tumours, *Cancer Res.* **13**:389.

TUBIANA, M., FRINDEL, E., AND MALAISE, E., 1968, La cinetique de proliferation cellulaire dans les tumeurs animales et humaines—influence d'une irradiation, in: *Effects of Radiation on Cellular Proliferation*, pp. 423–452, IAEA, Vienna.

VAAGE, J., DOROSHOW, J., AND DUBOIS, T. T., 1974, Radiation induced changes in established tumor immunity, *Cancer Res.* **34**:129.

VAN DER BRENK, H. A. S., BURCH, W. M., ORTON, C., AND SHARPINGTON, C., 1973, Stimulation of clonogenic growth of tumour cells and metastases in the lungs by local X-radiation, *Br. J. Cancer* **27**:291.

VAN PEPERZEEL, H. A., 1972, Effects of single doses of radiation on lung metastases in man and experimental animals, *Eur. J. Cancer* **8**:665.

VAN PUTTEN, L. M., 1968, Oxygenation and cell kinetics after irradiation in a transplantable osteosarcoma, in: *Effects of Radiation on Cellular Proliferation*, pp. 493–505, IAEA, Vienna.

VAN PUTTEN, L. M., AND KALLMAN, R. F., 1968, Oxygenation status of a transplantable tumor during fractionated radiation therapy, *J. Natl. Cancer Inst.* **40**:441.

VASSORT, F., WINTERHOLER, M., FRINDEL, E., AND TUBIANA, M., 1973, Kinetic parameters of bone marrow stem cells using *in vivo* suicide by tritiated thymidine or by hydroxyurea, *Blood* **41**:789.

VOS, O., 1968, Repopulation of the stem-cell compartment in hemopoietic and lymphatic tissues of mice after X-irradiation, in: *Effects of Radiation on Cellular Proliferation and Differentiation*, pp. 149–160, IAEA, Vienna.

WHITMORE, G. F., STANNERS, C. P., TILL, J. E., AND GULYAS, S., 1961, Nucleic acid synthesis and the division cycle in X-irradiated L-strain mouse cells, *Biochim. Biophys. Acta* **47**:66.

WINANS, L. F., DEWEY, W. C., AND DETTOR, C. M., 1972, Repair of sub-lethal and potentially lethal X-ray damage in synchronous Chinese hamster cells, *Radiat. Res.* **52**:333.

WITHERS, H. R., 1967, Recovery and repopulation *in vivo* by mouse skin epithelial cells during fractionated irradiation, *Radiat. Res.* **32**:227.

WITHERS, H. R., 1972, Cell renewal systems concept and the radiation response, in: *Frontiers of Radiation Therapy and Oncology*, Vol. 6 (J. M. VAETH, ed.), pp. 93–107, University Park Press, Baltimore.

WITHERS, H. R., 1975, The four R's of radiotherapy, *Adv. Radiat. Biol.* **5**:241.

WITHERS, H. R., AND MASON, K. A., 1974, The kinetics of recovery in irradiated colonic mucosa of the mouse, *Cancer* **34**:896.

WITHERS, H. R., AND MILAS, L., 1973, Influence of preirradiation of lung on development of artificial pulmonary metastases of fibrosarcoma in mice, *Cancer Res.* **33**:1931.

WITHERS, H. R., HUNTER, N., BARKLEY, H. T., JR., AND REID, B. O., 1974, Radiation survival and regeneration characteristics of spermatogenic stem cells of mouse testis, *Radiat. Res.* **57**:88.

YATVIN, M. B., CROUSE, D. T., AND CLIFTON, K. H., 1970, Studies on the mechanism of the stimulatory effect of lethally irradiated cells on tumor inocula, *Proc. Soc. Exp. Bio., Med.* **133**:1123.

8

High-LET Radiations

Eric J. Hall

1. Introduction

Radiation oncology, like most branches of medicine, is predominantly a clinical art, with the admixture of a small amount of science. Changes and improvements in this field may be empirical, based on a gradual evolution of accepted techniques, or they may be a direct result of laboratory-based research. While most advances in radiation oncology have been of the former kind, the introduction of high-LET radiations in undoubtedly one of the first concrete examples of the latter.

Much of the improvement in the results of treatment over the years has directly paralleled machine development. The push to higher accelerating energies and higher outputs produced the direct benefits of better depth doses and better localization of the high-dose region within the tumor. Physical solutions were found for what were essentially physical limitations. More recent developments have focused attention on overcoming biological limitations. Based on laboratory evidence, it is commonly believed that the effectiveness of conventional modalities such as X-rays and γ-rays is limited by the presence of hypoxic cells in the poorly vascularized regions of the tumor, which are resistant to X-irradiation and which provide a focus for the regrowth of the tumor. High-LET radiations represent one approach to overcoming this limitation; it is, historically, the first approach and was suggested by radiobiologists with a background in physics, who naturally thought in terms of physical solutions to biological problems. More recently, radiobiologists with a background in chemistry have looked to solving the same problem from a different viewpoint, and have developed the oxygen-mimicking drugs described in a previous chapter.

Eric J. Hall • Radiological Research Laboratory, College of Physicians and Surgeons of Columbia University, New York, New York 10032.

2. The Physics and Biology of High-LET Irradiations

ERIC J. HALL

2.1. The Absorption of Radiant Energy

Radiations may be classified as *directly* or *indirectly* ionizing. Fast-moving charged particles are *directly* ionizing; i.e., provided that the individual particles have sufficient kinetic energy, they can directly disrupt the atomic structure of the materials through which they pass. X- and γ-rays, together with neutrons, are *indirectly* ionizing. They do not themselves produce the chemical and biological damage, but when absorbed in the material through which they pass, they give up their energy to produce fast-moving charged particles. X-ray photons interact with the orbital electrons of atoms of the absorbing material to set in motion fast electrons. Neutrons interact with the nuclei of atoms of the absorbing material and set in motion fast-recoil protons, α-particles, and other nuclear fragments. These secondary charged particles are able to ionize and excite atoms of the absorber located along their tracks, which is the first step in the chain of events which ultimately leads to the expression of biological damage.

2.2. The Concept of Ionization Density

When ionizing radiations deposit energy in biological materials, ionizations and excitations occur which are not distributed at random but tend to be localized along the tracks of individual particles in a pattern dependent on the type of radiation involved. The average separation of primary events along the track of an ionizing particle decreases with increasing charge and mass. The tracks of energetic electrons, produced by the absorption of X- or γ-ray photons, will be traced by individual primary events which are well separated in space; hence X-rays are usually described as *sparsely ionizing.* At the other extreme, α-particles give rise to individual ionizing events which occur so close together that they tend to overlap, giving rise to tracks which consist of well-delineated columns of ionization. Figure 1 is an attempt to illustrate diagrammatically the density of ionization of a number of representative charged particles. The background of the picture shows the nucleus of a mammalian cell.

"Linear energy transfer" (LET) is a term introduced by Zirkle (1954) and was defined by the International Commission of Radiological Units as follows:

> The linear energy transfer (L) of charged particles in a medium is the quotient of dE/dl where dE is the average energy locally imparted to the medium by a charged particle of specified energy in traversing a distance of dl.
>
>   That is:

$$L = dE/dl$$

The traditional unit used for this quantity is keV per micrometer of unit-density material.

Most radiation modalities used in practice consist of a wide range of energies; this is certainly true for X-rays as well as for neutrons and pions. As a consequence,

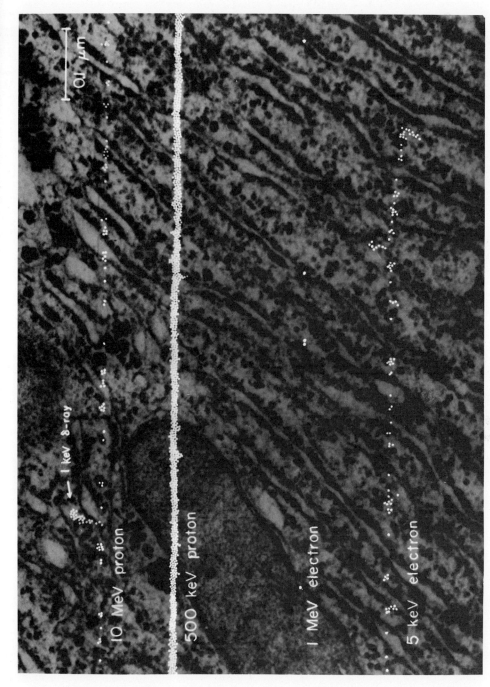

FIGURE 1. Representation of the density of ionization associated with various typical charged particles of interest in radiotherapy. For example, a 1 MeV electron may be set in motion when a photon of ⁶⁰Co γ-rays is absorbed, while a 10 MeV recoil proton may be set in motion by the high-energy fast neutrons used for radiotherapy. For scale purposes, the background is part of a mammalian cell. Courtesy of Dr. Albrecht Kellerer.

the charged particles set in motion by such radiations vary widely in ionization density, and the LET quoted can only be an average quantity. A further complication arises because it is possible to calculate the *average* in many different ways. The most commonly used are the *track average* and the *energy average*. The track average LET is calculated by dividing the particle track into equal lengths, calculating the energy deposited in each length, and finding the mean. The energy average LET is calculated by dividing the track into segments that have equal amounts of energy deposited, and finding the mean. These two methods of calculation may yield average LETs for the same radiation which differ by a large factor. By the same token, it is quite possible for different types of radiation which have the same average LET to produce quite diverse biological effects. As a result, LET is a quantity of limited significance except when dealing with particles of a well-defined energy.

Typical LET values for commonly used radiations are as follows: for ^{60}Co γ-rays, the track and energy average LETs are 0.27 and 0.32 keV/μm, respectively; the method of averaging makes very little difference in this case. For 14 MeV monoenergetic neutrons, the track average LET is about 12, while the energy average LET is about 75 keV/μm. Similar values would be typical of beams of π^- mesons. In the case of both of these radiation types, the charged particles set in motion span such a wide range of energy and LET that the track and energy averages differ significantly and the concept of LET is virtually meaningless. α-Particles of 2.5 MeV have a LET of about 120 keV/μm, while high-energy heavy nuclei may have a LET as high as 2000 keV/μm.

2.3. Cell Killing and Reproductive Integrity

Cell survival, or its converse, cell death, may mean different things to different people. For differentiated cells that do not proliferate, such as nerve, muscle, or secretory cells, death can be defined as the loss of a specific function. For proliferating cells, such as the stem cells in self-renewal tissues, loss of the capacity for sustained proliferation, i.e., loss of *reproductive integrity*, is an appropriate definition of cell death. A cell may still be physically present and apparently intact, it may be able to make proteins or synthesize DNA, and it may even be able to struggle through one or two mitoses, but if it has lost the capacity to divide indefinitely and produce a large number of progeny, it is by definition dead. The survivor which has retained its reproductive integrity and is able to proliferate indefinitely to produce a large colony is said to be "clonogenic."

This definition of cell death is generally relevant to the radiobiology of whole animals and plants and their tissues, and has a particular relevance to the radiotherapy of tumors. There are two reasons for this. First, it is an end point which can be scored readily and accurately by measuring the colony-forming ability of cells cultured *in vitro* or their ability to initiate tumor growth *in vivo*. Second, for a tumor to be eradicated, it is only necessary that cells be "killed" in the sense that they are rendered unable to divide and cause further growth and spread of the malignancy. In general, the loss of proliferative capacity can be brought about by quite modest doses of radiation. While a dose of tens of thousands of rads is necessary to destroy function in nonproliferating systems, the mean lethal dose for the loss of proliferative capacity is usually less than about 200 rads.

2.4. The Oxygen Effect

Many chemical and pharmacological agents have been discovered which modify the biological effects of ionizing radiations. The most dramatic of these is oxygen, and it is also the most important from a practical point of view. As early as the 1920s, it was noticed that simple biological systems such as *Ascaris* eggs and vegetable seeds were very much less sensitive to the effects of X-rays in the absence of oxygen (Holthusen, 1921; Petry, 1923). It was, however, the work of Mottram and his colleagues Gray and Read that led to a quantitative measurement of the oxygen effect and an appreciation of the potential importance of oxygen in radiotherapy (Mottram, 1936; Read, 1952; Gray *et al.*, 1953).

The effect of oxygen on cellular sensitivity to X-rays has been investigated for many different biological systems. It is generally found that oxygen is *dose modifying*; i.e., that the ratio of doses under hypoxic and aerated conditions is independent of the dose level and a constant for a given type of radiation. This ratio is known as the "oxygen enhancement ratio" (OER).

An important relationship exists between LET and the OER. Figure 2 shows mammalian cell survival curves for various types of radiation with widely different LETs, which consequently exhibit quite different oxygen enhancement ratios. Panel A refers to X-rays which are sparsely ionizing, have a low LET, and consequently exhibit a large OER of about 2.5. Panel B refers to 15 MeV neutrons, which are intermediate in ionizing density and characteristically show an OER of 1.6. Panel C relates to data for 4 MeV α-particles, which have a LET of about 100 keV/μm, corresponding to an OER of about 1.3. Panel D relates to densely ionizing radiations in the form of 2.5 MeV α-particles; survival estimates in the presence or absence of oxygen fall along a common line, so that the OER is unity. Barendsen and colleagues used mammalian cells cultured *in vitro* to investigate the OER for many different types of radiation (Barendsen *et al.*, 1960, 1966; Barendsen, 1964). The variation of OER with LET, calculated from their data, is shown in Fig. 3. In these investigations, the range of high LET values was obtained by using natural α-particles of different energies. In a comparable set of investigations, Todd covered a range of LETs by using heavy charged particles accelerated in the Berkeley HILAC (Todd, 1964, 1967). Particles of given LET were utilized by the so-called track segment method. The same range of LETs was covered by both Barendsen and Todd, but their methods of producing these high LETs were quite different. Consequently, the shape, and in particular the steepness, of the curve relating oxygen enhancement ratio to LET is not the same for the two sets of data. This probably reflects the different spatial patterns of energy deposition which surrounds the α-particles used by Barendsen compared with the faster-moving heavy charged particles used by Todd.

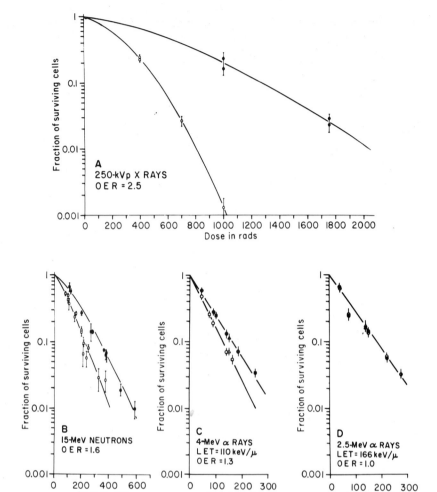

FIGURE 2. Survival curves for T1 kidney cells of human origin, determined for four different types of radiation. ○, Aerated conditions; ●, hypoxic conditions. Redrawn from Broerse *et al.* (1967) and Barendsen *et al.* (1966).

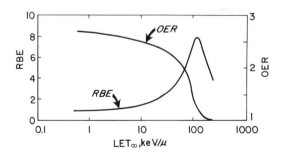

FIGURE 3. Variation of OER and RBE as a function of LET$_\infty$. α-Particles and deuterons were used to irradiate T1 kidney cells of human origin. Redrawn from Barendsen (1972).

The relative biological effectiveness (RBE) of some test radiation (r) compared
with 250 kVp X-rays is defined by the ratio D_{250}/D_r, where D_{250} and D_r are the
doses of 250 kV and the test radiation, respectively, required for equal biological
effect. As LET increases, the RBE of a radiation changes rapidly, as is illustrated in
Fig. 3. As the LET increases, the RBE increases slowly at first, and then more
rapidly until it reaches a maximum at about 100 keV/μm. Beyond this LET value,
the RBE again falls because of the phenomenon of overkill. The data shown are in
fact taken from the experiments of Barendsen and his colleagues, but closely
parallel those of Todd. There is no discrepancy in the data for the variation of
RBE with LET comparable to that which exists for the OER.

Following the demonstration of the oxygen effect with simple biological systems
in the 1930s and the 1940s, many clinical radiotherapists suspected that oxygen
influenced the radiosensitivity of tumors. It was, however, a paper by Thomlinson
and Gray (1955) which finally focused attention on oxygen as a major factor of
importance in radiotherapy. This paper reported a histological study of human
bronchial carcinoma. It was noted that large tumor cords always had a central area
of necrosis. In addition, however great the radius of the necrotic center, the
thickness of the sheath of actively growing tumor cells never exceeded about
180 μm, which coincided closely with the calculated diffusion distance of oxygen
in respiring tissue. This was evidence that oxygen exhaustion caused the development of areas of necrosis. It was then postulated that the presence of a small
proportion of hypoxic cells, perhaps a layer one or two cells thick surrounding the
necrotic areas, would be at an oxygen tension high enough for them to be
clonogenic, but low enough to protect them from the effects of X-rays. Such cells
could represent a focus for the regrowth of the tumor and limit the success of
radiotherapy with X-rays in at least some clinical situations.

While the arguments which stem from the work of Thomlinson and Gray are
credible and persuasive, they are based on qualitative observations from histological sections and do not include any conclusive proof that tumors contain viable
hypoxic cells. It was left to Powers and Tolmach (1963) to demonstrate unequivocally that a solid subcutaneous lymphosarcoma in the mouse contained clonogenic
hypoxic cells. Following this observation, many different investigators measured
the proportion of viable hypoxic cells in a wide range of experimental animal
tumors in the mouse and the rat, representing several histological types. The
results are summarized in Table 1. It is frequently found that approximately 15%
of the viable cells in experimental tumors are hypoxic. Indeed, this figure crops up
so consistently that it might be due simply to geometrical factors rather than
biological considerations.

Van Putten and Kallman (1968) determined the proportion of hypoxic cells in a
transplantable sarcoma in the mouse and found it to be about 15%. They went to
repeat this measurement in tumors that had received fractionated X-ray treatments and found that after 1000 rads the proportion of hypoxic cells was
unchanged at about 15%. This result argues strongly that during the course
of a fractionated regimen, cells moved from the hypoxic to the well-oxygenated compartment of the tumor, a phenomenon that has been termed

TABLE 1

Percentage of Hypoxic Cells in Experimental Tumors[a]

Authors	Host animal	Tumor type	Percent of hypoxic cells
Powers and Tolmach (1963)	Mouse	Lymphosarcoma	1
Hewitt and Wilson (1971)	Mouse	Round-celled sarcoma	≤50
Clifton *et al.* (1966)	Mouse	Adenosarcoma	21
Van Putten and Kallman (1968)	Mouse	Sarcoma	15
Hewitt *et al.* (1967)	Mouse	Squamous carcinoma	18
Howes (1969)	Mouse	Mammary carcinoma	12
Hill *et al.* (1971)	Mouse	Sarcoma	12
Van Putten (1968)	Mouse	Osteosarcoma	14
Suit and Maeda (1967)	Mouse	Mammary carcinoma	20–25
Kallman (1970)	Mouse	Mammary carcinoma	18–21
Reinhold (1966)	Rat	Rhabdomyosarcoma	15
Thomlinson (1971)	Rat	Sarcoma	17

[a] Based on data collected by Dr. R. Kallman in a review article on the phenomenon of reoxygenation and its implications for fractionated radiotherapy (Kallman, 1972).

"reoxygenation." The rate at which reoxygenation proceeds, and the extent to which it occurs, varies widely between different types of animal tumors studied (Thomlinson, 1969). In at least one animal tumor—an osteogenic sarcoma—reoxygenation is very slow, if it occurs at all (van Putten, 1968).

In the human situation, it is not known whether any or all tumors reoxygenate. In fact, it is not known with any certainty that human tumors contain viable hypoxic cells at all; however, based on histological evidence and by analogy with animal tumors, it is most likely that they do. The fact that in the clinic some tumors are eradicated with doses on the order of 6000–7000 rads, given in about 30 treatments, argues strongly in favor of reoxygenation taking place, since the presence of the smallest fraction of persistent hypoxic cells would make cures unlikely at these dose levels. It is an attractive hypothesis that tumors which do not respond well to radiotherapy are those which do not reoxygenate quickly and efficiently.

2.5. The Place and Need for High-LET Radiation in Radiotherapy

At the present time, a significant effort is being made to develop high-LET particle therapy facilities. The fact that it is considered to be worthwhile implies that there is a basic dissatisfaction with X- and γ-rays, the currently used modalities in radiotherapy. However, opinions are divided concerning the reason for this dissatisfaction. There is no doubt that, historically, the original rationale for the development of high-LET radiations was the desire to minimize the oxygen effect. However, the view has been voiced with increasing frequency that this may not represent the main advantage of particle therapy (Hall, 1967; Kaplan, 1970).

Some argue eloquently and persuasively that the principal advantage of charged particles is the depth-dose pattern which they produce, and that the lower oxygen effect is a bonus thrown in for good measure. The major improvements in radiotherapy since World War II have coincided with the introduction of megavoltage generators, and are probably a consequence of greatly improved depth-dose distributions. It is a compelling argument that further efforts to concentrate dose in the tumor, while sparing normal tissues, would be rewarded by a corresponding improvement in local tumor control. If this is the case, the main drawback of the present generation of X-ray machines is the dose distribution, which is limited by the approximately exponential absorption characteristics of photon beams. A major step forward would be the introduction of charged-particle beams, which have a limited range in tissue and which deposit a large proportion of their energy near the end of their range in the so-called Bragg peak region. Obvious contenders would include protons, α-particles, pions, and heavy ions; for any of these particle beams, enormously high energies are required, so that the Bragg peak can be located at a depth corresponding to a deep-seated tumor.

The ultimate choice of the optimum type of high-LET radiation to be used as a replacement for X- and γ-rays will depend on which of these various points of view turns out to be the most important. The rival merits of the various high-LET radiations are not necessarily mutually exclusive; there may well be a place and a need for more than one type of high-LET radiation, but this can only be decided after extensive long-term clinical trials. So far, neutrons are the only high-LET particles to have been tried extensively in the clinic, and it is already clear that, while they may have certain advantages, they are certainly not the cure-all for every problem in radiation therapy. There is also experimental evidence to alert us to the distinct possibility that these new treatment modalities might produce a striking benefit in only a limited number of tumor types, rather than a general "across-the-board" improvement in therapeutic ratio.

3. Neutrons

3.1. Nature and Production

A neutron is a particle having a mass approximately equal to that of a proton, but carrying no electrical charge. Because neutrons are electrically neutral, they cannot be accelerated in an electrical device. They are produced when a stream of charged particles, such as deuterons or protons, is accelerated to a very high energy and used to bombard a suitable target material such as beryllium. Neutrons are also emitted as by-products when heavy radioactive atoms undergo fission, i.e., split up to form two smaller atoms. In practical terms, there are three sources of fast neutrons that may be suitable for radiation therapy.

3.1.1. Fission Neutrons

Neutrons with a wide range of energies are produced in abundance inside a nuclear reactor by the fission of uranium-235. It is possible to extract a beam of fast neutrons from a reactor through an appropriate portal, but it is very poorly penetrating and of little use for external beam therapy. Some nuclides—in particular, californium-252—undergo spontaneous fission and give off a mixture of neutrons and γ-rays. Small sealed tubes containing this manmade nuclide represent the first available portable sources of neutrons. In this form, californium-252 is potentially an alternative to radium for use in interstitial and intracavitary therapy, in circumstances where the relatively low energy and penetrating power of fission spectrum neutrons do not constitute a serious limitation. Fission neutrons have a wide range of energies around 1 MeV.

3.1.2. Cyclotron-Produced Neutrons

A cyclotron is an electrical device capable of accelerating positively charged particles such as protons and deuterons to energies of many millions of volts. The most commonly used process is to accelerate deuterons, which are then made to impinge upon a beryllium target, as in the Hammersmith cyclotron, a wide leaving the neutron, which carries much of the kinetic energy of the incident particle. For example, when deuterons are accelerated to 15 MeV and made to impinge upon a beryllium target, as in the Hammersmith cyclotron, a wide spectrum of neutrons is produced, as shown in Fig. 4. In general, the modal neutron energy is about 40% of the energy of the deuteron beam that produced it; the total neutron spectrum covers a very wide range of energies. An alternative process that has only recently been investigated for possible applications in radiotherapy is to use protons on a target of beryllium or lithium. The disadvantage of this process is that the yield (and ultimately the dose rate) is lower than for the $d^+ \rightarrow$ Be process; however, it has the advantage that the neutron spectrum

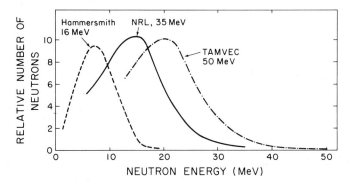

FIGURE 4. Spectra for three neutron beams used currently for radiotherapy. Since all used the $d^+ \rightarrow$ Be process, a wide range of neutron energies is present for each machine, with a modal energy about 40% of that of the accelerated deuteron. From Hall *et al.* (1975a).

contains more high-energy neutrons. It is possible that this process will come into favor in the near future.

3.1.3. 14 MeV d⁺ → T Neutrons

If a beam of deuterons, accelerated to a modest energy of 200–300 keV, is incident on a target containing tritium, neutrons are produced which are essentially monoenergetic at 14–15 MeV. The accelerated deuteron is "stripped" of its proton to become a fast neutron, while the target is slowly used up and converted to helium. The energy of the neutrons produced (14–15 MeV) is much greater than the energy of the incident deuteron; this extra energy is available because the internal binding energy of the helium atom is much lower than that of the tritium atom from which it is produced. This is, in theory, a most attractive method for generating neutrons, because in the first place it is relatively inexpensive (less so than a cyclotron), and in the second place the machinery involved is sufficiently compact to be accommodated in a treatment room of conventional size in a large urban hospital. At the present time, the serious drawback of this type of neutron generator is the low dose rate that is available. A neutron output of $3-5 \times 10^{12}$ n/sec is necessary to achieve a dose rate of about 9–15 rads/min at 1 m from the target, a treatment distance needed to result in percentage depth doses comparable to those of a conventional cobalt-60 unit. This cannot be achieved at the present time with the sealed tubes used in Europe because of technical difficulties in the design of the tritium target. There are a number of diverse approaches aimed at solving the problems. For example, Brennan *et al.* (1974) claimed to have attained a flux of over 5×10^{12} n/sec by using twin sources of a mixture of deuterons and tritons on opposite sides of a thin chromium target; a compact machine based on this principle will soon by available commercially.

3.2. Available Sources

Stone and his colleagues were the first to use neutrons for cancer therapy, utilizing a beam generated by a cyclotron at Berkeley during the years 1938–1943 (Stone and Larkin, 1942). This was a remarkable achievement in view of the fact that the neutron had only been discovered in the early 1930s (Chadwick, 1932). This effort was hampered by the lack of available radiobiological data and was interrupted by the entry of the United States into World War II. In reviewing their experience many years later, Stone concluded that "Neutron therapy as administered by us resulted in such bad late sequelae in proportion to the few good results that it should not be continued" (Stone, 1948).

The renewed interest in neutrons in the postwar years originated at the Hammersmith Hospital in London, where neutrons are generated by the 60-inch Medical Research Council Cyclotron. In this machine, 16 MeV deuterons incident on a beryllium target produce neutrons with a wide spectrum of energies having a modal value of around 6 MeV. The Hammersmith cyclotron was suggested and conceived by Gray, based on the notion that a lowered OER would be advantageous in radiotherapy; the earlier project at Berkeley had not been based on any particular radiobiological principle. While the dose rate from this machine is adequate (about 40 rads/min), the depth doses are only marginally so; at a treatment distance of 125 cm, the penetration of the beam is little better than that of 250 kV X-rays, which restricts the use of the beam to certain anatomical sites, mainly the head and neck. Patient treatment at Hammersmith was preceded by a long period of careful experimentation in radiological physics and radiobiology which laid a firm groundwork for the controlled clinical trials which are now under way.

Inspired by the early experiences of the Hammersmith group, which were described as "encouraging," additional clinical neutron facilities have been planned on both sides of the Atlantic. Table 2 is a summary of neutron facilities, existing and projected, as of June 1976. In Great Britain and continental Europe, the emphasis has been on the development of 14 MeV $d^+ \rightarrow T$ generators. The most attractive feature of a generator of this type is its compact form, which makes it suitable for installation in a treatment room of conventional size in a major cancer treatment center, together with the possibility of an isocentric mount. The British-built "Hiletron" is now commercially available and has been installed in two major radiotherapy centers in the United Kingdom (Greene and Jones, 1974). Phillips has also produced a generator based on this principle. Unfortunately, the development of $d^+ \rightarrow T$ generators has been slow and disappointing. At a treatment distance of 75 cm, the dose rate from the Hiletron is only 5 rads/min. For the depth doses from a machine of this type to equal those of a conventional cobalt unit, the treatment distance would need to be 125 cm, but this is ruled out by the low output. There will need to be rapid strides in the near future if $d^+ \rightarrow T$ generators are to be widely used in clinical practice.

TABLE 2

Neutron Facilities Used for or Proposed for Clinical Neutron Therapy, as of June 1976

	Process	Energy (MeV)
Cyclotrons		
Hammersmith Hospital, England	$d^+ \rightarrow Be$	16
Edinburgh, Scotland	$d^+ \rightarrow Be$	15
U.W.—Seattle, Washington, USA	$d^+ \rightarrow Be$	22
NRL—Washington, D.C., USA	$d^+ \rightarrow Be$	35
TAMVEC—Texas, USA	$d^+ \rightarrow Be$	50
Tokyo, Japan	$d^+ \rightarrow Be$	15
Chiba-Shi, Japan	$d^+ \rightarrow be$	30
Louvain, Belgium	$d^+ \rightarrow Be$	35
Linear accelerator		
Fermilab, Chicago, USA	$p^+ \rightarrow Be$	66
$d^+ \rightarrow T$ (MeV) machines		
Manchester, England		
Glasgow, Scotland		
Rijswik, Netherlands		
Amsterdam, Netherlands		
Hamburg, Germany		
Heidelburg, Germany		

Because of the limitations associated with 14 MeV d$^+$ → T generators, interest in a number of centers, particularly in the United States, has turned to the use of large cyclotrons which accelerate deuterons to energies in excess of 20 MeV. The cost of building such machines *de novo* would be too high to be contemplated for radiotherapy purposes, but a number of cyclotrons already exist which were built originally for high-energy physics research, and which can be modified for radiotherapy. This approach has been pursued in the United States and has led to the development of several high-energy neutron radiotherapy installations which have been treating cancer patients for a number of years. These are listed in Table 2. More recently, some centers in Europe, and notably in Japan, have also elected to turn to cyclotrons for the generation of neutrons.

3.3. Absorption Processes and Depth-Dose Patterns

Neutrons are uncharged particles and, for this reason, are highly penetrating compared with charged particles of the same mass and energy. They are indirectly ionizing, and are absorbed by elastic or inelastic scattering. In tissue, the former process gives rise predominantly to fast recoil protons which result from interactions of the fast neutrons with hydrogen atoms of the tissue. As the neutron energy is increased, inelastic scattering assumes more significance; for example, carbon nuclei in tissue split up into three α-particles, while oxygen nuclei split up into four α-particles (see Fig. 5). Although contributing a relatively small proportion of the total dose, the α-particles and heavier nuclei deposit energy at high LET, and have an important influence on the biological characteristics of the radiation. Figure 6 compares the percentage depth doses from conventional X- and γ-ray units with neutrons from a variety of sources. The important point to note is that the absorption of neutrons, like that of electromagnetic radiations, is approximately exponential with depth. By using neutrons of sufficiently high

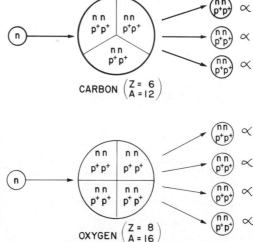

FIGURE 5. Production of spallation products. As the neutron energy rises, the probability increases of a neutron interacting with a carbon or oxygen nucleus to produce three or four α-particles, respectively.

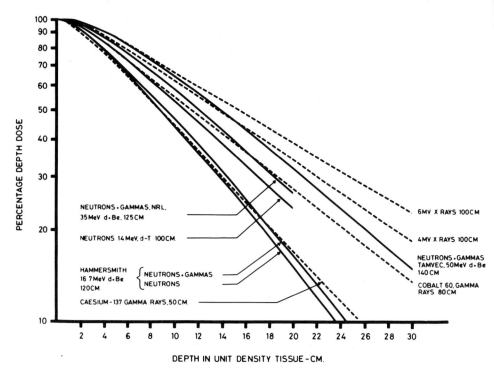

FIGURE 6. Percentage depth-dose curves for various neutron beams used or planned for radiotherapy, compared with conventional photon beams. Courtesy of Dr. John Parnell, Hammersmith Hospital, London.

energy and at an appropriately large treatment distance (125–150 cm), the percentage depth doses can be made comparable with those of a conventional cobalt-60 unit or linear accelerator. As far as dose distribution is concerned, however, neutrons can at best (and then only with difficulty) *equal* megavoltage X- and γ-rays; they certainly do not constitute an *improvement*. If it turns out that neutrons possess an inherent advantage over X- and γ-rays, it must stem from a difference in radiobiological properties, not from any improvement in dose distribution.

3.4. Biological Properties

The initial rationale for the introduction of neutrons into radiotherapy was undoubtedly their lowered OER. Neutrons are essentially a compromise; their OER is appreciably lower than that for X-rays, but it is still far from the ideal. They are used because it is possible to achieve a significant reduction in OER while retaining adequate penetration to treat deep-seated tumors.

The OER varies slowly with neutron energy over the whole range of fast-neutron energies available. The picture is complicated somewhat because some neutron beams are monoenergetic, while others, notably those produced by the $d^+ \rightarrow Be$ process, contain a wide spectrum of neutron energies. Low-energy monoenergetic neutrons of around 300 keV exhibit a low OER of around 1.3 because most of the recoil protons set in motion have an LET close to 100 keV/μm. As the neutron energy rises, the OER also increases because of the increasing range of the recoil protons set in motion when these neutrons are absorbed in tissue. 14 MeV $d^+ \to$ T neutrons are characterized by an OER of 1.6–1.8, which is about as large an OER as is possible with neutrons. At much higher neutron energies, the OER again decreases in value, presumably because of the presence of densely ionizing spallation products. Figure 7 shows the variation of OER as a function of the energy of the accelerated deuteron or proton used for the production of neutrons in high-energy cyclotrons. There may well be some move in the future to use higher energies for radiotherapy because the lower OER is combined with better percentage depth doses and a larger skin-sparing effect. A beam of fast neutrons, then, offers the possibility of a significant reduction in the OER, while maintaining a depth-dose pattern which is not very different from that characteristic of the present generation of large cobalt units and linear accelerators.

Broerse *et al.* (1968) made extensive measurements of human kidney (T1) cell survival for neutrons of several energies, namely, fission spectrum neutrons, 3 MeV neutrons, 16 MeV deuterons on beryllium, and 20 MeV tritons on beryllium. They found that RBE increases with neutron energy, although the RBE values did not correspond well with the RBE vs. LET relationship discussed in Section 2. They concluded that the concept of LET (whether track or energy

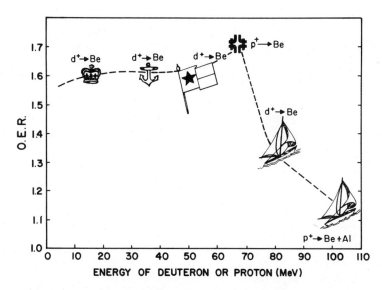

FIGURE 7. Oxygen enhancement ratio (OER) with *Vicia* for various neutron beams as a function of the energy of the deuteron or proton used to generate the beam. In order of increasing energy the sources are 16 MeV $d^+ \to$ Be, Hammersmith Hospital; 35 MeV $d^+ \to$ Be, Naval Research Laboratory, Washington, D.C.; 50 MeV $d^+ \to$ Be, Texas A & M Variable Energy Cyclotron; 67 MeV $p^+ \to$ Be, the National Accelerator Laboratory, Batavia (Fermilab); 80 $d^+ \to$ Be and 101 $p^+ \to$ Be, University of Maryland Cyclotron.

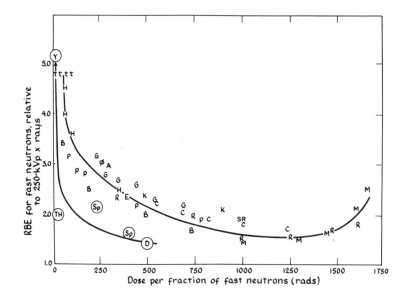

FIGURE 8. Relative biological effectiveness (RBE) values for various normal tissues irradiated with neutrons from the Hammersmith cyclotron as a function of the dose per fraction. H, Human skin reactions; P, pig skin reactions; G, 4-day gut death in mice; ϕ, leakage of protein from mouse gut; A, leakage of albumin from rat gut; B, stunting of tail growth in rats; K, observation of clones in rat bones; E, survival of chick embryos; R, rat skin reactions; SR, rat skin reactions; M, mouse skin reactions; C, clones in mouse skin; t, weight loss in mouse testes; Y, mouse lymphocytes; TH, weight loss in mouse thymus; Sp, mouse spleen colony assay; D, 30-day death in mice. Courtesy of Field (1969).

average LET) has limited significance for the interpretation of the biological effects of neutrons. For all neutron energies, RBE was found to be a strong function of neutron dose, decreasing with increasing dose. This is a direct consequence of the different survival curve shape characteristic of X-rays and neutrons; for neutrons, survival curves have a smaller initial shoulder and steeper slope than for X-rays.

As part of the extensive preclinical radiobiological measurements at the Hammersmith cyclotron, a wide range of RBE determinations were made for a variety of tumors and normal tissue in experimental animals (as well as for skin reactions in humans) using both single and fractionated treatment schedules. Experiments with normal tissue systems have included skin reactions in the pig, early skin reactions and late deformities in the feet of rodents, survival of hemopoietic stem cells using the colony-forming unit assay, survival of intestinal crypt stem cells, death due to esophageal damage, death due to lung fibrosis, damage to the capillary endothelium system, spinal cord damage, and acute and late reactions in the oral mucosa of monkeys. Tumor systems studied include the fibrosarcoma in rats, various mouse mammary tumors, the Lewis lung carcinoma

in mice, the rhabdomyosarcoma in rats, and pulmonary metastases in human
patients. Two striking and important facts emerge: (1) RBE varies with the dose
per fraction of neutrons. Figure 8 shows this variation for several normal tissue
end points and illustrates how important this effect can be; RBE increases rapidly
as the dose per fraction is reduced, reflecting directly the difference in survival
curves shape for X-rays and neutrons. (2) Even for a given dose, RBE varies a great
deal according to the tissue or endpoint studied.

For neutrons to be more effective than X-rays for clinical radiotherapy, the RBE
for tumors would need to be larger than for corresponding dose-limiting normal
tissues, i.e., the therapeutic gain factor, which has been defined as

$$\frac{\text{RBE tumor}}{\text{RBE normal tissue}}$$

should be larger than unity. Figure 9, taken from Field (1976), shows RBE values
for a range of normal tissues. While the single-dose RBE values obtained for

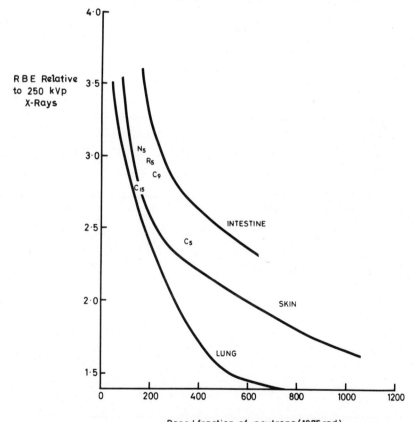

FIGURE 9. RBE values for five or more fractions as a function of dose per fraction of
fast neutrons produced by 16 MeV d^{+} → Be. Subscripts indicate the number of
fractions used. C, C3H carcinoma; R, RIB5 rat sarcoma; N, neck carcinoma. RBE
values for normal intestine, skin, and lung are shown for comparison. Courtesy of
Field (1976).

experimental tumors are in general higher than for normal tissues (probably reflecting the presence of hypoxic cell components in the tumors), for fractionated regimens the tumor RBEs fall between those for lung and intestine. It is conceivable, therefore, that fast neutrons may have a potential advantage for radiotherapy in situations where there are specific combinations of tumors and dose-limiting normal tissues, over and above the reduction in the importance of the oxygen effect.

As of June 1976, there are four cyclotrons in the world at which neutron beams are used to treat cancer patients; these will soon be joined by several more. All accelerate deuterons to different energies and consequently produce neutron beams which differ in biological effectiveness. There is an active program under way at present to make careful biological intercomparisons so that clinical data and dosage schedules can be compared between the various installations. Withers (1976) has used the jejunal crypt survival technique in the mouse to produce survival curves for all neutron energies presently in clinical use (Fig. 10). RBE decreases with neutron energy; Hammersmith neutrons generated at 16 MeV are more effective than Seattle (22 MeV) by 20%, more effective than NRL (35 MeV) by 30%, and more effective than TAMVEC (50 MeV) by about 40%. Using mammalian cells in culture, Hall *et al.* (1975*a*) found neutrons generated by 16 MeV d$^+\to$Be to be 20% more effective than 35 MeV d$^+\to$Be (TAMVEC). These studies clearly need to be augmented.

Since protocols used clinically almost always consist of a number of dose fractions rather than a single large exposure, the effect of fractionated neutron treatments is particularly relevant. Broerse and Barendsen (1969) performed

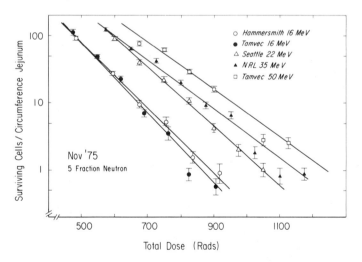

FIGURE 10. Dose–response curves for the survival of crypt cells in the mouse jejunum as a function of neutron dose. This elegant and repeatable biological test system has been widely used to compare the biological effectiveness of neutrons of different energies currently used for radiotherapy. The biological effect of a given dose *decreases* as the neutron energy *increases*. Courtesy of Dr. H. Rodney Withers.

fractionation studies with 15 MeV $d^+ \rightarrow T$ neutrons using human kidney cells, and found that the repair of sublethal damage between split doses was a factor of 2–3 smaller than for X-rays. Using the high-energy cyclotron-produced neutron at the Naval Research Laboratory (35 MeV $d^+ \rightarrow Be$), Hall *et al.* (1975*b*) found no detectable repair of sublethal damage between split doses of neutrons at the dose levels clinically used for daily dose fractions (about 140 rads). At higher neutron doses, repair does take place; indeed, it has been shown theoretically and experimentally that the repair of sublethal damage is quantitatively similar for X-rays and for neutrons at the *same dose level*. The lack of sublethal damage repair in the case of neutrons implies that the biological effectiveness of a multifraction regimen is much less dependent on the exact number of fractions than is the case for X-rays.

Another property in which neutrons differ from sparsely ionizing radiations is the ability to repair potentially lethal damage (PLD) subsequent to each. "PLD" is a term used to describe that component of the radiation damage that can be modified by changes in the postirradiation environment. PLD is not repaired following neutron irradiations, at least not to the extent that is characteristic of X-rays. This has been demonstrated for an animal tumor *in vivo* (Shipley *et al.*, 1975) and also for cells cultured *in vitro* (Hall and Kraljevic, 1976). Since PLD following X-irradiation is repaired in tumors but presumably not in normal tissues, this factor could detract from the therapeutic ratio for X-rays. The fact that PLD repair does not take place following neutron treatments could represent a therapeutic advantage for this densely ionizing radiation over and above the reduced oxygen effect.

3.5. Clinical Neutron Radiotherapy

In Great Britain, the use of fast neutrons in radiotherapy is being evaluated at the Hammersmith Hospital in London. This effort should soon be augmented by another small cyclotron at Edinburgh and $d^+ \rightarrow T$ generators at Manchester and Glasgow, but at the present time Hammersmith is the only significant clinical neutron facility in the United Kingdom. In the United States, three large cyclotrons have been used to generate neutrons for patient treatment for several years. The M. D. Anderson Hospital in Houston uses the Texas A&M cyclotron located 100 miles north in College Station; the radiotherapy group at the University of Washington at Seattle use the cyclotron in the physics department of the same university; a consortium of therapists, designated the Mid-Atlantic Neutron Therapy Association, use the Naval Research Laboratory in Washington, D.C. The U.S. effort will shortly be strengthened by the commission of a fourth high-energy facility at the Fermilab, near Chicago. Other clinical studies using neutrons have just started, or are about to start, in Holland, East and West Germany, Belgium, France, and Japan.

Patient treatment at Hammersmith was preceded by careful and extensive radiobiological experimentation. Following this, skin reactions were observed in volunteer patients to confirm the animal data (Morgan, 1967). During the years that followed, several hundred patients with a variety of advanced and radioresistant tumors were treated; these patients were thought to have a poor prognosis and to be unlikely to respond to conventional X-ray therapy. In this way, acceptable dose regimens were formulated and a great deal of neutron experience was accumulated. The results of these early studies could not be definitive because patients were neither randomized nor controlled, but the response of certain tumors (such as salivary gland tumors) was said to be "remarkable." It was also demonstrated clearly that neutron therapy could cause regression of advanced and radioresistant tumors, with acceptable early complications, in a manner comparable to that of more conventional treatment modalities (Catterall, 1974a,b; Catterall and Vonberg, 1974).

A prospective, randomized clinical trial to compare neutrons with X- and γ-rays was started in July 1971. Advanced tumors of the head and neck were chosen for the study, because tumor and normal tissue response could be readily observed, and because the relatively poor depth doses characteristic of the Hammersmith beam are suitable only for treating relatively superficial lesions.

Based on the first 100 or so patients treated in the random trial, Catterall *et al.* (1975) reported slightly more serious complications in the neutron-treated group, together with substantially better tumor regressions, compared with the control group treated with X- or γ-rays. The unavoidable weakness of this trial is that only about one-third of the control patients treated with photons received their therapy at Hammersmith; the remainder were treated at the various participating centers. A retrospective analysis of the data indicated that, on average, the patients receiving neutrons were treated more aggressively with higher effective doses than were the photon-treated controls. However, when only the most closely comparable photon-treated patients were considered, neutrons still appeared to produce significantly greater tumor control. Catterall and her colleagues concluded that the benefits of neutrons are real and suggested that patients with less advanced tumors should be included in the trial so that long-term effects on tumors and normal tissue could be observed.

The clinical experience to date at the three U.S. neutron therapy centers has been reviewed by Hussey *et al.* (1975). More than 400 patients with many different tumor types have been treated with nuetrons over the past 4 years, during which time there has been a gradual refinement of dose, time, and fractionation regimens. The clinical use of neutrons in the United States has not yet reached the stage of a prospective randomized trial, and the radiotherapists involved, who are dedicated and experienced clinicians, are rightly cautious and reluctant to make a premature assessment of the effectiveness of this new type of radiation. It is fair to say, however, that they are less encouraged and optimistic than their British colleagues at Hammersmith. What is clear is that the early results for neutron therapy of glioblastoma multiforme are disappointing; more than 50 patients have been treated at one or another of the U.S. centers, and the mean survival time of 7.5 months is virtually identical to that obtained with conventional radiation.

4.1. *Nature and Production*

π^- mesons, or pions as they are often called, are negatively charged particles having a mass 273 times that of an electron. Unlike other heavy charged particles of interest in radiotherapy, pions are unstable and have a mean life of only 2.54×10^{-8} sec. Pions can be produced in any nuclear interactions if the energy of the primary particle is sufficient to create the rest mass of the pion. For radiotherapy, pions with energies of about 40–90 MeV are of interest, since these particles have ranges in tissue of approximately 6–13 cm, respectively. In practice, either protons or electrons are accelerated to very high energy and used as projectiles to bombard a target in order to create pions. In either case, a substantial accelerator facility is required. For protons, a very-high-energy accelerator such as a synchrocyclotron or linear accelerator is necessary in order to accelerate protons to an energy of about 800 MeV. In the case of electrons, a more compact linear accelerator is possible; the problem in this case is the low yield of pions, and some elaborate focusing device is essential in order to harvest a greater proportion of the pions, which are produced isotropically in the source, and focus them into a target volume.

4.2. *Available Sources*

Facilities designed to produce pion beams are listed in Table 3. Much of the early experimental work, which provided the basis for the subsequent decisions to use pions clinically, was performed at the 180-inch cyclotron at Berkeley, California. The output from this machine is too low to be considered for clinical use. Later experimental work was performed on the NIMROD accelerator at Harwell in England; this machine could be adapted for clinical use if sufficient funds were available. Comparable experimental work was also performed at CERN, the European Organization for Nuclear Research located in Switzerland, and operated by 12 European countries.

TABLE 3
π^- *Meson Facilities*

	Particle accelerated
Experimental studies	
Berkeley, California, USA	p^+
Harwell, England	p^+
CERN—Zurich, Switzerland	p^+
Clinical machines	
Los Alamos, New Mexico, USA	p^+
Stanford, California, USA	e^-
TRIUMF—Vancouver, Canada	p^-
SIN—Switzerland	p^+

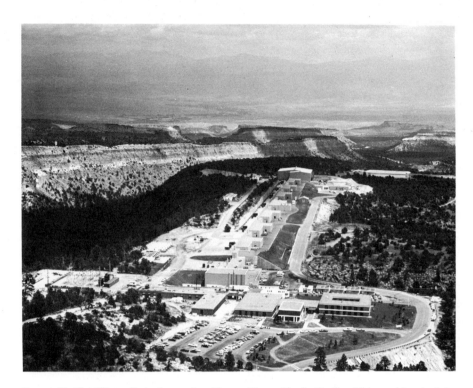

FIGURE 11. The Clinton P. Anderson Los Alamos Meson Physics Facility. This machine, built by the Energy Research and Development Administration, is over half a mile in length. Its enormous size and spectacular location high on a mesa in New Mexico are evident from the aerial photograph. Pions produced by this accelerator are used experimentally for the treatment of cancer. Photograph courtesy of Los Alamos Scientific Laboratory, New Mexico.

There are currently in the world four pion facilities that are scheduled to be used clinically for the treatment of cancer patients. The first is the huge proton linear accelerator sited at Los Alamos in New Mexico. A picture of this facility is shown in Fig. 11, which illustrates its enormous size and spectacular location high on a mesa in New Mexico. The first patient ever to receive pions for the treatment of cancer was treated at this facility in October 1973 (Kligerman *et al.*, 1975). The synchrocyclotron at Vancouver, British Columbia, is known as TRIUMF, and is a joint venture of a number of Canadian universities. It is nearing completion and will go into use shortly to treat patients at the British Columbia Cancer Institute. An accelerator at SIN (Schweizenisches Institut für Nuclearforschung), located near Zurich, Switzerland, is also being developed for clinical use, and a special vertical beam has been built for therapeutic applications. A noteworthy effort in the production of pion facilities will be at Stanford University in California where a different concept is involved. Instead of the huge accelerators associated with pion production at the other centers, it is the aim of the Stanford group to build a smaller and more compact machine which can be installed in or close to the existing radiotherapy facility. This accelerator will produce pions from accelerated electrons instead of from accelerated protons; this is made possible by the use of a cleverly conceived cryogenic focusing device (known as the SMPG or Stanford

Medical Pion Generator) which accepts pions from a large, solid angle and directs them through 60 treatment ports into the patients in a pseudorotation fashion (Kaplan *et al.*, 1973; Boyd *et al.*, 1973).

4.3. Absorption Processes and Depth-Dose Patterns

Pions travel through tissue in a manner similar to that of any other heavy charged particle, and stop after traveling a range that depends on their initial energy. The dose delivered by a beam of pions to a tissuelike medium increases very slowly with depth in the beginning, but gives rise to a sharply defined maximum near the end of the particle's range in the so-called Bragg peak region. This is a property which they have in common with all other heavy charged particles. Near the end of its range, a pion may be captured by one of the constituent atoms of the tissue, such as oxygen, carbon, or nitrogen. The pion cascades down the atomic levels, emitting characteristic X-rays (known as π^- mesic X-rays) in the process. The pion is eventually captured by the nucleus, which disintegrates or explodes into short-range densely ionizing fragments. This constitutes the so-called star production which is a unique feature of pions.

A depth-dose curve for negative pions in a water phantom is shown in Fig. 12; the curve exhibits a sharp peak at a depth corresponding to the maximum range of the particles. The pions behave like "overweight" electrons in passing through the first few centimeters of the absorbing material, but then produce densely ionizing heavy ions in a very localized region at the end of their track. A beam of this kind

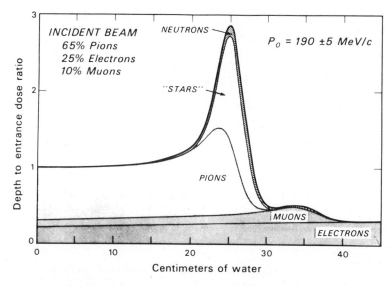

FIGURE 12. Depth-dose profile for a beam of π^- mesons. The dose reaches a maximum near the end of the particle's range, at a depth that depends on the initial energy of the particles. This figure also indicates the proportion of the dose resulting from the various primary and secondary particles. Courtesy of Curtis and Raju (1968).

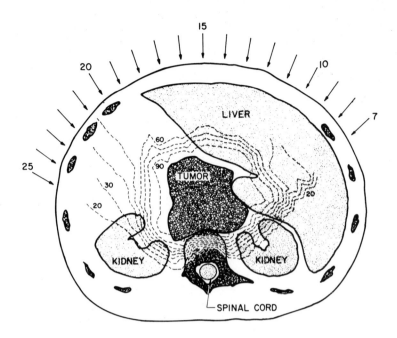

FIGURE 13. Calculated dose distribution for a tumor of the pancreas treated with the 60-channel Stanford Medical Pion Generator (SMPG). Because of the characteristic depth-dose patterns for pions, it is possible to achieve a high-dose region enclosing the tumor, while surrounding normal tissue is subject to a much lower dose. Courtesy of Dr. M. Bagshaw.

offers the attractive possibility to the radiotherapist of locating the tumor in a region where the absorbed dose is high, and where the radiation has the characteristics associated with high LET. At the same time, the normal tissues in the path of the incident beam are exposed to a lower dose of radiation, and the radiation involved has a lower biological effectiveness because it has a lower average LET.

As it stands, the depth-dose distributions shown in Fig. 12 would be quite unsuitable for clinical radiotherapy, because the Bragg peak is too sharply defined and not broad enough for most radiotherapeutic procedures. The peak region can be broadened to any extent desired by accepting a range of pion energies. Figure 13 illustrates the type of dose distribution that can be obtained with the 60-channel Stanford Medical Pion Generator. The high-dose region can be tailored to fit the tumor volume, while adjacent vital normal structures can be avoided. This is claimed to be the overwhelming advantage of pions over more conventional radiation modalities.

4.4. Biological Properties

Fowler and Perkins (1961) first advocated the potential of negative pions in radiotherapy. Their suggestion motivated several groups in different parts of the world to measure the physical and radiobiological properties of negative pions, although the dose rates available from the existing machines were several orders of magnitude smaller than those required for clinical use. While the available beams were adequate to demonstrate the physical characteristics and depth-dose patterns for pions, the low dose rates available severely hampered the biological investigations. Over a small field area of 3 by 3 cm, the dose rate at Berkeley was 5–60 rads/hr, at NIMROD in Harwell 20–180 rads/hr, and at CERN about 3 rads/hr. It is most probable that the accelerator at Los Alamos will be the first to achieve high dose rates which will be adequate not only for radiobiological studies but also for full-scale patient treatment.

The principal attraction of pions arises from the depth-dose pattern, which offers the radiotherapist the option of siting the tumor at the Bragg peak where the dose is high compared with adjacent normal tissue. The depth-dose curve in Fig. 12 shows the peak in absorbed dose only; the *biologically effective dose* in the peak may be even higher if the RBE of the densely ionizing star fragments is larger than that of the radiation absorbed in the incident plateau, which is virtually indistinguishable from X- or γ-rays. Unfortunately, this is an area of some dispute at the present time. Because of the low dose rates, most experiments to date have involved biological systems chosen for their radiosensitivity rather than their relevance to radiotherapy. This is true, for example; of the *Vicia faba* system. Pion experiments with *Vicia* have yielded some of the most credible OER data available, but RBE estimates with the same system, which range from 2.2 to 3.4 (Richman *et al.*, 1967; Gnanapurani *et al.*, 1972; Raju *et al.*, 1970; Winston *et al.*, 1973; Baarli and Bianchi, 1972), are meaningless because plant systems commonly exhibit higher RBEs than mammalian cells for densely ionizing radiations. For mammalian T1 cells in culture under aerated conditions, the RBE for pions at the Bragg peak is 1.6–2.4 (Burki *et al.*, 1969; Raju *et al.*, 1972), for human lymphocytes about 2 (Madhvanath, 1971), for HeLa cells 1.4–2.1 (Mill *et al.*, 1975), and for human skin about 1.5 (Kligerman *et al.*, 1976). The difficulty in these experiments is not only the low dose rate of the pions but also the dose rate of the reference low-LET radiation for which there is a marked dose-rate effect.

A second attraction and possible advantage of the pions is that the radiation in the peak region includes a high-LET component which should reduce the OER. Table 4 summarizes the OER determinations that have been made in the pion peak region. Values vary from 1.35 to 1.8, with perhaps more reliance to be placed on the higher figure, which is in good agreement with that predicted by calculation (Curtis and Raju, 1968). At first sight, it might have been anticipated that a lower OER would apply in the region of the peak. This is not the case, because the densely ionizing fragments from the star production are responsible for only a modest proportion of the total absorbed dose. As a consequence, the OER, even at the Bragg peak, is larger than for fast neutrons, and will be further increased when the peak is broadened and spread out to cover a tumor of 5–10 cm diameter.

It is probably fair to say that the radiobiological data obtained to date for pions, while of interest, are largely anecdotal, and will all have to be repeated when high-intensity, therapy-type beams become available.

TABLE 4
OER Values for π⁻ Mesons

Site	Biological system	Pion d/rate (rads/hr)	OER	Reference
Berkeley	*Vicia*, growth inhibition at 4°C	30	1.35–1.5	Raju *et al.* (1970)
	Vicia, chromosome aberrations	30	1.8	Gnanapurani *et al.* (1972)
	Arginine reversions in yeast	30–60	1.9	Raju *et al.* (1971)
	T1 cells	30	1.5	Raju *et al.* (1972)
NIMROD	*Vicia*, growth inhibition	20	1.8	Winston *et al.* (1973)
Los Alamos	T1 cells	300	1.5	Raju *et al.* (1975)

5. Heavy Ions

5.1. High-Energy Heavy Ions—Existing and Potential Sources

Until the summer of 1971, high-energy heavy nuclei were unique to the space environment. For a number of years following 1957, the HILAC accelerators at Yale and Berkeley had been used to accelerate nuclei as heavy as carbon and oxygen, but the maximum energy was limited (10 MeV/amu) and consequently the range in unit density material was only about 1 mm. These ions were used extensively for radiobiological studies with monolayers of cells, but were, of course, quite unsuitable for radiotherapy.

In July 1971, stripped nitrogen nuclei were successfully accelerated to 3.9 GeV at the Princeton Particle Accelerator (PPA), and soon afterward at the Berkeley Bevatron (White *et al.*, 1971; Grunder *et al.*, 1971). Subsequent to that date, beams of oxygen and neon were accelerated at both the PPA and the Bevatron, but neither machine was capable of accelerating nuclei of higher Z at intensities adequate for biological experiments. After about a year of radiobiological experimentation, PPA was closed down due to lack of funds. At the same time, substantial funds were made available at Berkeley to use the heavy-ion linear accelerator (the HILAC) as an injector for the Bevatron. The two machines were linked by a beam line, some 500 feet long, running down the hillside at Berkeley. This expensive and ambitious project has been completed and the combined facility is known as the Bevalac (Ghiorso *et al.*, 1973). In principle, this facility should be able to accelerate any ion of interest up to and including iron ions; so far, argon is the heaviest nucleus accelerated for biological experiments.

At the present time, this is a unique facility, the only machine in the world capable of accelerating high-energy heavy ions. There are a number of other physics accelerators in various countries which could be converted to this purpose

if a sufficient demand existed and funds were available. For example, there are
plans in both France and in the USSR to convert existing proton synchrotrons to
accelerate heavy ions.

5.2. Depth-Dose Profiles

Figure 14 shows depth-dose data for various nuclei. In all cases, the absorbed dose
is relatively constant in the entrance plateau, the length of which depends on the
energy of the incident particle; near the end of the particle's range, there is a
narrow Bragg peak region where a great deal of energy is deposited as the particle
comes to rest. As a general rule, the Bragg peak gets progressively narrower as the
Z of the particle increases; in addition, the ratio of peak-to-plateau absorbed dose
also gets larger and larger. The peak is too narrow to be used directly, and in order

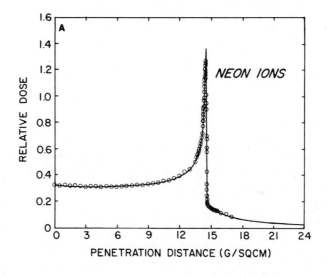

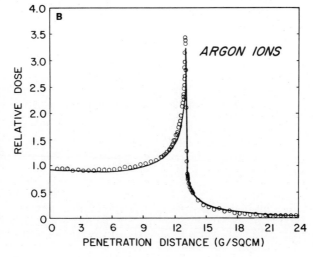

FIGURE 14. Depth-dose curves for high-energy neon ions (A) and argon ions (B). A large amount of energy is deposited at the end of the particle's range in the Bragg peak region. The depth at which the Bragg peak occurs is a function of the particle's initial energy. As the Z of the particle increases, the Bragg peak becomes narrower and taller. Courtesy of Dr. John Lyman.

to irradiate a tumor 5–10 cm in diameter, the peak must be "scanned," i.e., distributed over this region; this can be achieved either by using a ridge filter or by accepting particles with a range of energies. For very high Z particles, the dose absorbed in the peak will be at a very high LET, and consequently the RBE of the radiation will be low. Consequently, although there will be a sharp Bragg peak in the depth-dose curve, the biologically effective dose (i.e., absorbed dose × RBE) will not peak. At this stage, biological effect will simply be proportional to the particle flux. There will be no need to use a modulated beam or a ridge filter; biologically effective dose will remain virtually constant to the end of the particle's range. This situation is a matter of conjecture at the present time, since no biological measurements have been made on particles of sufficiently high Z for this to be observed.

5.3. Biological Properties

The use of ions heavier than helium in radiotherapy was proposed by Tobias as early as 1960 (Tobias and Todd, 1967). Despite the passing of so many years, the amount of radiobiological data for high-energy heavy ions is still meager, to say the least, largely because so few machines are capable of producing these particles and access to them is so limited. The potential of heavy ions in radiotherapy is still a matter of debate. It is generally agreed that the principal advantage of neutrons is their lowered OER, while pions promise an improved localization of dose within the target volume; these factors may or may not translate into a clinical gain in practice, but they are clearly *potential* advantages. By contrast, the benefit of heavy ions is not at all clear. They could prove to be the particle of choice *par excellence*, or it could turn out that they are not worth the trouble and expense of producing them; it remains for further experiments to determine this.

In early experiments at the HILAC accelerators, low-energy heavy ions were used to irradiate mammalian cells in thin monolayer cultures. OER values close to unity were obtained for carbon and for ions of higher Z (Todd, 1964). This, of course, referred to stopping ions. At a later date, when high-energy ions became available, extensive OER measurements were performed at the Princeton Particle Accelerator using 3.9 GeV nitrogen ions. The measurements were made with *Vicia* seedlings which occupied a volume 2 mm thick in the direction of the beam; this represented the limit of resolution in these experiments. Some of the data from the experiments are summarized in Fig. 15. Averaged over this thickness, the OER was found to be 1.55–1.65 at the Bragg peak, but only a few millimeters upstream of the peak the OER had a large value (close to 3) indistinguishable from that for X-rays (Hall and Kellerer, 1973). These experiments led to two conclusions: (1) Since the lowered OER is confined to such a narrow region at the Bragg peak, nitrogen ions are quite unsuitable for radiotherapy. (2) The large OER values immediately upstream from the Bragg peak were measured at positions of quite high LET values. Based on the OER vs. LET relationship measured with natural α-particles or slow heavy ions (Fig. 3), a lowered OER would have been

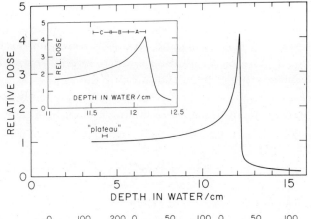

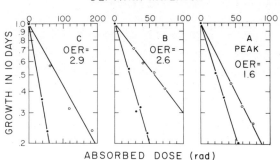

FIGURE 15. Upper panel: Depth-dose curve for 3.9 GeV nitrogen ions. The inset shows the Bragg peak on a larger scale and the three positions A, B, and C, at which radiobiological measurements were made. Lower panels: Response of *Vicia* seedlings to nitrogen ions under aerated and hypoxic conditions in three positions close to and upstream of the Bragg peak. From Hall and Kellerer (1973).

predicted for these positions. This discrepancy indicates that LET is not an adequate measure of quality for these high-energy heavy ions so far as the OER is concerned.

Extensive RBE measurements were also made for 3.9 GeV nitrogen ions, both at Princeton and at Berkeley, using mammalian cells in culture, *Vicia* seedlings, *Tradescantia* inflorescences, as well as mouse tumors and skin (Hall and Lehnert, 1973; Hall and Kellerer, 1973; Brown *et al.*, 1973; Underbrink *et al.*, 1973; Todd *et al.*, 1971). As expected, the RBE in the plateau region differs little from that of X-rays, but near the narrow Bragg peak, higher RBEs were obtained, the exact values depending on the biological system used and the dose range considered. As is frequently the case, plant materials yielded high RBE values, reaching 6.8 for *Vicia* and 18 for *Tradescantia*. For mammalian systems, the RBE in the peak region was in the range 1.5–4.5, depending on the dose level used.

Subsequently, some experiences have been performed at Berkeley with high-energy beams of oxygen, and also of neon, which looks the most promising particle to date. The data of Fu and Phillips (1976) for the 400 MeV nucleon neon beam indicate that the RBE is higher in the peak than in the plateau, although this advantage is practically lost when the Bragg peak is spread out to cover even a small simulated tumor of 4 cm in diameter. The OER in the terminal region of the spread-out Bragg peak is 1.4, a value which would presumably get larger if the peak were spread out over a larger volume.

Recent measurements with the 18 GeV argon beam at the Bevalac show that the RBE at the Bragg peak is almost identical to that in the entrance plateau. The OER was found to be 1.4 at the peak and 1.5 a few millimeters upstream from the peak. For these high-energy, high-Z particles, the LET in the region of the peak must exceed 1000 keV/μm, and yet the OER is significantly higher than unity and not much different from the values commonly reported for fast neutrons. LET is certainly not a good indicator of the biological properties of these particles, especially so far as OER is concerned, presumably because of the radial profile of energy deposition around the tracks and the long-range δ-rays set in motion.

6. Relative Merits of Neutrons, Pions, and High-Energy Heavy Ions

6.1. Patterns of Energy Deposition

The biological properties of the various particles are readily understood in terms of microdosimetric quantities. This is illustrated in Fig. 16. In the case of heavy ions, an overwhelming proportion of the absorbed dose at or close to the Bragg peak is associated with events of extremely high LET. For both pions and neutrons, on the other hand, the dose is spread out over a wide range of LET values, and only a small proportion is associated with LETs in excess of a few hundred keV/μm. The biological properties of these particles, therefore, have an intermediate value characteristic of a mixture of high- and low-LET radiations. The rival merits of the various heavy particles are summarized in Table 5. The principal differences compared with conventional photon radiations, which may be considered advantageous, are the lowering of the OER and an improvement in the depth-dose pattern.

6.2. The Particles Compared

Cyclotron-produced neutrons suitable for radiotherapy have an OER of about 1.6, which is much lower than for X-rays, although it is by no means unity and must be regarded as a compromise. As a consequence, neutrons are given three stars for OER in Table 5. As far as depth-dose pattern is concerned, neutrons can

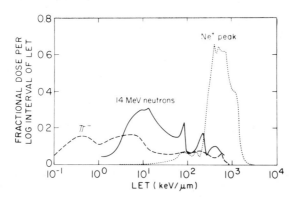

FIGURE 16. Fractional dose per log interval of LET plotted as a function of LET. Areas under the curves are proportional to the fraction of the dose in the corresponding range of LET. The dashed curve is the spectrum at the Bragg peak for 90 MeV π^- mesons. The solid curve corresponds to 14.6 MeV neutrons at a depth of 12 cm, while the dotted curve represents the spectrum for 5.7 GeV neon ions at the Bragg peak. I am indebted to Dr. J. Dicello for preparing this figure. From Hall (1973).

TABLE 5
Comparison of the Merits of Various Heavy Particles for Radiotherapy

Limitation X- or γ-rays	Neutrons	Pions	Heavy ions
Dose distribution limited by exponential absorption	—	★ ★ ★ ★	★ ★ ★ ★
Large OER	★ ★ ★	★ ★	★ ★ ★ ★

barely equal, much less improve upon, modern photon beams and certainly offer no advantage in this respect.

π^- mesons offer some improvement to both the depth-dose pattern and the OER. In a practical situation, with a spread-out Bragg peak and a high dose rate, their OER will probably turn out to be about 2.0, which is not as good as neutrons, and for this reason they receive two stars for OER in Table 5. However, their depth-dose distribution, particularly if the RBE should prove to be high in the region of the Bragg peak, is probably superior to that of any other available particle, and for this reason they are given a score of five stars. The unique characteristic of pions is the production of star fragments in the peak region, short-range, densely ionizing particles that raise the RBE in the peak relative to the plateau and help to preserve a peak-to-plateau ratio even when the peak is spread out to cover a tumor of realistic size. However, should a depth-dose distribution turn out to be the only advantage of pions, it would be difficult to make a compelling case for their use, since protons or α-particles can produce similar depth-dose patterns at a fraction of the cost.

For some years now, high-energy heavy ions have been thought to have great potential in radiotherapy. The promise was that a deep-seated tumor might be enclosed in a region of high dose, where the OER is close to unity and the RBEs are high because of the densely ionizing characteristics of the radiation; at the same time, the surrounding normal tissue would be subjected to a lower dose of radiation which is relatively sparsely ionizing and has a lower RBE. This expectation was based on the physical characteristics of charged particles which have a definite limited range in tissue and which, as they stop, deposit a lot of energy at high LET in the Bragg peak region. Although only limited data are available at present for high-energy heavy ions, it is already obvious that this utopian situation is unlikely to be achieved in practice.

The principal reason for using heavy ions might be the lowered OER. Low-energy beams of carbon and ions of higher Z had been shown to have an OER of 1.0, and it was hoped that a similar value might apply to high-energy heavy ions which also had enough penetration to be used in radiotherapy. However, the lowest OER value reported to date even for neon or argon, where the LET at the Bragg peak exceeds $1000 \, keV/\mu m$, is 1.4. This is, of course, lower than for neutrons or pions, and for this reason heavy ions are given four stars for OER in Table 5. These particles may also offer a depth-dose pattern which is an improvement over that of X-rays or neutrons, but it is unlikely that they can rival pions in this respect; consequently, they are given four stars for depth-dose pattern in Table 5. This may be somewhat disappointing, but the explanation is not hard to find. In order to achieve a lowered OER over an appreciable region close to the Bragg peak, it is necessary with these heavy ions to go to a high Z particle, such as neon. As a consequence, the peak-to-plateau ratio is lost, because of two factors. First, the Bragg peak gets progressively narrower as Z increases, and, second, the radiation in the peak becomes so densely ionizing that its RBE may be lower than in the entrance plateau. It is for these reasons that heavy ions cannot equal pions in terms of the depth-dose pattern.

It is not possible to choose which of these particles to favor in radiotherapy without first deciding which characteristic of X- and γ-rays limits their success in controlling localized malignant disease. If the large oxygen effect is the critical limitation of photons, then all three particles should result in an improvement, with heavy ions at the top of the list, followed by neutrons, and with pions in third place. This, of course, ignores the cost factor; heavy ions are much more expensive and less available than neutrons for a relatively modest gain in OER. On the other hand, if the major weakness of γ-rays is the dose distribution that can be obtained, then neutrons have no place and the solution would be to use charged particles of some kind, with pions having a distinct edge over heavy ions. In fact, protons or α-particles could achieve essentially the same result at a fraction of the cost.

Since it is not possible to choose between the heavy particles at the present time, there is obviously an urgent need for much more radiobiological data to be obtained with all of them, particularly for π^- mesons and high-energy heavy ions which are only now becoming available for the first time at intensities sufficient for detailed radiobiological investigations. In the course of the next decade, there is little doubt that all three types of heavy particles will be developed to the point where clinical trials may be conducted under favorable conditions. It is the earnest hope of everyone who has been associated with this development, regardless of his own partisan interests, that one or other of the new modalities will prove to be advantageous in a spectacular way and revolutionize the radiotherapy of human cancer.

ACKNOWLEDGMENTS

This investigation was supported by Contract E(11-1)-3243 from the Energy Research and Development Administration and by Grants CA-12536 and CA-18506, awarded by the National Cancer Institute, DHEW.

7. References

BAARLI, J., AND BIANCHI, M., 1972, Observed variations of RBE values in the stopping region of a 95 MeV negative pion beam, *Int. J. Radiat. Biol.* **22**:183.

BARENDSEN, G. W., 1964, Impairment of the proliferative capacity of human cells in culture by alpha particles with differing linear energy transfer, *Internat. J. Radiat. Biol.* **8**:453–466.

BARENDSEN, G. W., 1972, Radiobiological dose-effect relations for radiation characterized by a wide spectrum of LET; implications for their application in radiotherapy, in: *Proceedings of the Conference on Particle Accelerators in Radiation Therapy*, pp. 120–125, U.S. Atomic Energy Commission, Technical Information Center, LA-5180-c.

BARENDSEN, G. W., BEUSKER, T. L. J., VERGROESEN, A. J., AND BUDKE, L., 1960, Effects of different ionizing radiations on human cells in tissue culture. II. Biological experiments, *Radiat. Res.* **13**:841.

BARENDSEN, G. W., WALTER, H. M. D., FOWLER, J. F., AND BEWLEY, D. K., 1963, Effects of different ionizing radiations on human cells in tissue culture. III. Experiments with cyclotron accelerated alpha-particles and deuterons, *Radiat. Res.* **18**:106.

BARENDSEN, G. W., KOOT, C. J., VAN KERSEN, G. R., BEWLEY, D. K., FIELD, S. B., AND PARNELL, C. J., 1966, The effect of oxygen on impairment of the proliferative capcity of human cells in culture by ionizing radiations of different LET, *Int. J. Radiat. Biol.* **10**:317.

BOYD, D., SCHWETTMAN, H. A., AND SIMPSON, J., 1973, A large acceptance pion channel for cancer therapy, *Nucl. Instrum. Methods* **111**:315.

BRENNAN, J. T., BLOCH, P., HENDRY, G. O., HILTON, J. L., KIM, J., AND QUAM, W. M., 1974, Recent advances in the development of a 14 MeV neutron generator suitable for radiotherapy, *Br. J. Radiol.* **47**:912.

BROERSE, J. J., AND BARENDSEN, G. W., 1969, Recovery of cultured cells after fast neutron irradiation, *Int. J. Radiat. Biol.* **15**:335.

BROERSE, J. J., BARENDSEN, G. W., AND VAN KERSEN, G. R., 1967, Survival of cultured human cells after irradiation with fast neutrons of different energies in hypoxic and oxygenated conditions, *Int. J. Radiat. Biol.* **13**:559.

BROWN, D. Q., SEYDEL, H. G., AND TODD, P., 1973, Inactivation of cultured human cells and control of C_3H mammary tumors with accelerated nitrogen ions, *Cancer* **32**:541.

BURKI, H. J., BARENDSEN, G. W., RAJU, M. R., AMER, N. M., AND CURTIS, S. B., 1969, A method to determine acute radiation response of human cells to π mesons, in: *Semiannual Report, Biology and Medicine*, pp. 100–104, Bonner Laboratory and Lawrence Radiation Laboratory Report-UCRL-18793.

CATTERALL, M., 1974a, The treatment of advanced cancer by fast neutrons from the Medical Research Council's cyclotron at Hammersmith Hospital, London, *Eur. J. Cancer* **10**:343.

CATTERALL, M., 1974b, A report on three year's fast neutron therapy from the Medical Research Council's cyclotron at Hammersmith Hospital, London, *Cancer* **34**:91.

CATTERALL, M., AND VONBERG, D. D., 1974, Treatment of advanced tumors of head and neck with fast neutrons, *Br. Med. J.* **3**:137.

CATTERALL, M., SUTHERLAND, I., AND BEWLEY, D. K., 1975, First results of a clinical trial of fast neutrons compared with x or gamma rays in treatment of advanced tumors of the head and neck, *Br. Med. J.* **2**:653.

CHADWICK, J., 1932, Possible existence of a neutron, *Nature (London)* **129**:312.

CLIFTON, K. H., BRIGGS, R. C., AND STONE, H. B., 1966, Quantitative radiosensitivity studies of solid carcinoma *in vivo*: Methodology and effect of hypoxia, *J. Natl. Cancer Inst.* **36**:965.

CURTIS, S. B., AND RAJU, M. R., 1968, A calculation of the physical characteristics of negative pion beams—energy—loss distribution and Bragg curves, *Radiat. Res.* **34**:239.

FIELD, S. B., 1969, The relative biological effectiveness of fast neutrons for mammalian tissues, *Radiology* **93**:915.

FIELD, S. B., 1976, An historical survey of radiobiology and radiotherapy with fast neutrons, *Curr. Top. Radiat. Res. Q.* **11**:1.

FOWLER, P. H., AND PERKINS, D. H., 1961, The possibility of therapeutic applications of beams of negative π mesons, *Nature (London)* **189**:524.

FU, K., AND PHILLIPS, T. L., 1976, The relative biological effectiveness (RBE) and oxygen enhancement ratio (OER) of neon ions for the EMT6 tumor, work in progress, *Radiology* **120**:439.

GHIORSO, A., GRUNDER, H., HARTSOUGH, W., LAMBERTSON, G., LOFGREN, E., LOW, K., MAIN, R., MOBLEY, R., MORGADO, R., SALSIG, W., AND SELPH, R., 1973, The BEVALAC. An economical facility for very energetic heavy particle research. Presented at the Particle Accelerator Conference, San Francisco, March 5–7, 1973, Lawrence Berkeley Laboratory Report LBL-1386.

GNANAPURANI, M., RAJU, M. R., RICHMAN, C., AND WOLFF, S., 1972, Chromatid aberrations induced by π mesons in *Vicia faba* root meristem cells, *Int. J. Radiat. Biol.* **21**:49.

314

ERIC J. HALL

GRAY, L. H., CONGER, A. D., EBERT, M., HORNSEY, S., AND SCOTT, O. C. A., 1953, The concentration of oxygen dissolved in tissues at the time of irradiation as a factor in radiotherapy, *Br. J. Radiol.* **26:**638.

GREENE, D., AND JONES, R. E., 1974, The "Hiletron" neutron generator at Manchester, *Eur. J. Cancer* **10:**256.

GRUNDER, H. A., HARTSOUGH, W. D., AND LOFGREN, E. J., 1971, Acceleration of heavy ions at the Bevatron, *Science* **174:**1128.

HALL, E. J., 1967, The oxygen effect: Pertinent or irrelevant to clinical radiotherapy, *Br. J. Radiol.* **40:**874.

HALL, E. J., 1973, Radiobiology of heavy particle radiation therapy: Cellular studies, *Radiology* **108:**119.

HALL, E. J., AND KELLERER, A. M., 1973, The biophysical properties of 3.9 GeV nitrogen ions. III. OER and RBE determinations using *Vicia* seedlings, *Radiat. Res.* **55:**422.

HALL, E. J., AND KRALJEVIC, U., 1976, Potentially lethal radiation damage as a modifier of neutron RBE; implications for radiation therapy, *Radiology* **121:**731.

HALL, E. J., AND LEHNERT, S., 1973, The biophysical properties of 3.9 GeV nitrogen ions. IV. OER and RBE determinations using cultured mammalian cells, *Radiat. Res.* **55:**431.

HALL, E. J., ROIZIN-TOWLE, L. A., AND ATTIX, F. H., 1975a, Radiobiological studies with cyclotron-produced neutrons currently used for radiotherapy, *Int. J. Radiat. Oncol.* **1:**33.

HALL, E. J., ROIZIN-TOWLE, L., THEUS, R. B., AND AUGUST, L. S., 1975b, Radiobiological properties of high energy cyclotron-produced neutrons for radiotherapy, *Radiology* **117:**173.

HEWITT, H. B., AND WILSON, C. W., 1971, Survival curves for tumor cells irradiated *in vivo*, *Ann. N.Y. Acad. Sci.* **95:**818.

HEWITT, H. B., CHAN, D. P., AND BLAKE, E. R., 1967, Survival curves for clonogenic cells of a murine keratinizing squamous carcinoma irradiated *in vivo* or under hypoxic conditions, *Int. J. Radiat. Biol.* **12:**535.

HILL, R. P., BUSH, R. S., AND YEUNG, P., 1971, The effect of anaemia on the fraction of hypoxic cells in an experimental tumour, *Br. J. Radiol.* **44:**299.

HOLTHUSEN, H., 1921, *Pflügers Arch.* **187:**1.

HOWES, A. E., 1969, An estimation of changes in the proportions and absolute numbers of hypoxic cells after irradiation of transplanted C_3H mouse mammary tumours, *Br. J. Radiol.* **42:**441.

HUSSEY, D. H., PARKER, R. G., AND ROGERS, C. C., 1975, A preliminary report of the fast neutron therapy pilot studies in the United States, International Particle Radiation Therapy Workshop, Key Biscayne, Florida, Oct. 1–3, 1975, Proceedings (V. B. SMITH, ed.), American College of Radiobiology, Philadelphia.

KALLMAN, R. F., 1970, Oxygenation and reoxygenation of a mouse mammary carcinoma, in: *Proceedings of the Fourth International Congress of Radiation Research*, Evian, France, *Advances in Radiation Research*, Vol. 3 (J. F. DUPLAN AND A. CHAPIRO, eds.), pp. 1195–1204, Gordon and Breach, New York, 1973.

KALLMAN, R. F., 1972, The phenomenon of reoxygenation and its implications for fractionated radiotherapy, *Radiology* **105:**135.

KAPLAN, H. S., 1970, Radiobiology's contribution to radiotherapy: Promise or mirage? *Radiat. Res.* **43:**460.

KAPLAN, H. S., SCHWETTMAN, H. A., FAIRBANK, W. M., BOYD, D., AND BAGSHAW, M. A., 1973, A hospital-based superconducting accelerator for negative pi-meson beam radiotherapy, *Radiology* **108:**159.

KLIGERMAN, M. M., WEST, G., DICELLO, J. F., STERNHAGEN, C. J., BARNES, J. E., LOEFFLER, R. K., DOBROWOLSKI, F., DAVIS, H. T., BRADBURY, J. N., LANE, T. F., PETERSON, D. F., AND KNAPP, E. A., 1976, Initial comparative response to peak pions and x rays of normal skin and underlying tissue surrounding superficial metastatic nodules, *Am. J. Roentgenol.* **126:**261.

MADHVANATH, U., 1971, Effects of densely ionizing radiations on human lymphocytes cultured *in vitro*, Ph.D. thesis, University of California, Report UCRL-20680.

MILL, A., LEWIS, J. D., AND HALL, W. S., 1976, Radiation response of mammalian cells after irradiation with a beam of π^- mesons, *Br. J. Radiol.* **49:**166.

MORGAN, R. L., 1967, Fast neutron therapy-clinical applications, in: *Modern Trends in Radiotherapy* (T. J. DEELEY AND C. A. P. WOOD, eds.), pp. 171–186, Appleton-Century-Crofts, London.

MOTTRAM, J. C., 1936, Factor of importance in radiosensitivity of tumors, *Br. J. Radiol.* **9:**606.

PETRY, E., 1923, *Biochem. Z.* **135:**353.

POWERS, W. E., AND TOLMACH, L. J., 1963, A multicomponent x-ray survival curve for mouse lymphosarcoma cells irradiated *in vivo*, *Nature (London)* **197:**710.

RAJU, M. R., AMER, N. M., GNANAPURANI, M., AND RICHMAN, C., 1970, The oxygen effect of π mesons in *Vicia faba*, *Radiat. Res.* **41**:135.

RAJU, M. R., GNANAPURANI, M., STACKLER, B., MARTINS, B. I., MADHVANATH, U., HOWARD, J., LYMAN, J. T., AND MORTIMER, R. K., 1971, Induction of heteroallelic reversions and lethality in *Saccharomyces cerevisiae* exposed to radiations of various LET (^{60}Co rays, heavy ions, and π mesons) in air and nitrogen atmospheres, *Radiat. Res.* **47**:635.

RAJU, M. R., GNANAPURANI, M., RICHMAN, C., MARTINS, B. I., AND BARENDSEN, G. W., 1972, RBE and OER of π mesons for damage to cultured T-1 cells of human kidney origin, *Br. J. Radiol.* **45**:178.

RAJU, M. R., DICELLO, J. F., TRUJILLO, T. T., AND KLIGERMAN, M., 1975, Biological effects of the Los Alamos meson beam on cells in culture, *Radiology* **116**:191.

READ, J., 1952, The effect of ionizing radiations on the broad bean root. X. The dependence of the x-ray sensitivity on dissolved oxygen, *Br. J. Radiol.* **25**:89.

REINHOLD, H. S., 1966, Quantitative evaluation of the radiosensitivity of cells of a transplantable rhabdomyosarcoma in the rat, *Eur. J. Cancer* **2**:33.

RICHMAN, S. P., RICHMAN, C., RAJU, M. R., AND SCHWARTZ, B., 1967, Studies of *Vicia faba* root meristems irradiated with a π^- beam, *Radiat. Res. Suppl.* **7**:182.

SHIPLEY, W. U., STANLEY, J. A., COURTENAY, V. D., AND FIELD, S. B., 1975, Repair of radiation damage in Lewis lung carcinoma cells following *in situ* treatment with fast neutrons and γ rays, *Cancer Res.* **35**:932.

STONE, R. S., 1948, Neutron therapy and specific ionization, *Am. J. Roentgenol.* **59**:771.

STONE, R. S., AND LARKIN, J. C. JR., 1942, The treatment of cancer with fast neutrons, *Radiology* **39**:608.

SUIT, H. D., AND MAEDA, M., 1967, Hyperbaric oxygen and radiobiology of a C_3H mouse mammary carcinoma, *J. Natl. Cancer Inst.* **39**:639.

THOMLINSON, R. H., 1969, in: *Proceedings of the Carmel Conference on Time and Dose Relationship in Radiation Biology as Applied to Radiotherapy*, p. 242, BNL report 50203(C-57).

THOMLINSON, R. H., 1971, The oxygen effect and radiotherapy with fast neutrons, *Eur. J. Cancer* **7**:139.

THOMLINSON, R. H., AND GRAY, L. H., 1955, The histological structure of some human lung cancers and the possible implications for radiotherapy, *Br. J. Cancer* **9**:539.

TOBIAS, C. A., AND TODD, P. W., 1967, Heavy charged particles in cancer therapy, in: *Radiobiology and Radiotherapy*, pp. 1–21, National Cancer Institute Monograph No. 24.

TODD, P. W., 1964, Reversible and irreversible effects of ionizing radiations on the reproductive integrity of mammalian cells cultured *in vitro*, Ph.D. thesis, Lawrence Radiation Laboratory Report UCRL-11614, Berkeley, Calif.

TODD, P. W., 1967, Heavy ion irradiation of cultured human cells, *Radiat. Res. Suppl.* **7**:196.

TODD, P., SCHROY, C. B., VOSBURGH, K. G., AND SCHIMMERLING, W., 1971, Spatial distribution of biological effect in a 3.9 GeV nitrogen ion beam, *Science* **174**:1127.

UNDERBRINK, A. G., SCHAIRER, L. A., AND SPARROW, A. H., 1973, The biological properties of 3.9 GeV nitrogen ions. V. Determination of relative biological effectiveness for somatic mutations in *Tradescantia*, *Radiat. Res.* **55**:437.

VAN PUTTEN, L. M., 1968, tumor reoxygenation during fractionated radiotherapy: Studies with a transplantable mouse osteosarcoma, *Eur. J. Cancer* **4**:173.

VAN PUTTEN, L. M., AND KALLMAN, R. F., 1968, Oxygenation status of a transplantable tumor during fractionated radiotherapy, *J. Nat. Cancer Inst.* **40**:441.

WHITE, M. G., ISAILA, M., PRELEC, K. ALLEN, H. L., 1971, Acceleration of nitrogen ions to 7.4 GeV in the Princeton particle accelerator, *Science* **174**:1121.

WINSTON, B. M., BERRY, R. J., AND PERRY, D. R., 1973, Response of *Vicia faba* to irradiation with a beam of negative π mesons, under aeobic and hypoxic conditions, *Br. J. Radiol.* **46**:541.

WITHERS, H. R., 1976, personal communication.

ZIRKLE, R. E., 1954, in: *Radiation Biology*, Vol. 1 (A. HOLLAENDER, ed.), pp. 315–350, McGraw-Hill, New York.

9

Stem Cells, Nonproliferating Cells, and Their Kinetics in Normal and Neoplastic Tissues

MILAN POTMESIL, JOSEPH LoBUE, AND ANNA GOLDFEDER

Primum non nocere.
—a maxim of medicine

1. Introduction

At this time of increased efforts and promising results in the therapy of malignant neoplasias, it seems appropriate to review critically some principal aspects of cell and tissue kinetics as they relate to stem cells, to nonproliferating cells, and to cell recruitment into the mitotic cycle. Considering effective therapy, relatively slowly growing tumors possessing a large fraction of "nonproliferating" cells are of substantial concern. Such tumor cells, either "resting" or slowly cycling, may have an increased resistance to therapeutic agents, and some of them are probably potential stem cells. The contribution of cell kinetic data to planning and management of therapy of these types of cancer has not been fully adequate. Among the most likely reasons for this are the following: (1) most animal tumor systems used in cytokinetic investigations are not comparable to prevailing types of human

MILAN POTMESIL, JOSEPH LoBUE, AND ANNA GOLDFEDER ● Cancer and Radiobiological Research Laboratory and Laboratory of Experimental Hematology, Department of Biology, New York University, New York, New York 10003.

318

MILAN
POTMESIL,
JOSEPH
LOBUE,
AND
ANNA
GOLDFEDER

cancer; (2) applied methods have conceptual and technical limitations; and (3) experimental approaches have usually neither allowed for any correlation between the structure of neoplastic tissues and therapeutic responses nor revealed the kinetic status of various cell subpopulations during the course of treatment.

Numerous reviews containing analytical, critical, and speculative comments on subjects related to the topics of this chapter have recently appeared. These include, for example, evaluations of the effects of chemotherapeutic agents on bone marrow stem cells (Boggs and Chervenick, 1973); differences in proliferation kinetics of normal and malignant tissues and their exploitation in chemotherapy and radiotherapy (Brown, 1975); survival studies following chemotherapy or radiotherapy, including cell repair of therapeutic damage (Hahn, 1975); principles of cell kinetics as they relate to clinical radiation therapy (Hellman, 1975); various aspects related to the presence of hypoxic cells in human tumors and advantages or disadvantages of therapeutic approaches dealing with this problem (Kaplan, 1974); cell kinetics in tumors (Lamerton, 1973; 1974), methods of assay of stem cells in normal and malignant tissues (Lamerton and Blackett, 1974); cytokinetics of neutrophilic granulocytes (LoBue, 1973); cell kinetics in treated human acute leukemia (Mauer, 1975); methods used for studies of cytokinetics in normal and malignant tissues (Mendelsohn, 1975); cytokinetics of several experimental tumor lines treated by chemotherapeutics (Skipper and Schabel, 1973); some aspects of cytokinetics in neoplasias (Steel, 1973, 1975); cell population kinetics in irradiated tumors and repair of cellular damage (Tubiana, 1974); differential sensitivity of hematopoietic stem cells and tissue culture cells to cytotoxic effects of anticancer drugs (Valeriote and van Putten, 1975); applicability of cell kinetic data for successful chemotherapy (van Putten, 1974); effects of selected chemotherapeutics on the cell cycle (Wheeler and Simpson-Herren, 1973); and radiation therapy and cytokinetics (Withers, 1975)*. Since most of these reviews have stressed many although not all of the significant points related to cytokinetics of effective and potential stem cells, we feel that if additional attention were given to these subjects, this might lead to less orthodox and potentially productive approaches in cell kinetic studies.

2. Concept of Stem Cells

It is generally agreed that a rational approach to effective therapy of cancer should attempt to take advantage of any differential proliferative characteristics which may exist between normal and malignant cells. A comprehensive understanding of tumor-cell kinetic patterns is also essential for the intelligent use of fractionated irradiation or of chemotherapy combining several drugs. When considering responses of normal and tumor cells to various therapeutic agents, one should be primarily concerned with stem cells, as these cells retain the capacity to repopulate

---

* A monograph discussing identification, differentiation, cytokinetics and other topics related to stem cells in various normal tissues was published after this chapter was already in press [*Stem Cells of Renewing Populations* (A. B. Cairnie, P. K. Lala, and D. G. Osmond, eds.), Academic Press, New York, 1976].

the tissue. The number of stem cells and their kinetic characteristics (e.g., proliferative status, cell production rate, and life span) are relevant parameters reflecting changes that may occur during treatment. The concept of a stem cell fraction of a tumor-cell population seems to be more useful for cytokinetic studies than the idea of a growth fraction (see Section 3.4.1). The stem cell fraction would include all cells with clonogenic capacity. However, there are serious difficulties involved concerning a reasonably precise estimate of the size of this fraction. These and related problems have been discussed in numerous reviews; see, for example, Lamerton (1972, 1973, 1974), Boggs and Chervenick (1973), Lamerton and Blackett (1974), and van Putten (1974).

2.1. Basic Considerations

2.1.1. Definition of Stem Cells and Types of Stem Cell Populations

The term "stem cell" is used synonymously with "clonogen" or "progenitor cell" to mean a cell capable of extensive or "unlimited" self-replication and able to generate new cell lines by more or less progressive differentiation to mature cell types (Lajtha, 1967; Hellman *et al.*, 1969). The normal adult mammal retains many stem cell populations in a dynamic steady state in which population growth is balanced by some removal mechanism. Under certain conditions, cell populations may temporarily expand (e.g., embryogenesis, recovery from depopulation) or decrease (a differential cell population losing the capacity for further replication). Two extreme situations exist in the kinetic pattern of stem cells (Lajtha, 1967): (1) stem cell populations in which all cells participate in the cell cycle or (2) stem cell populations possessing a large proportion of cells not detectably participating in the cell cycle. In the former population, a fraction α of all cells divides and produces daughter cells which increase stem cell numbers, while a fraction $1 - \alpha$ is removed by differentiation or cell death. The value $\alpha = 0.5$ represents the dynamic steady-state condition, $\alpha > 0.5$ represents an expanding population, and $\alpha < 0.5$ represents a declining population. Excluding a reduction in intermitotic times, any recovery of a partially depleted cell population is possible only if the rate of differentiation is temporarily decreased. In steady-state stem cell populations with large numbers of nondividing cells, a balance exists between the removal of cells by differentiation or cell death and the production of cells. Cell depletion is compensated for either by nonproliferating cells being triggered into a cell cycle or by slowly proliferating cells being accelerated in their progression through the cell cycle. The simplest situation to consider in a growing stem cell population is exponential growth with some degree of random cell loss. A transient population of cells with a limited number of divisions or of nondividing maturing cells will retard population growth and may lead to the establishment of steady-state kinetics. It has been suggested (Bresciani, 1968) that variation in the stem cell compartment alone could easily result in continuous and unlimited growth of a polycompartmental system comprised of progenitor, expanding, and nonproliferating compartments. Theoretical analyses have shown that an

320

MILAN
POTMESIL,
JOSEPH
LOBUE,
AND
ANNA
GOLDFEDER

increased transit time through the expanding or the nonproliferating compartment cannot produce by itself the unlimited growth characteristic of neoplasia. Unlimited growth can be achieved only if the ratio between the fraction of stem cells remaining in the compartment and continuing to divide and the fraction of stem cells feeding into later sequential compartments exceeds 1. Moreover, a shift to unlimited growth does not require the involvement of the whole stem cell population. Such a change is usually considered to be a consequence of neoplastic transformation of stem cells, with loss of their attending sensitivity to regulatory mechanisms that in normal renewing tissue would keep the ratio constant (i.e., equal to 1).

2.1.2. Clonal Aging and Succession

A stem cell population could be maintained simply by cells proliferating for a very large number of generations. This tangential system provides for a pool of stem cells maintaining their number while at the same time continuously supplying cells entering the expanding or nonproliferating compartment. Alternatively, stem cells might have only a limited number of divisions at their disposal, with the form of their succession in a renewal system being clonal. Such an asynchronous-logarithmic system provides for a pool of stem cells consisting of a series of subpopulations with pedigrees of varying length. Stem cells are recalled asynchronously from a "resting" stage to form series of proliferating clones (Kay, 1965; Killman, 1968; reviewed by Gavosto, 1973). Killman's contention is that certain stem cells may enter a dormant state at various distances in lineage from the fertilized ovum ("sleepers"), while another fraction of stem cells remains actively proliferating ("feeders") and serves to maintain the "feeder" pool and supply progeny for the differentiating pool. When the "feeder" pool is exhausted, the "sleeper" cell is somehow activated and initiates a new clone of "feeders" replacing the old one. The size and function of such a system would depend on the rate of promotion of dormant cells and on the rate of proliferation and maturation in their daughter cells. The existence of an asynchronous-logarithmic system has been postulated for normal hematopoietic cells as well as for leukemic cells, but this hypothetical model might be applied to other systems as well. A predictable characteristic of neoplastic stem cell clones derived successively from a generation of dormant cells would be their heterogeneity.

There are experimental data available which support the concept of asynchronous-logarithmic multiplication of stem cells. Cytogenetic analyses have shown that human tumor cells are clonal in nature, and the presence of the same chromosome marker indicates their origin from a single cell. It has been suggested that some tumors consist of a single clone, others of two or more clones (reviewed by Atkin, 1970). However, tumor cells generally exhibit many common changes which may have occurred either coincidentally or sequentially. Studies of karyotype changes in human leukemias and experimental tumors (Ford and Clarke, 1963; Rovera and Pegoraro, 1968) have revealed a successive appearance of differing cell types which were variants of a single clone. Clonal development has been demonstrated as a feature of the history of many human leukemias. For example, in studies of chronic myeloid leukemia it was found that changes occurring at the time of the acute myeloblastic stage were superimposed upon the changes present in the chronic stage, each new line adding to previous chromosomal changes (DeGronchy *et al.*, 1968). Thus, in the history of a neoplasm, its stem cell population may be represented by several stem cell lines (clones). It has been suggested that the growth of stem lines rarely remains exponential for long, as each stem line gives rise to a short-lived transient population with a limited number of divisions. Asynchronous rise and fall of the stem line lead to clonal succession. Aging of cells in clones may be attributed to the process of differentiation, leading eventually to a loss of certain functions pertinent to the maintenance of clone size (reviewed by Smith, 1973). Asynchronous-logarithmic systems may operate not only at the level of stem cell pools but also at the level of differentiating, multiplicative progeny cells, at least in the thymic lymphocyte series (Potmesil and Goldfeder, 1973).

321
STEM CELLS,
NON-
PROLIFERATING
CELLS, AND
THEIR
KINETICS

2.2. Methods of Assay

2.2.1. Stem Cells of Normal Tissue

A variety of methods have been designed to investigate the properties of the stem cell pools in normal renewal tissues. Stem cells present in bone marrow, peripheral blood, spleen, or fetal liver of mice (Till and McCulloch, 1961; Goodman and Hodgson, 1962; Hands and Ainsworth, 1964; Till *et al.*, 1964), rat bone marrow or spleen (Comas and Byrd, 1967; Dunn, 1971), hamster bone marrow (Holloway *et al.*, 1968), and human peripheral blood (Chervenick and Boggs, 1971; Kurnick and Robinson, 1971) can be assayed as colony-forming units producing colonies *in vivo* in the spleen (CFU-s), by using the erythropoietin assay for erythropoietin-responsive cells (ERC) (Lajtha, 1970) or the plasma-clot and methyl cellulose techniques for erythroid stem cells (Till *et al.*, 1975), and by culture of myeloid-committed stem cells (CFU-c) (Metcalf, 1973; Stephenson *et al.*, 1971). The spleen colony method introduced by Till and McCulloch (1961) measures exogenous multipotential CFU-s of donor bone marrow, spleen, and blood injected into irradiated recipient mice or rats (Comas and Byrd, 1967). Recipient animals can also be treated with cytotoxic drugs instead of radiation (Santos and Haghshenass, 1968). In the endogenous spleen colony method, mice or rats are either whole-body irradiated (Till and McCulloch, 1963; Jenkins *et al.*, 1969), irradiated while partially shielded (Lajtha, 1970), or treated with cytotoxic drugs (Dunn and Elson, 1970), and spleen colonies arise from host CFU-s surviving the treatment. A modification of the endogenous assay for CFU is the technique of Withers and Elkind (1969), which measures the survival of crypt stem cells in the mouse jejunum. Two repopulation assays measuring the ability of transplanted progenitors to form mature progeny are erythroid-repopulating ability (ERA) based on radioactive iron uptake (reviewed by Blackett, 1968; Lajtha, 1970), and granulocyte-repopulating ability (GRA) based on the endotoxin-mobilization technique (review by Hellman *et al.*, 1970). *In vitro*

MILAN
POTMESIL,
JOSEPH
LOBUE,
AND
ANNA
GOLDFEDER

methods which assay the CFU-c of animal and human hematopoietic tissue using various culture media have been reviewed by Dunn (1971), Metcalf (1973), and Stohlman *et al.* (1974). The agar colony-forming assay estimates agar colony-forming units (CFU-a) mostly designated as CFU-c, yielding granulocytic, mononuclear, and granulocytic-mononuclear colonies in the presence of colony-stimulating factor (Pluznik and Sachs, 1965; Bradley and Metcalf, 1966; Metcalf *et al.*, 1967*a,b*; Metcalf and Foster, 1967). This assay has been discussed in a previous volume of this treatise, in which an abridged classification of hematopoietic stem cells is also tabulated (LoBue and Potmesil, 1975). CFU-c may be identical with some of the CFU-s (Stohlman *et al.*, 1974) and it represents a rather heterogenous population of cells. Different treatments of bone marrow donors and different conditions of cell cultures apparently allow different subpopulations of CFU-c to give rise to colonies (Dunn, 1971). Erythroid-committed stem cells may apparently be categorized as at least two age subgroups, the more primitive burst-forming units (BFU-E) and the more mature CFU-E (McLeod *et al.*, 1974; Tepperman *et al.*, 1974; Iscove and Sieber, 1975; Till *et al.*, 1975). In addition, techniques for culture of megakaryocytic stem cells (CFU-M) have been reported (e.g., see Nakeff and Daniels-McQueen, 1976).

2.2.2. Stem Cells of Neoplasms

Any meaningful evaluation of tumor responses to various therapeutic regimes should be concerned with the number and kinetic characteristics of cells which have the capacity to repopulate the tumor. There are a number of different techniques of tumor stem cell assay, testing either the capacity of a single-cell suspension of tumor cells to form clones *in vitro* and in recipient animals *in vivo* or the capacity to regrow the tumor *in situ*. A single-cell plating technique was introduced by Puck and Marcus (1950) and originally served as a tool in studies on the effects of ionizing radiation. The clonogenicity of cells in a suspension prepared from treated or untreated transplantable mouse or rat tumors can be assayed *in vitro* by their colony-forming ability (Frindel *et al.*, 1967; Barendsen and Broerse, 1969; Rockwell *et al.*, 1972; Dawson *et al.*, 1973; Thomson and Rauth, 1974; Lamerton and Blackett, 1974). Cells of some experimental tumors growing *in vivo* can be adapted to tissue culture conditions by a single passage (Hermens and Barendsen, 1969) or by repeated alternate passages (Rockwell *et al.*, 1972), or, conversely, adaptation to *in vivo* conditions can be achieved using cultured cell lines (Frindel *et al.*, 1967). This "adaptation" represents selections of stem cell lines growing under either condition. The method is suitable for sarcoma or sarcomalike tumors.

The end-point dilution technique was first applied as an *in vivo* colony-forming assay to mouse sarcoma and leukemia by Hewitt (1953) and Hewitt and Wilson (1959*a*). The method is based on earlier observations on quantitative tumor cell transplantations (Furth and Kahn, 1937; Kahn and Furth, 1938). The results are expressed as TD_{50} (number of injected tumor cells required to produce tumors at 50% of injected sites). Tumor cells are injected subcutaneously, mostly in axillary or inguinal regions, or intraperitoneally. This dilution assay has been used for studies of radiation effects on cell reproductive capacity in murine leukemias, sarcomas, and carcinomas (Hewitt and Wilson, 1959*b*; Berry and Andrews, 1961; Hewitt, 1966; Hewitt *et al.*, 1967; Maruyama *et al.*, 1967; Kallman *et al.*, 1967; Rockwell and Kallman, 1973), particularly in relation to different conditions of oxygenation in neoplastic tissue. The construction of radiation or drug dose–response curves is greatly facilitated by the use of TD_{50} data. The cloning efficiency of the assay, expressed as the number of tumor cells per single inoculum necessary to produce takes in 50% of injected sites, can be increased in some instances by an admixture of lethally irradiated cells of the same origin to the tested inoculum (Hewitt *et al.*, 1967, 1973). This effect is probably connected with thromboplastin release by lethally irradiated cells, leading to the production of a fibrin lattice at the site of inoculation (Peters and Hewitt, 1974). This process may provide anchorage and other favorable conditions for further proliferation of implanted cells. The accuracy of TD_{50} titration assays of solid tumors is usually lower than that of transplanted leukemias, lymphomas, or ascites tumors, and, besides low efficiency, a major problem is created by the seemingly random variations occurring from one experiment to another in the course of several passages of tumor transplants (Kallman *et al.*, 1967; Kallman, 1968). This may be attributed to technical factors, but biological changes in transplantability cannot be ruled out. In any event, simultaneous titrations of cell suspensions obtained from several untreated and treated tumors should be performed as part of one assay (Kallman *et al.*, 1967).

An alternative method applying the end-point dilution technique is the lung colony assay. Intravenous injection of a cell suspension of rat tumor or polyoma-transformed embryonic cells (van den Brenk *et al.*, 1973*a,b*; Williams and Till, 1966), mouse sarcoma (Hill and Bush, 1969), or adenocarcinoma (Shaeffer *et al.*, 1973) results in the formation of visible lung colonies, each presumably initiated by a single clonogenic cell. Thus the number of colonies is proportional to the number of injected cells with preserved, unlimited reproductive potential. Generally, this method requires a shorter time for completion of the experiment than the TD_{50} titration assay. One of the problems connected with this assay is its low cloning efficiency (number of lung colonies/number of injected cells, excluding vital dye). However, if lethally irradiated tumor cells are added to the suspension of tested cells, or if the lungs of the recipient animals are irradiated before the cell injections, then the efficiency can be increased by up to an order of magnitude. Whole-body irradiation is frequently applied to suppress the immune response in studies of antigenicity of tumor systems. The increased colony formation following this treatment is difficult to interpret since it could be due either to immunosuppression, to stimulatory effects of radiation on pulmonary colony formation, a phenomenon previously discussed (LoBue and Potmesil, 1975), or to a combination of the two (van den Brenk and Sharpington, 1972).

Another method used for quantitation of tumor stem cells is the spleen colony assay. Cells of the spontaneous thymic lymphoma of AKR mice (Bruce and van den Gaag, 1963), murine leukemia (Wodinsky *et al.*, 1967), or plasma-cell tumor

323
STEM CELLS,
NON-
PROLIFERATING
CELLS, AND
THEIR
KINETICS

324

MILAN
POTMESIL,
JOSEPH
LOBUE,
AND
ANNA
GOLDFEDER

(Bergsagel and Valeriote, 1968), when injected intravenously into recipients, lodge and grow in their spleens and form macroscopically detectable colonies. Each colony is presumably derived from a single cell, which is sometimes referred to as a tumor CFU. This assay has been used for the evaluation of different types of treatment (Bruce and Meeker, 1964, 1967; Bruce *et al.*, 1966), but it is considered less sensitive than other titration assays. Another end-point assay evaluates the reproductive potential of stem cells in a solid tumor remaining *in situ* after irradiation. Tested tumors are assigned at random to several different levels of local irradiation and the number of "cures" is scored in each group. The percentage of cured animals is recorded as a function of radiation dose, and the "tumor control dose" (TCD_{50}) is calculated (Suit, 1967; Gillette *et al.*, 1972; Suit *et al.*, 1972). TCD_{50} is defined as the radiation dose producing total regression in 50% of irradiated tumors. There is a theoretical correlation between the fraction of cells surviving the TCD_{50} dose and the number of cells required to reach the TD_{50} value (Reinhold and DeBree, 1968). However, in some instances the predicted value is in sharp contrast to that obtained experimentally for TCD_{50} (Rockwell and Kallman, 1973).

2.2.3. Reproducibility of Assays

There is at present no ideal method available for assaying tumor stem cells. It is certainly not surprising that data on cell survival assessed by exclusion of "vital" dyes, ^{51}Cr release, attachment of cells to glass, and plating efficiency did not correspond (Bhuyan *et al.*, 1976). This is apparently because each method relates to only one of several aspects of cellular activity. The dye exclusion technique, usually used for the counting of serially diluted cells, may overestimate the number of viable cells and cause an artificially low plating efficiency in a stem cell assay (Thomson and Rauth, 1974). There also are several other problems. The single-cell plating techniques were developed for tumors in which nearly all cells are stem cells, and it is therefore difficult to apply these tests to those differentiated tumors in which stem cells probably represent only a small fraction of the total population. The *in vitro* assay and *in vivo* lung colony assay give comparable results for an undifferentiated mouse fibrosarcoma (Thomson and Rauth, 1974); also, the TD_{50} dilution assay and the *in vitro* assay are comparable for an undifferentiated sarcomalike tumor (Rockwell and Kallman, 1973) maintained originally by alternate passages *in vivo* and *in vitro* (Rockwell *et al.*, 1972). Mouse melanoma (Lamerton and Blackett, 1974) gives comparable results using the *in vitro* plating technique, end-point dilution assay with inocula injected intramuscularly or subcutaneously, and lung colony production following an intravenous injection of a cell suspension. However, this tumor is rapidly growing, is anaplastic, and possesses a high clonic efficiency. The cloning efficiency of differentiated tumors is low, and, especially after more intensive treatment, the end-point dilution assays are impractical and unreliable for the high density of cell suspension required to meet the limit of end points. Also, certain tumor lines are incapable of growing from low inoculum levels. Moreover, assay techniques using

single-cell suspensions do not necessarily give a valid measure of the numbers of
tumor stem cells in unperturbed tumors and in treated tumors during the period
of damage and regrowth. The microenvironmental conditions of the cells isolated
and suspended during the assay procedures may differ substantially from conditions *in situ* (Lamerton and Blackett, 1974). Tumor cells are converted to
single-cell suspensions by mechanical means, trypsinization, or collagenase digestion. Thus cells are removed from their microenvironment, lose their contact with
each other and with connective tissue cells, and are subjected to various other
alterations. Marked toxic effects on viability of tumor cells have been observed in
mechanically and enzymatically prepared single-cell suspensions (Hofer *et al.*,
1974). The final yield of viable cells, as judged by transplantation tests, is as low as
5–30% after a mechanical dispersing of the tissues, 1–2% after trypsinization, and
10–15% after collagenase digestion. Different cultured tumor lines may display
large variations in their response to tissue disruption. A brief exposure to a trypsin
solution may lead to a limited digestion of certain membrane components and
may drastically affect the amounts of nuclear proteins. Consequently, there is a
6-hr delay in the onset of DNA synthesis in newly replated cells previously treated
with trypsin (Auer and Zetterberg, 1972; Maizel *et al.*, 1975). The plating
efficiencies of subcultured cell lines, their serum requirements, and the rate of
incorporation of labeled nucleotides and amino acids may be influenced even by
slight changes of pH which deviate from optimal values (Ceccarini, 1975). It can
be speculated that the number of tumor stem cells which would become effective
may depend on the capacity of stem cell clones to produce colonies under
different conditions of oxygenation and metabolic exchange, on their tolerance of
culture media, and so forth. It is possible that only a portion of the potential stem
cells are in a position to start focal repopulation, and under different experimental
conditions this portion may not necessarily be identical. This contention seems to
be supported by discrepancies between tumor cure-rate assay (TCD_{50}) performed
in situ and single-cell suspension assay TD_{50} (Rockwell and Kallman, 1973).
Further, no cell survival assay gives any information about the kinetic status of
tumor stem cells, i.e., whether they are "resting," arrested, or slowly or rapidly
progressing through the cell cycle. Quantitative results of stem cell responses in
most tumor systems subjected to treatments by cytotoxic drugs or irradiation are
only of relative value and reproducible under strict experimental conditions valid
only for the system employed. It also follows that many of the conclusions based
on comparison between results of transplantation or plating assays of neoplastic
cells and cells of normal tissues subjected to the same therapeutic protocol may
require careful reevaluation.

325

STEM CELLS,
NON-
PROLIFERATING
CELLS, AND
THEIR
KINETICS

2.3. Morphological Identification

2.3.1. Stem Cells of Normal Renewal Tissues

Purely functional terms such as hematopoietic "multipotential stem cell," "committed stem cells," "CFU-c," and "CFU-s" are based on cytokinetic and mor-

326

MILAN
POTMESIL,
JOSEPH
LOBUE,
AND
ANNA
GOLDFEDER

phological manifestations of their progeny and generally have no clear meaning in relation to cell morphology. Any attempt to identify bone marrow stem cells morphologically faces obvious difficulties. On the one hand, there is convincing evidence that—at least in man and in the mouse—a single compartment of bone marrow stem cells give rise to erythrocytic, granulocytic, and megakaryocytic precursors. On the other hand, cells of this type do not necessarily have to possess an identical morphological appearance. Moreover, the exact structure of the stem cell compartment is not presently known (reviewed by Boggs and Chervenick, 1973). As discussed in Section 2.2.1, CFU-c and CFU-s seem to represent rather heterogeneous populations. In addition, CFU-s exhibit differences related to their site of origin (Siminovitch et al., 1965; Lahiri and van Putten, 1969; Kretchmar and Conover, 1970). Experimental data also showed that CFU-s and CFU-c are not randomly distributed throughout the femoral bone marrow in mice. These data indicate that the process of differentiation and development of various hematopoietic cell lines probably has a well-defined spatial organization (Lord and Hendry, 1972; Lord et al., 1975). The "candidate stem cell' in bone marrow has been variously reported as identical to, or closely similar to, small and medium lymphocytes (Cudkowicz et al., 1964; Fliedner et al., 1970), hemocytoblasts (Thomas et al., 1965), monocytoid cells (Tyler and Everett, 1966; Tyler et al., 1972), or "transitional" lymphoid cells (Harris and Kugler, 1967; Moffatt et al., 1967). Transitional lymphoid cells comprise a continuous morphological spectrum from pachychromatic small cells to large leptochromatic blastoid cells, with different degrees of cytoplasmic basophilia. The evidence for the "candidate stem cell" is based on autoradiographic studies using [³H]TdR labeling of early progenitors with a follow-up of the progeny (DeGowin et al., 1972), combination of cytochemical and autoradiographic methods (Rosse and Trotter, 1974), and density gradient separation of hematopoietic cells yielding a high percentage of CFU (Van Bekkum et al., 1971), with or without additional [³H]TdR labeling in short-term cultures (Yoshida and Osmond, 1971; Moore et al., 1972). Conclusions of these and related studies support the contention that transitional lymphoid cells function as "committed stem cells" and are the precursors of bone marrow lymphocytes, granulocytes, and macrophages. Their small-sized, pale-stained subpopulation (Thomas, 1973; Dicke et al., 1973; Rubinstein and Trobaugh, 1973) or medium-to-large lymphoid cells (DeGowin and Gibson, 1976) have been suggested as the morphological equivalent of multipotential stem cells. These cells have a relatively slow rate of turnover (Rosse, 1970, 1973) and do not exhibit the rosette formation manifested by thymus-derived or bursa-equivalent lymphocytes (Barr et al., 1975). However, several objections must be raised at this point. Autoradiographic studies tracing the stem cell progeny cannot eliminate the possibility of [³H]-TdR reutilization. The disadvantage of purification procedures is that the characteristics of the enriched cell population may be no longer identical to those of normal steady-state hematopoietic cells. Pretreatment of donors, repeated density gradient separation, and subsequent incubation may by themselves have introduced changes of morphology. Moreover, these procedures may also alter the metabolic rate of cells under observation and trigger their proliferation, which in turn may influence cell size and overall morphology. It is a

well-established fact that "resting" cells of the lymphocytic series can be stimulated 327
STEM CELLS,
NON-
PROLIFERATING
CELLS, AND
THEIR
KINETICS
in vitro into proliferation, and this is accompanied by their morphological change
into transitional lymphocytes and lymphoid blast cells (Yoffey *et al.*, 1965; Astaldi
and Airo, 1967). Direct approaches such as time-lapse microcinematography may
be potentially more useful in dealing with these difficulties (e.g., see Cormack,
1976).

Stem cells of the epidermis and intestinal epithelium are confined to specific
regions in organs. The basal layer or statum germinosum of stratified squamous
epithelium is heterogeneous due to the presence of melanocytes, Langerhans
cells, early-differentiating epithelial cells (Christophers, 1971), and possibly stem
cells (Hamilton and Patten, 1972). A layer of columnar epithelial cells lines
intestinal crypts of Lieberkühn that invaginate into the lamina propria from the
base of each villus, and stem cells are probably located at some specific region of
these crypts. It is not clear whether the stem cell compartment comprises all cells in
the proliferative zone of the crypts or only those at the bottom (Lesher and
Bauman, 1969; Withers and Elkind, 1969; Hagemann *et al.*, 1972).

2.3.2. Neoplastic Stem Cells

Current methods cannot, with very few exceptions, identify tumor stem cells
morphologically and evaluate their kinetic behavior in tumors directly *in situ*.
Blast cells of human acute leukemias may develop a partial and usually abnormal
type of maturation. The most immature type of leukemic blast cell does not
behave as a self-maintaining system (Gavosto *et al.*, 1967*a,b*), and an influx of
leukemic stem cells from another compartment has been suggested. The large
blast cells with a leptochromatic nucleus and basophilic cytoplasm are metaboli-
cally active, their DNA content is 2–4c (Quaglino *et al.*, 1974), and these cells divide
in a rhythm very similar to that observed in normal bone marrow blast cells
(Gavosto *et al.*, 1960; Pileri *et al.*, 1964). In the course of successive divisions, large
blast cells give rise to small blasts with rather pachychromatic nuclei (Gavosto *et al.*,
1964; Killmann, 1965). The population of small leukemic blast cells may constitute as much as 95% of the leukemic cells in the bone marrow of some patients
(Saunders and Mauer, 1969). Based on cell kinetic studies, it has been suggested
that leukemic stem cells exist in two forms, either as proliferating large blasts or as
nonproliferating small blasts (Saunders and Mauer, 1969; Gabutti *et al.*, 1969).
Large- and medium-sized thymic lymphoma cells of AKR mice have a fine
chromatinic structure and basophilic cytoplasm and are engaged in active proliferation, whereas most small cells with a narrow rim of cytoplasm and dense nuclei
are either slowly cycling or "resting" (Omine and Perry, 1972). These small cells
are derived from the rapidly proliferating large-sized cells (Omine *et al.*, 1973).
Large leukemic cells and some of the small-sized cells have clonogenic properties
(Rosen *et al.*, 1970; Omine and Perry, 1973) and should be considered as stem
cells.

In a majority of solid tumors, a frustratingly monotonous mass of intermitotic
cells is offered for microscopic inspection. In addition to an unknown portion of
stem cells, these tumor cell populations include cells that are temporarily or

328

MILAN
POTMESIL,
JOSEPH
LOBUE,
AND
ANNA
GOLDFEDER

permanently nonproliferative, and also "doomed" cells, i.e., proliferating cells with a limited capacity for further division. The teratocarcinomas are included among the very few instances in which tumor stem cells can be identified. Pluripotential teratocarcinoma stem cells have been isolated and maintained *in vitro* as clonal cell lines (reviewed by Damjanov and Solter, 1974; Martin, 1975; Martin and Evans, 1975). There is strong evidence that chromosomal instability and high variability in chromosome number and structure exists in heteroploid cell populations of various solid tumors (reviewed by Kraemer *et al.*, 1972). Cells bearing the same array of chromosomes are considered as members of the same mutant clone of cells descended from a common ancestor. As most products of abnormal mitoses die after only a few more divisions, their chromosome constitutions being without any importance for the propagation of "immortal" cell lines, the selection from within is always for the fastest-growing mutant clone efficiently populating the tumor under existing microenvironmental conditions (reviews by Ford and Clarke, 1963; Ohno, 1971). Changes in the tumor environment may cause sequential clonal selection leading, for example, in experimental mammary tumors to progression from hormone dependency to autonomy (Kim and Depowski, 1975), and in chemically induced rat hepatocellular carcinomas from diversely aneuploid patterns seen in primary tumors to a relatively tight mode in further generations of transplants (Becker *et al.*, 1975). Some of the above observations have been highly confirmatory of the "stemline" theory (Makino, 1952; Hauschka, 1961). A stemline is defined as a particular cellular lineage characterized by a single mode in chromosome number with limited heterogeneity which has become adapted to existing conditions in tumors. The stemline theory has been subsequently further substantiated by studies on primary sarcomas induced by the Rous virus (Mark, 1969; Mitelman, 1971), transplantable tumors (Hsu, 1961), and Morris hepatomas (Nowell, 1975). There is always a central tendency toward a certain mode in chromosome number in tumors. It has been shown in transplantable murine tumors (e.g., Hauschka and Levan, 1951) that this central tendency drifts to new modes and forms with an increasing number of successive passages of transplants and that the chromosome number tends to concentrate in one or a few regions within the overall range. Cytophotometric studies have established a close correlation between the DNA content in heteroploid cells and their chromosome number. This correlation has been observed in a wide variety of human tumors (Atkin and Baker, 1966; Atkin *et al.*, 1966; Atkin, 1971; Stich and Steel, 1962) and mouse tumors (Richards, 1955; Freed and Hungerford, 1957; Meek, 1961). More recent studies of DNA distribution by flow microfluorometry have been completely confirmatory (Kraemer *et al.*, 1972). High heteroploid cell lines show high modal DNA values and low heteroploid lines exhibit modal DNA content close to that of diploid cells. In the abovementioned studies (Richards, 1955; Freed and Hungerford, 1957; Meek, 1961; Stich and Steel, 1962), DNA content was evaluated in interphase cells and in all four mitotic phases. These studies showed that the cellular heterogeneity of tumors is dynamic and competitive, and involves numerous cells that do not contribute to tumor growth. Some cells with high DNA content do not seem to continue beyond metaphase in the mitotic-cycle traverse. This failure appears to be related to the level of ploidy, and the portion of failing cells is large. Cells attaining anaphase and telophase have a significantly narrower range of DNA content than cells in metaphase or interphase, and a portion of these, with a prevailing mode of DNA content, is considered as representative of a stemline. The prevailing mode may be the same in primary tumors and in their metastases (Böhm *et al.*, 1971), or, sometimes, a new principal mode emerges in metastases (Zank and Krug, 1970; Granberg *et al.*, 1974). As a consequence of irradiation, a definite mode of DNA content may emerge in tumors with a poor response to therapy (Richards and Atkin, 1970). When the chromosome pattern alters, the behavior of the tumor may also change. In some instances, increasing aneuploidy accompanies increasing malignancy of human cervical, colonic, and bladder cancers (Granberg, 1971; Lamb, 1967; Lubs and Kotler, 1967). Changes in the karyotype composition were observed in Ehrlich ascites tumors during the development and again during the loss of resistance to daunorubicine (Hasholt *et al.*, 1971). A spontaneous transformation of a serially transplanted mouse mammary adenocarcinoma to a sarcomalike tumor (Goldfeder and Nagasaki, 1954) was accompanied by an increase in the aneuploidy (Goldfeder, 1965), and a sudden one-step increase in the ploidy of a transplantable hepatocellular carcinoma was accompanied by an accelerated growth pattern (Becker *et al.*, 1975). It has also been shown *in vitro* that cells with chromosomal anomalies have increased generation times when compared with euploid cells (Cure *et al.*, 1974), and that two ascites tumor lines with a different ploidy differ in kinetic parameters following irradiation (Lennartz *et al.*, 1970) or cyclophosphamide treatment (Habicht *et al.*, 1970). In conclusion, these studies indicate that the selection in solid tumors is always for the most efficiently growing mutant clone which represents the main mode of chromosome number or DNA content, and that cells bearing this prevailing mode represent the stemline. It can be speculated that most or all stem cells traversing the cell cycle belong to the cell cohort of the stemline.

329

STEM CELLS,
NON-
PROLIFERATING
CELLS, AND
THEIR
KINETICS

2.4. Principal Aspects of Stem Cell Kinetics

2.4.1. Control Mechanisms Relating to Stem Cell Kinetics

It has been postulated that leukemic cells with different degrees of leukemic involvement may coexist (Killmann, 1968). Some of these leukemic stem cells are defective in their differentiation potential, whereas others are apparently capable of full or abrupt differentiation. In addition, normal hematopoietic stem cells have also been found to be present during the course of leukemias (reviewed by Gavosto, 1973). A kinetic growth model for leukemia proposed by Gavosto and Pileri (1971) includes a group of stem cells maintaining unlimited growth and feeding into the multiplicative compartment. After a certain number of divisions, stem cells leave the multiplicative compartment and become "nonproliferating," being either confined to a mitotic resting stage, G_0 (Gavosto, 1973), or restricted in their slow progression through cell cycle to G_1 phase (Clarkson and Fried, 1971).

330

MILAN
POTMESIL,
JOSEPH
LOBUE,
AND
ANNA
GOLDFEDER

As subsequently discussed (Section 4.3.2), it has been suggested that temporarily nonproliferating stem cells may play an important kinetic role in the growth of the blast cell pool in human leukemias (Saunders and Mauer, 1969; Gabutti *et al.*, 1969). Although there is no direct proof of clonogenic capability of human leukemic cells *in vivo*, in AKR mice, thymic leukemic lymphoblasts and some of their nonproliferating or slowly proliferating progeny do seem to possess stem cell properties (Omine and Perry, 1973). It seems reasonable to assume that leukemic stem cells, as well as stem cells of differentiated tumors, may share some regulative properties of stem cells of normal tissues, which, under homeostatic control, produce cells for maturation (Lamerton, 1974). The normal homeostatic mechanism compensating for cell loss appears to be of two types: (1) a reduction of the intermitotic time in the stem cell compartment (Blackett, 1968); (2) in differentiated precursors, either a shortening of the intermitotic time or an extension of transit times through the various proliferating and differentiating compartments. In the latter case, more cell divisions can be inserted and the amplification of the pool of precursors will be increased (review by Boggs and Chervenick, 1973). As discussed in Sections 4.2.1 and 4.2.2, the homeostatic control mechanism may, for example, operate under conditions of irradiation or treatment with cell-cycle phase-nonspecific cytotoxic drugs. In differentiated tumors, a portion of the cell population may differentiate into more mature forms with some cellular function expressed (Section 3.4.3). This implies that a certain degree of homeostatic control has been preserved in these tumors. A fundamental question remains, namely, to what extent the rate of proliferation in various neoplasms is under the control of "poietins," chalones, or other humoral substances, and how far the growth is determined by population-size-dependent mechanisms of the neoplastic tissue (Lamerton, 1974). It has been shown in experiments with rat esophageal epithelium and mouse skin (Leblond *et al.*, 1967; Iversen *et al.*, 1968) that a full-size stem cell compartment is reached before cells are released for maturation. Observations on stem cell compartments of the bone marrow also seem to indicate an internal size control and proliferation-rate control related to bone marrow cellularity (Boggs and Chervenick, 1973). The maintenance of this compartmental size might be a self-limiting process, and thus low rate of stem cell proliferation could be explained by density-dependent inhibition of proliferation in cell populations confined to a particular anatomical area or to a certain volume (Lamerton, 1974). The feedback from the depletion of maturing cells would be expressed either as a proliferative stimulus overcoming the density-dependent inhibition or as a stimulus releasing cells for differentiation. Thus it may be that mechanical pressure, changes in cell density, and contact are all important factors which determine the proliferative status of stem cells in neoplasms.

2.4.2. Stem Cell Lines in Neoplasms

Solid tumors in man and experimental animals display a wide diversity of kinetic characteristics and histological patterns. Tumors of laboratory animals usually have larger growth fractions and higher rates of proliferation than most human tumors (Lamerton and Steel, 1968; Steel, 1972). Repeated passages of transplants probably influence not only the selection of tumor cell lines for those most efficient but also the entire tumor–host relationship. The growth rate often accelerates with increasing numbers of passages (Green, 1968). The tissue of a transplantable tumor, with a uniform histological pattern, lack of connective tissues, necrosis, and hemorrhage, constitutes suitable homogeneous material available for experimental purposes in a large number of comparable tumors. The DBA H tumor is a good example. This mouse mammary adenocarcinoma has been used for various radiobiological, biochemical, and cell-kinetic studies (Goldfeder, 1954; Goldfeder and Miller, 1963; Potmesil and Goldfeder, 1971). However, the histological and kinetic pattern of most transplantable tumors differs from that of the majority of tumors encountered clinically. In tumors in which nearly every cell may be a stem cell, the intermitotic time of the stem cell pool is close to that of the whole cell population and has only a small variance (Lamerton and Blackett, 1974). Slowly growing and differentiated tumors have a considerable spread in intermitotic and cycle-phase durations (Steel, 1972), with many cells having an intermitotic time undetectable by the technique of the fraction of labeled mitoses (FLM). These tumors probably have a small proportion of stem cells and are rather a mosaic of different rising and declining stem cell lines (see also Section 2.1.2). The production rate and size of a cell-line population can decline for various reasons, e.g., maturation, chromosomal abnormality, impaired exchange of nutrients and metabolites, or lack of oxygen. There are several model systems which are seemingly pertinent to studies of cell-line succession in neoplasms. It has been shown that human fibroblast cultures are extremely heterogeneous with respect to their growth potential. One group of clones has cells capable of a very limited number of divisions, whereas a second group of clones constitutes the proliferative pool (Martin et al., 1974). An increasing skewness develops in serial cultures, with prolongation of intermitotic times and decreasing rates of mitoses among cells of some still proliferating clones (Absher et al., 1974; Merz and Ross, 1969). Other examples of cell-line succession include different degrees of "stemness" and clonal senescence among populations of hematopoietic stem cells as well as lymphoid cells in vivo (Dunn, 1971; Worton et al., 1969; Siminovitch et al., 1964; Williamson and Askonas, 1972). Various stem cell lines of a tumor may differ from each other in, for example, their capacity to differentiate (Martin and Evans, 1975) and in hormone dependency (Noble and Hoover, 1975). It is also generally concluded that neoplastic stem cells, when propagated under favorable conditions, may exhibit an unlimited life span. On the contrary, most "normal" cell lines derived from various tissues are incapable of establishing long-term cultures. "Immortal" continuous cultures can be obtained by cultivation of neoplastic cells, cells transformed by oncogenic viruses, and cells spontaneously transformed in vitro (discussed by Cohen et al., 1974; Freedman and Slim, 1974; Nilsson and Pontén, 1975). The normal mammary gland has a limited ability to proliferate in vivo in serial transplant even under favorable conditions, but the preneoplastic gland has an unlimited life span when similarly propagated (Daniel et al., 1968). Many tumors that have been perpetuated in animals for years furnish convincing

332

MILAN
POTMESIL,
JOSEPH
LOBUE,
AND
ANNA
GOLDFEDER

evidence that neoplastic cells have an apparently unlimited life span when propagated *in vivo* under suitable conditions (e.g., anaplastic mammary carcinoma dbrB has been kept by serial transplant to mice of an inbred strain since 1918; Green, 1968). The observations support the clonal theory (Section 2.1.2) and indicate a distinction between normal and neoplastic stem cells, the latter being more responsive to the need to divide than to stimuli inducing differentiation (Kay, 1965). However, experiments with other systems of normal tissues are less consistent with this theory, and more difficult to interpret (Smith, 1973).

3. Concept of Nonproliferating Cells

Cells that apparently do not traverse different phases of the cell cycle (as shown by analytical techniques mentioned later) are referred to in the literature as "resting," "arrested," "quiescent," "nondividing," "noncycling," "nonproliferative," or "G_0 cells." In this chapter, the term "nonproliferating" has been chosen, and, by definition, these cells should either be restricted in their slow progression to one phase of the cycle or exhibit no apparent progression at all. This definition assumes the existence of "proliferating" and "nonproliferating" cells as more or less definitive subpopulations. The difference is by no means distinct when FLM analysis is applied. As discussed later, however, other analytical approaches are more discriminating. Since it has been strongly suggested that nonproliferating cells of neoplasms constitute a heterogeneous population, careful characterization of the various subpopulations according to age, drug sensitivity, repair potential, and clonogenicity would be of a considerable significance.

3.1. Basic Considerations

3.1.1. Nonproliferating Cells and G_0 or G_1 Phase

The essential feature of cell multiplication in many systems is the alternation of resting periods with periods of active proliferation. This alternation provides conditions necessary for size control of cell populations, cell differentiation, adaptation to changing environmental conditions, and interaction with other systems (Epifanova and Terskikh, 1969). According to generally accepted concepts, nonproliferating cells may reside in the G_0 phase (Lajtha, 1963; Quastler, 1963). This represents a reversible postmitotic and presynthetic state (Oehlert *et al.*, 1962); this state has been considered by some as the phase of "decision taking," that is, the interval during which it is determined whether the cell will differentiate or proliferate (Quastler and Sherman, 1959). Cells may also proceed through a long postmitotic and presynthetic G_1 phase. In some cases, the difference between G_0 and G_1 classes of cells seems to be established by the pattern of entry into the cell cycle upon appropriate stimulation. For instance, the sequence of events after partial hepatectomy includes a 15-hr lag period, followed by a burst of mitotic activity (Lajtha, 1963, 1964). It has been suggested that if parenchymal liver cells were in a prolonged G_1 phase instead of G_0, then a gradual increase in mitotic activity should start shortly after hepatectomy. There are several other *in vivo* and *in vitro* systems which, under normal conditions, seem to contain a high proportion of nonproliferating cells (reviewed by Baserga, 1968; Stein and Baserga, 1972). Synthesis of DNA and cell division can be triggered in these systems by various stimuli, and there is a prereplicative period varying in length from a minimum of 12–15 hr to a few days between the application of the stimulus and the initiation of DNA synthesis. Such systems include lymphocytes in short-term culture stimulated by phytohemagglutinin; organ cultures of skin stimulated by epidermal growth factor; liver, kidney, spleen, pancreas, salivary gland, mammary gland, or skeletal muscle stimulated by surgical procedures, chemical, or hormonal treatment, or by changed metabolic conditions. Cytokinetic behaviour of this kind has also been interpreted as indicating that those cells stimulated to divide were originally in G_0 state. Enzymes necessary for the process of DNA synthesis may decay with time in G_0 cells, and the interval between stimulation and initiation of DNA synthesis represents the time needed for a replenishment of the enzymatic equipment in the cell. The length of this preparatory period depends on the interval which has elapsed between the previous mitosis and "triggering" of the cell into preparation for DNA synthesis (Baserga, 1968). On the other hand, under certain cirumstances, a substantial increase in the percentage of [^{3}H]TdR-labeled cells and of mitotic figures occurs within a few hours following stimulation of the skin and bone marrow (Block *et al.*, 1963; Gidali and Lajtha, 1972; Lahiri and van Putten, 1972; reviewed by Lamerton, 1974). This suggests that cells either in G_1, in G_2, or in both phases are present and that these cells can relatively quickly complete preparation for DNA synthesis or mitosis. Another method designed to distinguish G_0 cells from G_1 cells compares the actual percentage of [^{3}H]TdR labeling following various time periods of continuous labeling with the theoretical proportion of labeling calculated for a G_1 or G_0 model (Brown, 1968). This and other models (Burns and Tannock, 1970; Fried, 1970) are based on specific assumptions, such as log-normal or uniform distribution of transit times and random probability per unit time for leaving G_0 phase. In general, most of these assumptions are without supportive experimental evidence. However, the "noncycle" model of cell kinetics includes G_0 cells and effectively simulates experimental results with a [^{14}C]TdR and [^{3}H]TdR label of hamster cheek pouch epithelium (Burns and Tannock, 1970).

In confluent monolayers of human WI-38 diploid fibroblasts, G_0 designates a specific state of cell arrest which differs from G_1 by several biochemical characteristics including chromatin template activity and serum requirements. Unlike G_0 cells, cells in G_1 phase do not require serum for stimulation and do not respond to it with an increase in chromatin template activity (Rovera and Baserga, 1973; Augenlicht and Baserga, 1974; Sander and Pardee, 1972). It has been proposed that cells in confluent monolayers are initially arrested in G_1, subsequently pass into G_0, and then continue deeper in G_0 as they remain quiescent. Thus G_0 seems to be composed of several different stages which can be distinguished by an

MILAN
POTMESIL,
JOSEPH
LOBUE,
AND
ANNA
GOLDFEDER

increasing lag time between stimulation and an increase in chromatin template activities (Augenlicht and Baserga, 1974). The mechanism underlying movement of G_1 cells into G_0, and subsequently into deeper levels of this stage, seems to be related to decreasing chromatin template activities. In stimulated cells, there is an increase in template activity due to synthesis of new species of nonhistone chromosomal proteins (reviewed by Baserga, 1973). The length of time required for a stimulated G_0 cell to enter DNA synthesis correlates with time spent in G_0 stage. A similar correlation has been found *in vivo* in rat liver after partial hepatectomy: the prereplicative phase is prolonged in older rats as compared to young ones (Bucher, 1963). The same effect has been reported after isoproterenol stimulation of rat salivary glands (Adelman *et al.*, 1972). This suggests that lengthening of the lag between stimulation and onset of DNA synthesis in G_0 cells correlates well with their time of quiescence, is comparable *in vivo* and in tissue culture, and demonstrates multiple levels of the G_0 state related to the biological age of the cell (Augenlicht and Baserga, 1974). There are also observations on cells kept in isoleucine-deficient media which support the aforementioned conclusions and indicate that the length of the prereplicative phase is determined not by the type of blocking agents but by the time period the cells have been quiescent (Pardee, 1974; Tobey, 1973). G_0 and G_1 cells also differ in their responses to treatment with hydroxyurea (Farber and Baserga, 1969). The initial steps leading to DNA synthesis in stimulated G_0 cells are insensitive to actinomycin D, which may be because of the presence of preexisting RNA templates, whereas there is an early actinomycin-sensitive period of RNA synthesis in cells proceeding through G_1 (reviewed by Stein and Baserga, 1972). In conclusion, the demonstration of G_0 cells in *in vivo* systems presents numerous problems. For example, it is often difficult to distinguish between cells residing in G_0 phase for a relatively short time from cells slowly progressing through the presynthetic G_1 (Epifanova and Terskikh, 1969). The fraction of "nonproliferating" cells in neoplasias is heterogeneous and may consist of several subpopulations, including both clonogenic and degenerating "sterile" cells, cells arrested in cycle, and cells cycling slowly. This heterogeneity obviously makes any attempt to differentiate G_0 and G_1 classes of cells even more troublesome.

3.1.2. Nonproliferating Cells and G_2 Phase

It has been found that cells may remain in G_2 phase, and there are indications that, at least in normal unstimulated tissue, such cells do not proceed slowly through a long G_2 phase but rather are blocked in a resting state somewhat comparable to a postmitotic-presynthetic G_0 phase. Cells enter this stage either after having completed DNA synthesis or prior to its completion, and may retain their capacity to divide after appropriate stimulation. It has been implied that cells may take the "decision" either to proliferate or to differentiate while in this suspended state, much as cells in G_0 do (review by Gelfant, 1966; Epifanova and Terskikh, 1969; Pederson and Gelfant, 1970). Cells blocked in G_2 have been described in mouse epidermis (Gelfant, 1962), mouse kidney and duodenum (Pederson and Gelfant,

1970), rat ileum and spleen (Post and Hoffman, 1969), chicken esophagus (Cameron and Cleffman, 1964), and a wide variety of other tissues of animal as well as plant origin (Gelfant, 1966). Cells blocked in G_2 phase are also present in a rat sarcoma (Post and Hoffman, 1967), in Ehrlich ascites tumors (DeCosse and Gelfant, 1968), and in several human carcinomas and sarcomas (Clarkson et al., 1965). In methylcholanthrene-induced rat sarcomas, there are a considerable number of nonproliferating cells retained in both G_1 and G_2 phases, and some of these cells have residency times of 1–2 weeks (Post et al., 1973; 1974). In certain tissues stimulated to proliferate, e.g., in the liver, nonproliferating G_2 cells do not enter the mitotic phase (Stocker, 1966). Since cells arrested in G_2 and stimulated to proliferate do not synthesize DNA but enter the mitotic phase directly, they are detectable as unlabeled mitoses in stimulated tissues continuously labeled with [^{3}H]TdR (Gelfant, 1966). Another method concurrently determines the mitotic and labeling indices in stimulated tissues. If the increase in the number of mitoses precedes the number of cells synthesizing DNA, this indicates that cells in mitoses were originally arrested in G_2 phase. There are several other procedures which may be used to detect G_2-arrested cells (Gelfant, 1966; DeCosse and Gelfant, 1968). In a more complex approach, the cell proliferation pattern can be investigated in single and serial samples of experimental tumors labeled continuously with [^{3}H]TdR, with a double label [^{3}H]TdR and [^{14}C]TdR, or with a single injection of [^{3}H]TdR. Statistical analysis of labeling indices and grain-count regression curves estimate variables, such as the size of the G_2 cell population and its transit times (Post et al., 1973). There is some indication based on experiments with mouse epidermis (Gelfant, 1963) that G_1 and G_2 "resting" periods might not cover all the possibilities of cell transition into the resting state (Epifanova and Terskikh, 1969).

3.2. Methods of Assay

3.2.1. Radioactive Thymidine and Iododeoxyuridine

A variety of techniques have been utilized to investigate cell proliferation kinetics and to distinguish "nonproliferating" from "proliferating" cells. Several tracer techniques applicable to microscopic studies and scintillation counting use [^{3}H]TdR, [^{14}C]TdR, or radioactive 5-iodo-2'-deoxyuridine (IUdR). There are also other labeled DNA precursors available such as [^{3}H]deoxycytidine, [^{3}H]deoxcytidine-5-monophosphate, and [^{14}C]formate, their rate of in vitro incorporation being comparable with that of [^{3}H]TdR (Hale et al., 1965; Hirt and Wagner, 1975). Thymidine can be used as an indicator and measure of DNA synthesis because it nearly exclusively incorporates into this nucleic acid. The label is nonexchangeable until death of the labeled cell (Perry and Gallo, 1970). Small quantities of [^{3}H]TdR may be found in biochemical fractions other than DNA (Counts and Flamm, 1966; Schneider and Greco, 1971), in the acid-soluble pool, or associated with RNA or with proteins (Reichard and Estborn, 1951; Marsh and Perry, 1964). In vivo uptake into cell nuclei is rapid, the first traces being

336

MILAN
POTMESIL,
JOSEPH
LOBUE,
AND
ANNA
GOLDFEDER

detectable within several seconds after application (Perry *et al.*, 1968); 95% of the label is incorporated within 25 min and the total labeling is completed within 1 hr (Rubini *et al.*, 1960; Staroscik *et al.*, 1964). Several factors may influence the rate of [^{3}H]TdR incorporation, such as the activity of thymidine kinase and other enzymes (Brent, 1971), the size of the endogenous thymidine pool (Stewart *et al.*, 1965), and the synthetic rate of other DNA precursors (Craddock and Nakai, 1962). Should the rate of incorporation of a labeled precursor be used as a direct measure of the nuclear DNA synthesis, these factors have to be taken into consideration and adequate precautions established (Hirt and Wagner, 1975; Dörmer *et al.*, 1975). Unexpectedly low incorporation has been found in some species of experimental animals (Adelstein and Lyman, 1968; Adelstein *et al.*, 1964; Das and Altman, 1971), and several possible explanantions of this phenomenon have been suggested (Nowakowski and Rakic, 1974). Approximately 2–6% of mice of different strains injected with [^{3}H]TdR do not appear to incorporate this labeled precursor into DNA of thymus, skin, and jejunum. This lack of incorporation is not, however, always generalized; the extent varies with time, and the mechanism involved is not completely known (Potten *et al.*, 1972). Extracts of human and bovine endometrium inhibit [^{3}H]TdR incorporation in various cell lines *in vitro* (Hinderer *et al.*, 1970; Chevalier and Verly, 1975). The inhibitory effect has been interpreted as a competitive inhibition caused by thymidine present in the extract, or by enzymatic activity converting thymidine into thymine. Reutilization of [^{3}H]TdR is of particular significance in cell populations with rapid turnover (Patt and Maloney, 1963; Steel and Lamerton, 1965) and can introduce errors in experiments with single labeling or time-limited labeling with consequent follow-up of the label. This includes the most common technique of labeled mitoses (Quastler and Sherman, 1959) designed to determine cell-cycle characteristics *in vivo* (Johnson *et al.*, 1967). While reutilization is not a problem when [^{3}H]TdR is applied in a continuous infusion or in repeated injections, the possibility of radiotoxicity is a major objection to any approach using large amounts of [^{3}H]TdR. Tritium incorporated into biological molecules can cause damage either from β-irradiation or from the local effects of transmutation. Radiation effects caused by emitted β-particles are the predominant factor in cell killing (Burki and Okada, 1968, 1970; Burki *et al.*, 1975), and ^{3}H toxicity is more effective within the nucleus than the cytoplasm (Marin and Bender, 1963*a,b*). Perturbation in cell-cycle progression and growth has been monitored by high-speed flow microfluorometry in cell cultures exposed to [^{3}H]TdR flash or continuous labeling, at precursor levels generally lower than that used in most cell kinetic studies (Ehmann *et al.*, 1975). Ideally, studies should be conducted at true tracer levels to obtain the distribution, incorporation, or elimination of radioactive precursors under conditions in which radiotoxicity, metabolic blocking, or stimulation can be minimized. The irregular thickness of biological samples results in energy absorption of emitted electrons. The influence of β-self-absorption is minimized if ^{3}H is replaced by ^{14}C. The latter tracer emits electrons with higher energies and negligible self-absorption (Dörmer and Brinkmann, 1972; Dörmer, 1973).

Grain-count density and labeling indices established autoradiographically may not correlate with the level of incorporation of the radioisotope as determined by liquid scintillation counting on the same sample of biological material (Chang and Looney, 1965; Oja *et al.*, 1967; Perry and Gallo, 1970). Self-absorption, type of biological material under study, methods of preparation, exposure time, and a variety of other factors influence any such comparison. There are also problems associated with the interpretation of autoradiograms, particularly the evaluation of lightly labeled cells in connection with background values. The grain count over a radioactive source always includes contributions from a variety of factors other than the radioactivity itself. Factors contributing to the overall background include mechanical pressure on the emulsion, irregular drying, prolonged exposure time of the emulsion, positive chemography above the specimen, contamination of the emulsion, conditions of development, and others (Rogers, 1973). All of the abovementioned factors, and other phenomena contributing to the background, may vary not only from one experiment to another but also within the same set, from one slide to another. Various rates of latent image formation and fading, positive and negative chemography present in the same preparation, and the influence of factors such as variation in emulsion thickness or in development time and temperature can also lead to considerable differences. To estimate background adequately, the emulsion should be exposed above a non-radioactive but otherwise identical specimen placed on the same slide, side by side with the active material. Background counts taken from areas of the nonradioactive specimen can be matched to counts obtained over areas of labeled tissue. A ratio of grain counts between both areas should be evaluated first (England and Miller, 1970; Rogers, 1973), and the required number of grains accumulated over the labeled source and over background area can be determined from an appropriate nomogram. This method is also applicable for photometric measurements of grain density in cases in which the measurement of integrated silver-grain reflectance replaces grain counting. In addition to factors discussed above, the overall background may also be increased by the "non-specific" labeling of proteins, carbohydrates, or lipids following administration of [^{3}H]TdR (Baserga and Malamud, 1969; Schneider and Greco, 1971). Control preparations should be prepared from tissues exposed to [^{3}H]TdR, but with incorporation of the label into DNA being prevented. This can be accomplished in some tissues, for example, by ovariectomy (Besciani, 1965). Further steps should correct grain counts observed over labeled specimens by subtracting the mean number of background grains. The distribution of background grain counts as well as the distribution of grain counts of labeled cells in technically satisfactory autoradiographs is Poisson in its character (England and Rogers, 1970; Rogers, 1973). The two distributions overlap, and several treatments of this problem have been developed. True labeling can be calculated by a method designed for "compatible" distribution of grain counts (Stillström, 1963) or by the "iterative" method (Benassi *et al.*, 1973), while a method designed by England *et al.* (1973) is recommended for levels of labeling near background. All these methods can be programmed for an advanced desk calculator. An arbitrary threshold grain count

338

MILAN
POTMESIL,
JOSEPH
LOBUE,
AND
ANNA
GOLDFEDER

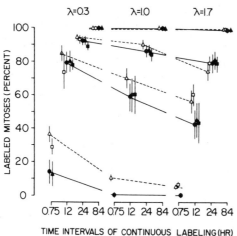

FIGURE 1. Comparison of various methods of subtracting autoradiographic background. Experimental data come from a line of mouse mammary carcinoma designated MT2 (Potmesil and Goldfeder, 1977). Tumor-bearing mice were injected either once (0.75-hr interval) or repeatedly at 4-hr intervals for 12, 24, and 84 hr. To obtain the fraction of labeled mitoses (FLM), 200 mitoses were examined in each set of histological sections. Background was subtracted (a) assuming either that cells with ≥ 1 grain, or with ≥ 2 grains, or with ≥ 3 grains were labeled ($\triangle$); (b) by the method of Shackney *et al.* (1973) ($\square$); (c) Benassi *et al.* (1973) ($\bullet$); (d) England *et al.* (1973) ($\blacktriangle$), and England and Miller (1970) ($\blacksquare$). For all methods listed under (b)–(d) assumed background values are expressed as a mean of silver-grain counts λ, and this corresponds either to 0.3, 1.0, or 1.7 grains per cell. Each point on the chart represents the mean FLM value of three tumors and its standard deviation is indicated by the bars. Solid and dashed lines connect identical sets of data which differ only in assumed values of λ.

differentiating background from true "labeling," has been widely discouraged (e.g., Cleaver, 1967; Moffatt *et al.*, 1971; Rogers, 1973), yet it is still sometimes used. Figure 1 shows that arbitrary background levels, as well as background mean grain counts either underestimated or overestimated because of an inappropriate evaluation, may lead to falsely positive or negative results, or to their substantial fluctuation (e.g., compare differences between FLM at background levels of $\lambda = 0.3$, 1.0, and 1.7). The levels of FLM sensitive to background subtraction are in the range of 0–90%. When the FLM is in excess of 90%, the variation of results obtained by different approaches is negligible. Furthermore, Fig. 1 indicates that the methods designed by Benassi *et al.* (1973), England *et al.* (1973), or England and Miller (1970) give consistently comparable results in the range of 12–90%. Stillström's method (Stillström, 1963) was not applied because the "incompatible" distribution of grain counts appeared in 75% of tested samples. Since, in our calculations, the method of England and Miller (1970) gives unrealistically low FLM at levels close to 100% (not shown in the figure), the two remaining approaches of Benassi *et al.* (1973) and England *et al.* (1973) seem to be the methods of choice.

The thymidine analogue 5-iodo-2′-deoxyuridine (IUdR) is a cytotoxic agent and a radiosensitizer (Mathias and Fisher, 1962; Berry and Andrews, 1962), but its reutilization is substantially lower than that of [³H]TdR (Hofer *et al.*, 1969; Dethlefsen, 1970; Clifton and Cooper, 1973). IUdR labeled with ¹²⁵I, ¹³¹I, or ⁵H has been used for cytokinetic studies (Hughes *et al.*, 1964; Porschen and Feinendegen, 1969; Hofer *et al.*, 1969; Hofer, 1970; Clifton and Yatvin, 1970; Hofer and Hofer, 1971; Burki *et al.*, 1971), and several reports indicate toxic effects caused by radiotracer doses of IUdR (Post and Hoffman, 1969; Dethlefsen, 1971; Hofer and

Hughes, 1971). These effects are primarily due to chemical toxicity *per se*. IUdR, at
doses of 0.013 μmol per mouse, significantly reduces both labeling index and
fraction of labeled mitoses in duodenal epithelial cells (Dethlefsen, 1974). Any
tracer method using IUdR is considered unsuitable for studies of therapeutically
perturbed tumors (Dethlefsen, 1971). Other methods of labeling, with clinical as
well as experimental application, utilize a non-DNA label diisopropylfluoro-
phosphate (DF-^{32}P) or chromium-51 for the study of leukocyte kinetics and are
not discussed in this chapter.

339
STEM CELLS,
NON-
PROLIFERATING
CELLS, AND
THEIR
KINETICS

3.2.2. Cytophotometry and High-Speed Cytophotometry

Rapid-scanning microspectrophotometers (Caspersson *et al.*, 1960; Caspersson
and Lomakka, 1962; Lomakka, 1965) and ultrarapid cytophotometers, such as
the flow microfluorometer (van Dilla *et al.*, 1969) and the impulse cytophotometer
(Dittrich and Göhde, 1969), can estimate the DNA content in large numbers
(several tens of thousands) of individual cells within a short time. This is done by
quantitative measurement of UV absorption of Feulgen-stained cells or fluorescent light emission from cells stained with fluorescent dyes (e.g., acriflavine,
propidium iodide, mithramycin, or ethidium bromide), which stain the double-
stranded DNA. Ultrarapid cytophotometry has been used to study drug-induced
perturbations of cell progression through the cell cycle in cell lines with well-
defined ploidy (Tobey and Crissman, 1972; Yataganas and Clarkson, 1974;
Yataganas *et al.*, 1974; Barlogie *et al.*, 1976; Krishan and Frei, 1976). If applied to
heteroploid cell populations, however, cytophotometry alone is not adequate to
obtain a clear picture of tumor-cell distribution in different phases of the cycle.
The results of cytophotometric measurements of DNA content in heteroploid
tumor cells, when performed serially, simply suggest certain particularities of cell
growth. Histograms cannot be interpreted correctly without a study of chromosome number to determine the possible extent of ploidy. The presence of
heteroploid cells having the potential to divide, cells which cannot divide, and cells
still proliferating but doomed to degenerate and die produces a system too
complex to be evaluated solely by the single criterion of cellular DNA content
(Vendrely, 1971). Cytophotometry, by itself, gives only limited information about
nonproliferating cells and their position ("arrest") in the cell cycle. Using a
combination of two criteria, that is, cells pulse-labeled with [^{3}H]TdR and subsequently subjected to cytophotometric and autoradiographic analysis, can be
highly informative. This method identifies cells in S phase (Frindel *et al.*, 1969;
Vendrely, 1971; Dombernowsky *et al.*, 1973), follows the progression of pulse-
labeled cells through the cell cycle (Fujota, 1974), or monitors changes in diploid
cell lines with increasing time in culture (Yamíshevsky *et al.*, 1974). Even with this
method, however, the uncertainty concerning identification of heteroploid cells in
G_1 or G_2 phase remains. Protracted labeling leads to some improvement. Continuous labeling of cells *in vitro* (Potter, 1970) or repeated injections of [^{3}H]TdR *in
vivo* (Lala and Patt, 1968; Bichel and Dombernowsky, 1973; Dombernowsky *et al.*,
1974) have demonstrated noncycling or slow-cycling cells with differing contents

MILAN
POTMESIL,
JOSEPH
LOBUE,
AND
ANNA
GOLDFEDER

of DNA, and reproducible results can be obtained in experiments conducted under carefully controlled conditions. A combination of flow microfluorometric analysis of DNA content in continuously [³H]TdR-labeled cells of a synchronized diploid line has produced good estimates of cell distribution within the cycle under various experimental conditions (Tobey, 1972a,b; Tobey and Crissman, 1972). Flow and impulse microfluorometric techniques have been applied primarily in systems with cells growing in a suspended state. However, the dispersal of solid tumors into a single-cell suspension creates substantial cellular debris causing technical problems and limitations in applicability of the method. Methods combining quantitative cytophotometry and autoradiography with different isotopes have been used, for example, for studies on interphase cells *in vitro* (Zetterberg and Killander, 1965). Other techniques applied in studies of G-phase fibroblasts include scanning microinterferometric and microspectrometric estimations of protein, total nucleotides, and DNA synthesis (Killander and Zetterberg, 1965b), time-lapse microcinematography, microspectrophotometry, and microinterferometry (Killander and Zetterberg, 1965a), or a combination of histochemistry, Feulgen cytophotometry, and [³H]TdR autoradiography (Vendrely *et al.*, 1968).

3.2.3. *Electronic Cell-Sorting and Cell-Separation Techniques*

Electronic cell sorting by size is applicable to cell populations in which cell volume and density are related to functional state. Principles of size-sorting instrumentation and its use have been described by Fulwyler (1970). Sizing of individual fractions of normal mouse thymic cells and thymic lymphoma cells has been performed with an automatic size-distribution plotter in conjunction with an electronic cell counter. Nonproliferating or slowly proliferating cells have been further identified by *in vitro* or *in vivo* labeling and autoradiography or scintillation counting (Rosen *et al.*, 1970; Omine and Perry, 1973; Omine *et al.*, 1973). In another approach, intracellular fluorescence served as a differentiating parameter for automated high-speed sorting of large numbers of cells (Hulett *et al.*, 1969; Gray and Mendelsohn, 1975). To isolate mammalian cells of a certain specific size and density from a heterogeneous cell population, a variety of physicochemical techniques have been developed (reviews by Leif, 1970b; Harwood, 1974). The method of cell separation by density gradient involves the application of various buoyant media such as sucrose, dextran, polyvinylpyrrolidone, the branched-chain copolymer Ficoll, or bovine serum albumin. A cell separation technique based on a continuous 1g sucrose density gradient sedimentation (Peterson and Evans, 1967; Mage *et al.*, 1968) has been used to analyze the cytokinetic behavior of cells in mouse thymic lymphoma (Omine and Perry, 1972; Omine *et al.*, 1973), and to isolate nonproliferating or slowly proliferating cells for transplantation studies (Rosen *et al.*, 1970). Still more complex multiparameter instrumentation techniques are available (Steinkamp *et al.*, 1973; Leif, 1970a).

3.3. Morphological Identification

341

STEM CELLS,
NON-
PROLIFERATING
CELLS, AND
THEIR
KINETICS

3.3.1. Cell Size and DNA Content

Nonproliferating or slowly proliferating cells of human acute leukemias have been differently described as blasts with some morphological indication of differentiation (Clarkson *et al.*, 1969), as "highly atypical" blasts (Killman, 1965), or as small-sized blast cells (Gavosto *et al.*, 1964; 1967*a*; Mauer and Fisher, 1966; Pileri *et al.*, 1967). *In vivo*, small-sized blasts accumulate [³H]TdR label very slowly (Karle *et al.*, 1973), some cells remaining unlabeled after 3 weeks of continuous [³H]TdR application (Clarkson *et al.*, 1969). Cell-size estimations from slide preparations, however, are subject to inherent errors and limitations. Blast cells of acute leukemias, particularly the myeloid and monocytic types, frequently have diploid chromosome complements (Sandberg *et al.*, 1964; Lampert and Gauger, 1968). As discussed in Section 3.2.2 and also later, this removes many of the difficulties of analysis encountered in cell populations with irregular ploidy, and facilitates separation of cells in the presynthetic phase by density gradient. Blast cells from the peripheral blood of patients with acute lymphoblastic and myeloblastic leukemia were labeled *in vitro* with [³H]TdR and then separated as to their size by 1*g* sucrose gradients. DNA contents was positively correlated with cell size, and the cell size corresponded to cell-cycle stages, small blasts being either slowly proliferating or possibly nonproliferating cells in G_1 (Sarna *et al.*, 1975). The spontaneous thymic lymphoma of AKR mice exhibits a marked variation in cell size comparable to that of human acute leukemias (Metcalf and Brumby, 1967). Small lymphoma cells with slightly pachychromatic nuclei (Metcalf and Wiadrowski, 1966) have a 2c DNA content and are either nonproliferating or slowly cycling (Rosen *et al.*, 1970; Omine and Perry, 1972, 1973). Several attempts have also been made to identify and quantitate nonproliferating cells of solid tumors using quantative cytophotometry (Kal, 1973*a*,*b*; Rajn *et al.*, 1974). Cells with a low content of DNA are regarded as nonproliferating or slowly proliferating (i.e., being in either G_0 or G_1 phase). This estimation can be used in diploid cell populations, although it overlooks the possiblity that cells in the post synthetic period with a 4c DNA content may also be "nonproliferating." Apart from some childhood cancers (Cox, 1968), solid malignant tumors in man are very rarely diploid and are generally characterized by varied and complex chromosomal changes. Their chromosome number varies from a very impressive hypodiploidy to triploid and tetraploid ranges in different percentages of cells, with additional multiple abnormalities being present. Large variations in chromosome number and in DNA content have also been observed in spontaneous and transplanted animal tumors and in tumors induced by chemical carcinogens (reviewed by Ohno, 1971; Kraemer *et al.*, 1972; Sandberg and Sakurai, 1974). Estimation of DNA content in cells of heteroploid tumors may provide an ambiguous correlation with cell distribution in the cell cycle. For example, a cell with 4c DNA content resulting from endomitosis is not distinguishable from a premitotic diploid cell

342

MILAN
POTMESIL,
JOSEPH
LOBUE,
AND
ANNA
GOLDFEDER

with doubled DNA content. Diploid cells with 2c DNA content, or cells containing an amount of DNA corresponding to the major mode of cells having completed a division, may represent cells progressing rapidly or slowly through G_1 phase, or cells "arrested" in this phase. Cells with DNA content between 2c and 4c may also include hypotetraploid cells not residing in S phase. Such circumstances may confuse any attempt to identify nonproliferating cells in solid tumors by their DNA content.

3.3.2. Morphology of the Interphase Chromatin

Manifestation of a continuous "chromosome cycle" in interphase cell nuclei has been reported, and this refers to changes of the chromatin structure taking place through various stages of the cell cycle. The amount of actinomycin D bound per unit of DNA (Pederson and Robbins, 1972), the sensitivity of chromatin to digestion by DNase (Pederson, 1972), circular dichroism spectra, and spectro-polarimetric analysis of chromatin binding with ethidium bromide (Nicolini et al., 1975) represent probes capable of detecting structural alterations of chromatin within various intermitotic phases. Changes of chromatin pattern in cell nuclei can also be studied microscopically. The distribution of chromatin densities of Feulgen-stained interphase cells has been measured by a scanning microden-sitometer (de la Torre and Navarrete, 1974). The integrated optical density per nucleus and the distribution of densities in individual nuclei suggest the position of cells during their cell-cycle progression. The efficiency of measurements can be largely improved by an image-analyzing computer. The results demonstrate cyclic changes in chromatin morphology and differences between cells with 2c DNA content, presumably in G_1 or G_0 phase, and cells with higher DNA values (Bibbo et al., 1973; Rowinski et al., 1972). The spread of measured values, however, is considerable (Sawicki et al., 1975), and therefore the method cannot be applied as a means of assigning individual cells to specific cell-cycle phases. Other histochem-ical techniques such as saffranin or indigopicocarmine stain (Alvarez and Valla-dares, 1972) or hematoxylin-eosin stain (Nešković, 1968) are also unreliable tools for distinguishing cell-cycle stages because of their inadequate consistency in measurements. Interphase nuclei of cultured human embryonic fibroblasts and synchronized HeLa cells stained with quinacrine dihydrochloride show a fluores-cent pattern that varies according to the stage of the cell cycle (Moser et al., 1975). The method demarcates three general fluorescent patterns in cell nuclei, one of them being typical for an early G_1. The ability of incorporated 5-bromo-deoxyuridine (BUdR) to alter staining properties of cell chromatin has permitted the detection of DNA synthesis in individual cells by light microscopy (Latt, 1973). Suppression of bis-benzimidarole or acridine-orange fluorescence by BUdR can be detected in fixed as well as unfixed cells replicating DNA (Hilwig and Gropp, 1973; Franceschini, 1974; Kato, 1974). These methods distinguish cells in S phase from cells in G_1 and G_2 phases. None of the abovementioned procedures, however, can differentiate cells with a short passage through G_1 from non-proliferating cells confined to this phase.

3.3.3. Morphology of Nucleoli

343

STEM CELLS,
NON-
PROLIFERATING
CELLS, AND
THEIR
KINETICS

Morphological "markers" distinguishing proliferating and nonproliferating cells are an essential aid in cytokinetic studies of solid tumors. Accumulated evidence points to the conclusion that the morphology of nucleoli in various cell types is related to the extent of their ribonucleoprotein biosynthesis, and this in turn in most systems relates to the capacity of cells to accomplish DNA replication and to divide. Nucleoli studied by electron and light microscopy show a characteristic distribution of RNA-containing structures which is dependent on the synthetic rate of ribosomal-RNA precursor (reviews by Busch and Smetana, 1970, 1974). Electron microscopic and biochemical investigations have revealed that the ribonucleoprotein structure of nucleoli is formed by a fibrillar component which is the site of rRNA-precursor formation, and by a granular component composed of 60 S ribosomal subunits in the process of maturation (Perry, 1962; Hay, 1968). Autoradiographic studies of tissue-culture cell lines, lymphocytes in short-term culture, and thymocytes and parenchymal tumor cells *in vivo* indicate that cells with large, dense nucleoli (compact nucleoli with a relatively uniform distribution of ribonucleoprotein components) show intensive labeling with [5-^{3}H]uridine ([^{3}H]UrR), whereas cells containing nucleoli with well-defined trabecular structure, ring-shaped nucleoli, and micronucleoli exhibit a very low incorporation of the label (Potmesil and Smetana, 1968, 1969, 1970; Smetana and Potmesil, 1970; Potmesil and Goldfeder, 1971, 1972). In electron micrographs of ring-shaped nucleoli, a peripheral ribonucleoprotein shell surrounds a central light core containing fine protein and chromatin filaments, and also chromatin clusters which are usually adjacent to the periphery of the nucleolus. Ring-shaped or trabeculate nucleoli are present in a variety of differentiated and mature cells (e.g., in mature lymphocytes and thymocytes, monocytes, maturing erythroblasts, highly differentiated smooth muscle cells, in lymphosarcoma and partially differentiated leukemic cells, and in mature plasmacytes in multiple myeloma; reviewed by Smetana, 1970; Busch and Smetana, 1970, 1974; Smetana *et al.*, 1975). Micrographs of neoplastic cells possessing different types of nucleoli are shown in Fig. 2(a–h).

Changes in nucleolar morphology reflect the kinetic status of cells during their respective periods of proliferation and "rest." Conversion of a cell from a hypofunctional, nonproliferative state to rapid growth requires increased synthesis of ribosomes and polysomes, and the stimulated cell exhibits a compensatory hypertrophy and reorganization of its nucleoli. The correlation between nucleolar function and structure studied in lymphocytes and thymocytes of human and murine origin can serve as an example. In "resting" mature lymphocytes possessing ring-shaped nucleoli (Smetana, 1961), RNA synthesis proceeds at a steady low rate (Cooper, 1969a). If this synthesis is blocked by addition of low concentrations of chromomycin A_3 to the culture medium, the nucleolar ring disappears and is replaced by nucleolar fragments (Potmesil and Smetana, 1969). However, upon addition of phytohemagglutinin to short-term cultures, ring-shaped nucleoli in mature lymphocytes are transformed into trabeculate nucleoli as early as 6 hr after

344
MILAN
POTMESIL,
JOSEPH
LOBUE,
AND
ANNA
GOLDFEDER

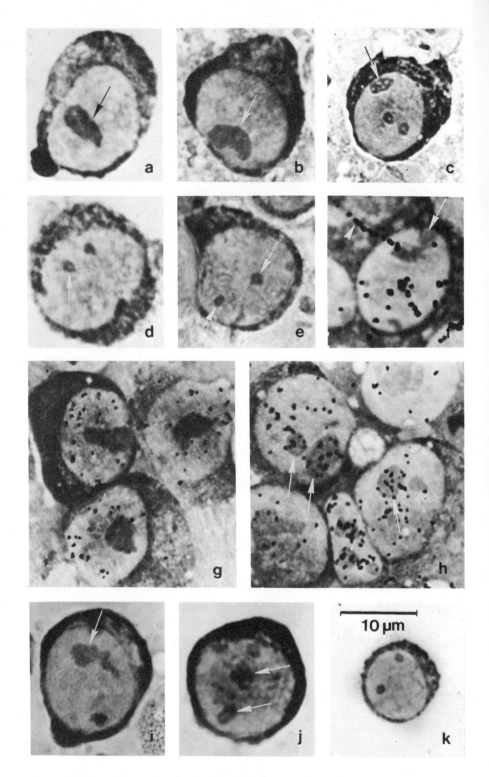

FIGURE 2. Photomicrographs of cells with different types of nucleoli. Transplantable mouse mammary carcinomas. Smear preparations: (a, b) cells with dense nucleoli (arrows), basophilic

345

STEM CELLS,
NON-
PROLIFERATING
CELLS, AND
THEIR
KINETICS

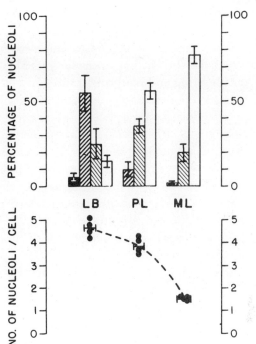

FIGURE 3. Types of nucleoli in thymic lymphocytes during maturation. Nucleoli were identified in smear preparations of six mouse thymuses, using 100 lymphoblasts (LB), 100 prolymphocytes (PL), and 200 mature lymphocytes (ML) in each sample. Upper panel: Percentages of dense nucleoli (■), large trabeculate nucleoli >4 μm in diameter (▨), trabeculate nucleoli (▧); and ring-shaped nucleoli (□). Vertical bars indicate standard deviation. Lower panel: Average number of nucleoli per cell. From Potmesil (unpublished).

initiation of stimulation. At this time, some small mature lymphocytes with dense nucleoli also appear for the first time (Potmesil and Smetana, 1970), and this is followed by the well-known blastogenic transformation of cultured lymphocytes into dividing blast-like cells, possessing prominent dense nucleoli incorporating [³H]UrR at a high rate (Potmesil and Smetana, 1969, 1970). A reverse sequence of events can be traced in cells of the lymphocytic series during their maturation. Most thymic lymphoblasts and prolymphocytes contain dense and large trabeculate nucleoli (Fig. 2i,j) and exhibit intensive incorporation of [³H]UrR (Potmesil and Goldfeder, 1972). These cells represent the proliferating pool that "feeds" into a large nonproliferating pool of mature lymphocytes, predominantly possessing ring-shaped nucleoli (Fig. 3). During maturation, at least some thymic cells proceed from the compartment of mature lymphocytes with trabeculate nucleoli

---

structures in nucleoli are relatively homogeneous in distribution and correspond to ribonucleoprotein; (c) cell with trabeculate nucleolus (arrow), basophilic structures are organized in well-defined trabecules separated by light areas; (d, e) cells with ring-shaped nucleoli (arrows), basophilic structures are present at the periphery of the nucleolus. Autoradiographs: (f) cell with dense nucleolus (arrow), β-track formation (point), [¹⁴C]TdR label; (g) cells with dense nucleoli, grains over nuclei, [³H] TdR label; (h) cells with dense nucleoli, grains over nucleoli (arrows) and nuclei, [³H]UrR label. Lymphocytes in mouse thymuses, smear preparations: (i) lymphoblast with dense nucleous (arrow); (j) lymphoblast with large trabulate nucleoli (arrows); (k) mature lymphocyte with ring-shaped nucleoli. All preparations stained with buffered toluidine blue (Smetana, 1967). (a, d, g, h) From Potmesil and Goldfeder (1971); with permission of *Cancer Research*; (i) from Potmesil and Goldfeder (1972), with permission of *Journal of Cell Biology*; (b, c, e, f) from Potmesil et al. (1975), with permission of *Cell and Tissue Kinetics*.

MILAN
POTMESIL,
JOSEPH
LOBUE,
AND
ANNA
GOLDFEDER

to the compartment of lymphocytes with ring-shaped nucleoli (Fig. 2k) (Potmesil and Goldfeder, 1973).

Studies using the demonstration of nucleoli and autoradiographic labeling of cells have shown that nucleolar morphology is applicable for classification of proliferating and nonproliferating cells in normal tissue, and for studies of their kinetics (Potmesil and Goldfeder, 1972, 1973). Quantitative data on two pools of parenchymal tumor cells assessed *in vivo* have also been presented (Potmesil and Goldfeder, 1971, 1977). The relative number of cells with trabeculate and ring-shaped nucleoli in tumor lines of mammary carcinomas is closely related to their growth rates and degree of differentiation. Both cell subpopulations increase steadily with increasing age of a tumor. A comparison of trabeculate and ring-shaped nucleoli with dense nucleoli revealed that nucleoli not only have a distinctly different structure but also differ in their size. Size-distribution curves suggest that this morphological distinction can be utilized in semiautomatic or automatic screening techniques. After mitosis, nucleoli are reorganized in late telophase figures and trabeculate or ring-shaped nucleoli can be distinguished. This demonstrates that cells with trabeculate or ring-shaped nucleoli are detected at the beginning of G_1 phase. In pulse-label experiments *in vivo*, 20–40% of tumor cells with dense nucleoli incorporate [^{3}H]TdR, whereas cells with trabeculate or ring-shaped nucleoli either do not incorporate the label at all or do so only in a very low percentage. Long exposure of autoradiograms with pulse-labeled cells (up to 9 weeks) predictably increased grain densities over cells with dense nucleoli, but did not change low grain densities over cells with trabeculate and ring-shaped nucleoli. Thus, even low levels of DNA synthesis, which would indicate residency of these cells in S phase, are not demonstrable. The incidence of few cells with trabeculate and ring-shaped nucleoli pulse-labeled with [^{3}H]TdR supports the contention of a random cell renewal in these two subpopulations. Microfluorometric measurements have revealed that cells with trabeculate and ring-shaped nucleoli have DNA content close to 2c, whereas cells with dense nucleoli have DNA content corresponding to 2c, 2–4c, and 4c. It can be concluded that cells with trabeculate and ring-shaped nucleoli do not traverse the whole cell cycle, but either proceed slowly through G_1 or are arrested in this phase.

Repeated injections of [^{3}H]TdR into tumor-bearing mice result in labeling of all cells with dense nucleoli and all mitotic figures at 36–60 hr, depending on the tumor line. Under these circumstances, newly generated cells with trabeculate and ring-shaped nucleoli and cells with nucleolar fragments are derived from labeled progenitor cells. Replacement of unlabeled cells of these types by their labeled counterparts indicates the rate of cell renewal. Cells with trabeculate nucleoli are replaced steadily, with an average transit time of 84 hr, whereas cells with ring-shaped nucleoli and with nucleolar fragments are replaced with a lag of 24 hr, the residency time for some of these cells being in excess of 84 hr. Since the survival time of mice implanted, for example, with DBA H tumors is approximately 24 days, these data indicate that a subpopulation of cells can reside in G_1 phase longer than one-sixth of this time without being lost via cell death. The conclusions drawn from these studies, namely, that cells with dense nucleoli represent the proliferating pool in tumors and cells with trabeculate and ring-shaped nucleoli represent the nonproliferating pool, have been applied in studies of cell kinetics in therapeutically treated tumors; this is further discussed in Section 4.3.3.

347
STEM CELLS,
NON-
PROLIFERATING
CELLS, AND
THEIR
KINETICS

3.4. Nonproliferating Cells in Leukemias and Solid Tumors

3.4.1. Growth Fraction

The concept of "growth fraction," based on experiments with spontaneous mouse mammary carcinomas, was first introduced by Mendelsohn (1960, 1962a). The growth fraction is defined as the proportion of cells participating in the cell cycle and can be calculated as the ratio between the pulse-labeling index and FLM, estimated at a time after a single injection of [^{3}H]TdR when the oscillations of the FLM curve have sufficiently dampened. Lamerton and Steel (1968) have pointed out that an assumed clear distinction between proliferating and nonproliferating cells may not be applicable in tumor-cell populations which manifest a wide distribution of cell-cycle times. Also, they have argued that the size of any cell fraction with a high rate of proliferation may substantially influence the level to which the curve of labeled mitoses damps out. However, the merit of this and similar concepts related to growth fraction (e.g., Kisieleski et al., 1961) is the indication that cell cycle does not account for all cytokinetic events, and that a certain fraction of cell populations may not proceed through the cycle at all. The size of this "nonproliferating" fraction may be suggested by the deficit between the growth fraction and the total cell population. An alternative method of estimating growth fraction is based on grain counts per cell at different time intervals after a single injection of [^{3}H]TdR (Baserga et al., 1963). The fraction of proliferating cells is calculated using the differences in variances of grain counts, but reutilization of the label (see Section 3.2.1), loss of labeled cells, and irregular distribution of the label between two daughter cells can influence the accuracy of this method. The technique of repeated injections of [^{3}H]TdR administered at intervals shorter than the duration of S phase may give information on the occurrence of proliferating cells in tumors (Baserga et al., 1960; Mendelsohn, 1962b, 1965). It has been pointed out that the size of growth fraction can be determined at the time when all mitotic figures are labeled, which indicates that the label was made available to all proliferating cells in the tumor. At such a time, however, the cumulative labeling index may easily be an overestimate of the proliferating pool, because a fraction of nonproliferating cells originating as daughter cells of labeled precursors would also become labeled. In still another approach, Steel and Hanes (1971) estimated growth fraction of tumor cells using computer analysis of data obtained by the technique of labeled mitosis. The proposed model assumes three different modes of cell loss, and the cell-cycle phases G_1, S, and G_2 are described by an independent log-normal distribution. The forms of the age distribution and theoretical continuous labeling curves are computed, and this permits calculation of growth fraction in a way which takes into account the distribution characteristic of expanding cell populations. Following this procedure, the calculated growth

348

MILAN
POTMESIL,
JOSEPH
LOBUE,
AND
ANNA
GOLDFEDER

fraction is a parameter of a model that may or may not be consistent with [³H]TdR-labeling data (Steel, 1972), and more reliable estimates of growth fraction can be obtained by matching the experimental and theoretical continuous-labeling curves. However, the model does not overcome the everpresent problem of where to draw the boundary between proliferating and nonproliferating cells in a population assessed by a method which does not allow for any sharp distinction among cycling, slowly cycling, and noncycling cells.

3.4.2. Nonproliferating Cells

Prolonged continuous infusions or repeated injections of [³H]TdR have been administered to patients with a variety of malignancies, including leukemias, lymphomas, and carcinomas (reviewed by Lamerton and Steel, 1968; Gavosto and Pileri, 1971; Clarkson, 1974). In every case, a significantly large proportion of neoplastic cells remained unlabeled and was considered to be "nonproliferating." Estimation of the growth fraction by Mendelsohn's method revealed that the fraction of nonproliferating cells corresponded to 23–59% in basal cell carcinomas and spindle cell epitheliomas (Frindel *et al.*, 1968), 57% in breast carcinoma, 44% and 42% in malignant melanoma (Young and De Vita, 1970), and 41–53% or 17–20% in two different regions of squamous carcinoma of the cervix (Bennington, 1969). Experimental data from FLM curves for some of the aforementioned, and for other neoplasms as well, were analyzed by the process of computer simulation indicated earlier (Steel and Hanes, 1971), and the growth fraction was estimated for a limited number of human tumors (Steel, 1972). The model indicated a wide range of nonproliferating cells in these tumors (24–82%). Using multiple labeling of cells with [³H]TdR, the cell-size distribution technique, DNA content determination in individual cells, and sucrose gradient separation techniques, Metcalf and co-workers, (Metcalf *et al.*, 1965; Metcalf and Wiadrowski, 1966; Metcalf and Brumby, 1967) and Perry and co-workers (Rosen *et al.*, 1970; Omine and Perry, 1972, 1973; Omine *et al.*, 1973) have convincingly demonstrated that thymic lymphomas of AKR mice possess a morphologically defined subpopulation of cells either residing in G_0 or moving through a long G_1 phase. Comparable results and conclusions were also reached for blast cells separated from peripheral blood of patients with acute lymphoblastic and myeloblastic leukemias (Sarna *et al.*, 1975). These and other studies on the kinetics of morphologically defined neoplastic cells have already been discussed in Section 3.3.1.

The proliferation of ascites tumors growing in the peritoneal cavity of mice gradually declines with time after inoculation, and this appears to be due mainly to a decrease in the growth fraction (Lala and Patt, 1966, 1968; Tannock, 1969; Frindel *et al.*, 1969; Dombernowsky and Hartmann, 1972; Dombernowsky *et al.*, 1973) and increasing prolongation of the cell-cycle time (Lala and Patt, 1966; Yankee *et al.*, 1967; Frindel *et al.*, 1969, Tannock, 1969; Hofer and Hofer, 1971). Feulgen microcytophotometry or pulse cytophotometry of single-cell DNA content and repeated [³H]TdR labeling have indicated the presence of nonproliferating cells with 2c and also 4c DNA content. The number of these cells was increased proportionally with the age of tumors (Lala and Patt, 1968; Frindel et al., 1969; Bichel and Dombernowsky, 1973; Dombernowsky and Bichel, 1975). This does not necessarily mean, however, that nonproliferating cells are arrested in a stage corresponding to G_2. The Ehrlich ascites tumor used for some of these experiments (Lala and Patt, 1968; Schiffer and Markoe, 1974) is considered to be a near-tetraploid line also containing highly polyploid cells. Histogram analysis of DNA content of NCTC fibrosarcoma cells in ascitic form (Frindel et al., 1969) has revealed the presence of cells with DNA content ranging from 2c to 16.5c. As discussed in Section 3.2.2, hyperploidy of cells may interfere with attempts to identify cells in different stages of the cell cycle by their DNA content. At least some proportion of "nonproliferating" ascitic cells consists of cells with slow progression through the cycle. Computed distribution curves of cell-cycle times in old ascitic tumors (Frindel et al., 1969) show a distinct "tail," indicating the presence of a slowly proliferating component (Steel, 1972). Reimplantation of ascites tumors approaching the plateau phase of growth drastically shortens cell-cycle time (Frindel et al., 1969; Peel and Fletcher, 1969; Dombernowsky et al., 1973; Schiffer and Markoe, 1974) and narrows the distribution of cell-cycle duration (Frindel et al., 1969). This suggests that after transplantation a fraction of slowly cycling cells was triggered into a fast proliferation and developed more uniform cell-cycle times. The growth fraction of a variety of animal tumors has been calculated by Steel (1972) as a variable derived from a model designed by Steel and Hanes (1971). The model suggests the highest growth fraction (42–100%) and the lowest portion of nonproliferating cells for serially transplanted experimental tumors, whereas the percentage of "nonproliferating" cells in tumors with a limited number of transplants ranged from 52% to 87%, and in autochthonous tumors from 41% to 90%. Among 33 tumors of different origin, the highest percentage of "nonproliferating" cells was found in carcinomas, either autochthonous or with a limited number of tansplants, and the lowest percentage was found in transplantable sarcomas. As a general rule, slowly growing tumors tend to have relatively long average intermitotic times with wide variations. Computation of the intermitotic time distributions based on the FLM method emphasizes the more rapidly dividing components of a cell population and tends to underestimate the size of slowly proliferating cell populations (Lamerton, 1972). The growth fraction of methylcholanthrene-induced rat sarcoma was 39%, and 23% of nonproliferating cells were confined to G_1 phase, whereas the remainder were in G_2 phase (Post et al., 1973). The transit time of the majority of cells in G_1 and G_2 was 13 and 7 days, respectively. These data were calculated from results of [^{3}H]TdR and [^{14}C]TdR labeling experiments. The volume doubling time of a rat mammary tumor and a fibrosarcoma differed by a factor of over 8 (Steel et al., 1966); approximately 5% of the cells in the fast-proliferating tumor and 70% of the cells in the slow-proliferating tumor were considered as slow or nonproliferating. As the growth rate of a mouse fibrosarcoma slowed, the growth fraction decreased, and thus the portion of nonproliferating cells increased (Frindel et al., 1967). This finding is consistent with comparable observations on human tumors (Laird, 1964; Steel and Lamerton, 1966).

349
STEM CELLS,
NON-
PROLIFERATING
CELLS, AND
THEIR
KINETICS

MILAN
POTMESIL,
JOSEPH
LOBUE,
AND
ANNA
GOLDFEDER

3.4.3. Cytodifferentiation and Cell Death

It has been suggested by Lajtha (1966) that certain cells may reveal their capacity for cytodifferentiation during the G_0 period. As reviewed by Epifanova and Terskikh (1969), it seems that in many normal tissues a single stimulus is sufficient to induce a G_0 cell to undergo differentiation. More often, however, these cells must pass through a mitotic cycle prior to differentiation. In the absence of adequate stimuli, cells may return to the G_0 state. Several of the attributes of differentiation proposed by Weiss (1953) and Dvořák (1971) seem to apply to malignant growth under specific circumstances (reviewed by Dustin, 1972). These include the following: discreteness (production of a definite number of discrete, distinct, discontinuous, and more or less defined cell types); stability and relative irreversibility; exclusiveness (differentiation in one direction excluding that in another one); and progressiveness (change leading to permanent gains or losses). Under experimental conditions and in biological processes, differentiation becomes less reversible as the cell becomes more specialized. Malignant cells retain a certain similarity to their normal counterparts and are often capable of varying degrees of biochemical and morphological differentiation. The simplest examples of this are acute myeloblastic leukemia with high percentage of neutrophilic promyelocytes (Undritz, 1973); the accumulation and storage of lipids, PAS-positive substances, and proteinaceous substances in the cytoplasm of some parenchymal cells in an anaplastic mouse mammary carcinoma dbrB (unpublished); production of IgM immunoglobin in multiple myeloma (Sullivan and Salmon, 1972) and in mouse plasmocytoma (Ghanta and Hiramoto, 1974); and the presence of granules typical of protein-secreting cells in the cytoplasm of small-cell bronchial carcinomas (Pariente and Brouet, in Dustin, 1972). The administration of erythropoietin (EP) in mice with erythroblastic Rauscher leukemia virus A (RLV-A) disease during the preleukemic phase significantly enhances erythroid differentiation (LoBue et al., 1972, 1974). Chronic administration of Ep to RLV-A anemic mice, if a proper dosage of Ep is used, results in amelioration of anemia and enhanced survival (LoBue et al., 1975). Administration of phenylhydrazine significantly elevates Ep levels in these mice and therefore the maturation block of RLV-A erythroblasts can also be overcome by phenylhydrazine as well as Ep "therapy" (LoBue et al., 1974; reviewed by LoBue and Potmesil, 1975). Similarly, erythroblasts of mice with Friend disease (Friend et al., 1971) and leukemic myeloblasts in mice and man (Sachs, 1974) can be induced to differentiate in vitro. Also, in a murine myeloma, in vitro differentiation toward "normal" plasmacytes has been reported (Saunders and Wilder, 1971). Hence malignant changes do not completely prevent cell differentiation, and such differentiation in malignant tumors may lead to specialized cells which are incapable of division and are therefore "nonmalignant" (Dustin, 1972).

Cell death may be age dependent (e.g., keratinized epithelium cells or polymorphonuclear leukocytes) or may be linked to a particular stage of the cell cycle, such as G_2 phase or mitosis, or may occur at any time in the cell replicative cycle. The intrinsic causes of cell death in tumor cells include irreversible cytodifferentiation, and instability of karyotype which may lead to lethal "errors." Two other major factors that play a role in cell death are impaired blood supply and immunological reactions. Well-differentiated tumors of the colon and skin lose differentiated cells in a manner similar to the usual loss of colonic epithelium and normal skin (reviewed by Cooper, 1973). It is also well known that with increasing size of solid tumors, the fraction of nonproliferating cells increases, as does cell loss. It has been suggested (Lala, 1972) that increased cell loss in old ascites tumors can be explained mainly by age-specific elimination of non-proliferating cells. Cell death in the nonproliferating compartment of tumors seems to be a random process with a wide distribution of cell survival times (Cooper, 1973).

351

STEM CELLS,
NON-
PROLIFERATING
CELLS, AND
THEIR
KINETICS

3.5. Resistance to Therapy

3.5.1. Plateau-Phase Cells

It has been pointed out (Valeriote and van Putten, 1975) that mammalian cells cultured *in vitro* can become nonproliferating for a number of reasons: they can be "contact inhibited," they can be inhibited by incubation at a low temperature or by hypoxia, or their nutrient sources and other metabolites such as isoleucine may be depleted. When a subculture of mammalian cells is incubated over an extended period of time, the rate of growth slows down so that a plateau phase is ultimately achieved. Plateau-phase cells may be maintained either in "fed" conditions in the absence of a slowly diffusible nutrient or in "unfed" conditions in media with depleted nutrients (Hahn and Little, 1972). There are some cell subpopulations capable of proliferating in "fed" cultures, but cell loss compensates for this proliferation, and the whole population is in steady state. In "unfed" cultures, there is a decrease in population numbers as a consequence of cell loss exceeding limited proliferation. Microfluorometric measurements have shown that most plateau-phase cells have a 2c DNA content, but some of them also a 4c DNA content. Upon subculture of these nonproliferating plateau cells at lower concentration in fresh medium, DNA synthesis is triggered and is followed by cell division (Hahn et al., 1968; Tobey and Ley, 1970; Hahn and Little, 1972; Glinos and Werrlein, 1972; Clarkson, 1974; Mauro et al., 1974a). The results of labeling experiments and grain-count analysis have suggested that cultured cells in a stationary growth phase either are slowly proliferating, with G_1 phase prolonged and highly variable, or are arrested in a G_0-like phase (Tobey and Ley, 1970; Hahn and Little, 1972). The plating efficiency (clonogenicity) of cells persisting in the plateau phase may decrease relatively slowly in one cell line and more rapidly in another (Hahn and Little, 1972). Human and rodent cell lines employed in this plateau-phase system have been either of normal origin (e.g., isolated from liver, kidney, ovaries, and peripheral blood) or malignant. The system is considered to resemble a tumor-cell population, while permitting the simplicity of *in vitro* manipulation (Hahn and Little, 1972; Clarkson, 1974). There are three different types of responses of cultured cells to chemotherapeutic agents: (1) killing of

352

MILAN
POTMESIL,
JOSEPH
LOBUE,
AND
ANNA
GOLDFEDER

proliferating cells in exponentially growing cultures and sparing of nonproliferating plateau-phase cells by cell-cycle phase-specific drugs (Borsa and Whitmore, 1969; Lloyd et al., 1972; Barranco and Novak, 1974; Clarkson, 1974; Krishan and Frei, 1976); (2) killing of both proliferating and nonproliferating plateau-phase cells by certain antitumor antibiotics and cell-cycle phase-nonspecific chemicals, with expressed greater cytotoxicity against proliferating cells (reviewed by Hahn and Little, 1972; Wilkoff et al., 1971; Clarkson, 1974; Barranco and Novak, 1974); or (3) a preferential killing of the plateau-phase cells over log-phase cells by bleomycin and nitrosourea (1-3-bis-2-chloroethyl-1-nitrosourea) in some systems (Barranco et al., 1973; Twentyman and Bleehen, 1973a). Preferential killing of the plateau-phase cells, however, has not been demonstrated in other systems (Mauro et al., 1974b; Twentyman and Bleehen, 1973b; van Putten et al., 1972), and discrepancies between these two series of experiments may be explained by the length of time cells have been allowed to stay in culture after treatment. Thus, the results indicate the importance of appropriate time intervals between the treatment and eventual subcultivation for survival of treated plateau-phase cells (Hahn, in van Putten, 1974). There is experimental evidence demonstrating that the expression of potentially lethal damage caused by various anticancer agents depends on the time of assay following the treatment (Hahn et al., 1973; Ray et al., 1973). Generally, the survival of single-dose irradiated plateau-phase cells is increased, at least in some systems, when the cells are not subcultured immediately after treatment, but are allowed to remain in the plateau-phase stage. This enhancement of survival is due to the repair of sublethal and potentially lethal damage, with both of these repair processes being independent and additive (Little, 1969; Hahn and Little, 1972; Little et al., 1973). Hypoxic plateau-phase cells accumulated in G_1 phase have significantly higher resistance to single-dose irradiation than synchronized proliferating cells progressing through G_1 (Koch et al., 1973). This may be explained in terms of a superior repair potential in the former type of cells.

Interpretation of recovery data is complicated by several additional factors. It has been suggested that both sublethal and potentially lethal lesions are similar, and involve alterations of the same subcellular components (Winans et al., 1972). These two types of lesions might differ quantitatively rather than qualitatively in various assay systems. Also, recovery from one kind of damage can be so enhanced that it masks cell response to the other type of damage (reviewed by Barranco et al., 1975). Such factors may account for conflicting reports on recovery from sublethal damage caused by various drugs (e.g., Hahn et al., 1968; Fox et al., 1969; Goldenberg, 1968). With increasing age of plateau-phase cells, the ability to repair sublethal radiation damage declines; this correlates well with age-dependent decreasing number of clonogens in the culture (Hahn, 1968) and with changes in cell kinetics (Twentyman et al., 1975). Another in vitro system has made use of spherical aggregates of normal hamster cells originally isolated from the lungs. As these spheroids grow larger, proliferative activity remains high at the peripheries while decreasing toward the centers, with necrosis eventually developing in the largest spheroids. Cells in the center of the aggregates are nonproliferating or slowly proliferating and exhibit a higher resistance to the effect of radiation than proliferating cells (Sutherland *et al.*, 1968, 1970; Durand and Sutherland, 1973). It has also been shown in this system that slow cycling G_1-like cells are relatively radiosensitive. A lack of time allowed for the repair of radiation damage may be a decisive factor even in this system.

3.5.2. Repair of Radiation Damage in Vivo

There are serious limitations inherent in any comparison of *in vitro* systems with *in vivo* conditions. However, some conclusions derived from experiments with plateau-phase cultures seem applicable, at least to some extent, to therapeutic responses of experimental ascitic and solid tumors. Both types of tumors are capable of repairing potentially lethal radiation damage (Belli *et al.*, 1971; Hahn *et al.*, 1974) as well as sublethal injury (Belli *et al.*, 1967; Suit and Urano, 1969). This repair capacity is attributed mainly to acutely and chronically hypoxic cells (Suit and Urano, 1969; Urano *et al.*, 1976). Cells in exponentially growing ascites tumors repair sublethal damage while showing no evidence of repair of potentially lethal damage. By contrast, old ascites tumors have a reduced ability to repair sublethal damage but show a considerable ability to repair potentially lethal damage (Belli *et al.*, 1971; Hahn and Frindel, in Hahn and Little, 1972; Little *et al.*, 1973). Cells in solid tumors have a reduced capacity for repair of sublethal damage (Kai and Barendsen, in Hahn and Little, 1972; Hill and Busch, 1973), but cells of old slow-growing mouse fibrosarcomas can repair potentially lethal radiation damage (Little *et al.*, 1973). The kinetics and amount of repair approximate that found in plateau-phase cultures (Belli *et al.*, 1970). Damage, lethal to tumor cells under different experimental conditions if repair is prevented, could be repaired within 4–6 hr in ascites tumors, and within a somewhat longer time period in solid tumors (Little *et al.*, 1973). These results suggest that *in vivo* repair of potentially lethal damage does occur in tumors with a large fraction of nonproliferating or slowly proliferating cells, some of them presumably hypoxic, and that an undisturbed *in situ* maintenance of irradiated tumors is an important factor for the repair processes. The observation that single-dose irradiation of mouse mammary carcinomas results in a depletion of proliferating cells and in an apparent sparing of morphologically defined nonproliferating or slowly proliferating cells seems to be consistent with the aforementioned conclusion (Potmesil *et al.*, 1975). Repair of potentially lethal damage influences the slope of survival curves in their linear region (Hahn and Little, 1972). The amount of repair in tumors treated with fractionated irradiation may depend not only on the size of the individual fractions but also on time intervals between successive doses (Little *et al.*, 1973). Lethal and sublethal radiation damage and repair phenomena in hypoxic cells are extensively discussed elsewhere in this volume.

3.5.3. Resistance to Chemotherapeutic Agents in Vivo

Differences in sensitivity to cytotoxic agents are mostly interpreted as a consequence of the proliferative state of the cell population in question (Bruce *et al.*,

354

MILAN
POTMESIL,
JOSEPH
LOBUE,
AND
ANNA
GOLDFEDER

1966). Generally, proliferating cells seem to be much more sensitive to anticancer agents than nonproliferating cells. Unstimulated B lymphocytes, precursors of humoral antibody-forming cells, normally reside in a nonproliferating state corresponding to G_0 (Syeklocha *et al.*, 1966). Following antigenic stimulation, cells are committed to producing antibodies and begin to proliferate (Perkins *et al.*, 1969). This constitutes a model of nonstimulated cells corresponding to the non-proliferating population, and stimulated cells corresponding to the proliferating pool. Cell-cycle phase-specific agents such as cytosine arabinoside (ara C), amethopterin, vincristine, and 5-fluorouracil have little or no effect on the survival of nonproliferating B cells *in vivo*, whereas proliferating B cells are sensitive to the action of these drugs. The smallest difference in sensitivity was noted with X-irradiation and with the cycle-nonspecific agent nitrogen mustard (Lin, 1973). Since the bone marrow is one of the critical dose-limiting tissues during courses of chemotherapy and since hematopoietic CFU can be readily manipulated to both proliferating and nonproliferating states, proliferation-dependent cytotoxicity has been extensively studied in this system (reviews by Valeriote and van Putten, 1975; Marsh, 1976). Numerous studies indicate that proliferating hematopoietic CFU are substantially more sensitive to vinblastine, 5-fluorouracil, mitomycin C, bleomycin, various alkylating agents, and other drugs than are CFU in a nonproliferating state. Proliferation-dependent cytotoxicity applies to CFU-s, CFU-c, and GRA, as well as ERA (see Section 2.2.1), for most chemotherapeutics assayed. As discussed by Valeriote and van Putten (1975), these observations and conclusions require two important qualifications. First, it is difficult to extrapolate drug effects from murine to human hematopoietic systems since, under normal conditions, substantially higher percentages of murine CFU-s than human CFU-s are nonproliferating; also, the kinetics of CFU recruitment after stem cell or progeny depletion might vary in both systems. Second, the length of time between the administration of the drug and the assay has a substantial influence on experimental results. The actual duration of cell exposure to a single dose of a cytostatic agent is uncertain *in vivo* and the decrease in CFU may be caused by cell death of stem cells both already proliferating and newly recruited from the nonproliferating pool; the decrease may also be caused by differentiation of CFU or by any combination of such events. Increasing time intervals between *in vivo* exposure and assay may allow for a delayed entry into the cell cycle and may lead to repair of chemically induced damage in nonproliferating CFU. Repair of damage in resting neoplastic cells, which has been demonstrated *in vivo*, is also discussed later.

The differential responses of nonproliferating and proliferating cells to the cytotoxic action of certain cell-cycle phase-specific agents seem to be well established, at least in some neoplastic systems. Treatment of thymic lymphomas in AKR mice with ara C in single or multiple doses leads to a marked depletion of proliferating large- and medium-sized blastic cells, whereas a significant number of small blasts appear to survive (Omine and Perry, 1973). As mentioned in Section 3.4.2, these small neoplastic cells are either nonproliferating or slowly proliferating cells, and at least some of them are clonogenic. Based on conclusions reached in experiments with AKR lymphomas, the relationship of blast size to therapeutic response has been further assessed in human leukemias (Sarna *et al.*, 1975) and the results are confirmatory. There is a preferential cell killing of large-size blasts by ara C and 6-thioguanine in acute myeloblastic leukemias. More examples indicating preferential killing of proliferating cells by some cytotoxic drugs can be found in the literature. Rapidly proliferating mouse leukemia L1210 (Yankee *et al.*, 1967) has been "cured" by administration of a single agent, ara C, using repeated treatments 4 days apart (Skipper *et al.*, 1970; Skipper and Schabel, 1973). This response is interpreted as an indication that there are only very few, if any, slowly proliferating or nonproliferating clonogenic cells in this type of neoplasia (Lamerton, 1972). Extensive experimental evidence supports this contention. The only experimental tumors "cured" by ara C alone are tumors with a short doubling time, high labeling indices, and a short median G_1 time (Skipper and Schabel, 1973). First or repeated passages of transplantable AK leukemia, and of L1210 leukemia in early stage, can be "cured" by optimally scheduled treatment by ara C or by a single dose of the cell-cycle nonspecific drug, cyclophosphamide (Bruce *et al.*, 1966; Schabel *et al.*, 1969; Skipper *et al.*, 1969, 1970), whereas more advanced forms of these two experimental leukemias can be cured only by ara C and cyclophosphamide together, or with other combinations of cytotoxic agents (Kline, 1974; Schabel *et al.*, 1974). Amethopterin is effective against proliferating cells of the L1210 and L5178Y ascites tumors and much less effective on "resting" cells (Hryniuk and Bertino, 1971). An advanced form of murine lymphocytic leukemia P38B can be cured by X-irradiation only if combined with chemotherapy (Wodinsky *et al.*, 1974). It has been commonly found that the growth rate of solid tumors decreases with their increasing volume and that the proliferating cell population decreases accordingly. The presence of a pool of nonproliferating cells increasing steadily with the increasing age of experimental solid tumors has been demonstrated directly (see Section 3.3.3; Potmesil and Goldfeder, 1977). It appears that nonproliferating or slowly proliferating cells seem to be resistant to cell-cycle-specific drugs, and also relatively insensitive to cycle-nonspecific agents such as cyclophosphamide (Bruce *et al.*, 1966; Skipper, 1971*b*; Bhuyan *et al.*, 1972). The early treatment of Lewis lung carcinoma in mice with cyclophosphamide, while the tumor was in a state of rapid proliferation, produced a favorable antitumor response. Treatment of developed tumors with a slow rate of proliferation, however, required progressively larger doses of the drug to achieve the desired antitumor response (DeWys, 1972). A mastocytoma, growing in either ascitic or solid form, was more sensitive to nitrosourea [1,3-bis(2-chloroethyl-)1-nitrosourea] in its early rather than in its late stage of growth (Hagemann *et al.*, 1973).

It should be stressed that the kinetic status of cells, by itself, is not an absolute criterion for determining cell sensitivity to drugs, but that there are various other factors involved as well (Valeriote and van Putten, 1975), such as uptake of drugs by cells, intracellular distribution of drugs, and efficiency of various enzyme systems in the catabolism of chemotherapeutics and in repair of cellular damage. Advanced L1210 leukemias are not curable by ara C, and this is not only the result

356

MILAN
POTMESIL,
JOSEPH
LOBUE,
AND
ANNA
GOLDFEDER

of the unfavorable kinetic condition of the clonogenic cell population but is also due to the presence of resistant leukemic cells lacking the enzymatic capacity to activate ara C (Schrecker et al., in Skipper and Schabel, 1973). Also, differences in therapeutic response to the same drug have been noted between different systems, e.g. between leukemias L1210 and AK (Razek et al., 1974). The mechanism by which cancer cells become resistant to chemotherapeutic agents, as well as therapeutic synergism, additive effects of drugs, and other related problems (e.g., classification of chemotherapeutic agents as cell-cycle phase-specific or nonspecific), are not within the scope of this chapter. Steel and Adams (1975) have shown that the survival fraction of tumor stem cells, following a dose of cyclophosphamide, was 10 times lower in small pulmonary metastases than in large intramuscular tumors. It has been suggested (Shipley et al., 1975) that this enhanced killing effect in small pulmonary metastases is caused by better drug availability to the tumor cells due to extensive microvasculature. This possibility, however, seems to be less likely for cyclophosphamide (Valeriote and van Putten, 1975) and the differential response may be better explained by the presence, in large tumors, of a sizable pool of nonproliferating clonogens, less sensitive to drug effects (see above). It has also been suggested that DNA replication in proliferating cells "fixes" the damage to DNA molecules caused by chemotherapeutics, whereas the delay in replication in nonproliferating cells allows for more time to repair the damage (Roberts et al., 1971). Hahn et al. (1973) have shown that repair of some potentially lethal damage in solid tumors exposed to bleomycin, cyclophosphamide, or 5-fluorouracil in vivo most satisfactorily explains increased survival of stem cells remaining in situ after drug administration for 24 hr rather than for 2 hr.

4. Recruitment of Cells into the Mitotic Cycle

Under normal conditions, stem cells of a renewal system are capable of self-replication, maintenance of the stem cell pool size, and also differentiation into more mature cell forms with specific functions. By analogy, tumor stem cells, in addition to their ability to expand the pool of clonogens and the pool of cells with limited proliferative potential, are capable of generating slowly proliferating or nonproliferating cells with a variable degree of maturity and a variable life span. Long time intervals between the first detection of a primary tumor and the development of secondaries (Willis, in Cooper, 1973), and the persistence of a small but significant fraction of leukemic cells as the cause of late relapses of the disease (Clarkson and Fried, 1971), indicate that neoplastic cells may persist in some privileged site in a state of "latency" but with their clonogenicity preserved. It seems likely that slowly proliferating or nonproliferating cells with preserved clonogenic potential are, upon appropriate stimulation, "recruited" or "triggered" into proliferation, and this leads to recurrences of the neoplastic disease. It is essential to determine whether nonproliferating cells in various neoplasms are truly resting cells capable of returning to proliferation, or whether these cells are destined to die without further cell division. At present, it is not feasible to answer the question of the kinetic status of "nonproliferating" leukemic and tumor cells by the methods outlined in Section 2.2.2, and new approaches to this problem are needed. It is also important to determine the mechanisms by which neoplastic cells are recruited from a resting to a proliferative state, and the inhibitory effects preventing recruitment of nonproliferating cells.

4.1. Basic Considerations

Many types of drug treatments, irradiation, or other manipulations may disturb random distribution of normal and neoplastic cells in different cell-cycle phases, and, as a consequence, larger-than-average fractions of cells passing simultaneously through various recognizable phases can be detected as temporary peaks in the mitotic or labeling indices, or as peaks in cell-distribution curves obtained by flow microfluorometry. Partial synchronization of cell progression through the cell cycle is a phenomenon which can be achieved in normal as well as in neoplastic cell populations, *in vivo* or *in vitro* (review by van Putten *et al.*, 1976). Treatments may lead to selective killing of cells in a sensitive phase of the cell cycle and to a predominance of cells in insensitive phases, to a slowdown of cell progression through certain parts of the cycle, or to a block of cell progression at a specific boundary. Synchronized populations may include stem cells as well as doomed cells. For example, cells accumulated at the G_2-M boundary as a consequence of treatment by various cytostatic drugs have only a limited proliferative capacity (Rao *et al.*, in van Putten *et al.*, 1976). The degree of synchrony achieved depends on the dosage of the drug and on the intervals between successive doses. This has been demonstrated, e.g., in an experimental melanoma treated with ara C (Gibson and Bertalanffy, 1972). It has also been shown that synchronization is detectable early after treatment *in vivo*, i.e., within 3–22 hr in various normal and neoplastic systems treated with hydroxyurea (Plager, 1975; review by van Putten *et al.*, 1976), 20 hr after the treatment of the bone marrow with bleomycin (Briganti *et al.*, 1975), and 6–8 hr after the last injection of ara C in experimental melanomas (Gibson and Bertalanffy, 1972). Changed conditions of treatment or its discontinuance leads to a rapid desynchronization, especially in neoplasms with a wide distribution of intermitotic times. Cell synchronization, however, is sometimes difficult to distinguish from other phenomena. The administration of 5-azacytidine to intact or to partially hepatectomized rats enhances thymidine incorporation into DNA of liver cells; this can be attributed either to a partial synchronization of proliferating hepatocytes or to changed levels of intracellular metabolites (Čihák *et al.*, 1972, 1976).

Cell depletion after therapy may also lead to recruitment of cells from a "resting" stage back into the cell cycle. "Recruitment" is a term designating both the induction of nonproliferating cells into proliferation and the acceleration of cell progression through a specific cell-cycle phase, followed by the traverse of

358

MILAN
POTMESIL,
JOSEPH
LOBUE,
AND
ANNA
GOLDFEDER

subsequent phases and cell division. Partial synchronization of cell progression through the cell cycle and cell recruitment might be simultaneous. Recruitment may be determined in neoplasms by current techniques under several basic conditions. The tumor-cell population must contain a large fraction of non-proliferating cells; recruitment should be achieved by an agent which kills cells rapidly over a limited and definable time period, and a significant fraction of recruited tumor cells leaves the resting phase over a short time interval. Cell populations becoming asynchronous during recruitment, small fractions of cells entering the cell cycle, recruited cells having a large variation in the intermitotic time, and survival of high numbers of doomed cells certainly represent circumstances unfavorably influencing the detection of cell recruitment. Time intervals between effective treatment and recruitment of nonproliferating cells into the mitotic cycle may depend on the extent of cell kill, on the efficiency of repair processes in damaged nonproliferating cells, and also on stimulatory effects leading to recruitment. Experimental data discussed later (Section 4.3.2) indicate that recruitment of nonproliferating cells may start several days after single-dose irradiation of experimental solid tumors. It has been reported that cells damaged by X-irradiation produce two to three generations of descendants but no long-term survivors (Trott and Hug, 1970), and this may also apply to some non-proliferating cells recruited into cell cycle.

Recruitment of nonproliferating cells into the cell cycle is desirable in neoplasms, since cycling cells are more sensitive to the killing effects of various chemical agents. Recruitment has been advocated as an important part of treatment schedules in clinical combination therapy. In the study of proliferation kinetics in normal as well as in neoplastic tissue, it is often useful to perturb the system by a single therapeutic agent, and to follow changes in the number of stem cells, cell-cycle time, cell production, and cell loss rates. Adverse effects of a single agent, such as acceleration of tumor growth rates, shortening of cell-cycle times, and increases in the fraction of proliferating cells or clonogens during the period of tumor recurrences may be at least partially attributable to recruitment of nonproliferating stem cells into cell cycle.

4.2. Therapy and Accelerated Neoplastic Growth

4.2.1. Irradiation

Clinical data have demonstrated accelerated growth of solid tumors subjected to single doses of therapeutical irradiation, a phenomenon also well recognized from numerous experimental studies. This includes clinical observations (Malaise et al., 1972) on lung metastases originating from a variety of different tumors, such as squamous cell carcinoma, adenocarcinoma, osteosarcoma, teratoma, and malignant melanoma. Diameters of lung loci were measured on radiographs in the posterior-anterior projection (Collins et al., 1956; Nathan et al., 1962), plotted as a function of time after irradiation with ^{60}Co, and the volume doubling time was calculated by the method of least squares. The mean volume doubling time was

reduced from 53.5 days before irradiation to 12.0 days after a single-dose
irradiation of 1000 rads. An acceleration of the growth rates was also noted in
metastases treated with two irradiations of 500 rads each delivered at 3-hr
intervals. These results are in accord with earlier studies of cutaneous (Rambert *et*
al., 1968) and lung metastases (Van Peperzeel, 1970), and also with a more recent
study by Van Peperzeel (1972). In the latter study, an accelerated growth of lung
metastases was observed after the initial reduction of tumor volume by X-
irradiation delivered to 11 patients with various types of solid tumors. In all
instances, with one exception, single-dose irradiation or a series of fractionated
irradiations with different regimes accelerated growth; this acceleration occurred
mostly on postirradiation days 3–6.

Stimulation of proliferation has also been repeatedly demonstrated in
irradiated experimental tumors. Effects of single doses of X-irradiation on lung
metastases were studied radiographically in dogs and mice (Van Peperzeel, 1972),
in which the size of lung tumor nodules was measured by using an enlarged
projection of radiograms. Lung metastases of spontaneous tumors in dogs
increased in size after a single dose of 150 or 300 rads. On day 6 and thereafter,
the volume doubling time of regrowing loci showed initial acceleration first, and
later a gradual return to preirradiation values. Lung "metastases" in mice were
induced by cell suspensions of an isogenic, poorly differentiated mammary
carcinoma injected intravenously. Following a single-dose irradiation of 105 or
210 rads, the mean volume doubling time in regrowing loci was 8 hr, as compared
to 24 hr in unirradiated loci. Subcutaneously implanted tumors irradiated with a
dose of 210 rads showed a distinct accleration at the beginning of regrowth. The
volume doubling time decreased from the preirradiation value of 24 hr to 12.1 hr,
the cell-cycle time was 23% shorter, the growth fraction increased from 0.87 to
1.0, and cell loss decreased. Cell-cycle parameters of a transplantable rat rhabdomyosarcoma irradiated with 2000-rad X-rays showed that, during tumor
regression, cells proliferated with a cell-cycle time of 12 hr instead of the 20 hr
measured in controls. This shortening of the cell cycle was due to a substantial
reduction of G_1 phase. Also, the growth fraction was probably increased (Hermens and Barendsen, 1969). Tubiana *et al.* (in Frindel and Tubiana, 1971) have
found a slight reduction of the cell cycle with shortening of G_1 phase and
prolongation of S phase in a fibrosarcoma irradiated with 600-rad X-rays 48 hr
earlier. Regarding cell-cycle variables in experimental tumors, the changes
induced by radiation can also include the following: prolongation of the cell cycle
(Frindel *et al.*, 1970); variation in S time and elongation of $G_2 + M$ phase (Brown
and Berry, in Frindel and Tubiana, 1971); slight shortening of S time (Hermens
and Barendsen, 1969); prolongation, or prolongation with consequent shortening, of S time (Frindel *et al.*, 1970; Tubiana *et al.*, in Frindel and Tubiana, 1971).
This may indicate a fluctuation of cell-cycle variables depending on the type of
tumor, applied dose of radiation, and time interval after irradiation. It can also be
calculated from experimental data of a transplantable mouse mammary
adenocarcinoma regrowing after a single dose of 470-rad X-irradiation that cell
doubling time is 40.1 hr and that it is 27.0 hr after 940 rads, and 26.8 hr after

360

MILAN
POTMESIL,
JOSEPH
LOBUE,
AND
ANNA
GOLDFEDER

1880 rads, as compared with 40.2 hr in unirradiated tumors (Potmesil *et al.*, 1975). When compared to unirradiated controls, the growth fraction is increased in regrowing tumors; the S time is slightly prolonged at the beginning of regrowth, and later shortened. Cell losses calculated from experimental data by the method of Steel (1968) decrease in regrowing irradiated tumors (approximately 30% decrease in cell loss can be observed in tumors irradiated with 940 or 1880 rads). As discussed later in Section 4.3.3, at this time of tumor regrowth, estimates derived by a modified method of Steel (1968) suggested recruitment of non-proliferating cells into the cell cycle. Malaise and Tubiana (1966) studied a fibrosarcoma irradiated *in situ* and cloned *in vitro*. The doubling time of cells surviving irradiation was shorter than in unirradiated controls, probably because of an increased growth fraction. Measurements of changes in the number of stem cells cloned *in vitro* in a rat rhabdomyosarcoma irradiated with a single dose of 1000 or 2000 rads of X-rays, or 600 rads of neutrons, indicated that surviving cells repopulated the tumor at a high rate (Barendson and Broerse, 1969). Their doubling time of 30 hr was about 3 times shorter than the doubling time in unirradiated tumors. When irradiated tumors were nearly repopulated, the growth rates decreased and became slower than those of control tumors. Moreover, at the end of fractionated irradiation, which was applied 15 times (5 times/week) with daily doses of 50, 70, or 100 rads of neutrons and 200 or 300 rads of X-rays, the surviving cells proliferated with the doubling time of approximately 2 days as compared with a doubling time of 4–5 days before irradiation (Barendsen and Broerse, 1970). The doubling time between fractions, calculated from Barendsen's data, was 2.5 days. The acceleration of tumor growth was partly related to the shortening of the cell-cycle time, but mostly to an increase in the growth fraction (Tubiana, 1973).

4.2.2. Chemotherapy and Surgery

Clinical studies indicate that the tumors which have been cured by aggressive chemotherapy are predominantly those with a high proliferative potential. Good examples of successful treatments are results obtained with several childhood tumors including Wilm's tumor, embryonal rhabdomyosarcoma, Burkitt's tumor stages I and II, and osteogenic sarcoma. Therapy combining several chemotherapeutic agents may result in long-term remission even in a disseminated neoplastic disease, as suggested by data obtained in children and adults suffering from Burkitt's tumor in advanced stages, metastatic Wilms' and Ewing's tumors, disseminated choriocarcinoma, Hodgkin's disease stages III and IV, metastatic testicular cancer, etc. (for reviews, see Burchenal, 1973; Halana, 1973; Perry, 1973; Metz, 1974). Excellent results have been achieved with intermittent combination therapy in acute lymphoblastic leukemias in children, leading to long-term survival; also, combinational therapy of nonlymphoblastic leukemias in adults has resulted in a relatively high percentage of complete remissions (Burchenal, 1973). Chemotherapeutic effects of several compounds used in some treatment protocols are of particular interest. Ara C, when given intravenously in doses of

361
STEM CELLS,
NON-
PROLIFERATING
CELLS, AND
THEIR
KINETICS

5 mg/kg body weight to children with acute lymphoblastic leukemia caused initial inhibition of cell proliferation, as indicated by decreased mitotic index and increased [^{3}H]TdR incorporation in leukemic cells. This was followed 48 hr later by an increase of both these variables (Lampkin et al., 1969). A similar effect was demonstrated in patients with acute lymphoblastic, myeloblastic, and myelomonocytic leukemia, the leukemic form of a lymphoma, and advanced medulloblastoma 24–48 hr after administration of this drug (Lampkin et al., 1971). An increase in [^{3}H]TdR labeling and mitotic indices was observed 48 hr after single or multiple injections of methotrexate (MTX) in patients with acute myeloblastic leukemia (Ernst and Killmann, 1971). Measurements of nuclear DNA content indicated an increasing predominance of cells in early S phase. Temporary "pile-up" of cells in S phase and subsequent increased flow through the cell cycle, resulting in elevated [^{3}H]TdR labeling and mitotic indices, indicated synchronization. This mechanism may also participate in the enhancement of proliferative activity observed after an injection of ara C. However, the long interval between injection and maximal effect (48–72 hr) seems to suggest some other mechanism, e.g., recruitment of proliferating cells from the nonproliferating cell pool (Vogler et al., 1974). A single dose of ara C reduced cell density in the ascitic fluid of a patient with recurrent ovarian carcinoma. The remaining viable cells grew more rapidly than unperturbed cells before treatment, the labeling and mitotic indices increased, and the cell-cycle time was shortened, most at the expense of G_1 phase (Sheehy et al., 1974).

Treatment of experimental tumors with cell-cycle phase-nonspecific drugs generally increases the growth fraction, thus making them more susceptible to subsequent regimes of cell-cycle phase-specific agents. For instance, when hamsters with plasmacytoma Pla 1 received a single dose (20 mg/kg) of the cell-cycle phase-nonspecific drug cytoxan, intracerebral implantation of counted cells from treated and control tumors showed that chemotherapy stimulated the rate of proliferation of viable cells. Their cell doubling time was 0.53 days as compared with about 3 days in untreated tumors (Griswold and Simpson-Herren, in Skipper, 1972). Four courses of ara C alone (a cell-cycle phase-specific drug) only slightly inhibited the growth of Pla 1. When administration of ara C followed treatment by cytoxan, there was a more significant delay in tumor recurrence as compared with results of treatment with a single dose of cytoxan alone. This observation suggests that perturbation of tumors by cytoxan left the tumor-cell populations temporarily more sensitive to ara C (Griswold, in Skipper, 1972). Similar experimental results have also been obtained with advanced Ca 755 in mice (Laster et al., 1969; Schabel, 1968). Mice bearing Ca 755 tumors were treated sequentially with cytoxan followed by 6-mercaptopurine in repeated (2, 3, and 4) courses. This resulted in 100% total tumor regressions and "cures." Treatment with cytoxan or 6-mercaptopurine alone on the same schedule as before, or even with higher doses, failed to "cure" (Schabel, 1968). These studies with two drugs are interpreted as indicating that the killing of nonproliferating cells can be achieved first by their recruitment into the cell cycle and then by reaching them in a drug-sensitive phase. It should be critically determined, however, whether good

362

MILAN
POTMESIL,
JOSEPH
LOBUE,
AND
ANNA
GOLDFEDER

results with combinations of various chemotherapeutics observed in clinical as well as experimental oncology are indeed caused by modification of cell kinetics and not by factors such as pharmacological interaction between drugs, enhanced penetration of one drug after pretreatment with the other, or potentiation of kill effects by some other mechanism (see discussion by van Putten *et al.*, 1976).

Since most current antitumor drugs act by interfering with proliferating cells, advanced tumors with a small fraction of proliferating and a large portion of noncycling cells are relatively refractory to this type of therapy. Available clinical evidence indicates that surgical removal of tumor masses increases the chances of chemotherapeutic cure of certain disseminated cancers (reviewed by Skipper, 1974). As tumor mass is substantially reduced by surgical treatment, the growth fraction of remaining viable tumor cells rises (Schabel, 1969). There is a large body of evidence available from a variety of human and animal tumors demonstrating changes in the growth rate of cells and their sensitivity to chemotherapeutic agents after they have been "uncrowded" and "adapted" to log-phase cultures *in vitro* (Eagle and Foley, 1956; Wheeler *et al.*, 1967, 1970; Cleaver, 1967; Skipper, 1968; Todo *et al.*, 1969). Under these conditions, the doubling time becomes considerably shorter, G_1 phase decreases, and [^{3}H]TdR labeling indices increase. All such tumor-cell cultures become sensitive to a variety of chemotherapeutic drugs. Similar situations arise under experimental conditions *in vivo*. Tumor cells of ascitic forms are sensitive to chemotherapy shortly after implantation when the growth is still exponential (Schmidt *et al.*, 1965; Tannock, 1969; Wiebel and Baserga, 1968). The available evidence suggests that surgical removal or *in situ* destruction of most cells in a tumor leaves the remaining cells temporarily stimulated to rapid growth (Schabel, 1969; Skipper, 1972, 1974). Surgically "perturbed" (i.e., dissected to 25 mg fragments) tumors of sarcoma 180 and adenocarcinoma Ca 755 were implanted into isogenic mice. Regardless of the doubling time of the donor tumors at the time of transplantation (between 1.2 and 9.7 days), each implanted tumor had an essentially identical growth rate, with initial doubling time of 0.9–1.5 days and gradual deceleration of growth. These results have been interpreted as an increase in the growth fraction stimulated by a decreased total tumor mass due to dissection (Schabel, 1969; Skipper, 1972).

4.3. Recruitment in Normal Tissues and Neoplasms

4.3.1. Recruitment in Normal Tissues

As discussed earlier (Section 3.1.1), cells in some, but not all, renewal tissues seem to be in a true G_0 state. Experimental results have shown that G_0 cells present in slowly proliferating tissues can be induced to enter the proliferating pool if appropriate stimulation is applied. Examples of G_0 recruitment have included liver stimulated either by partial resection or, in alloxan-diabetic rats, by insulin; salivary glands stimulated by treatment with isoproterenol; kidneys stimulated by contralateral nephrectomy, temporary ischemia, metabolic acidosis, mercuric chloride necrosis, or administration of folic acid; cartilage of hypophysectomized rats treated with growth hormone; mammary glands stimulated by estradiol-progesterone; estogen-stimulated uterus; skeletal muscle stimulated by wounding; pancreas of rats treated by ethionine; fibroblasts in tissue cultures stimulated by serum (reviewed by Baserga, 1968, 1973; Baserga and Wiebel, 1969; Stein and Baserga, 1972). A complex and interdependent series of biochemical events occurs in stimulated G_0 cells during their recruitment and prior to the onset of DNA synthesis. Pertinent to a variety of stimulated G_0-cell models (Baserga and Stein, 1971; Baserga, 1973) are, for instance, these findings: (1) stimulation of DNA synthesis in G_0 cells and preparation for mitosis are very sensitive *in vivo* and *in vitro* to even low concentrations of actinomycin D; (2) increases in the rate of RNA synthesis are detectable *in vivo* and *in vitro* in stimulated cells entering the early prereplicative phase; (3) new molecular species of RNA are detectable in stimulated but not in unstimulated G_0 cells; (4) stimulated cells bind increased amounts of actinomycin D or acridine orange; and (5) in several *in vitro* model systems there is an increase in chromatin template activity preceding DNA synthesis (see also Section 3.1.1). The increase in chromatin template activity is accompanied by structural changes detectable by circular dichroism as early as 2 hr after stimulation (Baserga *et al.*, in Nicolini and Baserga, 1975). An increase in the number of binding sites for ethidium bromide in isolated chromatin may be similarly explained (Lurguin, 1974). Other events related to those previously described include an early start (several hours after stimulation) in synthesis of nuclear acidic proteins; an increase of RNA polymerase activity and activity of uridine, uridylate, and cytidine kinase; increased synthesis of histones and nonhistone chromosomal proteins, their acetylation and phosphorylation; in later phases, an increased activity of enzymes associated with DNA synthesis and synthesis of their templates (review by Cooper, 1971; Baserga, 1973; Stein and Baserga, 1972).

The mammalian liver has a considerable capacity for compensatory regeneration of tissue either damaged by chemicals or removed by surgical ablation, and this aspect has been explored in numerous experiments (see reviews by Bucher, 1963, 1967a,b; Becker, 1973). Under physiological conditions, liver parenchymal cells in adults rarely divide. Following partial hepatectomy, increased mitotic activity reaches its peak at 28 hr (Carter *et al.*, 1956; Harkness, 1957), then falls gradually over the next several days. The increased mitotic activity is preceded by heightened DNA synthesis beginning at 16–18 hr (Grisham, 1962). Only a part of the nonproliferating cell population (55–60%) is triggered into the cell cycle during the first 24 hr (Bucher and Swaffield, 1964), and a total of 93% of hepatocytes may enter DNA synthesis over a span of 3 days after partial hepatectomy (Stocker, 1966). Approximately 20% of resting cells in folic acid-stimulated kidney, in regenerating pancreas, and in lactating mammary gland and 5% in contralateral kidney after nephrectomy enter DNA synthesis (reviewed by Baserga, 1968). This indicates that only a part of the nonproliferating cell population responds to the stimulus. Stimulated G_0 cells enter the cycle gradually

363
STEM CELLS,
NON-
PROLIFERATING
CELLS, AND
THEIR
KINETICS

MILAN
POTMESIL,
JOSEPH
LOBUE,
AND
ANNA
GOLDFEDER

and their degree of synchronization is relatively low (Nias and Fox, 1971). One of the most widely applied *in vitro* models of stimulated cell proliferation utilizes mature lymphocytes maintained in short-term cultures and triggered into cell cycle by various mitogens. Mature nonproliferating (presumably G_0) lymphocytes, following treatment with a mitogen, are induced to undergo a series of changes, leading to blastogenesis and ultimately to cell division (reviewed by Johnson and Rubin, 1970; Cooper, 1971). There is a very early increase in synthesis of low molecular weight RNA (Cooper and Rubin, 1965; Pogo *et al.*, 1966) which quickly appears in the cytoplasm of stimulated lymphocytes (Kay and Cooper, 1969). Within several hours after stimulation, the rate of ribosomal RNA-precursor synthesis increases and this continues for more than 20 hr (Cooper, 1969*a,b*). The percentage of cells synthesizing DNA reaches its peak at 72 hr (Cooper *et al.*, 1963), and the first mitotic wave appears at about 42 hr (Bender and Prescott, 1962).

Other tissues, such as epidermis and bone marrow, contain at least some cells in G_1 (or G_1 and G_2) that, upon stimulation, can be recruited relatively rapidly into proliferation. Nonproliferating CFU-s are triggered into the cell cycle when the number of proliferating CFU-s are reduced because of depletion. About 40% of CFU-s enter the cycle within 4 hr after stimulation; by 8 hr, about 50% have begun DNA synthesis; by 12 hr, there is an overshoot of the original value of cycling stem cells (reviewed by Tubiana *et al.*, 1974). Subtotal irradiation (one leg shielded) induces a continuous increase of CFU-s in S phase in the protected leg. This increase, stimulated abscopally, starts soon after irradiation and reaches its maximum 24 hr later (Croizat *et al.*, 1970). There are indications suggesting that the majority of mouse (Lajtha, 1972; Bruce *et al.*, 1966) and rat (Dunn and Elson, 1970; Haas *et al.*, 1971; Bohne *et al.*, 1970) bone marrow CFU-s are either nonproliferating or slowly proliferating with a long G_1, and may be stimulated into a rapid proliferation by endotoxin (Croizat *et al.*, 1970), by transplantation of CFU-s to irradiated recipients (Valeriote and Bruce, 1967), and by irradiation or chemotherapy (discussed earlier in Sections 4.2.1 and 4.2.2). The most apparent feature of these systems is the early recruitment of CFU-s into the cell cycle; this is in clear contrast to the onset of DNA synthesis in stimulated G_0 cells discussed in the preceding paragraph. Cellular subpopulations in a wide variety of normal tissues can be blocked in a resting state corresponding to G_2 phase. These "arrested" cells can be released into cycle in response to certain stimuli (review by Tobey *et al.*, 1971).

4.3.2. Recruitment in Leukemias and Tumors

Gavosto *et al.*, (1964, 1967*a,b*) and others (Mauer and Fisher, 1966) have observed that the proliferating blastic pool of human acute leukemia does not manifest self-maintaining kinetics, since the loss of blasts to the nonproliferating or slowly proliferating pool is greater than their birth rate. Recruitment of nonproliferating small blasts into the proliferating pool of large blasts has been suggested in two clinical studies. A patient with untreated acute lymphoblastic leukemia was repeatedly injected with [³H]TdR in two successive series 2 days apart (Saunders and Mauer, 1969). Only 10% of small blasts labeled in the first period, while 72% labeled in the second period. During the first period, proliferating large labeled blasts were rapidly replaced by unlabeled cells; in the second period, unlabeled proliferating blasts were replaced by labeled blasts and the proliferating pool maintained a high labeling index thereafter. The only identifiable source of replacement in both situations was small nonproliferating blasts. In another study (Gabutti *et al.*, 1969), patients with acute lymphoblastic leukemia were injected with a single dose of [³H]TdR and about 70 hr later treated with two doses of methotrexate. Bone marrow samples were analyzed for cellular DNA content and autoradiographic label. Following the second dose of methotrexate, the labeling index of small blasts (2c DNA) decreased, whereas the labeling index of large and medium blasts (2c–4c DNA) increased. The source of replacement of depleted proliferating blasts was identified as nonproliferating small blasts. These and related studies using ara C and 6-thioguanine treatments (Sarna *et al.*, 1975) suggest that under steady-state conditions, or after a treatment which depletes the proliferating pool, small blast cells are recruited into the S phase and establish a new proliferating pool. Label reutilization may have occurred in both experiments and influenced the percentages of labeled cells. Reutilization, however, is usually characterized by low levels of incorporation (Maruyama, 1964); high grain counts above some blasts and identical grain-count distribution above small and large blasts suggest that reutilization was not a serious factor in these studies. In more recent investigations, the recruitment of nonproliferating blast cells into the proliferative cycle was suggested in some patients treated with chemical agents (Lampkin *et al.*, 1971). The turnover rate of nonproliferating blasts in acute leukemia is slow (Fried, in Clarkson, 1974), and there are some indications of a potential for DNA repair in these cells (Stryckmans *et al.*, 1970).

It has been well established that the growth of experimental ascites tumors decreases with increasing tumor mass and time after inoculation (Klein and Révész, 1953; Patt *et al.*, 1953; Lala and Patt, 1966; Burns, 1968). With increasing age of tumors, "nonproliferating" cells accumulate at an increasing rate, and this is accompanied by increased cell loss, decreased growth fraction, and prolongation of the mean cell-cycle time (Lala and Patt, 1966, 1968; Peel and Fletcher, 1969; Dombernowsky *et al.*, 1973, 1974; Hartmann and Dombernowsky, 1974). Cytophotometric studies of hypotetraploid lines of ascites tumors at different stages of growth have demonstrated that nonproliferating cells had a 2c DNA content (Lala and Patt, 1968; Peel and Fletcher, 1969), or 2c and 4c DNA content (Frindel *et al.*, 1969; Dombernowsky *et al.*, 1974; Dombernowsky and Bichel, 1975). Indications that nonproliferating ascitic cells may be held up in a stage corresponding to G_2 have been discussed earlier (Section 3.1.2). It has been shown that reimplantation of ascites tumors with decelerated growth or withdrawal of tumor cells by aspiration is followed by a marked increase in the growth rate as determined by the mitotic and labeling indices (Burns, 1968; Bichel, 1970), and by a rapid increase in cell populations with 2c–4c DNA content (Dombernowsky and Bichel, 1975). Experimental data from mitotic and labeling indices, FLM

366

MILAN
POTMESIL,
JOSEPH
LOBUE,
AND
ANNA
GOLDFEDER

estimates in a cell population either continuously labeled or prelabeled before transplantation, and impulse cytophotometry may be interpreted as follows: (1) the "release" of nonproliferating cells starts 3–6 hr after implantation and the transition to the proliferating pool is probably terminated before 24 hr elapses (Dombernowsky *et al.*, 1974); (2) "decycling" and "recycling" of nonproliferating cells probably occur after mitoses and before DNA synthesis (Lala and Patt, 1968); (3) a major portion of nonproliferating cells move into the S phase after transplantation at a slow rate, whereas a small number enter S phase immediately after transplantation (Baserga and Gold, 1963; Wiebel and Baserga, 1968); (4) increased flux of cells through S phase is noticed 24–48 hr after transplantation or after partial removal of tumor cells by aspiration (Dombernowsky and Bichel, 1975). Reviewed data also suggest that some "nonproliferating" cells recruited into the cell cycle are already equipped with the machinery for DNA replication and therefore can be readily triggered into cell cycle when challenged by an appropriate stimulus (Wiebel and Baserga, 1968). This has been confirmed in Ehrlich ascites tumors treated with actinomycin D (Baserga *et al.*, 1965). Actinomycin D inhibits G_1-S transition, but only cells positioned "deeper" in G_1 are affected. Cells closer to the G_1/S boundary escape this inhibition. Based on such experimental results and on cytokinetic data discussed earlier (shortening of cell-cycle time and narrowing of the distribution of cell-cycle duration in reimplanted ascites tumors; Section 3.4.2), it can be concluded that nonproliferating cells in old ascites tumors are primarily cells slowly progressing through G_1, and that their recruitment into the proliferating pool, stimulated by reimplantation, starts with accelerated traverse through G_1. However, blockade of some nonproliferating cells in G_0 with random release cannot be completely excluded. It has also been shown that immunosuppression by mouse antilymphocytic serum releases some noncycling G_2-phase cells into mitoses in a heterologous tumor–host system (Ehrlich ascites tumors in DBA/2 mice) (DeCosse and Gelfant, 1968).

Spontaneous lymphoma in AKR mice (see also Sections 2.3.2, 3.2.3, 3.3.1, 3.4.2, and 3.5.3) has been widely used as an experimental model, especially for the evaluation of various chemotherapeutic agents (Schabel *et al.*, 1974). The primary site of this neoplasia is the thymus, and in the late stages of the disease the thymus, spleen, lymph nodes, and bone marrow become extensively infiltrated with neoplastic cells (reviewed by Omine and Perry, 1973). AKR lymphoma cells vary in size, with large and medium cells engaged in active proliferation. Small-sized cells with 2c DNA content, derived from the dividing cells, are constantly renewed and consist of both nonclonogenic and clonogenic cells residing either in G_0 or in a long G_1 phase (Omine *et al.*, 1973; Omine and Perry, 1973). Their clonogenicity has been directly demonstrated by separation of small nonproliferating or slowly proliferating cells in a $1g$ sucrose density gradient and by their inoculation into isogenic hosts, where these cells produced tumors as readily as the large proliferating cells (Rosen *et al.*, 1970; Omine and Perry, 1972). These experiments represent direct proof that in this neoplasia some nonproliferating stem cells, or stem cells slowly traversing G_1 phase, are recruited into the cell cycle. As mentioned earlier (Section 3.1.2), Post *et al.* (1973) interpreted their data on cell kinetics of a rat sarcoma in terms of recruitment from the nonproliferating cell pool to the cycle as an integral part of the tumor's life history. The clonogenic capacity of nonproliferating cells has also been tested in a transplantable rat rhabdomyosarcoma (Barendsen, 1974; Barendsen et al., 1973). Tumor cells were labeled in vivo with repeated injections of [³H]TdR to distinguish proliferating from nonproliferating cells. Cell suspensions were cultivated in vitro, and growing clones were examined autoradiographically for presence of the label. The unlabeled clones were considered as the progeny of unlabeled nonproliferating cells. However, since the duration of [³H]TdR labeling (16 hr) did not exceed the median cell-cycle time (20 hr), an alternative interpretation of these results would be that cells with slower progression through the cycle remained unlabeled. In a comparable experiment (Kallman, 1975), tumor-bearing mice were repeatedly injected with [³H]TdR during a 24-hr period, single-cell suspensions cultured in vitro, and colony formation screened. Labeled colonies were judged as descendents of proliferating cells and unlabeled colonies as descendants of clonogenic, nonproliferating cells. The interpretation suggested that in tumors irradiated with a single dose of 300 rads there is little if any recruitment of nonproliferating stem cells within 2–3 days after exposure. A marked increase in the growth fraction and a double peak (or a "dip" in the second peak) of a FLM curve were noticed in mouse adenocarcinomas on day 4 after a single-dose X-irradiation (von Szczepanski and Trott, 1975). This was intepreted as indicating that 4 days after irradiation of 1200 r there are at least two cell populations in treated tumors, one of them partially synchronized. This led to an assumption that some nonproliferating tumor cells were triggered into the cell cycle at that time. It should be pointed out, however, that the "fuzziness" and ambiguity of data based on analysis of FLM curves probably increase considerably in irradiated tumors, with numerous doomed cells being present and cell death occurring at various points in the cell cycle, including mitoses.

4.3.3. Mathematical Modeling

There are numerous mathematical approaches which have been used to construct kinetic models of nonproliferating cells and their recruitment in neoplasias. Some of them have been critically reviewed by Aroesty et al. (1973). A cytokinetic model of human acute lymphoblastic leukemia (Mauer et al., 1973) explores mechanisms controlling the growth of a leukemic cell population; some conclusions obtained by this model cannot be confirmed by experimental studies, but cell recruitment seems to be a phenomenon acceptable by the model system. Only two parameters derived from FLM data are required for a complete kinetic description in another model applicable to steady-state as well as exponentially growing cell populations (De Maertelaer and Galand, 1975); the resting stage is assumed to be constant in duration and cells leave this phase randomly. The basic hypothesis of another model (Burns and Tannock, 1970; see also Section 3.1.1) is that G_0 phase is entered by all dividing cells, the cells return to cell cycle with a constant probability per unit time, the remaining phases have approximately fixed durations. Only two

MILAN
POTMESIL,
JOSEPH
LOBUE,
AND
ANNA
GOLDFEDER

parameters are required to a complete kinetic description of such cell populations. This model has been further modified (Smith and Martin, 1973) and generalized to rapidly proliferating cells; according to this modification, cells leave the postmitotic resting stage at random, and enter their replicative cycle. Cell-population growth rate is determined by the probability with which cells leave their resting stage, by the duration of their replicative cycle, and by the rate of cell death. Data on the distribution of generation times of cells in tissue culture, obtained by time-lapse cinematography, fit predictions of this model. Another closely related model (Lebowitz and Rubinow, 1969; Rubinow et al., 1971) assumes that a fraction of cells may bypass G_0; that there is a constant cycle time and random loss, separately for cells in G_0 and for cells in cycle; and that cells leave G_0 and enter cell cycle with a uniform probability per unit time. It appears that model parameters approximate experimental data with varying precision. Of particular relevance are models suggesting the turnover rate of the relatively inaccessible compartment of nonproliferating cells in solid tumors. Mendelsohn and Dethlefsen (1973) estimated this turnover rate from the time-dependent relationship between labeling indices observed and expected for proliferating cells. The latter parameter is computed from FLM curve-derived variables. Steady-state kinetics has been simulated using matrix algebra (Roti Roti and Dethlefsen, 1975a,b). Several models of perturbed cellular kinetics were constructed, and the validity was tested by comparing simulated and experimentally obtained kinetic data. The best-fitting model showed that recruitment of nonproliferating cells participates in repopulation of the depleted proliferating pool. A model suggesting the size of the nonproliferating cell pool in treated tumors utilizes flow microfluorometric measurements (Kal and Hahn, 1976). The proportion of proliferating and nonproliferating cells in tumors before treatment should be known, and cell-cycle variables are assumed to be subjected only to minor alterations during treatments. The experimental results are interpreted as indicative of the recruitment of nonproliferating cells into cell cycle in tumors treated with radiation and hyperthermia. The kinetics of nonproliferating cells can also be studied in a more complex approach by computer simulation of growing populations of cells under various conditions, including therapeutic perturbations (see for example, Appleton et al., 1973; Valleron and Frindel, 1973; Chuang and Lloyd, 1975).

To determine whether recruitment of nonproliferating cells plays a role in the regrowth of irradiated tumors, the method of Steel (1968) was modified to estimate the loss rates from pools of morphologically defined "proliferating" and "nonproliferating" cells (Potmesil et al., 1975). Low-LET radiation was applied to a transplantable mouse mammary adenocarcinoma in a single subcurative dose at three different levels, 470, 940, and 1880 rads. Parenchymal tumor cells were classified according to their nucleolar morphology as either proliferating or nonproliferating (see Section 3.3.3), and their quantitative changes were followed at different time intervals after irradiation. Irradiation resulted in reduction of the number of cells in both pools, with apparent sparing of nonproliferating cells. The regenerative period started with a gradual increase in the number of cells in the proliferating pool, whereas the number of cells in the nonproliferating pool continued to fall in tumors irradiated with 940 rads (Fig. 4A) and 1880 rads (Fig. 4B). In the last phase of tumor regrowth, the increasing number of cells in the nonproliferating pool corresponded to its replenishment by cell transition from the proliferating pool. Other kinetic variables necessary for calculations of cell loss rates from the proliferating and nonproliferating pool, namely, the [^{14}C]TdR

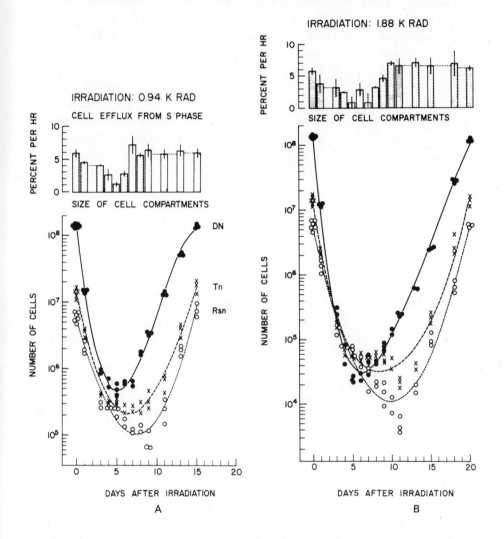

FIGURE 4A,B. Size of cell compartments as a function of time in mouse mammary carcinoma DBAH after single-dose irradiation (lower panels) and cell efflux from S phase at different time intervals after exposure (upper panels). Each point indicates compartmental size in a single tumor. DN, Cells with dense nucleoli (proliferating cell pool); Tn, cells with trabeculate nucleoli; Rsn, cells with ring-shaped nucleoli (nonproliferating cell pool). Columns represent the mean of cell effluxes in two to six samples; cell effluxes were obtained by double-labeling method with [^{3}H]TdR and [^{14}C]TdR and are expressed as number of cells per 100 cells per 1 hr. Vertical bars indicate standard deviation. From Potmesil *et al.* (1975), with permission of *Cell and Tissue Kinetics.*

370

MILAN
POTMESIL,
JOSEPH
LOBUE,
AND
ANNA
GOLDFEDER

labeling indices and the duration of DNA synthesis periods, were also estimated at various time intervals after irradiation. The cell loss rate from the nonproliferating pool was separated into cell loss rates for the compartment of cells with trabeculate nucleoli and the compartment of cells with ring-shaped nucleoli. In addition to losses from the tumor as a whole, the "net loss rate" of the nonproliferating pool reflects the rate of cell transition from the nonproliferating to the proliferating pool, minus the rate of transition in the opposite direction. A similar definition applies to the net loss rate from the proliferating pool and both compartments of the nonproliferating pool. The results presented in Fig. 5 have shown that (1) there are high losses in both pools, with excess losses in the proliferating pool during the early phase after irradiation; (2) in the early stage of regrowth after irradiation, the cell net loss rate for the nonproliferating pool increases, in contrast to the behavior of cell loss rate for the proliferating pool and the average cell loss rate for the tumor as a whole; and (3) in the late stage of regrowth, a decrease in net loss rate for the nonproliferating pool reflects the excess production of nonproliferating cells over control tumors. The sequence of transitions between the proliferating and nonproliferating pools was assumed in the following order: proliferating pool (P, cells with dense nucleoli)→ nonproliferating compartment I (Q', cells with trabeculate nucleoli)→ nonproliferating compartment II (Q", cells with ring-shaped nucleoli), and the transit in the opposite direction Q"→Q'→P. This assumption was based on the

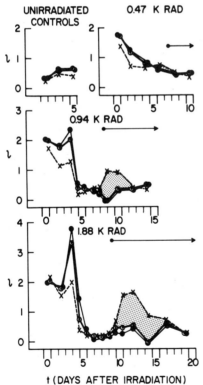

FIGURE 5. Net cell loss rates (l) of the proliferating pool (●—●), net cell loss rates of the nonproliferating pool (×---×), and the average cell loss rates (⊙—⊙) are plotted as a function of time for control unirradiated tumors and tumors irradiated with a single dose of 0.45, 0.94, or 1.88 krads. Dotted areas indicate the difference between net cell losses of the nonproliferating pool and average cell losses. Arrows indicate the time period of tumor regrowth. For explanation and interpretation of data, see text. From Potmesil *et al.* (1975), with permission of *Cell and Tissue Kinetics.*

371

STEM CELLS,
NON-
PROLIFERATING
CELLS, AND
THEIR
KINETICS

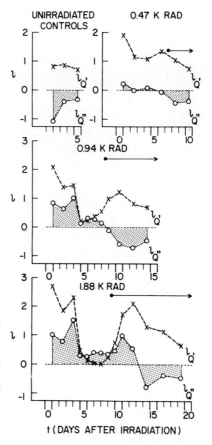

FIGURE 6. Net cell loss rates $l_{Q'}$ (cells with trabeculate nucleoli), and net cell loss rates $l_{Q'}$ (cells with ring-shaped nucleoli) calculated as a function of time for control unirradiated tumors and tumors irradiated with a single dose of 0.47, 0.94, or 1.88 krads. Dotted areas indicate positive or negative values of $l_{Q'}$. Arrows indicate the time period of tumor regrowth. For explanation and interpretation of data, see text. From Potmesil *et al.* (1975), with the permission of *Cell and Tissue Kinetics*.

following observations in normal and neoplastic cells: (1) maturation and differentiation of normal thymocytes are accompanied by cessation of their proliferation and by sequential changes of their nucleoli from dense to trabeculate to ring-shaped (Potmesil and Goldfeder, 1973); (2) cells with ring-shaped nucleoli represent not only the differentiated cell population of various malignant disorders (Smetana *et al.*, 1966, 1970), but also a subpopulation of blast cells in a "resting" state (Smetana *et al.*, 1966); there is evidence that certain "resting" neoplastic cells can be triggered into proliferation (Rosen *et al.*, 1970; Omine and Perry, 1972); (3) transformation of "resting" mature lymphocytes into proliferating blastoid cells by phytohemagglutinin is accompanied by changes of ring-shaped nucleoli into trabeculate and dense nucleoli (Potmesil and Smetana, 1970). Cell net loss rates calculated for cells with trabeculate nucleoli (Q') and cells with ring-shaped nucleoli (Q'') indicate net transition from Q'' to Q' before the onset of rapid regrowth (Fig. 6). This transition was followed 2–3 days later by transitions of Q' to the proliferating pool. The results, although crude, indicate the periods during which cell transitions between the nonproliferating and proliferating pools and between the pools of cells with trabeculate and cells with ring-shaped nucleoli seem to be significant, and the direction in which they occur. The

372

MILAN
POTMESIL,
JOSEPH
LOBUE,
AND
ANNA
GOLDFEDER

data suggest that cell transition from the nonproliferating to the proliferating cell pool takes place at the beginning of tumor regrowth after subcurative single-dose irradiation. These observations have been further substantiated by direct experimental demonstration of cell recruitment (Potmesil *et al.*, 1977). Tumor-bearing mice were repeatedly injected with [^{3}H]TdR, and the tumors were irradiated with a single dose of 2350 rads. A repeated administration of the label was continued thereafter, and tumors were sampled at various time intervals after irradiation. Ten hours before sacrifice, mice were injected with vincristine sulfate. The [^{3}H]TdR grain distribution over mitosis arrested in metaphase had a different pattern in tumors regrowing after irradiation when compared with unirradiated controls: two clearly delineated groups of mitoses emerged in irradiated tumors, one with grain counts corresponding to the background level and the other with a heavy label. As the only source of unlabeled mitoses at the beginning of regrowth were the remaining unlabeled cells with trabeculate and ring-shaped nucleoli belonging to the nonproliferating pool, this observation indicates that cell transition from the nonproliferating to the proliferating pool takes place in irradiated experimental mouse mammary carcinomas at the start of their regrowth.

5. Summary and Conclusions

It is well recognized that utilization of cytokinetics as a rational guide to cancer therapy should differentiate between responses of stem cells in normal critical tissues and neoplastic stem cells to various protocols of chemotherapy or radiation. Stem cells, defined as cells capable of "unlimited" self-replication, under steady-state conditions supply progeny for differentiation and maintain a pool of progenitors. They also respond to emergency conditions by enhanced proliferation and cytodifferentiation into progeny. There are several model system applicable to the characterization of the cytokinetics of tumor stem cells. A hypothetical polycompartmental system suggests the kinetics of tumor progression and remission, and the "feeder-and-sleeper" concept describes stem cells in two different states, either dormant or proliferating. The latter concept, corresponding to an asynchronous-logarithmic system, also accounts for heterogeneity of stem cell populations and their clonal development and succession (Section 2.1). A variety of methods have been designed to investigate clonogenic properties of the stem cell compartment of hematopoietic tissue. Hematopoietic stem cells can be assayed as endogenous or exogenous colony-forming units *in vivo* in the spleen (CFU-s) and also in culture (CFU-c, CFU-e, etc.). There are a number of assays evaluating responses of neoplasm to therapy, such as *in situ* inhibition of regrowth, tumor cure rate, or stem cell survival. The former two assays applied as either a "regrowth delay" or TCD$_{50}$ do not render any direct analysis of cell populations. Stem cell end-point dilution techniques test colony formation of single-cell suspensions *in vitro* or *in vivo* in recipient animals. However, marked toxic effects on tumor cells have been observed in mechanically and enzymatically prepared single-cell suspensions, and under these conditions only a part of the original stem cell population may retain its clonogenicity. Thus results of assays may vary substantially because of differing techniques and resulting experimental conditions. End-point clonogenic assays do not give any indication of the proliferative status of stem cells in the assayed tumor, i.e., whether stem cells were fast- or slow-proliferating or were arrested in some phase of the cell cycle. These assays are easily applicable for undifferentiated, fast-proliferating experimental tumors, whereas the clonogenic efficiency of differentiated tumors is low and the abovementioned assays may not be suitable (Section 2.2). Attempts have been made to identify hematopoietic CFU-s morphologically. Data from numerous experiments using separation and label techniques and other methods suggest that the "candidate" stem cell may be a member of a heterogeneous group known as the "transitional lymphocyte." Stem cells of other normal tissues, namely, of the epidermis and intestinal epithelium, are confined to specific regions in organs. With very few exceptions, current methods cannot identify tumor stem cells morphologically. There are indications that human leukemic stem cells exist in two forms, either as proliferating large blasts or as nonproliferating small blasts. This has its analogy in an experimentally demonstrable situation: stem cells in thymic lymphomas of AKR mice are among the large, proliferating cells and also among the small, nonproliferating cells. A large body of evidence indicates that in human as well as in experimental solid tumors, most products of abnormal mitoses die after having accomplished only a few divisions; that cells bearing the same array of chromosomes or the same mode of DNA content are considered as members of the same mutant clone, descendants from a common ancestor; and that the selection is always for the fastest or most efficiently growing mutant clone which represents the main mode of chromosome number or DNA content. It can be speculated that most or all stem cells traversing the cell cycle belong to the cell cohort of this stemline (Section 2.3). Stem cells, temporarily confined to the nonproliferating pool, may play an important kinetic role in the proliferative pattern of blast cells in human leukemia. It seems reasonable to assume that leukemic stem cells as well as stem cells of some differentiated tumors may retain a certain degree of homeostatic control, leading to differentiation into relatively mature forms with some function expressed. It is also proposed that mechanical pressure and changes in cell density and contact could be important factors in determining the rate of stem cell proliferation (Section 2.4). Available cytogenetic data show that human and experimental animal tumors are clonal in nature, with a successive appearance of differing stem cell lines which are variants of a predominant single clone. Stem cell lines may differ from each other, for example, in their capacity to differentiate (Sections 2.3 and 2.4).

The essential feature of cell multiplication in many systems is the alteration of resting periods with periods of active proliferation, which is a necessary prerequisite for size control of cell populations, cell differentiation, and adaptation to changing microenvironmental conditions. Nonproliferating cells are either restricted in their slow progression to one phase of the cycle or exhibit no apparent

MILAN
POTMESIL,
JOSEPH
LOBUE,
AND
ANNA
GOLDFEDER

progression at all. Differences between cells proceeding through a long G_1 phase and cells arrested in G_0 seem to be established in some systems by their pattern of entry into the cell cycle upon appropriate stimulation, by differences in some of the biochemical events leading to DNA synthesis (especially the actinomycin D resistant stage in the prereplicative period of G_0 cells), and by an increase in template activity due to synthesis of new species of nonhistone chromosomal proteins traced in stimulated G_0 cells. It has also been shown that cells in numerous normal and neoplastic tissues are suspended in the G_2 phase of the cell cycle (Section 3.1). A variety of different techniques have been utilized to investigate cell proliferation kinetics and to distinguish "nonproliferating" from "proliferating" cells. [³H]TdR autoradiography has often been employed. Several difficulties can make interpretation of labeling studies troublesome: reutilization of the label, radiotoxicity, unexpectedly low incorporation rate in some tissues, "self-absorption" of β-particles, the long-lived pool of labeled DNA precursors, the size of endogenous thymidine pool, and also the establishment of background levels for quantitative autoradiographic techniques. Cytophotometry is another technique which has been applied for localization of cells in different phases of the cell cycle. However, this method provides only limited information on the number and distribution of nonproliferating cells through the cycle, even when combined with autoradiography. The mean reason is irregular ploidy of cells in most human and animal tumors. The method also cannot discriminate between viable and dead cells. Combination of cytophotometry with continuous [³H]TdR labeling of cells of a diploid line in tissue culture gives a good estimate of cell distribution within the cycle. Electronic cell sorting by volume and cell separation techniques may isolate nonproliferating cells which differ in their volume and density from proliferating cells. Intracellular fluorescence can also serve as a differentiating parameter for high-speed sorting of large numbers of cells (Section 3.2). Cell size, or, in a more precise way, DNA content of cells can be used under specific conditions for morphological identification of nonproliferating cells. As discussed in some detail, the chromosome number in most solid tumors varies from an impressive hypodiploidy to triploidy, tetraploidy, and multiple abnormalities. Under these circumstances, estimation of DNA content provides rather ambiguous correlation with cell distribution in the cell cycle. Various biochemical and histochemical techniques can detect structural alterations of chromatin within cell-cycle phases, but none of these methods can differentiate cells with a short passage through a particular phase (e.g., G_1) from nonproliferating cells residing in that phase. The morphology of cell nucleoli is related to the extent of their ribonucleoprotein biosynthesis, and this in turn in most systems relates to the capacity of cells to trigger DNA synthesis and divide. Nucleoli can be used as morphological "markers" of proliferating and nonproliferating cells in a variety of normal tissues and also in neoplasms (Section 3.3). The "growth fraction" is defined as the proportion of cells participating in the cell cycle and can be calculated by several methods. The usefulness of some of these methods is limited by the reduced ability of labeled-mitoses curves to reflect the behavior of slowly proliferating cells. The size of the fraction of nonproliferating cells may be suggested by the deficit between the growth fraction and the total cell population. In a variety of human tumors, the number of nonproliferating cells is highly variable but usually quite high. Experimental tumors have various proportions of nonproliferating cells, the lowest in serially transplanted sarcomas and the highest in differentiated carcinomas, autochthonous or with limited number of transplants. A morphologically defined population of cells in G_0 or long G_1 phase was demonstrated in thymic lymphomas of AKR mice, and comparable results were also reached for human acute leukemia. Transplantation of "old" ascites tumors with a sizable portion of cells slowly progressing through G_1 drastically shortens the cell-cycle duration and narrows the distribution of cell-cycle times. This suggests that after transplantation a fraction of slowly proliferating cells is triggered to a fast proliferation. Cytodifferentiation is expressed in various degrees in leukemias and in a number of solid tumors. Differentiation of neoplastic cells can be enhanced in some systems by treatment *in vivo* or *in vitro*. This indicates that malignant changes do not completely prevent cell differentiation, and such differentiation may lead to specialized cells which are incapable of division and therefore "nonmalignant." Differentiation may be the prevailing intrinsic cause of cell death in some tumors (Section 3.4). Resistance to cell-cycle phase-specific drugs, and also to some extent to phase-nonspecific chemicals, is enhanced in plateau-phase cells in tissue cultures as compared with cells in exponential growth. Cells in a plateau phase, mostly slowly proliferating or nonproliferating, seem to have a capacity to repair sublethal and potentially lethal damage induced by chemicals and irradiation. Moreover, there are indications that slowly proliferating or nonproliferating cells in experimental ascitic and solid tumors can repair their potentially lethal damage, as well as sublethal injury. Viable hypoxic cells have been demonstrated in various tumors and represent the radioresistant component of the cell population. A major part of viable hypoxic cells is believed to be nonproliferating. It appears that nonproliferating or slowly proliferating cells of normal and malignant tissues *in vivo* are not only resistant to cell-cycle phase-specific agents but also relatively insensitive to cell-cycle nonspecific agents. It follows that differences in sensitivity to cytotoxic agents are, at least in some experimental systems, a consequence of the proliferative status of the cell population in question. It should be mentioned that the kinetic status of cells alone is not an absolute parameter determining their sensitivity to drugs. There are other factors involved, such as uptake of the drug by cells, drug distribution within a cell, efficiency of various enzyme systems participating in drug catabolism and in repair of induced damage (Section 3.4).

There is clinical evidence that neoplastic cells may persist for a considerable time in a state of "latency," but with their clonogenicity preserved. Upon appropriate stimulation, these cells may be recruited into proliferation, and this leads to recurrences of the neoplastic disease. "Recruitment" is a term designating both the induction of nonproliferating cells into proliferation and the acceleration of cell progression through a specific cell-cycle phase, followed by traverse of subsequent phases and by cell division. Cell depletion after therapy may trigger or enhance the extent of cell recruitment. Partial synchrony of cell progression

376

MILAN
POTMESIL,
JOSEPH
LOBUE,
AND
ANNA
GOLDFEDER

through the cell cycle and cell recruitment might be simultaneous, and cells recruited into the cell cycle may be clonogens as well as cells with a limited capacity for cell division (Section 4.1). Recruitment has been advocated as an important component of treatment schedules in clinical combination therapy. Adverse effects of a single therapeutic agent, such as acceleration of tumor growth rates, shortening of cell-cycle times, and increase in the fraction of proliferating cells and clonogens during the period of tumor recurrences, may be at least partially attributed to recruitment of nonproliferating stem cells into the cell cycle. It is of particular interest in clinical studies that tumors with a high proliferative potential, or tumors with a high proliferation induced by therapeutic manipulation, respond best to chemotherapy. The complexity of factors that determine the growth of tumors also influences their response to treatment. Slowly growing and differentiated tumors of man and experimental animals, with a small growth fraction and substantial portion of "resting" or slowly proliferating cells, are relatively resistant to treatment. It remains to be critically determined whether good results of combination therapy are caused by modification of cell kinetics or by other factors. "Uncrowding" of tissue-culture neoplastic cells and surgical dissection of experimental tumors accelerate growth and increase the proliferating pool, thus making cells more susceptible to various treatment regimes. It seems certain that the proliferation rate in human tumors is rarely higher than that observed in most critical normal tissues. However, selective responses based on differential cell proliferation can be obtained should the accelerated rate of tumor growth exceed that of normal tissue. Under these conditions, the tumor tissue would become more vulnerable to sequential therapy by cycle-phase specific drugs (Section 4.2). Cells in some renewal tissues seem to be in a true G_0 state and can be induced to enter the proliferating pool if appropriate stimulation is applied. A complex and interdependent series of biochemical events occurs in stimulated G_0 cells of normal tissue during their prereplicative phase before the onset of DNA synthesis. Stimulated G_0 cells enter the S phase gradually after a lag period. The most apparent feature of other renewal systems, such as bone marrow, is the early recruitment of stem cells into cell cycle. Upon stimulation, at least some of them may be released from a long G_1 traverse; cells arrested in G_2 phase can also be recruited into proliferation. It cannot be stated with assurance whether nonproliferating tumor cells are in a "resting" stage corresponding to G_0, or in a long G_1. Clear distinction between the kinetics of nonproliferating or slowly proliferating cells may not exist, at least not in tumors. Recruitment of nonproliferating ("potential") stem cells has been suggested in clinical studies of human acute leukemia, whereas clonogenic potential of nonproliferating neoplastic cells has been irrefutably demonstrated *in vivo* in only one experimental system. However, recruitment of nonproliferating cells may be detected under favorable conditions in some neoplasms after treatment, at the start of tumor regrowth. There are also indications based on mathematical analysis of experimental results that cell transition from the nonproliferating to the proliferating pool takes place at the beginning of tumor regrowth after subcurative single-dose irradiation. This conclusion has been further substantiated by direct experimental evidence (Section 4.3).

In conclusion, some aspects of the proliferating and slowly proliferating components of cell populations in both normal tissues and neoplasms have been summarized. In *normal renewal tissue*, under steady-state conditions, only a limited number of stem cells are involved in active proliferation, whereas the other part of the stem cell population is "resting." It is well established that stem cells of certain normal tissues enter a G_0 or G_1-prolonged phase, in which they retain proliferative capacity but do not enter S phase unless appropriately stimulated. Likewise, cells arrested in G_2 phase may be stimulated to division. Cells in G_0 or prolonged G_1 phase may retain their clonogenic potential for varying periods of time. Homeostatic mechanisms regulate pool size by controlling entry and exit of stem cells into G_0 or extended G_1, and this may lead, upon stimulation, either to a transition of G_0 cells into the proliferating pool or to acceleration of G_1 traverse. Other control mechanisms operate at different stages of cell maturation. In *undifferentiated, rapidly proliferating tumors* (e.g., most experimental tumors after numerous passages of transplants), the proliferating pool consists of a large fraction of tumor stem cells. Some of the proliferating cells may have a prolonged traverse through G_1, which becomes shortened upon stimulation. Such cells, which exhibit various degrees of differentiation, may also remain in G_1 phase before their death and removal. In *differentiated, slowly proliferating tumors* (most human and some experimental tumors), the proliferating pool consists of a small fraction of tumor stem cells and a large fraction of doomed but still proliferating cells. Cells of the latter fraction gradually slow their traverse through the cell cycle and eventually leave it. This diversity would account for the wide spread in intermitotic times observed in differentiated tumors. Just as stem cells in normal renewal tissue, tumor stem cells may be either proliferating, slowly proliferating, or nonproliferating. It is not clear whether a true G_0 phase exists in tumors, or whether "nonproliferating" tumor cells simply traverse G_1 phases of various duration. A low rate of rRNA-precursor synthesis estimated in cells residing in G_0 or G_1 phase correlates with nucleolar morphology of nonproliferating or slowly proliferating neoplastic cells. Thus this morphological marker is highly useful for kinetic studies of various cell populations. Malignant cells may retain some characteristics similar to those of the normal cells from which they originated. This holds true not only for their biochemical and morphological differentiation, but also for their kinetic pattern, which might be governed by partially preserved homeostatic regulatory mechanisms pertinent to the tissue of origin. It can then be speculated that one class of cells accelerates its G_1 traverse after stimulation and another releases cells into cell cycle with a delay comparable to G_0 transition in normal tissue. During the time of delay, repair of damage induced by therapeutic agents might have already been completed. The population of nonproliferating or slowly proliferating cells is probably heterogeneous, with various degrees of differentiation, age distribution, drug sensitivity, and with a potential for repair of therapeutically induced damage. Clonogenicity may be retained in some cells for a

378

MILAN
POTMESIL,
JOSEPH
LOBUE,
AND
ANNA
GOLDFEDER

variable period of time. These properties of nonproliferating cells might be strongly influenced by changing microenvironmental conditions in neoplastic tissues.

ACKNOWLEDGMENTS

The author wishes to thank Blanche Ciotti, Amando Roquillo, and Dennis M. Brown for their secretarial and technical assistance.

Preparation of this chapter and the original work reported were supported by research grants from NIH-DHEW (R01-CA 12076, R01-CA 12815, and R01–HL 03357), from the Mildred Werner League for Cancer Research, and from the National Leukemia Association, Inc.

6. References

ABSHER, P. M., ABSHER, R. G., AND BARNES, W. D., 1974, Genealogies of clones of diploid fibroblasts, *Exp. Cell Res.* **88:**95.

ADELMAN, R. C., STEIN, G., ROTH, G. S., AND ENGLANDER, D., 1972, Age-dependent regulation of mammalian DNA-synthesis and cell proliferation *in vivo, Mech. Ageing Dev.* 1:49.

ADELSTEIN, S. J., AND LYMAN, C. P., 1968, Pyrimidine nucleoside metabolism in mammalian cells: An *in vitro* comparison of two rodent species, *Exp. Cell Res.* **50:**104.

ADELSTEIN, S. J., LYMAN, C. P., AND O'BRIEN, R. C., 1964, Variation in the incorporation of thymidine into DNA in some rodent species, *Comp. Biochem. Physiol.* **12:**223.

ALVAREZ, Y., AND VALLADARES, Y., 1972, Differential staining of the cell cycle, *Nature (London) New Biol.* **238:**279.

APPLETON, D., MORLY, A. R., AND WRIGHT, N. A., 1973, Cell proliferation in the castrate mouse seminal vesicle in response to testosterone propionate. II. Theoretical Considerations, *Cell Tissue Kinet.* **6:**267.

AROESTY, J., LINCOLN, T., SHAPIRO, N., AND BOCCIA, G., 1973, Tumor growth and chemotherapy: Mathematical methods, computer simulations and experimental foundations, *Math. Biosci.* **17:**243.

ASTALDI, G., AND AIRO, R., 1967, Phytohaemagglutinin and human lymphocytes in short-term cell culture, in: *The Lymphocyte in Immunology and Haemopoiesis* (J. M. YOFFEY, ed.), Edward Arnold Publishers, London.

ATKIN, N. B., 1970, Cytogenetic studies on human tumors and premalignant lesions: The emergence of aneuploid cell lines and their relationship to the process of malignant transformation in man, in: *Genetic Concepts and Neoplasia*, 23rd Ann. Symp. Fund. Cancer Res., Williams and Wilkins, Baltimore.

ATKIN, N. B., 1971, Modal DNA values and chromosome number in ovarian neoplasia, *Cancer* **27:**1064.

ATKIN, N. B., AND BAKER, M. C., 1966, Chromosome abnormalities as primary events in human malignant disease, *J. Natl. Cancer Inst.* **36:**539.

ATKIN, N. B., MATTISON, G., AND BAKER, M. C., 1966, A comparison of the DNA content and chromosome number of fifty human tumors, *Br. J. Cancer* **20:**87.

AUER, G., AND ZETTERBERG, A., 1972, The role of nuclear proteins in RNA synthesis, *Exp. Cell Res.* **75:**245.

AUGENLICHT, L. H., AND BASERGA, R., 1974, Changes in G_0 state of WI-38 fibroblasts at different times after confluence, *Exp. Cell Res.* **89:**255.

BARENDSEN, G. W., 1974, Characteristics of tumor responses to different radiations and the relative biological effectiveness of fast neutrons, *Eur. J. Cancer* **10:**269.

BARENDSEN, G. W., AND BROERSE, J. J., 1969, Experimental radiotherapy of a rat rhabdomyosarcoma with 15 MeV neutrons and 300 kV X-rays. I. Effects of single exposures, *Eur. J. Cancer* **5:**373.

379

STEM CELLS,
NON-
PROLIFERATING
CELLS, AND
THEIR
KINETICS

BARENDSEN, G. W., AND BROERSE, J. J., 1970, Experimental radiotherapy of a rat rhabdomyosarcoma with 15 meV neutrons and 300 kV X-rays. II. Effects of fractionated treatments, applied five times a week for several weeks, *Eur. J. Cancer* **6**:89.

BARENDSEN, G. W., BROERSE, J. J., HERMENS, A. F., MADHUIZEN, H. T., VAN PEPERZEEL, H. H., AND RUTGERS, D. H., 1973, Clonogenic capacity of proliferating and nonproliferating cells of a transplantable rat rhabdomyosarcoma in relation to its readiosensitivity, *J. Natl. Cancer Inst.* **51**:1521.

BARLOGIE, B., DREWINKO, B. B., SCHUMANN, J., AND FREIREICH, E. J., 1976, Pulse cytophotometric analysis of cell cycle perturbation with bleomycin *in vitro*, *Cancer Res.* **36**:1182.

BARR, R. D., WHANG-PENG, J., AND PERRY, S., 1975, Hematopoietic stem cells in human peripheral blood, *Science* **190**:284.

BARRANCO, S. C., AND NOVAK, J. K., 1974, Survival responses of dividing and nondividing mammalian cells after treatment with hydroxyurea, arabinosylcytosine, or adriamycin, *Cancer Res.* **34**:1616.

BARRANCO, S. C., NOVAK, J. K., AND HUMPHREY, R. M., 1973, Response of mammalian cells following treatment with bleomycin and 1,3-bis-(2-chloroethyl)-1-nitrosourea during plateau phase, *Cancer Res.* **33**:691.

BARRANCO, S. C., NOVAK, J. K., AND HUMPHREY, R. M., 1975, Studies on recovery from chemically-induced damage in mammalian cells, *Cancer Res.* **35**:1194.

BASERGA, R., 1968, Biochemistry of the cell cycle: A review, *Cell Tissue Kinet.* **1**:167.

BASERGA, R., 1973, Control of cellular proliferation in mammalian cells, in: *Unifying Concepts of Leukemia* (R. M. DUTCHER AND L. CHIECO-BIANCHI, eds.), Karger, Basel.

BASERGA, R., AND GOLD, R., 1963, Uptake of tritiated thymidine by newly transplanted Ehrlich ascites tumor cells, *Exp. Cell Res.* **31**:576.

BASERGA, R., AND MALAMUD, D., 1969, *Autoradiography, Techniques and Applications*, Harper and Row, New York.

BASERGA, R., AND STEIN, G., 1971, Nuclear acidic proteins and cell proliferation, *Fed. Proc.* **30**:1752.

BASERGA, R., AND WIEBEL, F., 1969, The cell cycle of mammalian cells, *Int. Rev. Exp. Pathol.* **7**:1.

BASERGA, R., KISIELESKI, W. E., AND HALVORSEN, K., 1960, A study on the establishment and growth of tumor metastases with tritiated thymidine, *Cancer Res.* **20**:910.

BASERGA, R., TYLER, S. A., AND KISIELESKI, W. E., 1963, The kinetics of growth of the Ehrlich tumor, *Arch. Pathol.* **76**:9.

BASERGA, R., ESTENSEN, R. D., AND PETERSEN, R. O., 1965, Inhibition of DNA synthesis in Ehrlich ascites cells by actinomycin D. II. The presynthetic block in the cell cycle, *Proc. Natl. Acad. Sci. USA* **54**:1141.

BECKER, F. F., 1973, Humoral aspects of liver regeneration, in: *Humoral Control of Growth and Differentiation*, Vol. I (J. LOBUE and A. S. GORDON, eds.), Academic Press, New York.

BECKER, F. F., WOLMAN, S. R., ASOFSKY, R., AND SELLS, S., 1975, Sequential analysis of transplantable hepatocellular carcinomas, *Cancer Res.* **35**:3026.

BELLI, J. A., DICUS, J. G. AND BONTE, F. J., 1967, Radiation response of mammalian tumor cells. I Repair of sublethal damage *in vivo*, *J. Natl. Cancer Inst.* **38**:673.

BELLI, J. A., DICUS, J. G., AND NAGLE, W., 1970, Repair of radiation damage as a factor in preoperative radiation therapy, in: *The Interrelationship of Surgery and Radiation Therapy in the Treatment of Cancer* (J. M. VAETH, ed.), *Front. Radiat. Ther. Oncol.* **5**:40.

BENASSI, M., PAOLUZI, R., AND BRESCIANI, F., 1973, Computer subtraction of background in autoradiography with tritiated thymidine, *Cell Tissue Kinet.* **6**:81.

BENDER, M. A., AND PRESCOTT, D. M., 1962, DNA synthesis and mitosis in cultures of human peripheral leukocytes, *Exp. Cell Res.* **27**:221.

BENNINGTON, J. L., 1969, Cellular kinetics of invasive squamous carcinoma of human cervix, *Cancer Res.* **29**:1082.

BERGSAGEL, D. E., AND VALERIOTE, F. A., 1968, Growth characteristics of a mouse plasma cell tumor, *Cancer Res.* **28**:2187.

BERRY, R. J., AND ANDREWS, J. R., 1961, Quantitative studies of radiation effects on cell reproductive capacity in mammalian transplantable tumor system *in vivo*, *Ann. N.Y. Acad. Sci.* **95**:1001.

BERRY, R. J., AND ANDREWS, J. R., 1962, Modification of the radiation effect on the reproductive capacity of tumor cells *in vivo* with pharmacological agents, *Radiat. Res.* **16**:84.

BHUYAN, B. K., SCHEIDT, L. G., AND FRASER, T. J., 1972, Cell cycle phase specificity of antitumor agents, *Cancer Res.* **32**:398.

BHUYAN, B. K., LOUGHMAN, B. E., FRASER, T. J., AND DAY, K. J., 1976, Comparison of different methods of determining cell viability after exposure to cytotoxic compounds, *Exp. Cell Res.* **97**:275.

380

MILAN
POTMESIL,
JOSEPH
LOBUE,
AND
ANNA
GOLDFEDER

BIBBO, M., BARTELS, P. H., BAHR, G. F., TAYLOR, J., AND WIED, G. L., 1973, Computer recognition of cell nuclei from the uterine cervix, *Acta Cytol.* **17**:340.

BICHEL, P., 1970, Tumor growth inhibiting effect of JB-1 ascitic fluid. I. An *in vivo* investigation, *Eur. J. Cancer* **6**:291.

BICHEL, P., AND DOMBERNOWSKY, P., 1973, On the resting stages of the JB-1 ascites tumor, *Cell Tissue Kinet.* **6**:359.

BLACKETT, N. M., 1968, Investigations of bone marrow stem cell proliferation in normal, anemic and irradiated rats using methotrexate and tritiated thymidine, *J. Natl. Cancer Inst.* **41**:909.

BLOCK, P., SEITER, L., AND OEHLERT, W., 1963, Autoradiographic studies of the initial cellular response to injury, *Exp. Cell Res.* **30**:311.

BOGGS, D. R., AND CHERVENICK, P. A., 1973, Chemotherapy and leukokinetics, in *Cancer Chemotherapy II.*, The 22nd Hahnemann Symposium (I. BRODSKY, B. KAHN, AND J. H. MOYER, eds.), Grune and Stratton, New York.

BÖHM, N., SPRINGER, E., AND SANDRITTER, W., 1971, Fluorescence cytophotometric Feulgen-DNA measurements of benign and malignant human tumors, *Beitr. Pathol. Bd.*, **142**:210.

BOHNE, F., HASS, R. J., FLIEDNER, T. M., AND FACHE, I., 1970, The role of slowly proliferating cells in rat bone marrow during regeneration following hydroxyurea, *Br. J. Haematol.* **19**:533.

BORSA, J., AND WHITMORE, G. F., 1969, Cell kinetic studies on the mode of action of methotrexate on L-cells *in vitro*, *Cancer Res.* **29**:737.

BRADLEY, T. R., AND METCALF, D., 1966, The growth of mouse bone marrow cells *in vitro*, *Aust. J. Exp. Biol. Med. Sci.* **44**:287.

BRENT, T. P., 1971, Periodicity of DNA synthetic enzymes during the HeLa cell cycle, *Cell Tissue Kinet.* **4**:297.

BRESCIANI, F., 1965, Effect of ovarian hormones on duration of DNA synthesis in cells of the C3H mouse mammary gland, *Exp. Cell Res.* **38**:13.

BRESCIANA, F., 1968, Cell proliferation in cancer, *Eur. J. Cancer* **4**:343.

BRIGANTI, G., GALLOIN, L., LEVI, G., SPALLETA, V., AND MAURO, F., 1975, Effects of bleomycin on mouse bone marrow stem cells, *J. Natl. Cancer Inst.* **55**:53.

BROWN, J. M., 1968, Long G_1 or G_0 state: A method of resolving the dilemma for the cell cycle of an *in vivo* population, *Exp. Cell Res.* **52**:565.

BROWN, J. M., 1975, Exploitation of kinetic differences between normal and malignant cells, *Radiology* **114**:189.

BRUCE, W. R., AND MEEKER, B. E., 1964, Dissemination and growth of transplanted isologous murine lymphoma cells, *J. Natl. Cancer Inst.* **32**:1145.

BRUCE, W. R., AND MEEKER, B. E., 1967, Comparison of the sensitivity of hematopoietic colony-forming cells in different proliferative states to 5-fluorouracil, *J. Natl. Cancer. Inst.* **38**:401.

BRUCE, W. R., AND VAN DEN GAAG, H., 1963, A quantitative assay for the number of murine lymphoma cells capable of proliferation *in vivo*, *Nature (London)* **199**:79.

BRUCE, W. R., MEEKER, B. E., AND VALERIOTE, F. A., 1966, Comparison of the sensitivity of normal hematopoietic and transplanted lymphoma colony-forming cells to chemotherapeutic agents administered *in vivo*, *J. Natl. Cancer Inst.* **37**:233.

BUCHER, N. L. R., 1963, Regeneration of mammalian liver, *Int. Rev. Cytol.* **15**:245.

BUCHER, N. L. R., 1967a, Experimental aspects of hepatic regeneration, *New Engl. J. Med.* **277**:686.

BUCHER, N. L. R. 1967b, Experimental aspects of hepatic regeneration (concluded), *N. Engl. J. Med.* **277**:738.

BUCHER, N. L. R., AND SWAFFIELD, M. N., 1964, The rate of incorporation of labelled thymidine into deoxyribonucleic acid or regenerating rat liver in relation to the amount of liver excised, *Cancer Res.* **24**:1611.

BURCHENAL, J. H., 1973, The future of cancer chemotherapy, in: *Seventh National Cancer Conference Proceedings*, Lippincott, Philadelphia.

BURKI, H. J., AND OKADA, S., 1968, A comparison of killing of cultured mammalian cells induced by decay of incorporated tritiated molecules at $-196°C$, *Biophys. J.* **8**:445.

BURKI, H. J., AND OKADA, S., 1970, Killing of cultured mammalian cells by radition decay of tritiated thymidine, *Radiat. Res.* **41**:409.

BURKI, H. J., BUNKER, S., RITTER, M., AND CLEAVER, J. E., 1975, DNA damage from incorporated radioisotopes: Influence of the ⁵H location in the cell, *Radiat. Res.* **62**:299.

BURKI, K., SCHAER, J. C., GRIEDER, A., SCHINDLER, R., AND COTTIER, H., 1971, Studies on liver regeneration. I. ¹³¹Iododeoxyuridine as a precursor of DNA in normal and regenerating rat liver, *Cell Tissue Kinet.* **4**:519.

381

STEM CELLS,
NON-
PROLIFERATING
CELLS, AND
THEIR
KINETICS

BURNS, E. R., 1968, Initiation of DNA synthesis in Ehrlich ascites tumor in their plateau phase of growth, *Cancer Res.* **28**:1191.

BURNS, F. J., AND TANNOCK, I. F., 1970, On the existence of a G_0-phase in the cell cycle, *Cell Tissue Kinet.* **3**:321.

BUSCH, H., AND SMETANA, K., 1970, *The Nucleolus*, Academic Press, New York.

BUSCH, H., AND SMETANA, K., 1974, The nucleus of the cancer cell, in: *The Molecular Biology of Cancer*, Academic Press, New York.

CAMERON, I. L., AND CLEFFMAN, G., 1964, Initiation of mitoses in relation to the cell cycle following feeding of starved chickens, *J. Cell Biol.* **21**:169.

CASPERSSON, T., AND LOMAKKA, G., 1962, Scanning microscopic techniques for high resolution quantitative cytochemistry, *Ann N.Y. Acad. Sci.* **97**:449.

CASPERSSON, T., LOMAKKA, G., AND CASPERSSON, O., 1960, Quantitative cytochemical methods for the study of tumor cell populations, *Biochem. Pharmacol.* **4**:113.

CATER, D. B., HOLMES, B. E., AND MEE, L. K., 1956, Cell division and nucleic acid synthesis in the regenerating liver of the rat, *Acta Radiol.* **46**:655.

CECCARINI, C., 1975, Effect of pH on plating efficiency, serum requirement, and incorporation of radioactive precursors into human cells, *In Vitro* **11**:78.

CHANG, L. O., AND LOONEY, W. B., 1965, A biochemical and autoradiographic study of the *in vivo* utilization of tritiated thymidine in regenerating rat liver, *Cancer Res.* **25**:1817.

CHERVENICK, P. A., AND BOGGS, D. R., 1971, *In vitro* growth of granulocytic and mononuclear cell colonies from blood of normal individuals, *Blood* **37**:131.

CHEVALIER, S., AND VERLY, W. G., 1975, Identification of the inhibitor of labelled thymidine incorporation into HeLa cell DNA present in endometrial extract, *Eur. J. Cancer* **11**:657.

CHRISTOPHERS, E., 1971, Cellular architecture of the stratum corneum, *J. Invest. Dermatol.* **56**:165.

CHUANG, S.-N., AND LLOYD, H. H., 1975, Mathematical analysis of cancer chemotherapy, *Bull. Math. Biol.* **37**:147.

ČIHÁK, A., SEIFERTOVÁ, M., VESELÝ, J., AND ŠORM, F., 1972, Enhanced synthesis of DNA in liver of 5-azacytidine-treated rats subjected to partial hepatectomy, *Int. J. Cancer* **10**:20.

ČIHÁK, A., SEIFERTOVÁ, M., AND RICHES, P., 1976, Enhanced incorporation of thymidine into DNA in the liver of intact and partially hepatectomized rats pretreated with 5-azacytidine, *Cancer Res.* **36**:37.

CLARKSON, B. D., 1974, The survival value of the dormant state in neoplastic and normal cell populations, in: *Control of Proliferation in Animal Cells* (B. D. CLARKSON AND R. BASERGA, eds.), Cold Spring Harbor Laboratory, Cold Spring Harbor, N.Y.

CLARKSON, B. D., AND FRIED, J., 1971, Changing concepts of treatment in acute leukemia, *Med. Clin. North Am.* **55**:561.

CLARKSON, B. D., OTA, K., OHKITA, T., AND O'CONNOR, A., 1965, Kinetics of proliferation of cancer cells in neoplastic effusions in man, *Cancer* **18**:1189.

CLARKSON, B. D., FRIED, J., AND OGAWA, M., 1969, Magnitude of proliferating fraction and rate of proliferation of populations of leukemic cells in man, in: *Normal and Malignant Cell Growth* (R. M. J. FRY, M. L. GRIEM, AND W. H. KIRSTEN, eds.), Springer-Verlag, New York.

CLEAVER, J. E., 1967, *Thymidine Metabolism and Cell Kinetics*, Wiley, New York.

CLIFTON, K. H., AND COOPER, J. M., 1973, Reutilization of thymidine and iododeoxyuridine by mouse mammary carcinoma MTG-B, *Proc. Soc. Exp. Biol. Med.* **142**:1145.

CLIFTON, K. H., AND YATVIN, M. B., 1970, Cell population growth and cell loss in the MTG-B mouse mammary carcinoma, *Cancer Res.* **30**:658.

COHEN, L. A., TSUANG, J., AND CHAN, P.-C., 1974, Characteristics of rat normal mammary epithelial cells and dimethylbenzanthracene-induced mammary adenocarcinoma cells grown in monolayer culture, *In Vitro* **10**:51.

COLLINS, V. P., LOEFFLER, R. K., AND TIVEY, H., 1956, Observations on growth rates of human tumors, *Am. J. Roentgenol.* **76**:988.

COMAS, F. V., AND BYRD, B. L., 1967, Hemopoietic spleen colonies in the rat, *Radiat. Res.* **32**:355.

COOPER, E. H., 1973, The biology of cell death in tumors, *Cell Tissue Kinet.* **6**:87.

COOPER, E. H., BARKHAN, P., AND HALE, A. J., 1963, Observations on the proliferation of human leucocytes cultured with phytohaemagglutinin, *Br. J. Haematol.* **9**:101.

COOPER, H. L., 1969*a*, Ribosomal ribonucleic acid production and growth regulation in human lymphocytes, *J. Cell Biol.* **244**:1946.

COOPER, H. L., 1969*b*, Alternations in RNA metabolism in lymphocytes during the shift from resting state to active growth, in: *Biochemistry of Cell Division* (R. BASERGA, ed.), Charles C. Thomas, Springfield, Ill.

382

MILAN
POTMESIL,
JOSEPH
LOBUE,
AND
ANNA
GOLDFEDER

COOPER, H. L., 1971, Biochemical alterations accompanying initiation of growth in resting cells, in: *The Cell Cycle and Cancer* (R. BASERGA, ed.), Marcel Dekker, New York.

COOPER, H. L., AND RUBIN, A. D., 1965, RNA metabolism in lymphocytes stimulated by phytohemagglutinin: Initial responses to phytohemagglutinin, *Blood* **25**:1014.

CORMACK, D., 1976, Time-lapse characterization of erythrocytic colony-forming cells in plasma culture, *Exp. Hemat.* **4**:319.

COUNTS, W. B., AND FLAMM, W. J., 1966, An artifact associated with the incorporation of thymidine into DNA preparations, *Biochim. Biophys. Acta* **114**:628.

COX, D., 1968, Chromosome studies in 12 solid tumors from children, *Br. J. Cancer* **22**:402.

CRADDOCK, C. G., AND NAKAI, G. S., 1962, Leukemic cell proliferation as determined by *in vitro* deoxyribonucleic acid synthesis, *J. Clin. Invest.* **41**:360.

CROIZAT, H., FRINDEL, E., AND TUBIANA, M., 1970, Proliferation activity of the stem cells in the bone marrow of mice after single and multiple irradiations (total or partial body exposure), *Int. J. Radiat. Biol.* **18**:347.

CUDKOWICZ, G., BENNETT, M., AND SHEARER, G. M., 1964, Pluripotent stem cell function of the mouse "lymphocyte," *Science* **144**:866.

CURE, S., BOUÉ, J. G., AND BOUÉ, A., 1974, Growth characteristics of human embryonic cell lines with chromosomal anomalies, *Biomedicine* **21**:233.

DAMJANOV, J., AND SOLTER, D., 1974, Experimental teratoma, *Curr. Top. Pathol.* **59**:60.

DANIEL, C. W., DeOME, K. B., YOUNG, J. T., BLAIR, P. B., AND FAULKIN, L. J., JR., 1968, The *in vivo* life span of normal and preneoplastic mouse mammary glands: A serial transplantation study, *Proc. Natl. Acad. Sci. USA* **61**:53.

DAS, G. D., AND ALTMAN, J., 1971, Postnatal neurogenesis in the cerebellum of the cat and tritiated thymidine autoradiography, *Brain Res.* **30**:323.

DAWSON, K. B., MADOC-JONES, H., MAURO, F., AND PEACOCK, J. H., 1973, Studies on the radiobiology of a rat sarcoma treated *in situ* and assayed *in vitro*, *Eur. J. Cancer* **9**:59.

DeCOSSE, J. J., AND GELFANT, S., 1968, Noncycling tumor cells: Mitogenic response to antilymphocytic serum, *Science* **162**:698.

DeGOWIN, R. L., AND GIBSON, D. P., 1976, Pluripotential stem cell differentiation in hemopoietic colonies, *Blood* **47**:315.

DeGOWIN, R. L., HOAK, J. C., AND MILLER, S. H., 1972, Erythroblastic differentiation of stem cells in hemopoietic colonies, *Blood* **40**:881.

DeGRONCHY, J., deNAVA, L., FEINGOLD, J., BILSKI-PASQUIER, G., AND BOUSSER, J., 1968, Onze observations d'un modele precis d'evolution caryotypique au cours de la leucemie myeloide chronique, *Eur. J. Cancer* **4**:481.

DE LA TORRE, C., AND NAVARRETE, M. H., 1974, Estimation of chromatin patterns at G_1, S, and G_2 of the cell cycle, *Exp. Cell Res.* **88**:171.

DeMAERTELAER, V., AND GALAND, P., 1975, Some properties of the "G_0" model of the cell cycle. I. Investigation of the possible existence of natural constraints of the theoretical model in steady-state conditions, *Cell Tissue Kinet.* **8**:11.

DETHLEFSEN, L. A., 1970, Reutilization of ^{131}I-5-iodo-2′-deoxyuridine as compared to ^{3}H-thymidine in mouse duodenum and mammary tumor, *J. Natl. Cancer Inst.* **44**:827.

DETHLEFSEN, L. A., 1971, An evaluation of radioiodine-labeled 5-iodo-2′-deoxyuridine as a tracer for measuring cell loss from solid tumors, *Cell Tissue Kinet.* **4**:123.

DETHLEFSEN, L. A., 1974, ^{3}H-5-Iodo-2′-deoxyuridine toxicity: Problems in cell proliferation studies, *Cell Tissue Kinet.* **7**:213.

DeWYS, W. D., 1972, A quantitative model for the study of the growth and treatment of a tumor and its metastasis with correlation between proliferative state and sensitivity to cyclophosphamide, *Cancer Res.* **32**:367.

DICKE, K. A., VAN VOORD, M. J., MAAT, B., SHAEFER, U. W., AND VAN BEKKUM, D. W., 1973, Attempts at morphological identification of the haemopoietic stem cell in primates and rodents, in: *Haemopoietic Stem Cells*, Ciba Foundation Symposium 13 (New Series) (G. E. W. WOLSTENHOLME AND M. O'CONNOR, eds.), Elsevier, North-Holland, Amsterdam.

DITTRICH, W., AND GÖHDE, W., 1969, Impulsfluorametrie bei Einzelzellen in Suspensionen, *Z. Naturforsch.* **246**:360.

DOMBERNOWSKY, P., AND BICHEL, P., 1975, Cytokinetic variations during aging and regenerative growth in JB-1 ascites tumor studies by impulse cytophotometry, *Acta Pathol. Microbiol. Scand.* **83**:222.

383

STEM CELLS,
NON-
PROLIFERATING
CELLS, AND
THEIR
KINETICS

DOMBERNOWSKY, P., AND HARTMANN, N. R., 1972, Analysis of variations in cell population kinetics with tumor age in the L1210 ascites tumor, *Cancer Res.* **32**:2452.

DOMBERNOWSKY, P., BICHEL, P., AND HARTMANN, N. R., 1973, Cytokinetic analysis of the JB-1 ascites tumor at different stages of growth, *Cell Tissue Kinet.* **6**:347.

DOMBERNOWSKY, P., BICHEL, P., AND HARTMANN, N. R., 1974, Cytokinetic studies of the regenerative phase in the JB-1 ascites tumor, *Cell Tissue Kinet.* **7**:47.

DÖRMER, P., 1973, Quantitative autoradiography at the cellular level, in: *Micromethods in Molecular Biology* (V. NEUHOFF, ed.), Springer-Verlag, Berlin.

DÖRMER, P., AND BRINKMANN, W., 1972, Quantitative ^{14}C-Autoradiographie einzelner Zellen, *Histochemie* **29**:248.

DÖRMER, P., BRINKMANN, W., BORN, R., AND STEEL, G. G., 1975, Rate and time of DNA synthesis of individual Chinese hamster cells, *Cell Tissue Kinet.* **8**:399.

DUNN, C. D. R., 1971, The differentiation of haemopoietic stem cells, *Ser. Haematol.* **4**:1.

DUNN, C. D. R., AND ELSON, L. A., 1970, Quantitative studies of haemopoietic spleen colonies in rats treated with cytotoxic chemicals, *Br. J. Haematol.* **19**:755.

DURAND, R. E., AND SUTHERLAND, R. M., 1973, Dependence of the radiation response of an *in vitro* tumor model on cell cycle effects, *Cancer Res.* **33**:213.

DUSTIN, P., JR., 1972, Cell differentiation and carcinogenesis: A critical review, *Cell Tissue Kinet.* **5**:519.

DVOŘÁK, M., 1971, Submicroscopic cytodifferentiation, *Ergeb. Anat. Entwicklungsgesch.* **45**:4.

EAGLE, H., AND FOLEY, G. E., 1956, Cytotoxic action of carcinolytic agents in tissue culture, *Am. J. Med.* **21**:739.

EHMANN, U. K., WILLIAMS, J. R., NAGLE, W. A., BROWN, J. A., BELLI, J. A., AND LETT, J. T., 1975, Perturbations in cell cycle progression from radioactive DNA precursors, *Nature (London)* **258**:633

ENGLAND, J. M., AND MILLER, R. G., 1970, The statistical analysis of autoradiographs. II. Theoretical aspects including methods for optimal allocations of measurement effect, *J. Microsc.* **92**:167.

ENGLAND, J. M., AND ROGERS, A. W., 1970, The statistical analysis of autoradiographs. I. Grain count distributions over uniformly labelled sources, *J. Microsc.* **92**:159.

ENGLAND, J. M., ROGERS, A. W., AND MILLER, R. G., 1973, The identification of labelled structures on autoradiographs, *Nature (London)* **242**:612.

EPIFANOVA, O. I., AND TERSKIKH, V. V., 1969, On the resting period in the cell life cycle, *Cell Tissue Kinet.* **2**:75.

ERNST, P., AND KILLMANN, S. A., 1971, Perturbation of generation cycle of human leukemic myeloblasts *in vivo* by methotrexate, *Blood* **38**:689.

FARBER, E., AND BASERGA, R., 1969, Differential effects of hydroxyurea on survival of proliferating cells *in vivo*, *Cancer Res.* **29**:136.

FLIEDNER, T. M., CALVO, W., HAAS, R., FORTEZA, J., AND BOHNE, F., 1970, Morphologic and cytokinetic aspects of bone marrow stroma, in: *Hemopoietic Cellular Proliferation* (F. STOHLMAN, JR., ed.), Grune and Stratton, New York.

FORD, C. E., AND CLARKE, C. M., 1963, Cytogenic evidence of clonal proliferation in primary recticular neoplasms, *Can. Cancer Res. Conf.* **5**:129.

FOX, M., GILBERT, C. W., LAJTHA, L. G., AND NIAS, A. H. W., 1969, The interpretation of "split-dose" experiments in mammalian cells after treatment with alkylating agents, *Chem. Biol Interact.* **1**:241.

FRANCESCHINI, P., 1974, Semiconservative DNA duplication in human chromosomes treated with BUdR and stained with acridine orange, *Exp. Cell. Res.* **89**:420.

FREED, J. J., AND HUNGERFORD, D. A., 1957, DNA content of nuclei and chromosome number in sublines of the Ehrlich ascites carcinoma, *Cancer Res.* **17**:177.

FREEDMAN, V. H., AND SLIM, S., 1974, Cellular tumorigenicity in nude mice: Correlation with cell growth in semi-solid medium, *Cell* **3**:355.

FRIED, J., 1970, A mathematical model to aid in the interpretation of radioactive tracer data from proliferating cell populations, *Math. Biosci.* **8**:379.

FRIEND, C. W., SHER, W., HOLLAND, J. G., AND SATO, T., 1971, Hemoglobin synthesis in murine virus induced leukemic cells *in vitro*. Stimulation of erythroid differentiation by dimethylsulfoxide, *Proc. Natl. Acad. Sci. USA* **68**:379.

FRINDEL, E., AND TUBIANA, M., 1971, Radiobiology and the cell cycle, in: *The Cell Cycle and Cancer* (R. BASERGA, ed.), Marcel Dekker, New York.

FRINDEL, E., MALAISE, E. P., ALPEN, E., AND TUBIANA, M., 1967, Kinetics of cell proliferation of an experimental tumor, *Cancer Res.* **27**:1122.

384

MILAN
POTMESIL,
JOSEPH
LOBUE,
AND
ANNA
GOŁDFEDER

FRINDEL, E., MALAISE, E. P., AND TUBIANA, M., 1968, Cell proliferation kinetics in five human solid tumors, *Cancer* **22:**611.

FRINDEL, E., VALLERON, A. J., VASSORT, F., AND TUBIANA, M., 1969, Proliferation kinetics of an experimental ascites tumor of the mouse, *Cell Tissue Kinet.* **2:**51.

FRINDEL, E., VASSORT, F., AND TUBIANA, M., 1970, Effects of irradiation on the cell cycle of an experimental ascites tumor of the mouse, *Int. J. Radiat. Biol.* **17:**329.

FUJITA, S., 1974, Analysis of cytokinetics by means of Feulgen cytofluorometry combined with ^{3}H-thymidine autoradiography, *Exp. Cell Res.* **88:**395.

FULWYLER, M. J., 1970, Electronic cell sorting by volume, in: *Automated Cell Identification and Cell Sorting* (G. L. WIED AND G. F. BAHR, eds.), Academic Press, New York.

FURTH, J., AND KAHN, M. C., 1937, The transmission of leukemia in mice with a single cell, *Am. J. Cancer* **31:**276.

GABUTTI, U., PILERI, A., TAROCCO, R. P., GAVOSTO, F., AND COOPER, E. H., 1969, Proliferative potential of out-of-cycle leukaemic cells, *Nature (London)* **224:**375.

GAVOSTO, F., 1973, An outline of the objectives of the study of leukemic cell kinetics, in: *Unifying Concepts of Leukemia* (R. M. DUTCHER AND L. CHIECO-BIANCHI, eds.), *Bibl. Haemat.* **39:**968, Karger, Basel.

GAVOSTO, F., AND PILERI, A., 1971, Cell cycle of cancer cells in man, in: *The Cell Cycle and Cancer* (R. BASERGA, ed.), Marcel Dekker, New York.

GAVOSTO, F., MARAINI, G., AND PILERI, A., 1960, Nucleic acids and protein metabolism in acute leukemia cells, *Blood* **16:**1555.

GAVOSTO, F., PILERI, A., BACHI, C., AND PEGARRO, L., 1964, Proliferation and maturation defect in acute leukaemia cells, *Nature (London)* **203:**92.

GAVOSTO, F., PILERI, A., GABUTTI, V., AND MASERA, P., 1967a, Cell population kinetics in human acute leukemia. *Eur. J. Cancer* **3:**301.

GAVOSTO, F., PILERI, A., GABUTTI, U., AND MASERA, P., 1967b, Non-selfmaintaining kinetics of proliferating blasts in human actue leukemia, *Nature (London)* **216:**188.

GELFANT, S., 1962, Initiation of mitosis in relation to the cell division cycle, *Exp. Cell Res.* **26:**395.

GELFANT, S., 1963, Patterns of epidermal cell division. I. Genetic behaviour of the G_1 cell population, *Exp. Cell Res.* **32:**521.

GELFANT, S., 1966, Patterns of cell division: The demonstration of discrete cell populations, in: *Methods of Cell Physiology* (D. M. PRESCOTT, ed.), Academic Press, New York.

GHANTA, V. K., AND HIRAMOTA, R. N., 1974, Quantitation of total-body tumor cells (MOPC 104E). I. Subcutaneous tumor model, *J. Natl. Cancer Inst.* **52:**1199.

GIBSON, M. H. L., AND BERTALANFFY, F. D., 1972, In vivo synchrony of solid B16 melanoma by cytosine arabinoside, an inhibitor of DNA synthesis, *J. Natl. Cancer Inst.* **49:**1007.

GIDALI, J., AND LAJTHA, L. G., 1972, Regulation of haemopoietic stem cell turnover in partially irradiated mice, *Cell Tissue Kinet.* **5:**147.

GILLETTE, E. L., SUIT, H. D., AND MARSHALL, N., 1972, Redistribution and reoxygenation in a C3H mouse mammary carcinoma, *Radiat. Res.* **50:**574.

GLINOS, A. D., AND WERRLEIN, R. J., 1972, Density dependent regulation of growth in suspension cultures of L-929 cells, *J. Cell. Physiol.* **79:**79.

GOLDENBERG, G. J., 1968, Repair of sublethal damage of L5178Y lymphoblasts in vitro treated with dimethylmyleran and nitrogen mustard, *Biochem. Pharmacol.* **17:**820.

GOLDFEDER, A., 1954, Studies on radiosensitivity and "immunizing" ability of mammary tumors in mice, *Br. J. Cancer* **8:**320.

GOLDFEDER, A., 1965, Biological properties and radiosensitivity of tumors: Determination of the cell cycle and time of synthesis of deoxyribonucleic acid using tritiated thymidine and autoradiography, *Nature (London)* **207:**612.

GOLDFEDER, A., AND MILLER, L. A., 1963, Radiosensitivity and biological properties of two tumor types indigenous to the same host. VI. The effects of X-irradiation on subcellular units, *Int. J. Radiat. Biol.* **6:**575.

GOLDFEDER, A., AND NAGASAKI, F., 1954, Spontaneous transformation from carcinomatous to sarcomatous-like growth, *Cancer Res.* **14:**267.

GOODMAN, J. W., AND HODGSON, G. S., 1962, Evidence of stem cells in the peripheral blood of mice, *Blood* **19:**702.

GRANBERG, I., 1971, Chromosomes in preinvasive, microinvasive and invasive cervical carcinoma, *Hereditas* **68:**165.

385

STEM CELLS,
NON-
PROLIFERATING
CELLS, AND
THEIR
KINETICS

GRANBERG, I., GUPTA, A., JOELSSON, I., AND SPRENGER, E., 1974, Chromosomes and nuclear DNA. Study of a uterine adenocarcinoma and its metastases, *Acta Pathol. Microbiol. Scand.* (A) **82**:1.

GRAY, J. W., AND MENDELSOHN, M. L., 1975, A rapid technique of cell cycle analysis based on sorting cells in S phase, *Abst. 23rd Ann. Meet. Radiation Res. Soc. Gb.* **8**:64.

GREEN, E. L., 1968, *Handbook on Genetically Standardized JAX Mice*, The Jackson Laboratory, Bar Harbor, Me.

GRISHAM, J. W., 1962, A morphologic study of deoxyribonucleic acid synthesis and cell proliferation in regenerating rat liver: Autoradiography with thymidine-H³, *Cancer Res.* **22**:842.

HAAS, R. J., BOHNE, F., AND FLIEDNER, T. M., 1971, Cytokinetic analysis of slowly proliferating bone marrow cells during recovery from radiation injury, *Cell Tissue Kinet.* **4**:31.

HABICHT, W. K., LENNARTZ, K. D., SIMONEIT, K., BAHNTJE, U., EDER, M., AND GROSS, R., 1970, Cytophotometrische und autoradiographische Untersuchungen zur Wirkungen von Cyclophosphamid auf den Desoxyribonucleisäu regehalt und die Thymidineinbaurate bei Ehrlich-Ascitestumoren verschiedener Ploidie, *Arzneim. Forsch.* **20**:607.

HAGEMANN, R. F., SIGDESTAD, C. P., AND LESHER, S., 1972, Intestinal crypt survival and total and per crypt levels of proliferation and cellularity following irradiation: Role of crypt cellularity, *Radiat. Res.* **50**:583.

HAGEMANN, R. F., SCHENKEN, L. L., AND LESHER, S., 1973, Tumor chemotherapy: Efficacy dependent on mode of growth, *J. Natl. Cancer Inst.* **50**:467.

HAHN, G. M., 1968, Failure of Chinese hamster cells to repair sub-lethal damage when X-irradiated in the plateau phase of growth, *Nature (London)* **217**:741.

HAHN, G. M., 1975, Radiotherapy and chemotherapy: Some parallels and differences, *Radiat. Biol.* **114**:203.

HAHN, G. M. AND LITTLE, J. B., 1972, Plateau-phase cultures of mammalian cells, an *in vitro* model for human cancer, in: *Current Topics in Radiation Research* (M. EBERT AND A. HOWARD, eds.), North-Holland, Amsterdam.

HAHN, G. M., STEWARD, J. R., YANG, S. J., AND PARKER, V., 1968, Chinese hamster cell monolayer cultures. I. Changes in cell dynamics and modification of the cell cycle with the period of growth, *Exp. Cell Res.* **49**:285.

HAHN, G. M., RAY, G. R., GORDON, L. F., AND KALLMAN, R. F., 1973, Response of solid tumor cells exposed to chemotherapeutic agents *in vitro*: Cell survival after 2- and 24-hour exposure, *J. Natl. Cancer Inst.* **50**:529.

HAHN, G. M., ROCKWELL, S., KALLMAN, R. F., GORDON, L. F., AND FRINDEL, E., 1974, Repair of potentially lethal damage *in vivo* in solid tumor cells after X-irradiation, *Cancer Res.* **34**:351.

HALE, A. J., COOPER, E. H., AND MILTON, J. D., 1965, Studies of the incorporation of pyrimidines into DNA in single leukemic and other proliferating leukocytes, *Br. J. Haematol.* **11**:144.

HALNAN, K. E., 1973, Cancer—The future, *Br. J. Radiol.* **46**:793.

HAMILTON, E., AND PATTEN, C., 1972, Influence of hair plucking on the turnover time of the epidermis basal layer, *Cell Tissue Kinet.* **5**:505.

HANDS, G. E., AND AINSWORTH, E. J., 1964, Endotoxin protection and colony forming units, *Radiat. Res.* **32**:367.

HARKNESS, R. D., 1957, Regeneration of liver, *Br. Med. Bull.* **13**:87.

HARRIS, P. F., AND KUGLER, J. H., 1967, Transfusion of regenerating bone marrow into irradiated guinea pigs, in: *The Lymphocyte in Immunology and Haemopoiesis* (J. M. YOFFEY, ed.), Arnold, London.

HARTMANN, N. K., AND DOMBERNOWSKY, P., 1974, Autoradiographic and cytophotometric studies of the resting stages of the L1210 ascites tumor, *Cancer Res.* **34**:3296.

HARWOOD, R., 1974, Cell separation by gradient centrifugation, *Int. Rev. Cytol.* **38**:369.

HASHOLT, L., VISFELDT, J., AND DANØ, K., 1971, Karyotypic profile alterations in Ehrlich ascites tumour cells during development of resistance to Daunorubicine, *Acta Pathol. Microbiol. Scand.* (A) **79**:665.

HAUSCHKA, T. S., 1961, The chromosomes in ontogeny and oncogeny, *Cancer Res.* **21**:957.

HAUSCHKA, T. S., AND LEVAN, A., 1951, Characterization of five ascites tumors with respect to chromosome ploidy, *Anat. Rec.* **111**:467.

HAY, E. D., 1968, Structure and function of the nucleolus in developing cells, in: *The Nucleus* (A. J. DALTON AND F. HAGUENAU, eds.), Academic Press, New York.

HELLMAN, S., 1975, Cell kinetics, models and cancer treatment—Some principles for the radiation oncologist, *Radiology* **114**:219.

HELLMAN, S., GRATE, H. E., AND CHAFFNEY, J. T., 1969, Effects of radiation on the capacity of the stem cell compartment to differentiate into granulocytic and erythrocytic progeny, *Blood* **34**:141.

386

MILAN
POTMESIL,
JOSEPH
LOBUE,
AND
ANNA
GOLDFEDER

HELLMAN, S., GRATE, H. E., CHAFFNEY, J. T., AND CARMEL, R., 1970, Hemopoietic stem cell compartment: Patterns of differentiation following radiation or cyclophosphamide, in: *Hemopoietic Cellular Proliferation* (F. STOHLMAN, JR., ed.), Grune and Stratton, New York.

HERMENS, A. F., AND BARENDSEN, G. W., 1969, Changes of cell proliferation characteristics in a rat rhabdomyosarcoma before and after X-irradiation, *Eur. J. Cancer* **5:**173.

HEWITT, H. B., 1953, Studies of the quantitative transplantation of mouse sarcoma, *Br. J. Cancer* **7:**367.

HEWITT, H. B., 1966, The effect on cell survival of inhalation of oxygen under high pressure during irradiation *in vivo* of a solid mouse sarcoma, *Br. J. Radiol.* **39:**19.

HEWITT, H. B., AND WILSON, C. W., 1959a, Survival curve for mammalian leukaemia cells irradiated *in vivo* (implications for the treatment of mouse leukaemia by whole-body irradiation), *Br. J. Cancer* **13:**69.

HEWITT, H. B., AND WILSON, C. W., 1959b, The effect of tissue oxygen tension on the radiosensitivity of leukaemic cells irradiated *in situ* in the livers of leukaemic mice, *Br. J. Cancer* **13:**675.

HEWITT, H. B., CHAN, D. P.-S., AND BLAKE, E. R., 1967, Survival curves for clonogenic cells of a murine keratinizing squamous carcinoma irradiated *in vivo* or under hypoxic conditions, *Int. J. Radiat. Biol.* **12:**535.

HEWITT, H. B., BLAKE, E., AND PORTER, E. H., 1973, The effect of lethally irradiated cells on transplantability of murine tumors, *Br. J. Cancer* **28:**123.

HILL, R. P., AND BUSH, R. S., 1969, A lung-colony assay to determine the radiosensitivity of the cells of a solid tumor, *Int. J. Radiat. Biol.* **15:**435.

HILL, R. P., AND BUSH, R. S., 1973, The effect of continuous or fractionated irradiation on a murine sarcoma, *Int. J. Radiol.* **46:**167.

HILWIG, I., AND GROPP, A., 1973, Decondensation of constitutive heterochromatin in L cell chromosomes by a bisbenzimidazole compound (33258 HOECHST), *Exp. Cell Res.* **81:**474.

HINDERER, H., VOLM, M., AND WAYSS, K., 1970, Spizifische Hemmung der DNS Synthese von HeLa-Zellen durch Endometrium-Extrakt, *Exp. Cell Res.* **59:**464.

HIRT, A., AND WAGNER, H. P., 1975, Nuclear incorporation of radioactive DNA precursors and progression of cells through S: Combined radioautographic and cytophotometric studies on normal and leukaemic bone marrow and thoracic duct lymph cells of man, *Cell Tissue Kinet.* **8:**455.

HOFER, K. G., 1970, Radiation effect on death and migration of tumor cells in mice, *Radiat. Res.* **43:**663.

HOFER, K. G., AND HOFER, M., 1971, Kinetics of proliferation, migration, and death of L 1210 ascites cells, *Cancer Res.* **31:**402.

HOFER, K. G., AND HUGHES, W. L., 1971, Radioactivity of intranuclear tritium, ^{125}iodine and ^{131}iodine, *Radiat. Res.* **47:**94.

HOFER, K. G., PRENSKY, W., AND HUGHES, W. L., 1969, Death and metastatic distribution of tumor cells in mice monitored with ^{125}I-iododeoxyuridine, *J. Natl. Cancer Inst.* **43:**763.

HOFER, K. G., WARTERS, R. L., ROLFES, T. H., AND HOFER, M., 1974, Viability of tumor cells in mechanically and enzymatically prepared tissue suspensions, *Eur. J. Cancer* **10:**49.

HOLLOWAY, R. J., LARSEN, R. M., AND MITCHELL, F. E., 1968, Hemopoietic spleen colonies in the hamster, *Radiat. Res.* **35:**568.

HRYNIUK, W. M., AND BERTINO, J. R., 1971, Growth rate and cell kill, *Ann. N.Y. Acad. Sci.* **186:**330.

HSU, T. C., 1961, Chromosome evolution in cell populations, *Int. Rev., Cytol.* **12:**69.

HUGHES, W. L., COMMERFORD, S. L., GILTIN, D., KREUGER, R. C., SCHULTZE, B., SHAH, V., AND REILLY, P., 1964, Deoxyribonucleic acid metabolism *in vivo*. I. Cell proliferation and death as measured by incorporation of iododeoxyuridine, *Fed. Proc.* **23:**640.

HULETT, H. R., BOUMER, W. A., BARRETT, J., AND HARZENBERG, L. A., 1969, Cell sorting: Automated separation of mammalian cells as a function of intracellular fluorescence, *Science* **166:**747.

ISCOVE, N. N., AND SIEBER, F., 1975, Erythroid progenitors in mouse bone marrow detected by macroscopic colony formation in culture, *Exp. Hematol.* **3:**32.

IVERSEN, O. H., BJERKNES, R., AND DEVIK, F., 1968, Kinetics of cell removal, cell migration and cell loss in the hairless mouse dorsal epidermis, *Cell. Tissue Kinet.* **1:**351.

JENKINS, V. K., UPTON, A. C., AND ODELL, T. T., JR., 1969, Differences between exogenous and endogenous hemopoietic spleen colonies, *J. Cell Physiol.* **73:**141.

JOHNSON, L. I., AND RUBIN, A. D., 1970, Lymphocyte growth and proliferation in culture, in: *Regulation of Hematopoiesis* (A. S. GORDON, ed.), Appleton-Century-Crofts, New York.

JOHNSON, L. I., CHAN, P.-C., LOBUE, J., MONETTE, F. C., AND GORDON, A. S., 1967, Cell cycle analysis of rat lymphocytes cultured with phytohemagglutinin in diffusion chambers, *Exp. Cell Res.* **47:**201.

KAHN, M. C., AND FURTH, J., 1938, Transmission of mouse sarcoma with small numbers of counted cells, *Proc. Soc. Exp. Biol. Med.* **38**:485.

KAL, H. B., 1973*a*, Distributions of cell volume and DNA content of rhabdomyosarcoma cells growing *in vitro* and *in vivo* after irradiation, *Eur. J. Cancer* **9**:77.

KAL, H. B., 1973*b*, Proliferation behavior of P and Q cells in a rat rhabdomyosarcoma after irradiation as determined by DNA measurements, *Eur. J. Cancer* **9**:753.

KAL, H. B., AND HAHN, G. N., 1976, Kinetic responses of murine sarcoma cells to radiation and hyperthermia *in vivo* and *in vitro*, *Cancer Res.* **36**:1923.

KALLMAN, R. F., 1968, Methods for the study of radiation effects on cancer cells, in: *Methods in Cancer Research*, Vol. 4 (I. H. BUSCH, ed.), Academic Press, New York.

KALLMAN, R. F., 1975, The effect of irradiation on the ratio of cycling (P) to non-cycling (Q) cells in EMT6 tumors as determined by colony labeling, *Abst. 23rd Meet. Radiat. Res. Soc. Bd.*-4:6.

KALLMAN, R. F., SILINI, G., AND VAN PUTTEN, L. M., 1967, Factors influencing the quantitative estimation of the *in vivo* survival of cells from solid tumors, *J. Natl. Cancer Inst.* **39**:539.

KAPLAN, H. S., 1974, On the relative importance of hypoxic cells for the radiotherapy of human tumors, *Eur. J. Cancer* **10**:275.

KARLE, H., ERNST, P., AND KILLMANN, S. A., 1973, Changing cytokinetic patterns of human leukemic lymphoblasts during the course of the disease, studied *in vivo*, *Br. J. Haematol.* **24**:231.

KATO, H., 1974, Spontaneous sister chromatid exchanges detected by a BUdR labelling method, *Nature (London)* **251**:70.

KAY, H. E. M., 1965, How many cell generations? *Lancet* **2**:418.

KAY, J. E., AND COOPER, H. L., 1969, Rapidly labeled cytoplasmic RNA in normal and phytohaemagglutinin-stimulated human lymphocytes, *Biochim. Biophys. Acta* **186**:62.

KILLANDER, D., AND ZETTERBERG, A., 1965*a*, Quantitative cytochemical studies on interphase growth. I. Determination of DNA, RNA and mass content of age determined mouse fibroblasts *in vitro* and of intercellular variations in generation time, *Exp. Cell Res.* **38**:272.

KILLANDER, D., AND ZETTERBERG, A., 1965*b*, A quantitative cytochemical investigation of the relationship between cell mass and initiation of DNA synthesis in mouse fibroblasts *in vitro*, *Exp. Cell Res.* **40**:12.

KILLMANN, S.-A., 1965, Proliferative activity of blast cells in leukemia and myelofibrosis, morphological differences between proliferating and non-proliferating blast cells, *Acta Med. Scand.* **178**:263.

KILLMANN, S.-A., 1968, Acute leukemia: Development, remission, relapse pattern, relationship between normal and leukemic hemopoiesis, and the "sleeper-to-feeder" stem cell hypothesis, in: *Cell Kinetics in Human Leukemia, Ser. Haematol.* **1**:103.

KIM, U., AND DEPOWSKI, M. J., 1975, Progression from hormone dependence to autonomy in mammary tumors as *in vivo* manifestation of sequential clonal selection, *Cancer Res.* **35**:2068.

KISIELESKI, W. E., BASERGA, R., AND LISCO, H., 1961, Tritiated thymidine and the study of tumors, *Atompraxis* **7**:81.

KLEIN, G., AND RÉVÉSZ, L., 1953, Quantitative studies on the multiplication of neoplastic cells *in vivo*. I. Growth curves of the Ehrlich and MC1M ascites tumors, *J. Natl. Cancer Inst.* **14**:229.

KLINE, J., 1974, Potentially useful combinations of chemotherapy detected in mouse tumor systems, *Cancer Chem. Rep.* Part I. **4**:33.

KOCH, C. J., KRUUV, J., FREY, H. E., AND SNYDER, R. A., 1973, Plateau phase in growth induced by hypoxia, *Int. J. Radiat. Biol.* **23**:67.

KRAEMER, P. M., DEAVEN, L. L., CRISSMAN, H. A., AND VAN DILLA, M. A., 1972, DNA constancy despite variability in chromosome number, in: *Advances in Cell and Molecular Biology*, Vol. 2 (E. J. DuPRAW, ed.), Academic Press, New York.

KRETCHMAR, A. L., AND CONOVER, W. R., 1970, A difference between spleen derived and bone marrow derived colony forming units in ability to protect lethally irradiated mice, *Blood* **36**:772.

KRISHAN, A., AND FREI, E., III, 1976, Effect of adriamycin on the cell cycle traverse and kinetics of cultured human lymphoblasts, *Cancer Res.* **36**:143.

KURNICK, J. E., AND ROBINSON, W. A., 1971, Colony growth of human peripheral white blood cells *in vitro*, *Blood* **37**:136.

LAHIRI, S. K., AND VAN PUTTEN, L. M., 1969, Distribution and multiplication of colony forming units from bone marrow and spleen after injection in irradiated mice, *Cell Tissue Kinet.* **2**:21.

LAHIRI, S. K., AND VAN PUTTEN, L. M., 1972, Location of the G_0-phase in the cell cycle of the mouse haemopoietic spleen colony forming cells, *Cell Tissue Kinet.* **5**:365.

LAIRD, A. K., 1964, Dynamics of tumor growth, *Br. J. Cancer* **18**:490.

MILAN
POTMESIL,
JOSEPH
LOBUE,
AND
ANNA
GOLDFEDER

LAJTHA, L. G., 1963, On the concept of the cell cycle, *J. Cell. Comp. Physiol.* **62**:143.

LAJTHA, L. G., 1964, Recent studies in erythroid differentiation and proliferation, *Medicine* **43**:625.

LAJTHA, L. G., 1966, Cytokinetics and regulation of progenitor cells, *J. Cell. Comp. Physiol.* **67**:133.

LAJTHA, L. G., 1967, Stem cells and their properties, *Can. Cancer Res. Conf.* **7**:31.

LAJTHA, L. G., 1970, Stem cell kinetics, in: *Regulation of Hematopoiesis* (A. S. GORDON, ed.), Appleton-Century-Crofts, New York.

LAJTHA, L. G., 1972, Kinetics of proliferation and differentiation, in: *Regulation of Erythropoiesis* (A. S. GORDON, M. CONDORELLI, AND C. PESCHLE, eds.), Il Ponte, Milan.

LALA, P. K., 1972, Evaluation of the mode of cell death in Ehrlich ascites tumor, *Cancer* **29**:261.

LALA, P. K., AND PATT, H. M., 1966, Cytokinetic analysis of tumor growth, *Proc. Natl. Acad. Sci. USA* **56**:1735.

LALA, P. K., AND PATT, H. M., 1968, A characterization of the boundary between the cycling and resting states in ascites tumor cells, *Cell Tissue Kinet.* **1**:137.

LAMB, D., 1967, Correlation in chromosome counts with histologic appearance and prognosis in transitional-cell carcinoma of the bladder, *Br. med. J.* **1**:273.

LAMERTON, L. F., 1972, Cell proliferation and the differential response of normal and malignant tissues, *Br. J. Radiol.* **45**:161.

LAMERTON, L. F., 1973, Tumor cell kinetics, *Br. Med. Bull.* **29**:23

LAMERTON, L. F., 1974, The mitotic cycle and cell population control, *J. Clin. Pathol.* **27**: Suppl. 7, 19.

LAMERTON, L. F., AND BLACKETT, N. M., 1974, A comparison of proliferative characteristics of bone marrow and tumors and response to cytotoxic agents, in: *Control in Proliferation of Animal Cells* (B. D. CLARKSON AND R. BASERGA, eds.), Cold Spring Harbor Laboratory, Cold Spring Harbor, N.Y.

LAMERTON, L. F., AND STEEL, G. G., 1968, Cell population kinetics in normal and malignant tissues, in: *Progress in Biophysics and Molecular Biology* (J. A. V. BUTLER AND D. NOBLE, eds.), Pergamon Press, New York.

LAMPERT, F., AND GAUGER, J. W., 1968, Chromosomen der Zellen der akuten Leukämie im Kindesalter, *Wochenschr. Klin.* **46**:882.

LAMPKIN, B. C., NAGAO, T., AND MAUER, A. M., 1969, Drug effect in acute leukemia, *J. Clin. Invest.* **48**:1124.

LAMPKIN, B. C., NAGAO, T., LICHTENBERG, A., AND MAUER, A., 1971, Synchronization and recruitment in acute leukemia, *J. Clin. Invest.* **50**:2204.

LASTER, W. R., JR., MAYO, J. G., AND SIMPSON-HERREN, L., 1969, Success and failure in the treatment of solid tumors. II. Kinetic parameters and "cell cure" of moderately advanced carcinoma 755, *Cancer Chem. Rep.* **53**:169.

LATT, S. A., 1973, Microfluorometric detection of deoxyribonucleic acid replication in human metaphase chromosomes, *Proc. Natl. Acad. Sci. USA* **70**:3395.

LATT, S. A., STETTEN, G., JUERJENES, L. A., WILLARD, H. F., AND SHER, C. D., 1975, Recent developments in the detection of deoxyribonucleic acid synthesis by 33258 HOECHST fluorescence, *J. Histochem. Cytochem.* **23**:493.

LEBLOND, C. P., CLERMONT, Y., AND NADLER, N. I., 1967, The pattern of stem cell removal in three epithelia (oesophagus, intestine, and testis), *Can. Cancer Res. Conf.* **7**:3.

LEBOWITZ, J. L., AND RUBINOW, S. I., 1969, Grain count distributions in labelled cell populations, *J. Theor. Biol.* **23**:99.

LEIF, R. C., 1970a, A proposal for an automatic multiparameter analyzer for cells, (AMAC), in: *Automated Cell Identification and Cell Sorting* (G. L. WIED AND J. F. BAHR, eds.), Academic Press, New York.

LEIF, R. C., 1970b, Buoyant density separation of cells, in: *Automated Cell Identification and Cell Sorting* (G. J. WIED AND J. F. BAHR, eds.), Academic Press, New York.

LENNARTZ, K. J., ADLER, D., BLANKENSTEIN, L., EDER, M., AND FRIEDMANN, G., 1970, Änderung der Wachstumskinetik von Ehrlich-Ascitestumoren verschiedneer Ploidie nach Röntgenbestrahlung, *Experientia (Basel)* **26**:897.

LESHER, S., AND BAUMAN, J., 1969, Cell proliferation in the intestinal epithelium, in: *Normal and Malignant Cell Growth* (R. J. M. FRY, M. L. GRIEM, AND W. H. KIRSTEN, eds.), Springer-Verlag, New York.

LIN, H., 1973, Differential lethal effect of cytotoxic agents on proliferating and nonproliferating lymphoid cells, *Cancer Res.* **33**:1716.

LITTLE, J. B., 1969, Repair of sub-lethal and potentially lethal radiation damage in plateau phase cultures of human cells, *Nature (London)* **224**:804.

LITTLE, J. B., HAHN, G. M., FRINDEL, E., AND TUBIANA, M., 1973, Repair of potentially lethal radiation damage *in vitro* and *in vivo*, *Radiobiology* **106**:689.

LLOYD, H. H., DULMADGE, E. A., AND WIELKOFF, L. G., 1972, Kinetics of the reduction in viability of cultured L1210 leukemia cells exposed to 5-azacytidine (NSC-102816), *Cancer Chem. Rep.* **56**:585.

LOBUE, J., 1973, Stem cell and neutrophilic granulocyte kinetics, *Med. Clin. North Am.* **57**:265.

LOBUE, J., AND POTMESIL, M., 1975, Stimulation, in: *Cancer: A Comprehensive Treatise*, Vol. 3 (F. F. BECKER, ed.), Plenum Press, New York.

LOBUE, J., ALEXANDER, P., JR., FREDRICKSON, T. N., SCHULTZ, E. F., GORDON, A. S., AND JOHNSON, L. I., 1972, Erythrokinetics in normal and disease states. Virally-induced murine erythroblastosis: A model system, in: *Regulation of Erythropoiesis* (A. S. GORDON, M. CONDORELLI, AND C. PESCHLE, eds.), Il Ponte, Milan.

LOBUE, J., GORDON, A. S., WEITZ-HAMBURGER, A., FERDINAND, P., CAMISCOLI, J. F., FREDRICKSON, T. N., AND HARDY, W. D., JR., 1974, Erythroid differentiation in murine erythroleukemia, in: *Control of Proliferation in Animal Cells* (B. Clarkson and R. Baserga, eds.), Cold Spring Harbor Laboratory, Cold Spring Harbor, N.Y.

LOBUE, J., FREDRICKSON, T. N., GALLICHIO, V., RONQUILLO, A., AND GORDON, A. S., 1975, Exogenous and endogenous erythropoietin in the treatment of the fatal anemia of RLV disease, in: *Erythropoiesis* (K. NAKAO, J. W. FISHER, AND F. TAKAKU, eds.), Tokyo University Press, Tokyo.

LOMAKKA, G., 1965, A rapid scanning and integrating cytophotometer, *Acta Histochem.* **6**:47.

LORD, B. I., AND HENDRY, J. H., 1972, The distribution of haemopoietic colony-forming units in the mouse femur and its modification by X-rays, *Br. J. Radiol.* **45**:110.

LORD, B. I., TESTA, N. G., AND HENDRY, J. H., 1975, The relative spatial distributions of CFU-s and CFU-c in the normal mouse femur, *Blood* **46**:65.

LUBS, H. A., AND KOTLER, S., 1967, The prognostic significance of chromosome abnormalities in colon tumors, *Am. Intern. Med.* **67**:328.

LURGUIN, P. F., 1974, The use of intercalating dye molecules in the study of chromatin structure, *Chem. Biol. Interact.* **8**:303.

MAGE, M. J., EVANS, W. H., AND PETERSON, E. A., 1968, Enrichment of antibody plaque-forming cells of spleen by sedimentation at unit gravity, *Proc. Soc. Exp. Biol. Med.* **127**:478.

MAIZEL, A., NICOLINI, C., AND BASERGA, R., 1975, Effect of cell trypsinization on nuclear proteins of WI-38 fibroblasts in culture, *J. Cell. Physiol.* **86**:71.

MAKINO, S., 1952, A cytological study on the Yoshida sarcoma, an ascites tumor of white rats, *Chromosoma* **4**:649.

MALAISE, E., AND TUBIANA, M., 1966, Croissance des cellules d'un fibrosarcome expérimental irradié chez la souris C3H, *C. R. Acad. Sci.* **263D**:292.

MALAISE, E., CHARBIT, A., CHAVAUDRA, N., COMBES, P. F., DOUCHER, J., AND TUBIANA, M., 1972, Change in volume of irradiated human metastases. Investigation of repair of sublethal damage and tumour repopulation, *Br. J. Cancer* **26**:43.

MARIN, G., AND BENDER, M. A., 1963a, Survival kinetics of HeLa S-3 cells after incorporation of ^{3}H-thymidine or ^{3}H-uridine, *Int. J. Radiat. Biol.* **7**:221.

MARIN, G., AND BENDER, M. A., 1963b, A comparison of mammalian cell-killing by incorporated ^{3}H-thymidine and ^{3}H-uridine, *Int. J. Radiat. Biol.* **7**:235.

MARK, J., 1969, Rous sarcoma in mice: The chromosomal progression in primary tumors, *Eur. J. Cancer* **5**:307.

MARSH, J. C., 1976, The effects of cancer chemotherapeutic agents on normal hematopoietic precursor cells: A review, *Cancer Res.* **36**:1853.

MARSH, J. C., AND PERRY, S., 1964, Thymidine catabolism by normal and leukemic human leukocytes, *J. Clin. Invest.* **43**:267.

MARTIN, G. R., 1975, Teratocarcinomas as model system for the study of embryogenesis and neoplasia, *Cell* **5**:229.

MARTIN, G. R., AND EVANS, M. J., 1975, Multiple differentiation of clonal teratocarcinoma stem cells following embryoid body formation *in vitro*, *Cell* **6**:467.

MARTIN, G. M., SPRAGUE, C. A., NORWOOD, T. H., AND PENDERGRASS, W. R., 1974, Clonal selection, attenuation and differentiation in an *in vivo* model of hyperplasia, *Am. J. Pathol.* **74**:137.

MARUYAMA, Y., 1964, Re-utilization of thymidine during death of cells, *Nature (London)* **201**:93.

MARUYAMA, Y., BRIESE, F. W., AND BROWN, B. W., 1967, X-irradiation response by TD-50 and survival time assays for a murine lymphoma, *Radiat. Res.* **30**:96.

390

MILAN
POTMESIL,
JOSEPH
LOBUE,
AND
ANNA
GOLDFEDER

MATHIAS, A. P., AND FISHER, G. A., 1962, The metabolism of thymidine by murine leukemic lymphoblasts (L51 78 Y), *Biochem. Pharmacol.* **11**:57.

MAUER, A. M., 1975, Cell kinetics and practical consequences for therapy of acute leukemia, *N. Engl. J. Med.* **293**:389.

MAUER, A. M., AND FISHER, V., 1966, Characteristics of cell proliferation in four patients with untreated acute leukemia, *Blood* **28**:428.

MAUER, A. M., EVERT, C. F., LAMPKIN, B. C., AND McWILLIAMS, N. B., 1973, Cell kinetics in human acute lymphoblastic leukemia: Computer simulation with discrete modeling techniques, *Blood* **41**:141.

MAURO, F., FALPO, B., BRIGANTI, G., ELLI, R., AND ZUPI, G., 1974a, Effects of antineoplastic drugs on plateau-phase cultures of mammalian cells. I. Description of the plateau-phase system, *J. Natl. Cancer Inst.* **52**:705.

MAURO, F., FALPO, B., BRIGANTI, G., ELLI, R., AND ZUPI, G., 1974b, Effects of antineoplastic drugs on plateau-phase cultures of mammalian cells. II. Bleomycin and hydroxyurea, *J. Natl. Cancer Inst.* **52**:715.

McLEOD, D. L., SHREEVE, M. M., AND AXELRAD, A. A., 1974, Improved plasma culture system for production of erythrocytic colonies *in vitro*: Quantitative assay method for CFU-e, *Blood* **44**:517.

MEEK, E. S., 1961, Deoxyribonucleic acid content of mouse ascites tumor cells in interphase and mitoses, *Br. J. Cancer* **15**:162.

MENDELSOHN M. L., 1960, The growth fraction: A new concept applied to tumors, *Science* **132**:1496.

MENDELSOHN, M. L., 1962a, Autoradiographic analysis of cell proliferation in spontaneous breast cancer of C3H mouse. III. The growth fraction, *J. Natl. Cancer Inst.* **28**:1015.

MENDELSOHN, M. L., 1962b, Chronic infusion of tritiated thymidine into mice with tumors, *Science* **135**:213.

MENDELSOHN, M. L., 1965, The kinetics of tumor cell proliferation, in: *Cellular Radiation Biology*, Williams AND Wilkins, Baltimore.

MENDELSOHN, M. L., 1975, Cell cycle kinetics and raditation therapy, in: *Radiation Research. Biomedical, Chemical and Physical Perspectives* (O. F. NYGAARD, H. I. ADLER, AND W. K. SINCLAIR, eds.), Academic Press, New York.

MENDELSOHN, M. L., AND DETHLEFSEN, L. A., 1973, Cell kinetics of breast cancer: The turnover of nonproliferating cells, in: *Recent Results in Cancer Research*, Vol. 42 (M. L. GRIEM, E. V. JENSEN, J. E. ULTMANN, AND R. W. WISSLER, eds.), Springer-Verlag, New York.

MERZ, G. S., JR., AND ROSS, J. D., 1969, Viability of human diploid cells as a function of *in vitro* age, *J. Cell. Physiol.* **74**:219.

METCALF, D., 1973, The colony stimulating factor, in: *Humoral Control of Growth and Differentiation* Vol. 1 (J. LOBUE AND A. S. GORDON, eds.), Academic Press, New York.

METCALF, D., AND BRUMBY, M., 1967, Coulter counter analysis of lymphoma differentiation patterns in AKR mice with lymphoid leukaemia, *Int. J. Cancer* **2**:37.

METCALF, D., AND FOSTER, R., JR., 1967, Behavior on transfer of serum stimulated bone marrow colonies, *Proc. Soc. Exp. Biol. Med.* **126**:758.

METCALF, D., AND WIADROWSKI, M., 1966, Autoradiographic analysis of lymphocyte proliferation in the thymus and in thymic lymphoma tissue, *Cancer Res.* **26**:483.

METCALF, D., NAKAMURA, K., AND WIADROWSKI, M., 1965, Patterns of cellular differetiation in spontaneous and transplanted lymphoma in mice, *Aust. J. Exp. Biol. Med.* **43**:413.

METCALF, D., BRADLEY, T. R., AND ROBINSON, W., 1967a, Analysis of colonies developing *in vitro* from mouse bone marrow cells stimulated by kidney feeder layers or leukemic serum, *J. Cell. Physiol.* **69**:93.

METCALF, D., FOSTER, R., AND PALLARD, M., 1967b, Colony stimulating activity of serum from germ free normal and leukemic mice, *J. Cell. Physiol.* **70**:131.

METZ, W. D., 1974, Cancer chemotherapy: Now a promising weapon, *Science* **184**:970.

MITELMAN, F., 1971, The chromosomes of fifty primary Rous sarcomas, *Hereditas* **69**:155.

MOFFATT, D. J., ROSSE, C., AND YOFFEY, J. M., 1967, Identity of the haemopoietic stem cell, *Lancet* **2**:547.

MOFFATT, D. J., YOUNGBERG, S. P., AND METCALF, W. K., 1971, The validity of autoradiographic labeling, *Cell Tissue Kinet.* **4**:293.

MOORE, M. A. S., WILLIAMS, N., AND METCALF, D., 1972, Purification and characterization of the *in vitro* colony forming cell in monkey hemopoietic tissue, *J. Cell. Physiol.* **79**:283.

391

STEM CELLS,
NON-
PROLIFERATING
CELLS, AND
THEIR
KINETICS

Moser, G. C., Müller, H., and Robbins, E., 1975, Differential nuclear fluorescence during the cell cycle, *Exp. Cell Res.* **91**:73.

Nakeff, A., and Daniels-McQueen, S., 1976, *In vitro* colony assay for a new class of megakaryocyte precursors: colony-forming unit megakaryocyte (CFU-M), *Proc. Soc. Exp. Biol. Med.* **151**:587.

Nathan, M. H., Collins, V. P., and Adams, R. A., 1962, Differentiation of benign and malignant pulmonary nodules by growth rate, *Radiology* **79**:221.

Nešković, B. A., 1968, Developmental phases in intermitosis and the preparation for mitosis of mammalian cells *in vitro*, *Int. Rev. Cytol.* **24**:71.

Nias, A. H. W., and Fox, M., 1971, Synchronization of mammalian cells with respect to the mitotic cycle, *Cell Tissue Kinet.* **4**:375.

Nicolini, C., and Baserga, R., 1975, Circular dichroism and ethidium bromide binding studies of chromatin from WI-38 fibroblasts stimulated to proliferate, *Chem. Biol. Interact.* **11**:101.

Nicolini, C., Ajiro, K., Borun, T., and Baserga, R., 1975, Chromatin change during cell cycle of HeLa cells, *J. Biol. Chem.* **250**:3381.

Nilsson, K., and Pontén, J., 1975, Classification and biological nature of established human hematopoietic cell lines, *Int. J. Cancer* **15**:321.

Noble, R. L., and Hoover, L., 1975, A classification of transplantable tumors in NC rats controlled by estrogen from dormancy to autonomy, *Cancer Res.* **35**:2935.

Nowell, P. C., 1975, Cytogenetics, in: *Cancer: A Comprehensive Treatise*, Vol. 1 (F. F. Becker, ed.), Plenum Press, New York.

Nowakowski, R. S., and Rakic, P., 1974, Clearance rate of exogenous ^{3}H-thymidine from the plasma of pregnant rhesus monkeys, *Cell Tissue Kinet.* **7**:189.

Oehlert, W., Lauf, P., and Seemayer, N., 1962, Autoradiographische Untersuchungen über den Generationszyklus der Zellen des Ehrlichschen Mäuse-Aszites carcinoms, *Naturwissenschaften* **49**:137.

Ohno, S., 1971, Genetic implication of karyological instability of malignant somatic cells, *Physiol. Rev.* **51**:696.

Oja, H. K., Oja, S. S., and Hasan, J., 1967, Calibration of stripping film autoradiography on sections of rat liver labeled with tritium, *Ex. Cell Res.* **45**:1.

Omine, M., and Perry, S., 1972, Use of cell separation at 1 *g* for cytokinetic studies in spontaneous AKR leukemia, *J. Natl. Cancer Inst.* **48**:697.

Omine, M., and Perry, S., 1973, Perturbations of leukemic cell population in AKR mice due to chemotherapy, *Cancer Res.* **33**:2596.

Omine, M., Sarna, G. P., and Perry, S., 1973, Composition of leukemic cell population in AKR leukemia and effects of chemotherapy, *Br. J. Cancer* **9**:557.

Pardee, A. B., 1974, A restriction point for control of normal animal cell proliferation, *Proc. Natl. Acad. Sci. USA* **71**:1286.

Patt, H. M., and Maloney, M. A., 1963, An evaluation of granulocytopoiesis, in: *Cell Proliferation* (L. F. Lamerton and R. J. M. Fry, eds.), F. A. Davis, Philadelphia.

Patt, H. M., Blackford, M. E., and Drallmeier, J. L., 1953, Growth characteristics of Krebs ascites tumor, *Proc. Soc. Exp. Biol. Med.* **83**:520.

Pederson, T., 1972, Chromatin structure and the cell cycle, *Proc. Natl. Acad. Sci. USA* **69**:2224.

Pederson, T., and Gelfant, S., 1970, G_2-population cells in mouse kidney and duodenum and their behavior during the cell division cycle, *Exp. Cell Res.* **59**:32.

Pederson, T., and Robbins, E., 1972, Chromatin structure and the cell division cycle: Actinomycin binding in synchronized HeLa cells, *J. Cell Biol.* **55**:322.

Peel, S., and Fletcher, P. A., 1969, Changes occurring during the growth of Ehrlich ascites cells *in vivo*, *Eur. J. Cancer* **5**:581.

Perkins, E. H., Sado, T., and Makinodan, T., 1969, Recruitment and proliferation of immunocompetent cells during the log phase of the primary antibody response, *J. Immunol.* **103**:668.

Perry, R. P., 1962, The cellular sites of synthesis of ribosomal and 45 S RNA, *Proc. Natl. Acad. Sci. USA* **48**:2179.

Perry, S., 1973, Cancer chemotherapy: A broad overview, in: *Seventh National Cancer Conference Proceedings*, Lippincott, Philadelphia.

Perry, S., and Gallo, R. C., 1970, Physiology of human leukemic leukocytes: Kinetic and biochemical considerations, in: *Regulation of Hematopoiesis* (A. S. Gordon, ed.), Appleton-Century-Crofts, New York.

392

MILAN
POTMESIL,
JOSEPH
LOBUE,
AND
ANNA
GOLDFEDER

PERRY, S., GODWIN, H., AND ZIMMERMAN, T., 1968, Physiology of granulocytes, *J.A.M.A.* **203**:937.

PETERS, L. J., AND HEWITT, H. B., 1974, The influence of fibrin formation on the transplantability of murine tumor cells: Implications for the mechanism of the Révécz effect, *Br. J. Cancer* **29**:279.

PETERSON, E. A., AND EVANS, W. H., 1967, Separation of cells by sedimentation at unit gravity, *Nature (London)* **214**:824.

PILERI, A., GABUTTI, V., MASERA, P., AND GAVOSTO, F., 1967, Proliferative activity of the cells of acute leukaemia in relapse and in steady state, *Acta Haematol.* **38**:193.

PILERI, A., PEGARARO, L., BACHI, C., AND GAVOSTO, F., 1964, Pouvoir proliferant des éléments blastiques leucèmiques, *Sangre* **9**:320.

PLAGER, J., 1975, The induction of transient increases in mitotic rate in murine tissues following prolonged intravenous infusion of hydroxyurea, *Cell Tissue Kinet.* **8**:517.

PLUZNICK, D. H., AND SACHS, L., 1965, The cloning of normal cells in tissue culture, *J. Cell. Comp. Physiol.* **66**:319.

POGO, B. G. T., ALLFREY, V. G., AND MIRSKY, A. E., 1966, RNA synthesis and histone acetylation during the course of gene activation in lymphocytes, *Proc. Natl. Acad. Sci. USA* **55**:805.

PORSCHEN, W., AND FEINENDEGEN, L., 1969, In-vivo-Bestimmung der Zellverlustrate bei Experimentaltumoren mit markiertem Jododeoxyuridin, *Strahlentherapie* **137**:718.

POST, J., AND HOFFMAN, J., 1967, Late effects of H^3TdR as a DNA label on liver cell replication, *Radiat. Res.* **30**:748.

POST, J., AND HOFFMAN, J., 1969, A G_2 population of cells in autogenous rodent sarcoma, *Exp. Cell Res.* **57**:111.

POST, J., SKLAREW, R. J., AND HOFFMAN, J., 1973, Cell proliferation patterns in an autogenous rat sarcoma, *J. Natl. Cancer Inst.* **50**:403.

POST, J., SKLAREW, R. J., AND HOFFMAN, J., 1974, Immediate and delayed effects of nitrogen mustard on cell replication in an autogenous rat sarcoma, *J. Natl. Cancer Inst.* **52**:1897.

POTMESIL, M., AND GOLDFEDER, A., 1971, Nucleolar morphology, nucleic acid syntheses, and growth rates of experimental tumors, *Cancer Res.* **31**:789.

POTMESIL, M., AND GOLDFEDER, A., 1972, Nucleolar morphology and maturation of thymic lymphocytes, *J. Cell. Biol.* **53**:832.

POTMESIL, M., AND GOLDFEDER, A., 1973, Nucleolar morphology and cell proliferation kinetics of thymic lymphocytes, *Exp. Cell Res.* **77**:31.

POTMESIL, M., AND GOLDFEDER, A., 1977, Identification and kinetics of G_1 phase-confined cells in experimental mammary carcinomas, *Cancer Res.* **37**:857.

POTMESIL, M., AND SMETANA, K., 1968, The effect of chromomycin A_3 on the formation of ring shaped nucleoli and incorporation of H^3 uridine in cell cultures, *Folia Biol. (Prague)* **14**:132.

POTMESIL, M., AND SMETANA, K., 1969, Significance of ring shaped nucleoli and micronucleoli in human lymphocytes, *Folio Biol. (Prague)* **15**:300.

POTMESIL, M., AND SMETANA, K., 1970, Studies on nucleoli of lymphocytes in human peripheral blood. Transformation of nucleoli and incorporation of H^3-uridine in phytohaemagglutinin stimulated lymphocytes and reversibility of induced changes after chromomycin A_3 treatment, *Folia Haematol. (Leipzig)* **94**:264.

POTMESIL, M., LUDWIG, D., AND GOLDFEDER, A., 1975, Cell kinetics or irradiated experimental tumors: Relation between the proliferating and the nonproliferating pool, *Cell Tissue Kinet.* **8**:369.

POTMESIL, M., GOLDFEDER, A., BROWN, D. M., AND RICE, L., 1977, Cell kinetics of irradiated experimental tumors: Cell transition from the nonproliferating to the proliferating pool, in preparation.

POTTEN, C. S., HAGEMANN, R. F., AND REILAND, J. M., 1972, Temporary localized depression of tritiated thymidine incorporation in mouse tissues after pulse labelling, *Cell Tissue Kinet.* **5**:193.

POTTER, C. G., 1970, Microspectrophotometry and autoradiography in the study of DNA values of cells in tissue culture, *Exp. Cell. Res.* **61**:141.

PUCK, T. T., AND MARCUS, P. I., 1955, A rapid method for viable cell titration and clone production with HeLa cells in tissue culture: The use of X-irradiated cells to supply conditioning factors, *Proc. Natl. Acad. Sci. USA* **41**:432.

QUAGLINO, D., DePASQUALE, A., AND TANIN, G., 1974, Autoradiographic and cytophotometric investigations on blast cells from acute leukemia, *Haematologica* **59**:141.

QUASTLER, H., 1963, The analysis of cell population kinetics, in: *Cell Proliferation* (L. F. LAMERTON AND R. J. M. FRY, eds.), F. A. Davis, Philadelphia.

393

STEM CELLS,
NON-
PROLIFERATING
CELLS, AND
THEIR
KINETICS

QUASTLER, H., AND SHERMAN, F. G., 1959, Cell population kinetics in the intestinal epithelium of the mouse, *Exp. Cell Res.* **17**:420.

RAJN, M. R., TURJILLO, T. T., MULLANEY, P. F., ROMERO, B. S., AND WALTERS, R. A., 1974, The distribution in the cell cycle of normal cells and of irradiated tumor cells in mice, *Br. J. Radiol.* **47**:405.

RAMBERT, P., MALAISE, E., LAUGIER, A., SCHLENGER, M., AND TUBIANA, M., 1968, Données sur la vitesse de croissance de tumeurs humaines, *Bull cancer* **55**:323.

RAY, G. R., HAHN, G. M., BAGSHAW, M. A., AND KURKJIAN, S., 1973, Cell survival and repair of plateau-phase cultures after chemotherapy, relevance to tumor therapy and to the *in vitro* screening of new agents, *Cancer Chem. Rep.* **57**:473.

RAZEK, A., VIETTI, T., AND VALERIOTE, F., 1974, Optimum time sequence for the administration of vincristine and cyclophosphamide *in vivo*, Cancer Res. **34**:1857.

REICHARD, P., AND ESTBORN, B., 1951, Utilization of deoxyribotides in the synthesis of polynucleotides, *J. Biol. Chem.* **188**:839.

REINHOLD, H. S., AND DEBREE, C., 1968, Tumour cure rate and cell survival of a transplantable rat rhabdomyosarcoma following X-irradiation, *Eur. J. Cancer* **4**:367.

RICHARDS, B. M., 1955, Deoxyribose nucleic acid values in tumor cells with reference to the stem-cell theory of tumor growth, *Nature (London)* **175**:259.

RICHARDS, B. M., AND ATKIN, N. B., 1970, DNA content of human tumors: Change in uterine tumors during radiotherapy and their response to treatment, *Br. J. Cancer* **13**:788.

ROBERTS, J. J., BRENT, T. P., AND CRATHORN, A. R., 1971, Evidence for the inactivation and repair of the mammalian DNA template after alkylation by mustard gas and half mustard gas, *Eur. J. Cancer* **7**:515.

ROCKWELL, S., AND KALLMAN, R. F., 1973, Cellular radiosensitivity and tumor radiation response in the EMT6 tumor cell system, *Radiat. Res.* **53**:281.

ROCKWELL, S., KALLMAN, R. F., AND FAJARDO, L. F., 1972, Characteristics of a serially transplanted mouse mammary tumor and its tissue-culture adapted derivative, *J. Natl. Cancer Inst.* **49**:735.

ROGERS, A. W., 1973, *Techniques of Autoradiography*, Elsevier, New York.

ROSEN, P. J., PERRY, S., AND SCHABEL, F. M., JR., 1970, Proliferation capacity of leukemic cells in AKR leukemia, *J. Natl. Cancer Inst.* **45**:1169.

ROSSE, C., 1970, Two morphologically and kinetically distinct populations of lymphoid cells in the bone marrow, *Nature (London)* **227**:73.

ROSSE, C., 1973, Precursor cells to erythroblasts and to small lymphocytes of the bone marrow, in: *Haemopoietic Stem Cells*, Ciba Foundation Symposium 13 (New Series) (G. E. W. WOLSTENHOLME AND M. O'CONNOR, eds.), Elsevier, North-Holland, Amsterdam.

ROSSE, C., AND TROTTER, J. A., 1974, Cytochemical and radioautographic identification of cells induced to synthesize hemoglobin, *Blood* **43**:885.

ROTI ROTI, J., AND DETHLEFSEN, L. A., 1975a, Matrix simulation of duodenal crypt cell kinetics. I. The steady state, *Cell Tissue Kinet.* **8**:321.

ROTI ROTI, J., AND DETHLEFSEN, L. A., 1975b, Matrix simulation of duodenal crypt cell kinetics. II. Cell kinetics following hydroxyurea, *Cell Tissue Kinet.* **8**:335.

ROVERA, G., AND BASERGA, R., 1973, Effect of nutritional changes on chromatin template activity and non-histone chromosomal protein synthesis in WI-38 and 3T6 cells, *Exp. Cell. Res.* **78**:116.

ROVERA, G., AND PEGORARO, L., 1968, Evoluzione clonale e caratteri stiche della distribuzione degli extracromosomi in tre casi di leucemia mieloide cronica acutizzata, *Haematol. Arch.* **53**:465.

ROWINSKI, J., PIEŃKOWSKI, M., AND ABRAMEZUK, J., 1972, Area representation of optical density of chromatin in resting and stimulated lymphocytes as measured by means of Quantimet, *Histochemie* **32**:75.

RUBINI, J. R., CRONKITE, E. P., BOND, V. P., AND FLIEDNER, T. M., 1960, The metabolism and fate of tritiated thymidine in man, *J. Clin. Invest.* **39**:909.

RUBINOW, S. I., LEBOWITZ, J. L., AND SAPSE, A. M., 1971, Parameterization of *in vivo* leukemic cell populations, *Biophys. J.* **11**:175.

RUBINSTEIN, A. S., AND TROBAUGH, F. E., 1973, Ultrastructure of presumptive hemopoietic stem cells, *Blood* **42**:61.

SACHS, L., 1974, Differentiation of hematopoietic cells, in: *Control of Proliferation in Animal Cells* (B. D. CLARKSON AND R. BASERGA, eds.), Cold Spring Harbor Laboratory, Cold Spring Harbor, N.Y.

SANDBERG, A. A., AND SAKURAI, M., 1974, Chromosomes in the causation and progression of cancer and leukemia, in: *The Molecular Biology of Cancer* (H. BUSCH, ed.), Academic Press, New York.

394

MILAN
POTMESIL,
JOSEPH
LOBUE,
AND
ANNA
GOLDFEDER

SANDBERG, A. A., ISHIHARA, T., KIKUCHI, Y., AND CROSSWHITE, L. H., 1964, Chromosomal differences among the acute leukemias, *Ann. N.Y. Acad. Sci.* **113:**663.

SANDER, G., AND PARDEE, A. B., 1972, Transport changes in synchronously growing CHO cells and L cells, *J. Cell. Physiol.* **80:**267.

SANTOS, G. W., AND HAGHSHENASS, M., 1968, Cloning of syngeneic hematopoietic cells in the spleens of mice and rats pretreated with cytotoxic drugs, *Blood* **32:**629.

SARNA, G., OMINE, M., AND PERRY, S., 1975, Cytokinetics of human acute leukemia before and after chemotherapy, *Eur. J. Cancer* **11:**483.

SAUNDERS, E. F., AND MAUER, A. M., 1969, Reentry of nondividing leukemic cells into a proliferative phase in acute childhood leukemia, *J. Clin. Invest.* **48:**1299.

SAUNDERS, G. C., AND WILDER, M., 1971, Repetitive maturation cycles in a cultured mouse myeloma, *J. Cell Biol.* **51:**344.

SAWICKI, W., ROWINSKI, J., AND SWENSON, R., 1975, Change of chromatin morphology during the cell cycle detected by means of automated image analysis, *J. Cell. Physiol.* **84:**423.

SCHABEL, F. M., JR., 1968, *In vivo* leukemic cell kill kinetics and "curability" in experimental systems, in: *The Proliferation and Spread of Neoplastic Cells*, Williams and Wilkins, Baltimore.

SCHABEL, F. M., JR., 1969, The use of tumor growth kinetics in planning "curative" chemotherapy of advanced solid tumors, *Cancer Res.* **29:**2384.

SCHABEL, F. M., JR., SKIPPER, H. E., TRADER, M. W., LASTER, W. R., JR., AND SIMPSON-HERREN, L., 1969, Spontaneous AK leukemia as a model system, *Cancer Chem. Rep. Part 2* **53:**329.

SCHABEL, F. M., JR., SKIPPER, H. E., TRADER, M. W., LASTER, W. R., JR., AND CHEEKS, J. B., 1974, Combination chemotherapy for spontaneous AKR lymphoma, *Cancer Chem. Rep. Part 1* **4:**53.

SCHIFFER, L. M., AND MARKOE, A. M., 1974, Cytokinetic stability of an Ehrlich ascites tumor, *Cell Tissue Kinet.* **7:**305.

SCHMIDT, L. H., FRADKIN, R., SULLIVAN, R., AND FLOWERS, A., 1965, Comparative pharmacology of alkylating agents, part II, *Cancer Chem. Rep.* **403:**1015.

SCHNEIDER, W. D., AND GRECO, A. E., 1971, Incorporation of pyrimidine deoxyribonucleosides in liver lipids and other components, *Biochim. Biophys. Acta.* **228:** 610.

SHACKNEY, S. E., FORD, S. S., AND WITTIG, A. B., 1973, The effects of counting threshold and emulsion exposure duration on the percent labeled mitosis curve and their implication for cell cycle analysis, *Cancer Res.* **33:**2726.

SHAEFFER, J., EL-MAHDI, A. M., AND CONSTABLE, W. C., 1973, Lung colony assays of murine mammary tumor cells irradiated *in vivo* and *in vitro*, *Radiology* **109:**703.

SHEEHY, P. F., FRIED, J., WINN, R., AND CLARKSON, B. D., 1974, Cell cycle changes in ovarian cancer after arabinosylcytosine, *Cancer* **33:**28.

SHIPLEY, W. V., STANLEY, J. A., AND STEEL, G. G., 1975, Tumor size dependency in the radiation response of the Lewis lung carcinoma, *Cancer Res.* **35:**2488.

SIMINOVITCH, L., TILL, J. E., AND MCCULLOCH, E. A., 1964, Decline in colony-forming ability of marrow cells subjected to serial transplantation into irradiated mice, *J. Cell. Comp. Physiol.* **64:**23.

SIMINOVITCH, L., TILL, J. E., AND MCCULLOCH, E. A., 1965, Radiation responses of haemopoietic colony-forming cells derived from different sources, *Radiat. Res.* **24:**482.

SKIPPER, H. E., 1968, Biochemical, biological, pharmacologic, toxicologic, kinetic, and clinical (subhuman and human) relationships, *Cancer* **21:**600.

SKIPPER, H. E., 1971*a*, Kinetics of mammary tumor cell growth and implications for therapy, *Cancer* **6:**1479.

SKIPPER, H. E., 1971*b*, The cell cycle and chemotherapy of cancer, in: *The Cell Cycle and Cancer* (R. BASERGA, ed.), Marcel Dekker, New York.

SKIPPER, H. E., 1972, Kinetic behavior versus response to chemotherapy, *Natl. Cancer Inst. Monogr.* **34:**2.

SKIPPER, H. E., 1974, Combination therapy: Some concepts and results, *Cancer Chem. Rep. Part 2* **4:**137.

SKIPPER, H. E., AND SCHABEL, F. M., JR., 1973, Quantitative and cytokinetic studies in experimental tumor models, in: *Cancer Medicine* (J. F. HOLLAND AND E. FREI, III, eds.), Lea and Febiger, Philadelphia.

SKIPPER, H. E., SCHABEL, F. M., JR., TRADER, M. W., AND LASTER, W. R., JR., 1969, Response to therapy of spontaneous, first passage and long passage lines of AK leukemia, *Cancer Chem. Rep.* **53:**345.

SKIPPER, H. E., SCHABEL, F. M., JR., MELLETT, L. B., MONTGOMERY, J. A., WILKOFF, L. J., LLOYD, H. H., AND BROCKMAN, R. W., 1970, Application of biochemical, cytokinetic, pharmacologic, and toxicologic relationships in the design of optimal therapeutic schedules, *Cancer Chem. Rep.* **56:**431.

SMETANA, K., 1961, A further contribution to the question of the incidence of nucleoli in the nuclei of mature lymphocytes in man, *Folia Biol. (Prague)* **7**:268.

SMETANA, K., 1967, Basic histochemical and cytochemical methods, in: *Methods in Cancer Research*, Vol. 2 (H. BUSCH, ed.), Academic Press, New York.

SMETANA, K., 1970, Electron microscopy of lymphocytes, in: *Methods in Cancer Research*, Vol. 5 (H. BUSCH, ed.), Academic Press, New York.

SMETANA, K., AND POTMESIL, M., 1970, A further contribution on the evidence of ring shaped nucleoli and micronucleoli in mature human lymphocytes, *Folio Haematol. (Leipzig)* **93**:16.

SMETANA, K., LANE, M., AND BUSCH, H., 1966, Studies on nucleoli of leukemic agranulocytes and plasmacytes in multiple myeloma, *Exp. Mol. Pathol.* **5**:236.

SMETANA, K., GYORKEY, F., GYORKEY, P., AND BUSCH, H., 1970, Comparative studies on the ultrastructure of nucleoli in human lymphosarcoma cells and leukemic lymphocytes, *Cancer Res.* **30**:1149.

SMETANA, K., GYORKEY, F., GYORKEY, P., AND BUSCH, H., 1975, Studies on nucleoli of maturing human erythroblasts, *Exp. Cell Res.* **91**:143.

SMITH, J. A., AND MARTIN, L., 1973, Do cells cycle? *Proc. Natl. Acad. Sci. USA* **70**:1263.

SMITH, J. M., 1973, Cells and aging, in: *Cell Biology in Medicine* (E. E. BITTAR, ed), Wiley, New York.

STAROSCIK, R. N., JENKINS, W. H., AND MENDELSOHN, M. L., 1964, Availability of tritiated thymidine after intravenous administration, *Nature (London)* **202**:456.

STEEL, G. G., 1968, Cell loss from experimental tumors, *Cell Tissue Kinet.* **1**:193.

STEEL, G. G., 1972, The cell cycle in tumors: An examination of data gained by the technique of labelled mitosis, *Cell Tissue Kinet.* **5**:87.

STEEL, G. G., 1973, Cytokinetics of neoplasia, in: *Cancer Medicine* (J. F. HOLLAND and E. FREI, III, eds.), Lea and Febiger, Philadelphia.

STEEL, G. G., 1975, The growth kinetics of tumors in relation to their chemotherapeutic response, *Laryngoscope* **85**:359.

STEEL, G. G., AND ADAMS, K., 1975, Stem-cell survival and tumor control in the Lewis lung carcinoma, *Cancer Res.* **35**:1530.

STEEL, G. G., AND HANES, S., 1971, The technique of labelled mitosis: Analysis by automatic curve-fitting, *Cell Tissue Kinet.* **4**:93.

STEEL, G. G., AND LAMERTON, L. F., 1965, The turnover of tritium from thymidine in tissues of the rat, *Exp. Cell Res.* **37**:117.

STEEL, G. G., AND LAMERTON, L. F., 1966, The growth of human tumors, *Br. J. Cancer* **20**:74.

STEEL, G. G., ADAMS, K., AND BARRETT, J. C., 1966, Analysis of the cell population kinetics of transplanted tumors, *Br. J. Cancer* **20**:784.

STEIN, G., AND BASERGA, R., 1972, Nuclear proteins and the cell cycle, in: *Advances in Cancer Research*, Vol. 15 (G. KLEIN AND S. WEINHOUSE, eds.), Academic Press, New York.

STEINKAMP, J. A., FULWYLER, N. J., AND COULTER, J. R., 1973, A new multiparameter separator for microscopic particles and biological cells, *Rev. Sci. Instrum.* **44**:1310.

STEPHENSON, J. R., AXELRAD, A. A., MCLEOD, D. L., AND SHREEVE, M. M., 1971, Induction of colonies of hemoglobin-synthesizing cells by erythropoietin in vitro, *Proc. Natl. Acad. Sci. USA* **68**:1542.

STEWART, P. A., QUASTLER, H., SKOUGAARD, M. R., WIMBER, D. R., WOLFSBERG, M. F., PERROTTA, C. A., FERBEL, B., AND CARLOUGH, M., 1965, Four-factor model analysis of thymidine incorporation into mouse DNA and the mechanism of radiation effects, *Radiat. Res.* **24**:521.

STICH, H. F., AND STEEL, H. D., 1962, DNA content of tumor cells. III. Mosaic composition of sarcomas and carcinomas in man, *J. Natl. Cancer Inst.* **28**:1207.

STILLSTRÖM, J., 1963, Grain count corrections in autoradiography, *Int. J. Appl. Radiat.* **14**:113.

STOCKER, R., 1966, Der Proliferationsmodus im Niere und Leber, *Verh. Deutsch. Ges. Pathol.* **50**:53.

STOHLMAN, F., JR., QUESENBERRY, P. J., AND TYLER, W. S., 1974, The regulation of myelopoiesis as approached with in vivo and in vitro techniques, in: *Progress in Hematology*, Grune and Stratton, New York.

STRYCKMANS, P., DELALIEUX, G., AND MANASTER, J., 1970, The potentiality of out-of-cycle acute leukemia cells to synthesize DNA, *Blood* **36**:697.

SUIT, H. D., 1967, Effects of radiation on tumors in animals, *Can. Cancer Res. Conf.* **7**:387.

SUIT, H. D., AND URANO, M., 1969, Repair of sublethal radiation injury in hypoxic cells of a C3H mouse mammary carcinoma, *Radiat. Res.* **37**:423.

SUIT, H. D., MARSHALL, N., AND WOERNER, D., 1972, Oxygen, oxygen plus carbon dixoide, and radiation therapy of a mouse mammary carcinoma, *Cancer* **30**:1154.

395

STEM CELLS,
NON-
PROLIFERATING
CELLS, AND
THEIR
KINETICS

MILAN
POTMESIL,
JOSEPH
LOBUE,
AND
ANNA
GOLDFEDER

SULLIVAN, P. W., AND SALMON, S. E., 1972, Kinetics of tumor growth and repression in IgG multiple myeloma, *J. Clin. Invest.* **51**:1697.

SUTHERLAND, R. M., McCREDIE, J. A., AND INCH, W. R., 1968, Growth of multicell spheroids in tissue culture as a model of modular carcinomas, *Br. J. Cancer* **22**:258.

SUTHERLAND, R. M., INCH, W. R., McCREDIE, J. A., AND KRUUV, J., 1970, A multi-component radiation survival curve using an *in vitro* model, *Int. J. Radiat. Biol.* **18**:491.

SYEKLOCHA, D., SIMINOVITCH, L., TILL, J. E., AND McCULLOCH, E. A., 1966, The proliferative state of antigen-sensitive precursors of hemolysin producing cells determined by the use of the inhibitor vinblastine, *J. Immunol.* **96**:472.

TANNOCK, I. F., 1969, A comparison of cell proliferation parameters in solid and ascites Ehrlich tumors, *Cancer Res.* **29**:1527.

TEPPERMAN, D., CURTIS, J. E., AND McCULLOCH, E. A., 1974, Erythropoietic colonies in cultures of human marrow, *Blood* **44**:659.

THOMAS, E. D., FLIEDNER, T. M., THOMAS, D., AND CRONKITE, E. P., 1965, The problem of the stem cell: Observations in dogs following nitrogen mustard, *J. Lab. Clin. Med.* **65**:794.

THOMAS, D., 1973, The radiation chimera as an experimental model for the study of haemopoietic stem cell populations, in: *Haemopoietic Stem Cells*, Ciba Foundation Symposium 13 (New Series) (G. E. W. WOLSTENHOLME AND M. O'CONNOR, eds.), Elsevier, North-Holland, Amsterdam.

THOMSON, J. E., AND RAUTH, A. N., 1974, An *in vitro* assay to measure the viability of KHT tumor cells not previously exposed to culture conditions, *Radiat. Res.* **58**:262.

TILL, J. E., AND McCULLOCH, E. A., 1961, A direct measurement of the radiation sensitivity of normal mouse bone marrow cells, *Radiat. Res.* **14**:213.

TILL, J. E., AND McCULLOCH, E. A., 1963, Early repair processes in marrow cells irradiated and proliferating *in vivo*, *Radiat. Res.* **18**:105.

TILL, J. E., McCULLOCH, E. A., AND SIMINOVITCH, I., 1964, Isolation of variant cell lines during serial transplantation of hematopoietic cells derived from fetal liver, *J. Natl. Cancer Inst.* **33**:707.

TILL, J. E., PRICE, G. B., MAK, T. W., AND McCULLOCH, E. A., 1975, Regulation of blood cell differentiation, *Fed. Proc.* **34**:2279.

TOBEY, R. A., 1972a, Arrest of Chinese hamster cells in G_2 following treatment with the anti-tumor drug bleomycin, *J. Cell. Physiol.* **79**:259.

TOBEY, R. A., 1972b, Effects of cytosine arabinose, daunomycin, mithramycin, aracytidine, adriamycin and amenoptherin on mammalian cell cycle traverse, *Cancer Res.* **32**:2720.

TOBEY, R. A., 1973, Production and characterization of mammalian cells reversibly arrested in G_1 by growth in isoleucine-deficient medium, in: *Methods in Cell Biology*, Vol. 6 (D. M. PRESCOTT, ed.), Academic Press, New York.

TOBEY, R. A., AND CRISSMAN, H. A., 1972, Use of flow microfluorometry in detailed analysis of effects of chemical agents on cell cycle progression, *Cancer Res.* **32**:2726.

TOBEY, R. A., AND LEY, K. D., 1970, Regulation of initiation of DNA synthesis in Chinese hamster cells. I. Production of stable, reversible G_1-arrested populations in suspension culture, *J. Cell. Biol.* **46**:151.

TOBEY, R. A., PETERSON, D. F., AND ANDERSON, E. C., 1971, Biochemistry of G_2 and mitosis, in: *The Cell Cycle and Cancer* (R. BASERGA, ed.), Marcel Dekker, New York.

TODO, A., FRIED, J., AND CLARKSON, B., 1969, Kinetics of proliferation of human hematopoietic cells in suspension culture, *Proc. Am. Cancer Res.* **10**:93.

TROTT, K. R., AND HUG, O., 1970, Intraclonal recovery of division probability in pedigrees of single X-irradiated mammalian cells, *Int. J. Radiat. Biol.* **17**:483.

TUBIANA, M., 1973, Clinical data and radiobiological basis for radiotherapy, *Curr. Top. Radiat. Res.* **9**:109.

TUBIANA, M., 1974, Achievements to be expected from new developments in tumour radiotherapy, *Eur. J. Cancer* **10**:373.

TUBIANA, M., FRINDEL, E., CROIZAT, H., AND VASSORT, F., 1974, Study of some of the factors influencing the proliferation and differentiation of the multipotential hemopoietic stem cell, in: *Control in Proliferation of Animal Cells* (B. D. CLARKSON, AND R. BASERGA, eds.), Cold Spring Harbor Laboratory, Cold Spring Harbor, N.Y.

TWENTYMAN, P. R., AND BLEEHEN, N. M., 1973a, The sensitivity to bleomycin of spleen colony-forming units in the mouse, *Br. J. Cancer* **28**:66.

TWENTYMAN, P. R., AND BLEEHEN, N. M., 1973b, The sensitivity of cells in exponential and stationary phases of growth to bleomycin and to 1,3-bis(2-chloroethyl)-1-nitrosourea, *Br. J. Cancer* **28**:500.

397
STEM CELLS,
NON-
PROLIFERATING
CELLS, AND
THEIR
KINETICS

TWENTYMAN, P. R., AND BLEEHEN, N. M., 1975, Changes in sensitivity to radiation and to bleomycin occurring during the life history of monolayer cultures of a mouse tumor cell line, *Br. J. Cancer* **31**:68.

TWENTYMAN, P. R., WATSON, J. V., BLEEHEN, N. M., AND ROWLES, P. M., 1975, Changes in cell proliferation kinetics occurring during the life history of monolayer cultures of a mouse tumor cell line, *Cell Tissue Kinet.* **8**:41.

TYLER, R. W., AND EVERETT, N. B., 1966, A radioautographic study of hemopoietic repopulation using irradiated parabiotic rats, *Blood* **28**:873.

TYLER, R. W., ROSSE, C., AND EVERETT, N. B., 1972, The hemopoietic repopulating potential of inflammatory exudate cells, *J. Reticuloendothel. Soc.* **11**:617.

UNDRITZ, E., 1973, *Sandoz Atlas of Haematology*, 2nd ed., Sandoz, Basel.

URANO, M., NESUMI, N., ANDO, K., KOIKE, S., AND OHNUMA, N., 1976, Repair of potentially lethal radiation damage in acute and chronically hypoxic tumor cells *in vivo*, *Radiology* **118**:447.

VALERIOTE, F. A., AND BRUCE, W. R., 1967, Comparison of the sensitivity of hematopoietic colony-forming cells in different proliferative states to vinblastine, *J. Natl. Cancer Inst.* **38**:393.

VALERIOTE, F. A., AND VAN PUTTEN, L., 1975, Proliferation-dependent cytotoxicity of anticancer agents: A review, *Cancer Res.* **35**:2619.

VALLERON, A. J., AND FRINDEL, E., Computer simulation of growing cell populations, *Cell Tissue Kinet.* **6**:69.

VAN BEKKUM, D. W., VAN NOORD, M. J., MAAT, B., AND DICKE, K. A., 1971, Attempts at identification of hemopoietic stem cell in mouse, *Blood* **38**:547.

VAN DEN BRENK, H. A. S., AND SHARPINGTON, C., 1972, Effect of local x-irradiation of a primary sarcoma in the rat on dissemination and growth of metastases: Dose–response characteristics, *Br. J. Cancer* **25**:812.

VAN DEN BRENK, H. A. S., BURCH, W. M., ORTON, C., AND SHARPINGTON, C., 1973*a*, Stimulation of clonogenic growth of tumor cells and metastases in the lungs by local X-irradiation, *Br. J. Cancer* **27**:291.

VAN DEN BRENK, H. A. S., SHARPINGTON, C., AND ORTON, C., 1973*b*, Macrocolony assays in the rat of allogeneic Y-P388 and W-256 tumor cells injected intravenously: Dependence of colony forming efficiency on age of host and immunity, *Br. J. Cancer* **27**:134.

VAN DILLA, M. A., TRUJILLO, T. T., MULLANEY, P. F., AND COULTER, J. R., 1969, Cell microfluorometry: A method for rapid fluorescence measurement, *Science* **163**:1213.

VAN PEPERZEEL, H. A., 1970, Patterns of tumor growth after irradiation, Ph.D. Thesis, Groningen, Drukkerij van Denderen.

VAN PEPERZEEL, H. A., 1972, Effects of single doses of radiation on lung metastases in man and experimental animals, *Eur. J. Cancer* **8**:665.

VAN PUTTEN, L. M., 1974, Are cell kinetic data relevant for the design of tumour chemotherapy schedules? *Cell Tissue Kinet.* **7**:493.

VAN PUTTEN L. M., LELIEVELD, P., AND KRAM-IDSENGA, L. K. J., 1972, Cell cycle specificity and therapeutic effectiveness of cytostatic agents, *Cancer Chem. Rep.* **56**:691.

VAN PUTTEN, L. M., KRIZER, H. J., AND MULDER, J. H., 1976, Perspectives in cancer research, Synchronization in tumour chemotherapy, *Eur. J. Cancer* **12**:79.

VENDRELY, C., 1971, Cytophotometry and histochemistry of the cell cycle, in: *The Cell Cycle and Cancer* (R. BASERGA, ed.), Marcel Dekker, New York.

VENDRELY, C., LAPERON, A., AND TOURNIER, P., 1968, Etude de variations d'activités enzymatiques au cours des différentes phases du cycle de génération de cellules en cultures, *Bull. Cancer* **55**:31.

VOGLER, W. R., COOPER, L. E., GROTH, D. P., 1974, Correlation of cytosine arabinoside-induced increment in growth fraction of leukemic blast cells with clinical response, *Cancer* **33**:603.

VON SZCZEPANSKI, L., AND TROTT, K.-R., 1975, Post-irradiation proliferation kinetics of serially transplanted murine adenocarcinoma, *Br. J. Radiol.* **48**:200.

WEISS, P., 1953, Some introductory remarks on the cellular basis of differentiation, *J. Embryol. Exp. Morphol.* **1**:181.

WHEELER, G. P., AND SIMPSON-HERREN, L., 1973, Effects of purines, pyrimidines, nucleosides and chemically related compounds on the cell cycle, in: *Drugs and the Cell Cycle*, Academic Press, New York.

WHEELER, G. P., BOWDON, B. J., AND WILKOFF, L. J., 1967, The cell cycle of leukemia L1210 cells *in vivo* and *in vitro*, *Proc. Soc. Exp. Biol. Med.* **126**:903.

WHEELER, G. P., BOWDON, P. J., AND ADAMSON, D. J., 1970, Effects of 1,3-bis(2-chloroethyl)-1-

398

MILAN
POTMESIL,
JOSEPH
LOBUE,
AND
ANNA
GOLDFEDER

nitrosourea and some chemically related compounds upon the progression of cultured H.Ep. 2 cells through the cell cycle, *Cancer Res.* **30**:1817.

WIEBEL, F., AND BASERGA, R., 1968, Cell proliferation in newly transplanted Ehrlich ascites tumor cells, *Cell Tissue Kinet.* **1**:273.

WILKOFF, L. J., LLOYD, H. H., AND DULMADGE, E. A., 1971, Kinetic evaluation of the effect of actinomycin D, daunomycin and mitomycin C on proliferating cultured leukemic L1210 cells, *Chemotherapy* **16**:44.

WILLIAMS, J. F., AND TILL, J. E., 1966, Formation of lung colonies by polyoma-transformed rat embryo cells, *J. Natl. Cancer Inst.* **37**:177.

WILLIAMSON, A. R., AND ASKONAS, B. A., 1972, Senescence of an antibody-forming cell line, *Nature (London)* **238**:337.

WINANS, L. F., DEWEY, W. C., AND DETTOR, C. M., 1972, Repair of sublethal and potentially lethal X-ray damage in synchronous Chinese hamster cells, *Radiation Res.* **52**:333.

WITHERS, H. R., 1975, Cell cycle redistribution as a factor in multifraction irradiation, *Radiology* **114**:199.

WITHERS, H. R., AND ELKIND, M. M., 1969, Radiosensitivity and fractionation response of crypt cells of mouse jejunum, *Radiol. Res.* **38**:598.

WODINSKY, J., SWINIARSKI, J., AND KENSLER, C. J., 1967, Spleen colony studies of leukemia L1210. I. Growth kinetics of lymphocytic L1210 cells *in vivo* as determined by spleen colony assay, *Cancer Chem. Rep.* **51**:415.

WODINSKY, L., SWINIARSKI, J., KENSLER, C. J., AND VENDITTI, J. N., 1974, Combination radiotherapy and chemotherapy for P388 lymphocytic leukemia *in vivo*, *Cancer Chem. Rep. Part 1* **4**:73.

WORTON, R. G., McCULLOCH, E. A., AND TILL, J. E., 1969, Physical separation of hematopoietic stem cells differing in their capacity for self-renewal, *J. Exp. Med.* **130**:91.

YAMÍSHEVSKY, R., MENDELSOHN, M. L., MAYALL, B. H., AND CRISTOFALO, V. J., 1974, Proliferative capacity and DNA content of aging human diploid cells in culture. A cytophotometric and autoradiographic analysis, *J. Cell. Physiol.* **84**:165.

YANKEE, R. A., DEVITA, V. T., AND PERRY, S., 1967, The cell cycle of leukemia L1210 cells *in vivo*, *Cancer Res.* **27**:2381.

YATAGANAS, X., AND CLARKSON, B. D., 1974, Flow microfluorometric analysis of cell killing with cytotoxic drugs, *J. Histochem. Cytochem.* **22**:651.

YATAGANAS, X., STRIFE, A., PEREZ, A., AND CLARKSON, B. D., 1974, Microfluorometric evaluation of cell kill kinetics with 1-β-D-arabinofuranosylcytosine, *Cancer Res.* **34**:2795.

YOFFEY, J. N., WINTER, G. C. B., OSMOND, D. G., AND MEEK, E. S., 1965, Morphological studies in the culture of human leucocytes with phytohaemagglutinin, *Br. J. Haematol.* **11**:488.

YOSHIDA, Y., AND OSMOND, D. G., 1971, Identity and proliferation of small lymphocyte precursors in cultures of lymphocyte-rich fraction of guinea-pig bone marrow, *Blood* **37**:73.

YOUNG, R. C., AND DEVITA, V. T., 1970, Cell cycle characteristics of human solid tumors *in vivo*, *Cell Tissue Kinet.* **3**:285.

ZANK, M., AND KRUG, H., 1970, Zytophotometrische DNA-Bestimmungen an Primärtumoren und Metastasen, *Geschwulstforsch.* **36**:343.

ZETTERBERG, A., AND KILLANDER, D., 1965, Quantitative cytophotometric and autoradiographic studies on the rate of protein synthesis during interphase in mouse fibroblasts *in vitro*, *Exp. Cell Res.* **40**:1.

Surgery

10

The Changing Role of Surgery in the Treatment of Cancer

Bernard Fisher

1. Introduction

When consideration is given to recent advances and progress made in the treatment of cancer, little attention is directed toward those changes taking place that are probably as profound and as far reaching in consequence as are any in our time. To many—particularly those in other disciplines—the surgical approach to cancer is deemed anachronistic in concept. While categorically such may be true, the leading edge of that specialty is attempting to redefine the basis for cancer surgery so that it is in keeping with present understanding of tumor biology.

Just as repair of a hernia is based on anatomical considerations and operations for duodenal ulcer on physiological principles, so must there be a firm rationale for the surgical management of cancer. For almost a century, those precepts on which cancer surgery was and still is based have been almost entirely without opposition—perhaps for want of viable alternatives, or perhaps because of the dominance of those in positions of leadership. Within the last decade, partially because of dissatisfaction with results obtained, but more importantly because of new information coming from a variety of sources, old "unchallengeable" concepts have been and are being reassessed. In many instances, they have been found lacking. Consequently, there has resulted the present period of clinical

BERNARD FISHER ● University of Pittsburgh School of Medicine, Pittsburgh, Pennsylvania 15261.

uncertainty which will persist until a firm new basis for cancer surgery has evolved and its new position in the "family" of modalities available for the treatment of cancer has been established. Operation no longer employs the distinction of being "an only child" in that regard.

What has been the basis for cancer surgery in the past? What factors are modifying those principles? What in the future is likely to be the role of operation for the management of cancer? This brief overview will present vignettes of information directed toward answering these and similar questions. Obviously it cannot help but reflect the opinions of this author which have been developed during two decades of involvement with certain aspects of oncology at both the laboratory and the clinical level. Despite such shortcomings, perhaps it will promote an awareness of and an insight into the changes occurring in the primary management of patients with solid tumors—changes which are more exciting and holding more promise for accomplishment than any others which have been documented over the centuries.

2. Evolution of the Operative Treatment of Cancer

Just as it is foolish to judge a person's achievements out of context of his time, so is it improper to evaluate the positive or negative accomplishments of an era without an appreciation of the circumstances which gave rise to them. In tracing the evolution of cancer surgery through the ages, it is of importance to know how those who formulated and influenced the course of action of a particular time conceived of the disease. For it was (and still is) those conceptions which have provided the reasons for what was done.

2.1. Prior to the Twentieth Century

Several publications document in detail the early history of oncology and are worthy of examination by those interested in the subject (Hayward, 1965a,b,c; Haagensen, 1933). Hippocrates, 2400 years ago, described many forms of cancer and indeed originated the term "carcinoma." Unfortunately, there is little or no information to indicate his perception of the disease. Galen in the second century A.D. elaborately classified tumors and considered cancer a systemic disease related to an excess of black bile and therefore beyond cure by operation. His teachings held sway until the eighteenth century, and consequently until that time there existed no firm justification for the use of surgery in the treatment of cancer.

The first surgeon to consider cancer a local and curable disease is not known (Hayward, 1965b). A number of eighteenth-century surgeons made an effort to develop a rationale for cancer surgery. Valsalva (1704) from the beginning of the eighteenth century ignored the Galenic teaching that cancer was only a local manifestation of a generalized serological excess of black bile. He believed that it was at first a local lesion capable of cure by surgery, that it spread by lymphatics to regional nodes, and that it tended to recur. Others continued to develop such a thesis. The French surgeon LeDran (1757) and the Italian Morgagni (1769) were most influential in that regard. Their thoughts are best summarized by the following, written by LeDran concerning breast cancer:

> The writers who have treated this subject have represented a cancer as a sordid spreading ulcer and have looked on it as incurable; but—every cancer begins by the obstruction of one or more glands and is at first only a tumor formed by obstruction; but afterwards it becomes schirrous and then carcinomatous . . . . If a schirrous is once arrived to a certain degree of size and hardness we have no medicines sufficiently powerful to dissolve it. If the patient is only incommoded by its weight it may be left to itself. But if it increases, surgery afforded no other remedy but extirpation and where that is practicable we may be assured of success. Also, if just becoming painful, provided the operation is not delayed, we may hope for a perfect cure.
>
> In some more advanced cases palliative surgery may relieve symptoms and prolong life, though recurrence may be certain.
>
> If only a few axillary glands are found involved, be sure to remove them along with the breast or it might give rise to a fresh cancer.

Thus originated the assumption that cancer was a local disease which was curable if found sufficiently early.

2.2. From Halsted to the Present

The principles on which present-day cancer surgery is based were formulated almost 100 years ago (Halsted, 1890/1891). No one was more influential in conditioning the minds of generations of surgeons relative to the management of patients with neoplasms than was the American surgeon William S. Halsted. While his name is most closely associated with the operation for breast cancer popularly referred to as "radical mastectomy," the same precepts promulgated by him for that procedure have served as an enduring basis for all cancer surgery. In order to understand Halsted's rationale for the type of surgery he advocated, it is important to appreciate his concept of the biology of cancer—and particularly how he thought tumors disseminated. Some insight relative to that is gleaned from his publication of 1907 (Halsted, 1907). He apparently placed little significance on the bloodstream as a mechanism for the development of metastases, as is indicated by his following statement:

> Although it undoubtedly occurs, I am not sure that I have observed from breast cancer, metastasis which seemed definitely to have been conveyed by way of the blood vessels; and my views as to the dissemination of carcinoma of the breast accord so fully with Handley's that I may in justice to him, who has formulated and expressed them so well, quote now and again from his admirable chapters. "In showing that cancer cells in the blood excite thrombosis, and that the thrombosis as it organizes usually destroys or renders them harmless, Goldman and Schmidt seem to have established a fact of primary importance and one which is strongly opposed to the embolic theory as applied to carcinoma" (Handley, 1922). We believe with Handley that cancer of the breast in spreading centrifugally preserves in the main continuity with the original growth and before involving the viscera may become widely diffused along surface planes.

Halsted also believed that bone metastases occurred in cases of breast cancer very rarely in areas not actually invaded by subcutaneous nodules. It was his opinion that there was a significant relationship between the bone deposits and the subcutaneous nodules and that "it [tumor] permeates to the bone rather than metastasizes to it, and this via the lymphatics along fascial planes." Thus his concepts were really those of W. Sampson Handley, who, unfortunately, wrongly influenced the thinking of several generations of surgeons and, more importantly, gave rise to surgical procedures that were basically unsound. It was not until 1938, when Gray (1939) demonstrated that the mode of spread to lymph glands was by lymphatic emboli and that cancer cells did not remain for any length of time within the lumen of lymphatic vessels, that Handley's influence terminated.

Halsted's understanding of tumor dissemination is best summarized when he wrote the following: "There is then a definite more or less interrupted or quite uninterrupted connection between the original focus and all the outlying deposits of cancer . . . the centrifugal spread annexing by continuity a very large area in some cases. Thus, the liver may be invaded by way of the deep fascia, the linea alba and the round ligament, the brain by the lymphatics accompanying the middle meningeal artery."

The following quote from Halsted's publication concerning breast cancer is presented because it so clearly set the stage for an era of surgery which must be viewed as incredible in terms of both its longevity and its freedom from criticism. It thus deserves careful consideration.

> Though the area of disease extend from cranium to knee, breast cancer in the broad sense is a local affection, and there comes to the surgeon an encouragement to greater endeavor with the cognition that the metastases to bone, to pleura, to liver, are probably parts of the whole, and that the involvements are almost invariably by process of lymphatic permeation and not embolic by way of the blood. Extension, the most rapid, taking place beneath the skin along the fascial planes, we must remove not only a very large amount of skin and a much larger area of subcutaneous fat and fascia, but also strip the sheaths from the upper part of the rectus, the serratus magnus, the subscapularis, and at times from parts of the latissimus dorsi and the teres major. Both pectoral muscles are, of course, removed.
> A part of the chest wall should, I believe, be excised in certain cases, the surgeon bearing in mind always that he is dealing with lymphatic and not blood metastases and that the slightest inattention to detail, or attempts to hasten convalescence by such plastic operations as are feasible only when a restricted amount of skin is removed, may sacrifice his patient.
> It must be our endeavor to trace more definitely the routes traveled in the metastases to bone, particularly to the humerus, for it is even possible in case of involvement of this bone that amputation of the shoulder joint plus a proper removal of the soft parts might eradicate the disease. So, too, it is conceivable that ultimately when our knowledge of the lymphatics traversed in cases of femur involvement becomes sufficiently exact, amputation at the hip joint may seem indicated.

Two other precepts harmonized with the "Halstedian" concept in giving rise to "modern" cancer surgery. First, it was (and still is by many) supposed that a growing tumor remains localized at its site of origin for a period of time, but at some instant during its growth tumor-cell invasion of lymphatics and dissemination of regional nodes takes place. After a further interval during which time the tumor is locoregional only, and during which time there is an increase in tumor size, systemic dissemination ensues. Second, as a result of the theory first formulated by Virchow in 1860 (1863), there has existed the belief that lymph nodes provide an effective barrier to the passage of tumor cells.

As a consequence of the above considerations and in keeping with the understanding of the disease at the time, there arose an *anatomical* basis for cancer surgery. The "proper" cancer operation consisted of removal of the primary tumor together with regional lymphatics and lymph nodes by *en bloc* dissection. Since it was deemed that there was a certain "orderliness" about tumor spread and that clinically recognizable cancer was in many instances a locoregional disease, it was considered to be more curable if the surgeon would only be more *expansive* in his interpretation of what constituted the "region" and if, above all, he utilized better technique so that he could eradicate the last cancer cell. Locoregional recurrences were more often than not considered to be the result of inadequate application of surgical skill rather than a manifestation of systemic disease. The hope was held high that "one more lymph node dissection would cure more cancers." Radical cancer surgery based on those anatomical considerations has persisted for 75 years.

With the advent of better supportive measures to improve patient survival, i.e., blood transfusions, anesthesia, correction of physiological deficits resulting from operation, and development of technical skills, super-radical cancer surgery came into being. Not too long ago (and still occasionally) such procedures as extended radical mastectomy, hemipelvectomy, forequarter amputation, partial evisceration, and even hemicorpectomy were being carried out and written about.

Other nuances of surgical technique, for the most part mechanical and simplistic in concept, have been from time to time introduced by the surgeon in an attempt to "trap" and eliminate the "stray" tumor cell. A prime impetus to such procedures was the demonstration by Fisher and Turnbull (1955) of tumor cells in the mesenteric venous blood of patients undergoing operation for colorectal carcinoma and the subsequent observations by others (Delarue, 1960; Long *et al.*, 1960; Ritchie and Webster, 1961; Roberts *et al.*, 1962) of showers of cancer cells in the blood during operation. To meet the challenge of those findings, there followed the "no-touch technique," the employment of "preliminary venous ligation," the use of "taping" of segments of intestine above and below tumors, the washing of operative wounds, and/or the intraluminal instillation with a variety of cytocidal agents. As an aside, it is of historic interest that while Ashworth (1869) first demonstrated bloodborne tumor cells in 1869, aside from a few sporadic reports (Ward, 1913) of abnormal cells in blood of isolated patients with tumors and the finding by Pool and Dunlop (1934) of abnormal cells in the blood of 17 of 40 cancer patients, the true nature of which was uncertain, little interest in tumor cells in blood was entertained until the late 1950s.

The past quarter of a century has seen the zenith and the beginning decline of cancer surgery based on anatomical principles. Despite, in some instances, extraordinary feats of skill and daring, noteworthy gains in terms of patient survival and disease-free life have eluded the surgeon. To the contrary, much physical and mental trauma has been inflicted without those dividends. Partially as a result of disappointment with results obtained and more significantly as a consequence of conceptual changes that have resulted from new information concerning tumor biology, a new basis for cancer surgery is undergoing synthesis.

405

CHANGING
ROLE OF
SURGERY IN
CANCER
TREATMENT

What considerations are leading to a redefinition of the role of operation in the treatment of cancer? The following section touches upon some of those which seem most pertinent to this reviewer.

3. Factors Prompting Redefinition of the Rationale for Surgery in Cancer Management

3.1. Cancer as a Systemic Disease

Information from a variety of sources indicates that most if not all patients with solid tumors have disseminated disease by the time a clinical diagnosis is established. This is not surprising when it is appreciated that a 1-cm tumor, which is usually the minimal size capable of physical diagnosis (e.g., breast) and which is looked upon as an "early" tumor, has already progressed through 30 of its 40 doublings; that number which is lethal to the patient. Considering that relatively few tumors are detected when they are less than 1 cm, it is appropriate that they may be considered "advanced" at the time of diagnosis. Data (Fisher *et al.*, 1975*a*) regarding the percent of treatment failures 10 years following radical mastectomy for what were considered to be clinically "curable" breast cancers strikingly emphasize the systemic nature of that cancer (Table 1). The finding that three out of four patients with positive axillary nodal involvement and almost nine out of ten with four or more of such nodes containing tumor become treatment failures indicates the inadequacy of extensive locoregional surgery. Treatment failure rates of other common and lethal cancers, i.e., pancreas (99%), lung (90%), prostrate (70%), and bowel (60%), similarly indicate the probability of metastases at the time of diagnosis.

Correlating information concerning the fate of patients having breast cancer with what is known about growth rates and other features regarding the kinetics of cells from such tumors, and employing certain assumptions, Skipper (1974) has provided estimates of the residual tumor-cell burden that might be expected to be present in a host following primary tumor removal, i.e., the number of viable cancer cells that are beyond the reach of surgery (Table 2). Zero viable tumor cells

TABLE 1
Treatment Failures 5 and 10 Years after Radical Mastectomy

Nodal status (histological)	5 years (%)	10 years (%)
Positive and Negative (all patients)	40	50
Negative	18	24
Positive	65	76
1–3	50	65
≥4	79	86

407

CHANGING
ROLE OF
SURGERY IN
CANCER
TREATMENT

TABLE 2
Residual Tumor-Cell Burden following Primary Tumor Removal[a]

| Viable breast cancer cells beyond the reach of surgery | Percent of operable patients bearing the numbers of tumor cells indicated presuming an overall median doubling time of of 30 or 40 days (and other stated assumptions) | | | | | |
| | Negative nodes | | 1 or more positive nodes | | 4 + positive nodes | |
	30-day	40-day	30-day	40-day	30-day	40-day
0 or "1" slow cell	65[b]	65[b]	36[b]	36[b]	14[b]	14[b]
"1" (with median DT) or <	80	74	56	47	22	17
10^1 or <	82	77	59	51	26	18
10^2 or <	85	80	63	56	30	22
10^3 or <	88	82	69	59	39	26
10^4 or <	90	86	73	65	45	33
10^5 or <	93	89	78	70	52	42
10^6 or <	95	93	83	78	63	53
10^7 or <	97	96	89	85	76	67
10^8 or <	99	99	94	92	88	85
10^9 or <	"100"	"100"	"100"	"100"	"100"	"100"

[a] From Skipper (1974).
[b] 5-year tumor-free survivors *observed*.

in that chart refers to none above some relatively small number with which host immune mechanisms may be able to cope. He has also provided some "reasonable" estimates of the body burden of tumor cells present at detection of a recurrence (Table 3). As a result of such "modelling," there arises some insight

TABLE 3
Seemingly Reasonable Estimates of the Body Burden on Tumor Cells at Detection of Recurrence[a]

| Number of tumor cells | Weight | If in a single spherical clone or mass | | |
		Diameter (mm)		Palpable (depending on site)
10^1	0.01 μg	0.025	<	No
10^2	0.1 μg	0.025	<	No
10^3	1.0 μg	0.12	<	No
10^4	10 μm	0.25	<	No
10^5	100 μg	0.6	∘	No
10^6	1 mg	1.2	◯	No
10^7	10 mg	2.5	◯	No
10^8	100 mg	6	◉	?
10^9	1 g	12		Yes [b]
10^{10}	10 g	25	>	Yes
10^{11}	100 g	60	>	Yes
10^{12}	1 kg	120	>	Yes

[a] From Skipper (1974). The volume of a sphere $= 0.5236d^3$. Subcutaneous solid animal tumors are usually first palpable and measurable at about 60 mg.
[b] Reasonable range: the average is likely to be somewhere between 1 and 10 g.

into the prevalence of cancer as a systemic disease at diagnosis and the numbers of cells which need to be eradicated by systemic therapy to enhance the curability of surgery.

The fact that some patients are apparently "cured" by operation alone is no indication that the surgical procedure eradicated every last cancer cell, that the disease was completely locoregional in extent, and that dissemination had not taken place. Such a concept is most difficult for the surgeon to accept. There is failure to appreciate that the residual tumor-cell burden may have been sufficiently minimal for its eradication by host factors which play a significant role in the success or failure of the operative procedure. It is impossible to estimate the number of micrometastases which may have been aborted by removal of a primary tumor. That removal of a primary tumor is not equivalent to the removal of a "foreign body" is apparent from the increasing number of reports describing a variety of changes in the host and in residual tumor cells. The following sections consider those alterations.

3.2. Consequences of Removal of a Primary Tumor

Not only are host immunological mechanisms affected by a growing tumor, but its removal may so further alter those host functions as to influence the course of a patient. The consequences of both the tumor removal and the surgical procedure itself seem important in that regard. In addition, there is evidence to indicate that removal of a primary tumor may alter the growth pattern of micrometastases.

3.2.1. Immunological Effects

In general, it is accepted that tumors are antigenic and are capable of eliciting a host immune response which is both cell and serum mediated. Peripheral blood lymphocytes from patients with a variety of tumors have been found to be capable of killing tumor cells of the same tumor type growing in tissue culture. Removal of a primary tumor has diverse effects on the various aspects of the host immune response.

3.2.1a. On Serum Blocking Activity. Serum from patients with a variety of tumor types has been shown to be capable of interfering with the cytotoxic effects of lymphocytes. Whatever the mechanism(s) responsible, i.e., "blocking antibody" hindering lymphocyte/tumor-cell interaction by coating the latter, antigen–antibody complexes in the serum interfering with cell-mediated responses, or antigen released from tumor cells interfering with lymphocyte action by binding to their surface, evidence has accumulated to indicate that the surgical removal of a tumor diminishes the inhibitory activity of serum directed toward cellular immunity.

A lessening of such "blocking" activity was noted by Hellström *et al.* (1970) within 4 days after removal of an experimentally induced tumor. Those findings were confirmed by Heppner (1972), who found that the inhibitory activity progressively decreased following tumor excision. Our own experience in that regard utilizing a spontaneous C3H mammary carcinoma has indicated that by 14 days following tumor removal there was a complete loss of serum blocking factor (Fisher, unpublished) in animals whose immunity persisted.

409

CHANGING
ROLE OF
SURGERY IN
CANCER
TREATMENT

Data obtained by Currie and Basham (1972) from a series of cancer patients are in keeping with those acquired in animal model systems. Not only were they able to demonstrate a specific inhibition of lymphocyte function by serum from such patients, but also their findings served to implicate tumor antigen as the serum component responsible for inhibiting lymphocyte cytotoxicity. Particularly germane to this discussion was their inability to detect a serum inhibitory effect in patients with a minimal tumor burden.

3.2.1.b. On Cell-Mediated Immunity. Removal of a primary tumor has been observed to affect cells involved in the immune process in a variety of ways. Barski and Youn (1969) observed that peritoneal macrophages from a host with a growing tumor inhibited growth of tumor cells *in vitro* (colony inhibition). With progressive tumor growth, the peritoneal cells became inert, but following removal of the primary tumor they regained their former ability to impair tumor-cell growth. Mikulska *et al.* (1966) noted that spleen cells from a tumor-bearing host, when mixed *in vitro* with tumor cells, failed to suppress growth of the tumor cells following their injection into syngeneic recipients. Three weeks following tumor removal, spleen cells were capable of inhibiting growth of tumor cells.

In the same vein, Whitney *et al.* (1974) have noted that mice exposed to an inoculum of tumor cells developed tumor-specific immunity before the appearance of a palpable tumor. This persisted until tumors reached 10% of the animal's body weight, after which there was a rapid decline and loss of such immunity. Lymphoid cell competence as measured by mitogen stimulation was also lost. Following surgical resection of the primary tumor, immunity increased and mitogen responses were restored.

Of pertinence to surgeons are the findings of Alexander and Hall (Alexander, 1972; Alexander and Hall, 1970). They observed that a paralysis of regional lymph nodes occurred with progressive tumor growth. Propagation of specific cell-mediated responses from the nodes, i.e., release of immunoblasts into the efferent lymphatics, ceased. Following tumor removal, however, that activity was resumed.

Our own observations (B. Fisher *et al.*, 1974*a*) utilizing two different syngeneic tumor–host systems revealed that even after tumors had been present for a prolonged period of time, regional lymph node cells displayed *in vitro* cytotoxicity against cells from the immunizing tumor and were capable of interfering with (neutralizing) the *in vivo* growth of tumor cells. Only when animals approached death from their tumors did such cells demonstrate loss of their cytotoxicity. Following removal of primary tumors (B. Fisher *et al.*, 1974*b*) at times when lymph node cells displayed cytotoxicity, that quality of the lymph node cells was rapidly lost. The *in vitro* cytotoxicity displayed by macrophages obtained following culture of bone marrow cells from animals bearing a tumor disappeared following tumor removal (B. Fisher *et al.*, 1976).

That operation may affect the cell-mediated immune responsiveness of patients with cancer is evident from the observations of Watkins (1973). She observed impaired lymphocyte transformation in those whose disease was limited in extent as well as in those with carcinomatosis. The PHA response returned to normal in most cases after successful removal of tumor, but remained low when malignant tissue persisted after palliative surgery. Reversal of a depressed tuberculin response after surgery has also been demonstrated in some patients with cancer (Hughes and McKay, 1965; Israel *et al.*, 1973).

3.2.1c. On Tumor-Specific Antibodies. Circulating antitumor antibodies, specific for a particular immunizing tumor, were detected in an immune host by Pilch and Riggins (1966) only after surgical removal of a tumor. The presence of these antibodies correlated with increased resistance to subsequent isologous tumor transplants. Graham and Graham (1955) detected circulating antibodies in a number of patients only after primary tumors had been surgically excised. Others have more recently recorded a similar experience (Odili and Taylor, 1971).

3.2.1d. On Spontaneous Regressions. Spontaneous regression of metastases in man was reported following removal of primary tumors (Everson and Cole, 1966), particularly those of renal origin. Unfortunately, no immunological information was available from such patients, but the mechanism of regression was in all probability immunological in nature.

3.2.1e. Adverse Immunological Effects. It must be noted that at least two investigations suggest that removal of a primary tumor might adversely affect tumor immunity. Stjernswärd (1968) reported that following removal of tumors there was a loss of immunity, as evidenced by the response to a challenge of cells from the same tumor. In another model system, Gershon and Carter (1969) observed that tumor resection resulted in a rapid decrease in immunity, accompanied by an increased number of metastatic deposits. Reinoculation of tumor cells was followed by a return of immunity.

3.2.1f. Nonspecific Effects of the Surgery Itself. It has been noted elsewhere in this chapter that extensive removal of a tumor mass, while failing to eradicate all tumor present in a host, may reduce the residual tumor burden to a level which might be eradicated by host mechanisms. The operation employed may, however, nonspecifically interfere with such defense mechanisms and reduce that capability of the host. Thus the benefit of putting the residual tumor burden within the "rejection potential" of the patient may be negated.

While surprisingly little information exists concerning the nonspecific effects of surgery and of anesthesia on systemic immunity in tumor and non-tumor-bearing hosts, there is evidence to suggest that cell-mediated but not necessarily humoral antibody responses may be altered by those modalities. In that regard, several investigators (Riddle, 1967; Park *et al.*, 1971) observed that following a variety of surgical operations, human lymphocyte transformation in response to phytohemagglutinin (PHA) stimulation was significantly depressed. Similarly, the number of antibody-producing cells in experimental animals was lessened by surgical trauma and anesthesia under some circumstances (Humphrey *et al.*, 1969, 1970) and was enhanced under others (Humphrey *et al.*, 1970). Heppner (1972) also found that surgery *per se* could serve as a stimulus for cell-mediated immunity in tumor-bearing hosts. Other effects of operation on host defense are depression of the activity of the reticuloendothelial system and phagocytosis in humans as well as animals and also of circulating opsonins (Donovan, 1967; Saba and DiLuzio, 1969; Saba, 1970; Scovill and Saba, 1973).

411

CHANGING
ROLE OF
SURGERY IN
CANCER
TREATMENT

3.2.2. *Effect of Removal of Primary on Residual (Metastatic) Tumor-Cell Kinetics*

Numerous studies (Frindel *et al.*, 1967; Laird, 1964; McCredie *et al.*, 1965; DeWys, 1972) have demonstrated that as tumors increase in mass there is a slowing of their growth rate. This growth pattern of solid tumors has been described mathematically by means of the Gompertzian equation which expresses the rate of tumor growth and the effect of a retarding factor that fits the decreasing rate of growth as the tumor increases in size. Thus solid tumor growth has been characterized as "Gompertzian." A variety of explanations have been utilized to account for the decreasing growth rate. Inadequacy of local blood supply (McCredie *et al.*, 1965), immunological factors (Laird, 1964; McCredie *et al.*, 1965), competition for nutrition (McCredie *et al.*, 1965), and others (DeWys, 1972) have all received consideration. Whatever the mechanism(s), of prime importance is how the presence or removal of a primary tumor influences the kinetics of metastatic tumor cells, for such information has direct therapeutic implication. According to Schabel (1969), when tumors increase in size the growth fraction of the viable tumor cells in cell division cycle decreases. Large tumors are apt to contain a preponderance of resting tumor cells, i.e., those with a prolonged G_1 time. DeWys (1972) has reported a synchronous slowing of the rate of growth of an implanted tumor as well as of its metastases even though the latter were microscopic in size. With removal of the primary tumor, the slowing of metastatic tumor growth was reversed. Thus a significant reduction of a large viable tumor-cell population by operation or radiation or subcurative chemotherapy probably results in an increase in the growth fraction and shortening of the tumor-cell generation time in the metastases. Temporarily nondividing or noncycling cells comprising metastatic foci may once again become actively cycling and dividing and thus become more vulnerable to chemotherapeutic agents (Schabel, 1975). In a study by Simpson-Herren *et al.* (1974), it was shown that small cell populations in distant metastases have a higher growth fraction than do those in the primary tumor from which they originated. In the Lewis lung tumor system, the metastatic tumors had a shorter doubling time than did primary tumors except in those surviving well past the median time of death. The cell cycle and S phase were shorter and the labeling index was higher in the metastatic tumors. Such findings again have important therapeutic implications. They suggest that metastases may display greater sensitivity than a primary tumor to chemotherapeutic agents and that the use of a large primary tumor as an index of drug effectiveness may be misleading. Further information correlating the growth characteristics of a primary tumor with its metastases is urgently needed.

3.3. Reassessment of the Role of the Lymphatics and Lymph Nodes in Cancer

There has been renewed concern with the role of lymph, lymph nodes, and the lymph vascular system in the biology of malignancy (B. Fisher and E. R. Fisher, 1968). Contrary to Sampson Handley's and Halsted's beliefs, it is now well appreciated that tumor cells, on gaining access to lymphatics, may be carried as emboli directly to a lymph node, where they are arrested in the subcapsular sinus of one or more lobules, at which point early growth occurs (Fig. 1). Likewise, it is accepted that additional cells from a primary tumor may traverse collateral or alternative lymphatic pathways to lodge in more distal nodes when those more proximal are already involved. That lymphatic metastases may appear in distant rather than proximal nodes, even when the latter are not involved, has been recognized since Paget's time (1870) (Patey, 1967) but is consistently ignored in surgical thinking. This phenomenon of skip metastases is related to direct lymphatic communication and the dynamics of the lymph flow in the area involved. Such bypasses can explain the noninvolvement of individual lymph nodes and atypical distribution of lymphogenous metastases.

The concept originally expressed by Bartels (1909) that lymph does not reach the blood without passing through at least one lymph node still prevails, despite evidence to the contrary. It has been established that, in addition to being carried

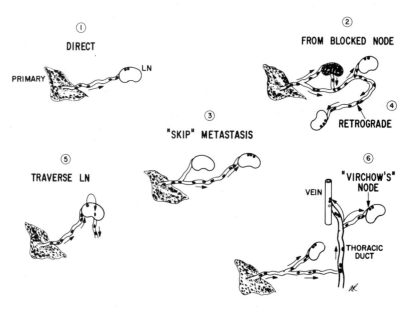

FIGURE 1. Pathways of lymphatic tumor-cell dissemination.

to regional lymph nodes, tumor-cell emboli may bypass such nodes to enter **413**

CHANGING
ROLE OF
SURGERY IN
CANCER
TREATMENT
directly into the thoracic duct and be conveyed directly to veins at the base of the
neck, from which point they are blood borne. Controversy has existed concerning
the magnitude and significance of other lymphaticovenous pathways throughout
the body. This has been particularly so relative to the presence of such connections
in lymph nodes and the part they play in the entry of tumor cells into the
bloodstream. Studies from our laboratory support the existence and possible
importance of such communications in tumor-cell dissemination. Evidence by
others seems to substantiate such an event.

Recently, we have challenged the concept that lymph nodes act as an effective
barrier to tumor-cell dissemination. Virchow (1863) first formulated the theory
that the lymph node effectively trapped particulate matter in the lymph. Over the
years, the effectiveness of nodes in trapping inanimate particles, bacteria, viruses
and red blood cells has been evaluated repeatedly. As a result of opinion and
inference from such investigations, there exists, with few exceptions, the generally
held belief that lymph nodes provide an effective barrier to the passage of tumor
cells. It is remarkable, however, that this conclusion was reached without ever
employing tumor cells to test the integrity of the lymph node relative to the
transmigration of such cells. Data obtained by us in that regard support the
conclusion that the lymph node is not so effective a barrier to tumor cells as
formerly believed (B. Fisher and E. R. Fisher, 1966a, 1967a,b). The majority of
tumor cells entering the node may fail to maintain permanent residence.
Moreover, information obtained with erythrocytes or other particulate matter has
little relevance to the fate of tumor cells. In addition, there is evidence to suggest
that tumor cells themselves could be as much a determinant of their residence as
are the biological and mechanical properties of the node.

As a result of the foregoing, it no longer seems tenable to believe that tumor cells
in lymphatics have only one final destination—lymph nodes. There is sufficient
evidence that tumor cells that are primarily lymph borne may reach the blood
vascular system, through which they become further dispersed. Only recently,
however, has it been demonstrated that tumor cells circulating in the blood
vascular system may likewise find their way into the lymphatics and hence the
thoracic duct (B. Fisher and E. R. Fisher, 1966b). Thus the two vascular systems
may be so unified insofar as tumor-cell dissemination is concerned that it is no
longer realistic to consider them independently as routes of neoplastic dissemination.

Evidence implicating immunological mechanisms in the fate of tumors pro-
vokes other considerations. Should a human neoplasm contain tumor antigens
that evoke a host immune response—a situation no longer to be considered
remote—it would seem reasonable to anticipate that when cells from such a tumor
become disseminated via lymphatics they may be destroyed by the immune node.
Experimental evidence obtained both *in vivo* and *in vitro* in support of the tumor-
cell-destructive properties of sensitized lymphocytes supports such a possibility.

The cell population of a tumor may consist of both a proliferating and a
nonproliferating pool of cells. The latter may consist of those cells that are

permanently nonreplicating and those that are capable of subsequent proliferative activity. Might it not be possible that small numbers of disseminated nonproliferative cells (either type) may find their way to a lymph node, where they lodge to remain nonproliferative and unobserved for varying periods?

As a consequence of all of these findings and considerations, it is our opinion that it is unrealistic to continue to accept the finding of negative lymph nodes as indicative *only* of the fact that a given tumor has been removed prior to its lymphatic dissemination. Although such an event may have occurred, it is also possible that anatomical factors have permitted tumor cells to bypass nodes, or they could have lodged and failed to proliferate, remaining dormant (Fig. 2).

Similar considerations may be given to positive regional lymph nodes (RLNs) (Fig. 3). Conventionally, the presence of a tumor-containing node is considered simply to be the result of tumor cells having disseminated via lymphatics, with their subsequent lodgment and growth in nodes. This may represent an oversimplification of the phenomenon. Perhaps only when the number of disseminated cells, i.e., the challenge dose, exceeds the capability of the node for cell destruction or, alternatively, there is a reduction of the immune capabilities of the node and/or possibly a change in the biological nature of the tumor cell, does tumor grow in the lymph node. It has been well demonstrated in animal systems that tumor immunity can be overcome when the challenge dose is of sufficient size.

Recently, we carried out a series of investigations that utilized lymph nodes from patients with operable breast and colon cancers. Findings (B. Fisher *et al.*, 1972) support the possibility that the reason why some nodes in a group harbor metastatic tumor and others do not is that such metastases are more likely to be

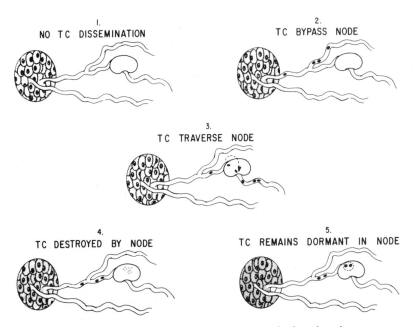

FIGURE 2. Alternative reasons for a tumor-negative lymph node.

415

CHANGING
ROLE OF
SURGERY IN
CANCER
TREATMENT

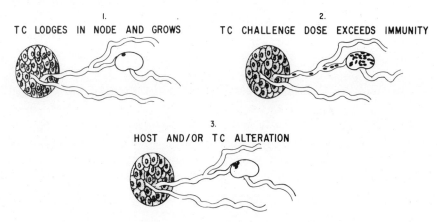

FIGURE 3. Alternative reasons for a tumor-positive lymph node.

related to biological differences between nodes than to anatomical happenstance (i.e., transport of tumor cells to some nodes but not to others), as is conventionally believed. Our studies also suggest that cells of RLNs continue to possess immunological capabilities, despite the presence of growing tumors. Observations in two different syngeneic tumor–host systems utilizing *in vivo* neutralization and *in vitro* cytotoxicity have revealed that even after tumors had been present for a prolonged period of time, RLN cells were capable of interfering with the growth of tumor cells (B. Fisher *et al.*, 1974*a*). Neither distant lymph node cells nor spleen cells ever fully displayed that characteristic. Only when animals approached death from their tumors did RLN cells demonstrate loss of their neutralizing capability.

Other investigations were carried out by us to determine whether functional characteristics of lymph cells, i.e., lymphocyte transformation and thymidine uptake, correlated with histopathological discriminants of RLNs and of the tumor present (E. R. Fisher *et al.*, 1973; B. Fisher *et al.*, 1974*c*). In general, no clear relationship was found to exist.

Thus the presence or absence of tumor in lymph nodes may not be of as great significance as was believed in the determination of lymphatic tumor-cell dissemination. Since, as is well known, there is a better prognosis in cancer patients when lymph nodes are not involved, on cursory consideration such a hypothesis may seem untenable. It may be, however, that positive lymph nodes merely denote that disseminated tumor cells that produced such growth, as a result of intrinsic cell properties and/or host factors, are capable of developing metastases in other parts of the body as well. Negative nodes may merely reflect conditions that, in addition to preventing nodal growth of tumor, inhibit metastases from occurring in other places. Moreover, perhaps those cells that traverse lymph nodes are more readily destroyed when they are dispersed via the blood vascular system than when they are retained in significant numbers in nodes. Might it not be possible that the patient with negative lymph nodes is the one whose immune competence is entirely adequate to eliminate disseminated tumor cells, thereby preventing secondary tumor growth and that this is the reason for a more favorable prognosis?

Extensive evidence that further negates the outmoded, simplistic, mechanistic consideration of a tumor as a foreign body has accumulated from experimental studies with increased rapidity in recent years. Such information conclusively demonstrates that a tumor and its metastases are not autonomous of the host but are intimately related to a variety of the functions of the latter. Although such studies may be justifiably criticized for their impertinence to clinical situations, nevertheless, clinical corollaries are not infrequent. Our own investigations in this regard over a 15-year period have demonstrated the effects on tumor growth of such a wide spectrum of factors as blood flow alterations, trauma, rheological changes, diet, reticuloendothelial activity, endocrine interrelationships, and others. Many of the host factors investigated exhibit opposing effects on the growth of metastases. The possible combinations and permutations that may be operative in any particular instance may provide an explanation for the difficulty in expressing host–tumor relationships more succinctly in the patient. The interested reader is referred to several reviews of the findings (B. Fisher and E. R. Fisher, 1965; E. R. Fisher and B. Fisher, 1974).

3.5. The Significance of Multicentric Cancers

That cancers of some organs and tissues may be multicentric in origin has long been recognized (Cheatle and Cutler, 1931). Particular attention has recently been directed toward the multicentricity of breast cancer which has been shown to occur not only in humans (Foote and Stewart, 1945; Gallager and Martin, 1969; Nicholson, 1921) but also in certain animals (Bosner, 1945; Willis, 1953). The impetus for such concern has been the consideration that segmental resections of the breast with or without radiation may be equally as effective in terms of curability as a more radical procedure, and cosmetically more acceptable. One of the major deterrents to the acceptability of such a limited resection is the realization that it may ignore clinically and pathologically undetected *de novo* cancers at sites within the breast remote from the dominant mass.

Similarly, there has appeared evidence to indicate that the incidence of cancer in the contralateral breast may be *much* greater than previously supposed (Urban, 1967, 1969). The disturbing fact is that despite the significance incidence of multifocal lesions in both breasts of a woman with a primary breast cancer only extremely rarely will there be evidence of two or more clinically overt primary cancers in the same breast. Similarly, the presence of synchronous bilateral tumors is uncommon and the incidence of a second asynchronous primary tumor in the involved breast fails to approach the incidence of occult lesions detected by random biopsy or autopsy (Slack *et al.*, 1973). For example, Kramer and Rush (1973) noted the incidence of clinically latent intraductal carcinomas in breasts of women over the age of 70 who died from causes other than mammary carcinoma to be 19 times greater than the reported incidence of clinical breast cancer. Such findings are highly suggestive that all cancers do not progress to overt lesions or may even undergo regression. That such a possibility is not remote comes from the knowledge that neuroblastomas of the adrenal in children, thyroid carcinomas, and carcinomas of the prostate are found more frequently in random pathological material examined than they are found clinically in comparable populations (Burnet, 1967).

It is of the utmost urgency that the clinical significance of occult multicentric cancers be ascertained in order to define correct surgical strategies relative to them. At present, it is difficult for surgeons resorting to orthodox principles of cancer management to accept the possibility that "a cancer may not be a cancer!" From a basic biological point of view, it seems to this reviewer that there is need for information relating the kinetics of growth of such tumor foci to those of the primary tumor. Does the presence or absence of a primary tumor influence their growth? Are their kinetics similar to those of distant metastatic foci (see Section 3.2.2)? Will they become more susceptible to destruction by antitumor agents following removal of the primary?

4. A Biological Basis for Cancer Surgery

As a result of the foregoing data and comments, it would seem that if patient curability were dependent on the surgical removal of "every last cancer cell," the outlook would indeed be bleak and operative intervention would at best be looked upon as a palliative procedure. The primary aim of oncological surgery at present seems to this reviewer to be directed toward reducing the tumor burden of the patient to a number of viable cells which are entirely destroyable (1) by host immunological (and other) factors alone, (2) by systemically administered anticancer agents, or (3) by a combination of both. The increasing evidence indicating that primary tumor removal may result in a variety of beneficial host changes and may by increasing the growth fraction of residual tumor cells make them more susceptible to anticancer agents is of profound importance and provides a rational basis for cancer surgery.

5. Surgery in Conjunction with Other Therapeutic Modalities

There are two aims in the management of patients with cancer. In order of importance the first is related to achieving a disease-free life, and the second is directed toward attaining the best cosmesis and quality of life possible without compromising the patient's chance for cure. Until the present, arguments relative to the merits of less radical operative procedures have been directed toward testing the null hypothesis, i.e., that such procedures are as good as but no better than more extensive operations relative to survival. Operations such as segmental or total mastectomy for breast cancer have been advocated essentially for improvement of cosmesis rather than for the prolongation of disease-free survival.

It has been hoped that the improvement is cosmesis could be achieved with a disease-free interval equal to that obtained by a more radical procedure, i.e., as good or as bad depending on one's satisfaction or dissatisfaction with results obtained by the radical operation.

As the worth of combined-modality therapy, i.e., adjunctive chemo-, immuno-, and/or hormonal therapy, is demonstrated, all treatment (surgery and radiation) directed toward local and regional tumor control will require reappraisal. For example, the worth of 1-phenylalanine mustard (L-PAM) (or other chemotherapeutic regimens) reported (B. Fisher *et al.*, 1975*b*) when administered following radical mastectomy is related to its effect on systemic disease. That same systemic effect should be observed if L-PAM is given following total or segmental mastectomy. Moreover, the possibility exists that such systemic therapy may be equally effective against minimal residual local and/or regional disease. As a consequence, all modalities which have been considered for local and regional control must be evaluated and reevaluated in the light of findings indicating the effectiveness of a systemic agent. If, for example, even should total mastectomy not be so effective as radical mastectomy, the possibility remains that with effective systemic therapy the procedures could produce equivalent results. Similarly, even if segmental mastectomy is at this time not so efficacious as total or radical mastectomy, the addition of chemotherapy could make it an equivalent procedure. In essence, as systemic therapy becomes more effective, the more likely it becomes that lesser operative procedures could be comparable. As a consequence, increased disease control may be accomplished together with better cosmesis and quality of life. It is not unreasonable to anticipate that the use of systemic therapy will make more remote the chance that a lesser surgical procedure will be putting the patient at a disadvantage. In fact, it is not heretical or unreasonable to speculate that at some time in the not too distant future, when diagnostic methodology has improved so that earlier cancers are detected, and when there is better understanding regarding the proper use of anticancer agents in concert so as to obtain maximum effectiveness, surgery may play a subsidiary role in the management of solid tumors and may be entirely supplanted by other modalities. Most urgently needed for the proper synchronization of available therapeutic modalities in order to make such a concept a reality is the availability of a biological assay which can indicate with precision the amount and the location of residual tumor that is present following operation.

6. Conclusion and Summary

A prime goal of surgical science is to establish all operative procedures on a firm basis relative to anatomical, physiological, and biological information of the time. Since such knowledge is constantly changing, it stands to reason that certain operations may become obsolete, may need revision, or may become more firmly established. For three-quarters of a century, surgery for cancer has been based almost entirely on anatomical considerations. The aquisition of new information such as has been presented in this chapter and elsewhere has tended to undermine the validity of those often presumed infallible principles. As a result, there has occurred great confusion regarding the proper type of surgery to employ for neoplastic disease. It would seem that this is a result of the fact that, while prior considerations have lost validity, knowledge is only beginning to allow synthesis of a *new* basis for cancer surgery which is biological rather than anatomical in character. Immunological and other effects resulting from removal of a primary tumor are now beginning to be appreciated. The primary aim of surgery for cancer is to decrease the tumor burden of the host to that level which is vulnerable to destruction by host factors alone and/or in conjunction with a variety of anticancer agents having different modes of action.

419

CHANGING
ROLE OF
SURGERY IN
CANCER
TREATMENT

No longer will surgery serve as the sole treatment for cancer with its prime mission the eradication of every last cancer cell. It will make its contribution in concert with other modalities.

7. References

ALEXANDER, P., 1972, Tumor immunology in perspective, in: *Frontiers of Radiation Therapy and Oncology* (J. M. VAETH, ed.), pp. 213–222, Karger, New York.

ALEXANDER, P., AND HALL, J. G., 1970, The role of immunoblasts in host resistance and immunotherapy of primary sarcomata, *Adv. Cancer Res.* **13**:1.

ASHWORTH, R. T., 1869, A case of cancer in which cells similar to those in the tumours were seen in the blood after death, *Aust. Med. J.* **14**:146.

BARSKI, G., AND YOUN, J. K., 1969, Evolution of cell-mediated immunity in mice bearing an antigenic tumor: Influence of tumor growth and surgical removal, *J. Natl. Cancer Inst.* **43**:111.

BARTELS, F., 1909, *Das Lymphgefässystem*, Gustav Fischer, Jena.

BOSSON, G. M., 1945, Microscopical study of evolution of mouse mammary cancer—Effect of milk factor and comparison with human disease, *J. Pathol. Bacteriol.* **57**:413.

BURNET, F. M., 1967, Immunological aspects of malignant disease, *Lancet* **1**:1171.

CHEATLE, G. L., AND CUTLER, M., 1931, *Tumours of the Breast—Their Pathology, Symptoms and Diagnosis and Treatment*, Lippincott, Philadelphia.

CURRIE, G. A., AND BASHAM, C., 1972, Serum mediated inhibition of the immunological reactions of the patient to his own tumour: A possible role for circulating antigen, *Br. J. Cancer* **26**:427.

DELARUE, N. C., 1960, The free cancer cell, *Can. Med. Assoc. J.* **82**:1175.

DEWYS, W. D., 1972, Studies correlating the growth rate of a tumor and its metastases and providing evidence for tumor related systemic growth retarding factors, *Cancer Res.* **32**:374.

DONOVAN, A. J., 1967, The effect of surgery on reticuloendothelial function, *Arch. Surg. (Chicago)* **94**:247.

EVERSON, T. C., AND COLE, W. H., 1966, *Spontaneous Regression of Cancer*, Saunders, Philadelphia.

FISHER, B., AND FISHER, E. R., 1965, The biology of metastasis, in: *Current Concepts in Surgery* (J. H. DAVIS, ed.), pp. 321–351, McGraw-Hill, New York.

FISHER, B., AND FISHER, E. R., 1966a, Transmigration of lymph nodes by tumor cells, *Science* **152**:1397.

FISHER, B., AND FISHER, E. R., 1966b, Interrelationship of hematogenous and lymphatic tumor cell dissemination, *Surg. Gynecol. Obstet.* **122**:791.

FISHER, B., AND FISHER, E. R., 1967a, The barrier function of the lymph node to tumor cells and erythrocytes. I. Normal nodes, *Cancer* **20**:1907.

FISHER, B., AND FISHER, E. R., 1967b, The barrier function of the lymph node to tumor cells and erythrocytes. II. Effect of X-ray, inflammation, sensitization and tumor growth, *Cancer* **20**:1914.

FISHER, B., AND FISHER, E. R., 1968, Role of the lymphatic system in dissemination of tumor, in: *Lymph and the Lymphatic System*, pp. 324–347, Charles C Thomas, Springfield, Ill.

FISHER, B., SAFFER, E. A., AND FISHER, E. R., 1972, Studies concerning the regional lymph node in cancer. III. Response of regional lymph node cells from breast and colon cancer patients to PHA stimulation, *Cancer* **30**:1202.

FISHER, B., SAFFER, E. A., AND FISHER, E. R., 1974a, Studies concerning the regional lymph node in cancer. IV. Tumor inhibition by regional lymph node cells, *Cancer* **33**:631.

FISHER, B., WOLMARK, N., AND COYLE, J., 1974b, Effect of *Corynebacterium parvum* on cytotoxicity of regional and non-regional lymph node cells from animal with tumors present and removed, *J. Natl. Cancer Inst.* **53**:1793.

FISHER, B., SAFFER, E., AND FISHER, E. R., 1974c, Studies concerning the regional lymph node in cancer. VII. Thymidine uptake by cells from nodes of breast cancer patients relative to axillary location and histopathologic discriminants, *Cancer Res.* **34**:1668.

FISHER, B., SLACK, N., KATRYCH, D. L., AND WOLMARK, N., 1975a, Ten year follow-up of breast cancer patients in a cooperative clinical trial evaluating surgical adjuvant chemotherapy, *Surg. Gynecol. Obstet.* **140**:528.

FISHER, B., CARBONE, P., ECONOMOU, S. G., FRELICK, R., GLASS, A., LERNER, H., REDMOND, C., ZELEN, M., KATRYCH, D. L., WOLMARK, N., BAND, P., FISHER, E. R., AND OTHER COOPERATING INVESTIGATORS, 1975b, 1-Phenylalanine mustard (L-PAM) in the management of primary breast cancer: A report of early findings, *N. Engl. J. Med.*, **292**:117.

FISHER, B., WOLMARK, N., COYLE, J., AND SAFFER, E. A., 1976, Effect of a growing tumor and its removal on the cytotoxicity of macrophages from cultured bone marrow cells, *Cancer Res.* **36**:2302.

FISHER, E. R., AND FISHER, B., 1974, Some theoretical and practical considerations of metastases, *Contemp. Surg.* **4**:85.

FISHER, E. R., AND TURNBULL, R. B., JR., 1955, Cytologic demonstration and significance of tumor cells in the mesenteric venous blood in patients with colorectal carcinoma, *Surg. Gynecol. Obstet.* **100**:102.

FISHER, E. R., SAFFER, E. A., AND FISHER, B., 1973, Studies concerning the regional lymph node in cancer. VI. Correlation of lymphocyte transformation of regional node cells and some histopathologic discriminants, *Cancer* **32**:104.

FOOTE, F. W., AND STEWART, F. W., 1945, Comparative studies of cancerous versus noncancerous breasts, *Ann. Surg.* **121**:5.

FRINDEL, E., MALAISE, E. P., ALPEN, E., AND TUBIANA, M., 1967, Kinetics of cell proliferation of an experimental tumor, *Cancer Res.* **27**:1122.

GALLAGER, H. S., AND MARTIN, J. E., 1969, The study of mammary carcinoma by mammography and whole organ sectioning, *Cancer* **23**:855.

GERSHON, R. D., AND CARTER, R. L., 1969, Factors controlling concomitant immunity in tumor bearing hamsters: Effect of prior splenectomy and tumor removal, *J. Natl. Cancer Inst.* **43**:533.

GRAHAM, J. B., AND GRAHAM, R. M., 1955, Antibodies elicited by cancer in patients, *Cancer* **8**:409.

GRAY, H. J., 1939, Relation of the lymphatic vessels to the spread of cancer, *Br. J. Surg.* **26**:462.

HAAGENSEN, C. D., 1933, An exhibit of important books, papers, and memorabilia illustrating the evolution of the knowledge of cancer, *Am. J. Cancer* **18**:42.

HALSTED, W. S., 1890/1891, The treatment of wounds with especial reference to the value of the blood clot in the management of dead spaces, *Johns Hopkins Hosp. Rep.* **2**:255.

HALSTED, W. S., 1907, The results of radical operations for the cure of carcinoma of breast, *Ann. Surg.* **46**:1.

HANDLEY, W. S., 1922, *Cancer of the Breast and Its Operative Treatment*, A. Murray, London.

HAYWARD, O. S., 1965a, The history of oncology. I. Early oncology and the literature of discovery, *Surgery* **58**:460.

HAYWARD, O. S., 1965b, The history of oncology. II. The society for investigating cancer, London, *Surgery* **58**:586.

HAYWARD, O. S., 1965c, The history of oncology. III. America and the cancer lectures of Nathan Smith, *Surgery* **58**:745.

HELLSTRÖM, I., HELLSTRÖM, K. E., AND SJÖGREN, H. O., 1970, Serum mediated inhibition of cellular immunity to methylcholanthrene-induced murine sarcomas, *Cell. Immunol.* **1**:18.

HEPPNER, G. H., 1972, *In vitro* studies on cell-mediated immunity following surgery in mice sensitized to syngeneic mammary tumors, *Int. J. Cancer* **9**:119.

HUGHES, L. E., AND McKAY, W. D., 1965, Suppression of the tubercular response in malignant disease, *Br. Med. J.* **2**:1346.

HUMPHREY, L. J., WINGARD, D. W., AND LANG, R., 1969, The effect of surgery and anesthesia on the immunologic responsiveness of the rat, *Surgery* **65**:946.

HUMPHREY, L. J., FREDERICKSON, E. L., AND AMERSON, J. R., 1970, Effect of anesthesia and amputation on tumor and general immunity of the mouse, *J. Surg. Res.* **10**:265.

ISRAEL, L., MUGICA, J., AND CHAHINIAN, P., 1973, Prognosis of early bronchogenic carcinoma: Survival curves of 451 patients after resection of lung cancer in relation to the results of the preoperative tuberculin skin test, *Biomedicine* **19**:68.

KRAMER, W. M., AND RUSH, B. F., 1973, Mammary duct proliferation in the elderly—A histopathologic study, *Cancer* **31**:130.

LAIRD, A. K., 1964, Dynamics of tumor growth, *Br. J. Cancer* **18**:490.

LeDRAN, H. F., 1757, Mémoires avec un précis de plusieurs observations sur le cancer, *Mem. Acad. R. Chic.* **3**:1.

LONG, L., JONASSON, O., ROBERTS, S., McGRATH, R., McGREW, E., AND COLE, W. H., 1960, Cancer cells in the blood; results of simplified isolation technique, *AMA Arch. Surg.* **80**:910.

McCREDIE, J. A., INCH, W. R., KRUUV, J., AND WATSON, T. A., 1965, The rate of tumor growth in animals, *Growth* **29**:331.

MIKULSKA, A. B., SMITH, C., AND ALEXANDER, P., 1966, Evidence for an immunological reaction of the host directed against its own actively growing primary tumor, *J. Natl. Cancer Inst.* **36**:29.

MORGAGNI, G. G., 1769, *The Seats and Causes of Diseases Investigated by Anatomy*, Miller and Cadell, London (translated by B. Alexander, reprinted by Hafner, 1960, for New York Academy of Medicine).

NICHOLSON, G. W., 1921, Carcinoma of breast, *Br. J. Surg.* **8**:527.

ODILI, J. L., AND TAYLOR, G., 1971, Transience of immune responses to tumour antigens in man, *Br. Med. J.* **4**:584.

PARK, S. K., BRODY, J. I., WALLACE, H. A., AND BLAKEMORE, W. S., 1971, Immunosuppressive effect of surgery, *Lancet* **1**:53.

PATEY, D. H., 1967, A review of 146 cases of carcinoma of the breast operated on between 1930 and 1943, *Br. J. Cancer* **21**:260.

PILCH, Y. H., AND RIGGINS, R. S., 1966, Antibodies to spontaneous and MC-induced tumors in inbred mice, *Cancer Res.* **26**:871.

POOL, E. H., AND DUNLOP, R. R., 1934, Cancer cells in bloodstream, *Am. J. Cancer* **21**:99.

RIDDLE, P. R., 1967, Distributed immune reactions following surgery, *Br. J. Surg.* **54**:882.

RITCHIE, A. C., AND WEBSTER, D. R., 1961, Tumor cells in the blood, in: *Proceedings of the Fourth Canadian Cancer Conference*, Academic Press, New York.

ROBERTS, S., JONASSON, O., LONG, L., McGREW, E. A., McGRATH, R., AND COLE, W. H., 1962, Relationship of cancer cells in the circulating blood to operation, *Cancer* **15**:232.

SABA, T. M., 1970, Mechanism mediating reticuloendothelial system depression after surgery, *Proc. Soc. Exp. Biol. Med.* **133**:1132.

SABA, T. M., AND DiLUZIO, 1969, Surgical stress and reticuloendothelial function, *Surgery* **65**:802.

SCHABEL, F. M., JR., 1969, The use of tumor growth kinetics in planning "curative" chemotherapy of advanced solid tumors, *Cancer Res.* **29**:2384.

SCHABEL, F. M., JR., 1975, Concepts for systemic treatment of micrometastases, *Cancer* **35**:15.

SCOVILL, W. A., AND SABA, T. M., 1973, Humoral recognition deficiency in the etiology of reticuloendothelial depression induced by surgery, *Ann. Surg.* **178**:59.

SIMPSON-HERREN, L., SANFORD, A. H., AND HOLMQUIST, J. P., 1974, Cell population kinetics of transplanted and metastatic Lewis lung carcinoma, *Cell. Tissue Kinet.* **7**:349.

SKIPPER, H. E., 1974, *Combination Therapy*, p. 1, Booklet 13, Southern Research Institute, Birmingham, Ala., December 23, 1974.

SLACK, N. H., BROSS, E. J., NEMOTO, T., AND FISHER, B., 1973, Experience with bilateral primary carcinoma of the breast in a cooperative study, *Surg. Gynecol. Obstet.* **136**:433.

STJERNSWÄRD, J., 1968, Immune status of the primary host toward its own methylcholanthrene induced sarcomas, *J. Natl. Cancer Inst.* **40**:13.

URBAN, J. A., 1967, Bilaterality of cancer of the breast: Biopsy of the opposite breast, *Cancer* **20**:1867.

URBAN, J. A., 1969, Biopsy of the "normal" breast in treating breast cancer, *Surg. Clin. N. Am.* **49**:291.

VALSALVA, A. M., 1704, *Deaure Humana Troatatus*, C. Pisarii, Bononrae.

VIRCHOW, R., 1863, *Cellular Pathology*, Lippincott, Philadelphia.

WARD, G. R., 1913, The blood in cancer with bone metastases, *Lancet* **1**:676.

WATKINS, S. M., 1973, The effects of surgery on lymphocyte transformation in patients with cancer, *Clin. Exp. Immunol.* **14**:69.

WHITNEY, R. B., LEVY, J. G., AND SMITH, A. G., 1974, Influence of tumor size and surgical resection on cell mediated immunity in mice, *J. Natl. Cancer Inst.* **53**:111.

WILLIS, R. A., 1953, *Pathology of Tumors*, 2nd ed., Butterworth, London.

421

CHANGING
ROLE OF
SURGERY IN
CANCER
TREATMENT

Immunotherapy

11

Immunotherapy of Human Cancer

EVAN M. HERSH, G. M. MAVLIGIT, J. U. GUTTERMAN, AND S. P. RICHMAN

1. Introduction

The efficacy of the conventional modalities of cancer treatment—surgery, radiotherapy, and chemotherapy—has been reasonably well defined. There is also sufficient experience to permit one to predict the nature of future improvements in efficacy for these conventional modalities. For surgery, it is likely that the limit of efficacy has been reached, and while surgery can effectively cure a proportion of patients with apparent local disease, it is clear that disseminated, microscopic tumor deposits are present in at least half the operable cases at the time of surgery, ultimately eventuating in metastatic disease. A limited but important additional role for surgery will be the debulking of metastatic disease in an attempt to reduce the tumor burden and thus to improve the efficacy of subsequent systemic treatment with chemotherapy, immunotherapy, and other possible approaches.

Similar conclusions can be drawn with regard to radiotherapy. Thus radiotherapy is a local form of cancer treatment, and with certain limited exceptions (such as the treatment of chronic lymphocytic leukemia with whole-body irradiation) it is unlikely that major advances in the control of systemic disease will be made. In contrast to surgery, however, the current local cure rate may be improved by the use of newer particles such as fast neutrons and π^-

EVAN M. HERSH, G. M. MAVLIGIT, J. U. GUTTERMAN, AND S. P. RICHMAN • Department of Developmental Therapeutics, The University of Texas System Cancer Center, M. D. Anderson Hospital and Tumor Institute, Houston, Texas 77030.

EVAN M. HERSH,
G. M. MAVLIGIT,
J. U. GUTTERMAN,
AND
S. P. RICHMAN

mesons, which may have an improved degree of tumor specificity and a higher fraction tumor-cell kill.

Predictions are more difficult to make for chemotherapy. During the last 30 years, and particularly during the last 10 years, major progress has been made in the control of several hisotological types of disseminated and metastatic malignancy with chemotherapy. Complete remission rates in several lymphomas and leukemias approach 100%, and cure rates in some of these diseases are approaching 50%. Recently, in certain solid tumors such as breast cancer and testicular cancer, the addition of newer chemotherapeutic agents such as adriamycin and cis-platinum, particularly in various combinations, has resulted in response rates of 75% or higher. However, in other metastatic solid tumors such as lung cancer and colon cancer, response rates in patients with disseminated disease still range between 20% and 40% in spite of the application of a variety of new chemotherapeutic agents, even when administered in combination. Also, when responses are achieved, response durations are short, involving intervals of less than 1 year. An area of very encouraging recent results in chemotherapy is adjuvant chemotherapy. In sarcoma and breast cancer, there is now strong evidence that postsurgical chemotherapy will increase the cure rate. Thus, based on past experience, one can anticipate for chemotherapy a relatively slow introduction of new chemotheraputic agents with increased efficacy and decreased toxicity. However, because of the relatively close similarity between normal and tumor cells, the current approaches to chemotherapy may not be destined to result in cure for the majority of disseminated tumors (see Volume 5 of this series). It should also be pointed out that not only in chemotherapy but also in surgery and radiotherapy, immunological reactivity, both general and tumor directed, seems to influence the outcome of treatment and that the three major modalities of cancer treatment are themselves immunosuppressive.

This then is the setting in which the new field of immunotherapy is developing. The basic characteristic of immunotherapy, which offers the hope that it will ultimately come to play an important and even curative role, is that its objective is to restore or augment normal mechanisms of host defense against tumor. These are the mechanisms presumed to play a decisive role in the curative effects of the conventional modalities of surgery and radiotherapy by eliminating residual local and disseminated foci of tumor cells. Also, because it is designed to restore or augment normal mechanisms, toxicity of immunotherapy should be minimal relative to the often severe toxicity and morbidity associated with surgery, radiotherapy, and chemotherapy. Finally, because of its limited toxicity, immunotherapy can be added at full dose to the three conventional modalities of cancer treatment. This is in contrast to other approaches of combination therapy (such as radiation plus chemotherapy or the simultaneous use of two or more chemotherapeutic agents), where additive toxicity is an important dose-limiting factor.

On the other hand, our enthusiasm for the potential of immunotherapy must be placed in the context of the potential impact of other scientific advances on cancer. There are several developments in our understanding of the tumor cell which indicate that several new systemic approaches to cancer treatment may be

developed over the next decade. These include improved understanding of the
biochemical basis of cellular proliferation and its regulation, improved understanding of the biochemical characteristics of the transformed vs. the normal cell,
improved understanding of the characteristics of the tumor cell vs. the normal cell
surface, as well as newer knowledge regarding the immunological factors involved
in the etiology, pathogenesis, and course of malignant disease in experimental
systems and in man. These developments not only make it likely that there will be
advances in the areas of chemotherapy and immunotherapy, but also suggest that
there may be new approaches to cancer treatment based neither on the use of
cytotoxic and antiproliferative drugs not on immunological manipulations. These
would include control of tumor-cell proliferation by manipulation of cyclic
nucleotide metabolism (Braun *et al.*, 1974), control of tumor-cell proliferation by
use of chalones (Bullough and Lawrence, 1968), the biochemical induction of
differentiation among undifferentiated tumor cells (Monard *et al.*, 1973), and the
inhibition of tumor-cell infiltration of tissues by interference with cell surface
serine proteases (Hynes, 1973).

A variety of immunological characteristics of cancer form the basis for the
developing field of immunotherapy. Since many of these have been discussed in
detail in preceding chapters, they need only to be discussed in a logical and
relevant sequence in this introduction. Immunological factors are involved in
most aspects of the etiology, pathogenesis, and course of malignant disease. That
host defence failure is involved in cancer etiology is based on a variety of
observations. These include experimental data that immunosuppression results
in increased takes and an increased final incidence and death rate among animals
with strongly antigenic virus- and carcinogen-induced tumors (Allison *et al.*,
1967). Immunosuppressive treatments may also result in increased metastases
among usually nonmetastasizing tumors (Balner and Dersjant, 1969). Clinically,
there is an increased incidence of lymphoma and leukemia among individuals
with immunodeficiency diseases, and among individuals receiving chronic
immunosuppressive therapy for renal transplants or other clinical indications
(Waldmann *et al.*, 1972; Penn and Starzl, 1972). This is partial support for the
concept of immunosurveillance (Burnett, 1970), although the pattern of histological types of malignant tumors in these patients is quite different than the pattern
of malignant tumors among the general population. There is a strong relationship
between immunocompetance and prognosis in cancer, with immunocompetent
patients having a relatively good prognosis and immunoincompetent patients
having a relatively poor prognosis (Hersh *et al.*, 1975). Conventional modalities of
cancer treatment are immunosuppressive (Hersh and Freiriech, 1968). Tumor
antigens and tumor-specific host immune responses to these antigens have been
observed in the majority of animal and human tumors studied (Hellström *et al.*,
1968). If there is vigorous tumor immunity the prognosis is relatively good, while
if there is weak tumor immunity the prognosis is relatively poor (Gutterman *et al.*,
1973*a*). Evidence of spontaneous antitumor activity also supports these concepts.
Thus infiltration of the primary tumor with lymphocytes, macrophages, or

EVAN M. HERSH,
G. M. MAVLIGIT,
J. U. GUTTERMAN,
AND
S. P. RICHMAN

plasma cells, sinus histiocytosis in regional lymph nodes, and perivascular round-cell infiltration in the region of the tumor are all associated with a good prognosis (Black *et al.*, 1956). Recently, several non-tumor-specific host defense factors have been shown to have potent antitumor activity. The most important of these is the selective killing of tumor cells and relative sparing of normal cells by activated macrophages (Hibbs *et al.*, 1972).

The above observations have established the rationale for human cancer immunotherapy. Thus, if tumor antigens and tumor immunity exist, if generalized immunodeficiency or deficiency of specific host defense factors occurs in cancer and is associated with a poor prognosis, and if activation of various host defense components to or even above the normal level can result in the killing of tumor cells, then a variety of immunological manipulations can be anticipated to have potent antitumor activity. There are some data to indicate that this is indeed the case. In experimental animals and in the clinical setting, immunotherapy can be demonstrated to have significant activity. Several major approaches to immunotherapy have been developed. These include active-nonspecific immunotherapy, active-specific immunotherapy, adoptive immunotherapy, immunorestorative immunotherapy, passive immunotherapy, local immunotherapy, and combinations thereof. Tumor types which have been shown to benefit from immunotherapy in man include skin cancer, breast cancer, colon cancer, lung cancer, head and neck cancer, urogenital cancer, malignant melanoma, acute and chronic leukemia, malignant lymphoma, and sarcoma. In general, the most striking result of immunotherapy in these disease categories has been prolongation of the disease-free interval and survival after remission has been induced by the conventional modalities of treatment. At present, there are only a few examples in which immunotherapy has increased the response rate.

There are a variety of problems associated with the current status and future development of immunotherapy. Tumor antigens on human tumors have not been well defined, in terms of either their precise localization, their immunogenicity and antigenicity, their precise localization, their immunogenicity and antigenicity, their cross-reactivity with normal tissue components, or their interaction with host defense factors—and they certainly have not been well defined in terms of their biochemical characteristics. An improved understanding of these problems is obviously fundamental to the development of this field, at least for active-specific immunotherapy. Similarly, the mechanism of effective tumor immunity is not understood, and, while a variety of specific components have been identified, mainly by *in vitro* studies (lymphocyte-mediated cytotoxicity, macrophage-mediated cytotoxicity, antibody-dependent cell-mediated cytotoxicity, complement-dependent antibody-mediated cytotoxicity, etc.), it is not known which of these factors are important *in vivo* in the host control of the tumor. This knowledge is important if we are to identify those factors most important to augment with immunotherapy and to identify the factors to study during the evaluation of new approaches to immunotherapy.

The mechanism of host defense failure in malignancy is also not well understood. Again, a variety of factors such as general failure of cell-mediated immunity, decline in specific antitumor immunity of either the cell-mediated or humoral type, development of circulating blocking factors, and a variety of genetic, age-related, and nutrition-related factors have all been identified individually (Hersh *et al.*, 1975). However, which play the critical role in determining progression of the tumor is not clear at this time. Furthermore, whether the immunodeficiency associated with the progression of tumors precedes or follows tumor growth has not been determined unequivocally. Since a major objective of immunotherapy is to restore these deficient host defense factors, it is essential that their precise *in vivo* role be defined.

The nature of the circulating blocking factors which interfere with general immunocompetence or specific tumor immunity is also not well defined. For example, whether the specific factors consist of circulating antigen, circulating antigen–antibody complex, antitumor antibody, or even anti-idiotypic antibody is not clear (Jose and Seshidri, 1974). It is also possible that the nature of these blocking factors may vary from one tumor type to another. If an objective of immunotherapy is to reduce these blocking factors, it is clear that their nature must be better understood. The mechanism of action of the immunopotentiators is only partially understood; it is complex, and involves effects on the number, location, and function of T and B lymphocytes and macrophages, on the size and function of the reticuloendothelial system, and on the antibody response. Immunopotentiators may also modify the function of other relevant organs such as the liver and bone marrow. Preparation of the active components of these immunopotentiators will depend on an improved understanding of their mechanism of action and, in addition, an improved approach to evaluation of their relevant effects and an improved understanding of their potential for the production of immune enhancement. Thus immunotherapeutic agents may suppress as well as augment host defense mechanisms, or they may augment an undesired component of the immune system (such as antibody which might be involved in blocking factors) (Flannery *et al.*, 1973).

In spite of these problems, significant empirical progress has been made both in experimental animal models and at the clinical level during the last few years. A number of effective active-nonspecific immunotherapy agents of the bacterial adjuvant type have been described, including bacillus Calmette Guérin (BCG), methanol extraction residue (MER), BCG cell-wall skeleton, and *Corynebacterium parvum*. There are also chemical immunorestorative agents such as levamisole and biological immunorestorative agents such as thymic hormones and extracts. In addition, successful immunotherapy trials have been conducted involving the use of immunization with tumor cells or tumor antigens. Thus, in spite of poor understanding of the mechanisms involved, considerable clinical progress has been made, and this offers an optimistic prospect for more significant development of this field in the future.

2. Principles of Immunotherapy and Approaches to Immunotherapy

In order to establish and discuss the principles of immunotherapy, it is necessary to define the approaches to immunotherapy and the expected results of these

EVAN M. HERSH,
G. M. MAVLIGIT,
J. U. GUTTERMAN,
AND
S. P. RICHMAN

430 approaches (Table 1). There are seven major approaches to immunotherapy. They are active-nonspecific immunotherapy, active-specific immunotherapy, adoptive immunotherapy, immunorestorative immunotherapy, passive immunotherapy, local immunotherapy, and combinations of these. Some difficulties or uncertainties in classification exist. The chemical agent levamisole, which acts (presumably through the cyclic nucleotide system of lymphocytes) to restore the expression of immune responsiveness of the cell-mediated type in sensitized individuals, is the prototype of chemical manipulation of the immune system. Some investigators have classified this drug in the category of active-nonspecific immunotherapy agents or immunorestorative agents, but perhaps it should be considered the first in a unique class of chemical immunological modulators. Finally, a possible approach to immunotherapy is the depletion of undesirable immune reactants from the circulation. These would include blocking antibody and antigen–antibody complex.

"Active-nonspecific immunotherapy" refers to the use of adjuvants, usually of microbial origin, which have one or more of the following immunological effects: increase of general immunocompetence, augmentation of cell-mediated or humoral immune reponses, expansion of the T-lymphocyte population, activa-

TABLE 1
Approaches to the Immunotherapy of Malignant Disease

Approach	Mechanisms of action	Commonly used reagent	Diseases where activity demonstrated
Active nonspecific (immunostimulation)	Increase general immune competence, activate macrophages, possible cross-immunogenicity with tumor antigens	BCG *C. parvum* MER	Melanoma Leukemia Colon Cancer Lung Cancer Breast Cancer
Immunorestoration	Restore immunocompetence of subjects	Levamisole Thymosin	Lung Cancer Breast cancer
Active specific	Increase specific cell-mediated and humoral antitumor immunity	Tumor cells Tumor antigen	Leukemia Lung cancer
Adoptive	Transfer tumor immunity from immune or hypo-immune subjects, active molecules from immune cells	Immune cells Transfer factor Immune RNA Lymphokines	None with certainty ? Sarcoma ? Melanoma
Passice	Transfer cytotoxic, deblocking, opsonizing, ADCC, or drug- or isotope-transporting antibody	Allogeneic or xenogeneic natural or-induced antibody	None with certainty
Local-regional	Locally activate macrophages, kill tumor by bystander effect of DTH, induce specific tumor immunity	BCG *C. parvum* PPD DNCB	Lund cancer Melanoma Breast cancer

tion of macrophases, and increase of reticuloendothelial system function. "Active-specific immunotherapy" refers to immunization procedures with tumor cells, tumor antigens, modified tumor cells, or modified tumor antigens, which are designed to selectively increase antitumor, cell-mediated, or humoral immunity. "Adoptive immunotherapy" refers to the transfer—with cells or cell products from an immunocompetent donor or from a donor specifically immune against the tumor—of the donor's general immunocompetence or specific tumor immunity, to an unresponsive or hyporeponsive tumor-bearing recipient. "Immunorestorative immunotherapy" refers to the use of agents such as levamisole or thumus hormones which increase the number of mature functional T lymphocytes. "Passive immunotherapy" refers to the transfer of antitumor antibody from an immune donor to a tumor-bearing recipient. This antibody may be cytotoxic, deblocking, opsinizing for the tumor cells, cytophilic for macrophages, or active in antibody-dependent cell-mediated cytotoxicity. The antibody may also be a carrier for cytotoxic drugs or radionuclieds. Passive immunotherapy might also include the administration of other serum factors with direct or indirect antitumor activity such as complement components, properdin, lymphokines, or tumor necrosis factor. "Local immunotherapy" refers to the introduction directly into the tumor of active-nonspecific or adoptive immunotherapeutic reagents. These may induce not only killing of the locally injected tumor but also augmentation of specific tumor resistance throughout the body. Finally, combinations of these approaches have been used with presumed, but not proven, greater effectiveness than the individual modalities alone.

There is a good rationale for the use of combination approaches. Active-specific immunotherapy should be more effective if used in combinations with an adjuvant such as BCG, which would increase the specific immune response. Active-specific immunotherapy and active-nonspecific immunotherapy should both be more effective if immunocompetence and immune responsiveness are normalized by immunorestorative therapy. Activation of the reticuloendothelial system and activation of macrophages with antitumor properties should be more effective if specific antitumor antibody of either the cytophilic or opsinizing type is given concurrently. However, it is not yet proven in human or animal immunotherapy that such combination approaches are more effective than the individual approaches alone.

What are the immunological defects to be treated and the host defense functions to be activated by immunotherapy? A variety of general non-tumor-specific and tumor-specific immunological defects have been observed in a fraction of the cancer patient population. Those patients are the ones who usually have a poor prognosis, in terms of reduced disease-free interval after surgery or radiotherapy, reduced remission rates after systemic therapy, and shortened survival compared to subjects without those defects. For example, in patients with solid tumors, impaired ability to develop primary delayed hypersensitivity to dinitrochlorobenzene (DNCB) is associated with either inoperability or a short disease-free interval after potentially curative surgery (Eilber and Morton, 1970). Persistence of diminished or declining DNCB reactivity after surgery is associated

EVAN M. HERSH,
G. M. MAVLIGIT,
J. U. GUTTERMAN,
AND
S. P. RICHMAN

with impending relapse (Eilber *et al.*, 1975). Diminished recall antigen reactivity or conversion from positive to negative recall antigen reactivity is associated with a poor prognosis during chemotherapy (Hersh *et al.*, 1976a) whereas patients who show improved recall antigen reactivity during chemotherapy have a relatively good prognosis (Hersh *et al.*, 1976a). Similar observations have been made in a variety of solid tumors in association with lymphocyte blastogenic responses to nonspecific mitogens such as phytohemagglutinin (PHA) and in the mixed lymphocyte reaction (MLR) (Catalona *et al.*, 1974). Patients with solid tumors also have diminished antibody responses to primary antigens such as *Salmonella adelaide flagellin* (Lee *et al.*, 1970), and those patients with a poor antibody response have a poor prognosis. Recently, attention has been focused on enumeration of circulating peripheral blood leukocytes. Lymphopenia, monocytopenia, and reduced levels of T and B lymphocytes are all associated with progressive tumor growth, dissemination of tumor, and a poor prognosis (Hersh *et al.*, 1976a).

In acute leukemia, the intensity of primary delayed-type hypersensitivity responses to keyhole limpet hemocyanin (KLH), *in vivo* delayed hypersensitivity responses to a variety of recall antigens (particularly fungal antigens such as dermatophytin), and *in vitro* lymphocyte blastogenic responses to mitogens such as PHA and antigens such as streptolysin O all predict for prognosis (Hersh *et al.*, 1974). The level of B lymphocytes at the termination of remission-induction chemotherapy is also quite important (Hersh *et al.*, 1976a). In the malignant lymphomas, DNCB reactivity and the development of delayed hypersensitivity to purified protein derivative (PPD) after BCG have proven predictive (Eltringham and Kaplan, 1973).

In the area of specific tumor immunity, cell-mediated and humoral immune responses, both *in vivo* and *in vitro*, have been useful in evaluating the stage of disease and the patient's prognosis. Thus *in vitro* lymphocyte blastogenic responses to autologous tumor cells, in both solid tumors and acute leukemia, predict for prognosis in terms of remission rate, remission duration, and survival (Gutterman *et al.*, 1973a). Patients with very vigorous responses have an improved prognosis. In contrast, patients with advanced disease may have absent blastogenic responses to autologous tumor cells. *In vivo* delayed hypersensitivity responses to tumor antigen may be measured in several disease categories, such as malignant melanoma, lung cancer, and acute leukemia (Hollinshead *et al.*, 1974). Patients with limited disease usually have positive skin tests, whereas patients with advanced disease have negative skin tests. While the specificity of lymphocyte-mediated or mononuclear cell-mediated cytotoxicity to tumor target cells is debated, there is general agreement that patients with localized disease or with a good prognosis have more vigorous cytotoxic activity than patients with advanced disease (Hellström *et al.*, 1971). In several disease categories, for example, in sarcoma and melanoma, circulating antibody measured by cytotoxicity or immunofluorescence is associated with remission (Morton *et al.*, 1971a). There is usually a striking decline in the antibody level preceding or associated with relapse. Finally, the local inflammatory response (as measured by the skin-window technique) is usually normal in patients with early malignancy and declines progressively as the malignancy advances. Patients with advanced cancer usually have a diminished or absent mononuclear phase of the inflammatory response (Dizon and Southam, 1963; Penny *et al.*, 1971). Of great importance, all conventional modalities of cancer treatment including surgery, radiotherapy, and chemotherapy may be markedly immunosuppressive.

From this brief description, it is obvious that there are many specific immunological defects in the cancer patient, particularly the patient with progressive disease or the patient under treatment. These can be the subject of immunological manipulation. Since correlations between the extent of disease and immunological deficiency and between immunological deficiency and a poor prognosis have been made, it seems logical to assume that if these immunological abnormalities were corrected, prognosis would improve. Prognosis might also improve if selected host defense factors were augmented above the normal level. However, one must be cautioned that all of these abnormalities including those involving specific tumor immunity are, at present, only indirectly related to the course of the malignant process. A cause-and-effect relationship has not been established. Also, the precise mechanisms of *in vivo* host control of tumor-cell proliferation and dissemination are not known. Therefore, it is conceivable that all of the immunological abnormalities observed in cancer patients, both tumor specific and not tumor specific, are related to independent factors and are therefore not directly related to tumor progression. Also, it is known that tumor progression and the circulating products produced by tumors suppress measurable host defense mechanisms. Thus abnormal host defense is the result, rather than the cause, of the tumor progression (Occhino *et al.*, 1973). However, these two possibilities do not entirely explain host defense failure in cancer, nor do they preclude effective immunotherapy. It has already been demonstrated in animal systems and in man that immunological manipulations directed at restoring general immunocompetence or boosting specific tumor immunity can improve the measurable host defense defects and the prognosis of the tumor-bearing subject. Immunological manipulations directed at restoring delayed-type hypersensitivity *in vivo*, increasing the levels of circulating monocytes, T cells, or B cells, increasing the cytotoxic antibody response, decreasing blocking factors, increasing specific tumor immunity, increasing the inflammatory response, and increasing particle clearance by the reticuloendothelial system all should have antitumor benefit.

It is also possible that normal host defense mechanisms may not be adequate and that a hyperfunctional state of the normal host defense mechanisms may be necessary for an immunotherapeutic effect. For example, it is known that in leukemia a good prognosis is associated with a supranormal PHA response but not with a normal PHA response (Hersh *et al.*, 1976a) and with a very vigorous blastogenic response to autologous tumor cells (stimulation index greater than 10 but not stimulation index between 3 and 10), and that in patients with melanoma receiving immunotherapy a very vigorous delayed hypersensitivity response to either recall or primary antigens (dermatophytin or KLH, with induration at 48 hr measuring greater than 15 mm but not 5–15 mm) is associated with

EVAN M. HERSH,
G. M. MAVLIGIT,
J. U. GUTTERMAN,
AND
S. P. RICHMAN

prolonged survival (Gutterman *et al.*, 1976). These data are indirect evidence that the normal host defense mechanisms and the normal level of tumor immunity may not be vigorous enough to destroy tumor cells with relatively weak tumor antigens. Augmentation of immune responses and other host defense mechanisms above the normal level may be necessary. Thus repeated immunization may increase antibody activity and affinity, may create heightened levels of delayed hypersensitivity, and may activate macrophages to the point where they can effectively kill tumor cells. Although it has only been measured to a limited degree, reticuloendothelial system (RES) function in cancer patients is either normal or slightly elevated (Sterm, 1960). Since circulating antigen–antibody complexes are hypothesized to be an important mechanism of tumor resistance to host defense mechanisms (Jose and Seshadri, 1974), it seems likely that hyperactivation of the RES may be required to clear these complexes and change the balance of the tumor–host relationship in favor of the host.

On the basis of the host defense mechanisms in cancer and the defined defects in these mechanisms in some cancer patients and on the basis of the approaches to immunotherapy, what are the major objectives of immunotherapy? The first objective must be the restoration of general immunologically incompetent. This may be approached via adoptive immunotherapy or by the administration of immunorestorative immunotherapy with thymic hormones (Goldstein *et al.*, 1970) or by administration of chemical agents such as levamisole (Tripodi *et al.*, 1973). It may also be achieved in the malnourished or vitamin-deficient individual by appropriate nutrition (Law *et al.*, 1973). A second objective of immunotherapy is to induce heightened specific tumor immunity or to restore tumor immunity if absent or weak. This may be achieved by active-specific and adoptive immunotherapy and also as a concomitant effect of active-nonspecific immunotherapy. A third objective of immunotherapy is to hyperactivate various components of the general or non-tumor-specific host defenses including T- and B-cell levels and activity, and macrophage and RES activity in various organs and in the tumor itself. This may be referred to as "immunopotentiation" and may be accomplished by the administration of active-nonspecific immunotherapeutic reagents or perhaps by the administration of macrophage-activating factors. Finally, a fourth objective of immunotherapy is specific immune modulation. This may be defined as the selective manipulation of the immune system to achieve a particular objective. One may wish to selectively activate T-cell-mediated immunity; one may wish to selectively increase the levels of circulating cells (T lymphocytes or macrophages); one may wish to selectively suppress production of antibody of certain classes (blocking antibody); or one may wish to selectively augment the antibody response of a certain class such as cytotoxic antibody. These objectives may be accomplished by a variety of immunological maneuvers.

3. Multimodality Cancer Therapy

Intimately involved with the development of cancer immunotherapy is the concept of multimodality cancer treatment. This applies to the patient with limited disease which is surgically "curable," as well as to the patient with advanced

metastatic disease. In multimodality cancer treatment, all appropriate forms of cytoreductive and host resotrative therapy must be brought to bear in a logical sequence against both evident or detectable tumor and suspected nonevident microscopic foci of tumor cells. This approach is currently practiced in a restricted fashion in certain disease categories. For example, radiotherapy to the chest wall after surgical extirpation of primary mammary cancer will prevent local recurrence of disease, although it does not increase the cure rate (Cuttler and Heise, 1969). Combined surgery and radiotherapy in head and neck cancer does increase the cure rate (Fletcher *et al.*, 1970). Adjuvant chemotherapy (Fisher *et al.*, 1975) or immunotherapy (Gutterman *et al.*, 1976) prolongs the disease-free interval and survival after surgical extirpation of certain malignant tumors.

However, this concept is currently being broadened. Thus, for patients with disseminated or metastatic malignant disease and for patients with a probability of recurrence of at least 15% after definitive remission-induction therapy, we must apply all appropriate modalities of treatment that could further reduce the tumor burden, whether or not there is evident or microscopic disease remaining after definitive therapy. For example, the patient with advanced metastatic disease should undergo surgical debulking of accessible tumor, radiotherapy for local nonremovable radiosensitive tumor, chemotherapy to affect widely disseminated microscopic and evident foci of metastatic disease, and immunotherapy to augment host defense mechanisms against the tumor. Nutritional or vitamin therapy may also be appropriate. Patients whose disease the surgeon would at present consider inoperable and patients to whom the radiotherapist is not anxious to apply palliative therapy must be reconsidered for this type of additive therapy. The systemic modalities of cancer treatment, namely, chemotherapy and immunotherapy, become more effective as the tumor burden is reduced. Therefore, surgical debulking and local tumor destruction by radiotherapy may be very important components of combined-modality treatment and may greatly augment the effects of systemic therapy.

The combined-modality approach also applies to immunotherapy. Thus the combination of multiple immunotherapeutic modalities should at least have additive and might even have synergistic effects. Combined-modality immunotherapy would cover the entire spectrum of potentially modifiable components of the tumor–host interaction from the antigenicity and immunogenicity of the tumor cells to the terminal effector mechanisms. For example, one might be able to modify tumor cells, converting them from a nonimmunogenic to an immunogenic state. One might be able to break tolerance to tumor cells if this exists. After maneuvers relating to the immunogenicity of the tumor, one might attempt to reverse the non-tumor-specific immune deficiency associated with cancer, and to then selectively activate those components of the host defense system which are most relevant to the tumor. This would include activation of macrophages and of cell-mediated immunity, increase of cytotoxic or other antitumor antibodies, and clearing of circulating antigen–antibody complexes. If several of these effects such as activation of macrophages and increase of

436

EVAN M. HERSH,
G. M. MAVLIGIT,
J. U. GUTTERMAN,
AND
S. P. RICHMAN

lymphocyte-mediated immunity could be achieved simultaneously, the antitumor effects should be additive and might be synergistic. This, however, is an approach for the future. There are no good examples of combined-modality immunotherapy at present.

4. Problems in Monitoring and Evaluation of Immunotherapy

The conventional modalities cancer treatment are relatively easy to evaluate and monitor. The completeness of surgical extirpation of tumor can be readily evaluated pathologically, and by conventional clinical testing. Similarly, radiotherapy can easily be monitored by the measurement of tumor regression, and by relatively rapid evaluation of dose-limiting tissue toxicity. Chemotherapy can also be evaluated and monitored with relative ease. Thus the antitumor activity of a drug or drug combination is usually manifest by measurable tumor regression within a few months. The maximally tolerated dose of a drug is almost always equivalent to the most effective dose, and toxicity is readily measured by determining the degree of myelosuppression, the degree of acute gastrointestinal toxicity, the degree of chronic gastrointestinal toxicity, and the degree of other dose-limiting toxicities such as peripheral neuropathy and cardiomyopathy. Measurement of this acute and chronic toxicity helps not only in determining dose but also in determining route and schedule of administration. Since most cancer is systemic, the systemic or intravenous administration of antitumor agent is desirable. This is almost always possible with antitumor chemotherapeutic agents but is just in its earliest stages of development and evaluation for immunotherapeutic agents.

In contrast to the relative ease of determining both efficacy and toxicity and thus dose, route, and schedule for the conventional modalities of cancer treatment, it is extremely difficult to make the same determinations for immunotherapy. For active-nonspecific immunotherapy with adjuvants or active-specific immunotherapy with tumor cells or tumor antigen, for adoptive immunotherapy, or for immunorestorative immunotherapy, there is no clear-cut dose-limiting toxicity, nor is there any evident schedule dependency. This applies to the oral, cutaneous, subcutaneous, intramuscular, intracavitary, or even intravenous route of administration. For example, for active-nonspecific immunotherapy with BCG given by the scarification route, one could administer a very low dose of viable organisms, such as 10^5 with an an interval as long as 1 year between treatments, or one could administer very high doses of organisms, such as 10^9 with a frequency as intensive as every 2–3 days. Both extremes of schedule and dose would be well tolerated, and even the low dose might well elicit some degree of local immunological reactivity.

Dose–response studies of immunological effects also present serious problems in both conduct and interpretation, for the following reasons: We do not know which immunological functions that we can measure or which immunological effects that we observe are relevant in terms of host control of tumor. None of our tests may measure that host defense mechanism by which the tumor is actually controlled by the host *in vivo*. The maximum immunostimulating dose may not be the optimal one. In other words, the maximal attainable degree of immunological activation or augmentation may not be optimal in terms of host control of tumor, and excessive immune responses may actually be detrimental (Piessens *et al.*, 1970). Furthermore, while low doses of immunopotentiating agents will not be effective and moderate doses may be effective, high doses may actually be immunosuppressive (Geffard and Orbach-Arbouys, 1976). They may also suppress some functions while stimulating others, further confusing the issue. These factors make dose–response studies very difficult.

Another important difficulty in evaluating immunotherapy relates to the therapeutic end point. While a valid end point for immunotherapy is indeed the observation of tumor regression, the most common end point is prolongation of remission duration, disease-free interval, duration of stabilization of tumor growth, and duration of survival. It can take 2–5 years to measure some of these durations or intervals. Therefore, it is almost impossible to do adequate dose, schedule, and therapeutic response studies that are relatively easy to carry out for surgery, radiotherapy, and chemotherapy.

Now there are a variety of tests available to monitor the immunotherapy of human cancer. It must be borne in mind, however, that all of these, including those which are claimed to be tumor specific, can at present only be interpreted to be indirectly related to host control of tumor and to the effects of immunotherapy. The tests available to monitor immunotherapy include measurement of primary delayed hypersensitivity responses to antigens such as KLH or haptenes such as DNCB, established delayed hypersensitivity responses to recall antigens such as candidin, *in vitro* lymphocyte blastogenic response to mitogens, antigens, and allogeneic tissues, the primary antibody response, the secondary antibody response, the levels of circulating lymphocytes and monocytes in the peripheral blood, the levels of circulating immunoglobulins or isoantibodies, the levels of circulating T and B lymphocytes in the peripheral blood, and lymphocyte or monocyte cytotoxicity to target cells *in vitro*, either direct or antibody dependent. One can also measure the inflammatory response *in vivo* by the skin-window technique and measure the activity of the RES *in vivo* by particle clearance.

In regard to specific tumor immunity, depending on the availability and suitability of various target cells, either freshly collected from the patient or growing in the form of tissue-culture cell lines, one can measure lymphocyte- or monocyte-mediated cytotoxicity, antibody-mediated or antibody-dependent cell-mediated cytotoxicity, lymphocyte blastogenic responses to cells or antigens, and migration inhibitory responses to cells or antigens. One can also measure *in vivo* delayed hypersensitivity, either to the tumor cells themselves or to antigen extracted from the tumor cells.

Several general observations have been made with regard to the immunological effects of immunotherapy. For example, for the microbial adjuvants there is some evidence that administration of an agent such as BCG, MER, or *C. parvum* can result in increased delayed-type hypersensitivity responses to primary antigens

438

EVAN M. HERSH,
G. M. MAVLIGIT,
J. U. GUTTERMAN,
AND
S. P. RICHMAN

(Gutterman *et al.*, 1973*b*) and to recall antigens (Hersh *et al.*, 1976*a*), and can result in increased lymphocyte blastogenic responses to mitogens or antigens (Hersh *et al.*, 1976*b*). The numbers of circulating T and B cells have not been altered by adjuvant therapy. Monocyte or macrophage activity, RES activity, and the antibody response have not been studied to a significant degree in patients receiving these agents. Both adjuvant immunotherapy and active-specific immunotherapy have been studied in terms of cell-mediated cytotoxicity to target cells, and both have been shown to have some degree of an increase of this type of reactivity (Weiss *et al.*, 1976). Adoptive immunotherapy with immune RNA or transfer factor has also been studied. Both cytotoxicity to target cells (Pilch *et al.*, 1974) and increased blastogenic response to target cells or target-cell antigens (Pilch *et al.*, 1976) have been observed. However, none of these studies has been adequately controlled in terms of the use of control tissue, nor do they take into account the wide fluctuations observed in lymphocyte reactivity when followed serially with time. Patients receiving transfer factor have also been studied extensively for transfer of delayed hypersensitivity. In general, specific transfer has been observed, under the appropriate clinical circumstances (Lawrence, 1974). However, nonspecific effects such as increased MLC reactivity (Dupont *et al.*, 1974) and increased numbers of rosette-forming cells (Spitler *et al.*, 1972) have been observed, and there is also some evidence for immunosuppression (Kirkpatrick and Gallin, 1975). Finally, the immunorestorative agents such as levamisole and thymosin have been studied. After the administration of these agents, increased delayed-type hypersensitivity to recall antigens (Tripodi *et al.*, 1973), increased lymphocyte blastogenic responses to antigens (Schafer *et al.*, 1976), and increased numbers of circulating lymphocytes or circulating T cells as measured by the rosette method (Schafer *et al.*, 1976) have been reported.

The weakness of all of these observations is that it is not clear that the immunotherapy which results in augmentation of an immune response is what also results in a therapeutic effect, and furthermore it is not clear that there is a concordance between the immunological alteration and the therapeutic efficacy. This is particularly difficult to determine when the immunotherapy extends over many months or years, and the end point, namely, response duration or survival duration, is distal from the time of onset of immunotherapy. Furthermore, no long-term studies of immunotherapy extending over years have been reported, and therefore it is possible that there are critically important immunotherapy-induced changes in immunological reactivity at one point, which have their clinical manifestation in terms of remission or relapse months or years in the future. No rational experimental design to deal with this type of problem and to answer these questions even exists at the present time.

5. Animal Models of Immunotherapy

Animal models have been useful in identifying reagents with immunotherapeutic activity. Animal models also play an important role in studies of host–tumor interaction of the mechanism of action of immunotherapy and in guiding the development of clinical trials. Well-designed animal models are essential for rapid progress in the development of the field of immunotherapy. Ideally, animal models should be used both to identify new modalities of immunotherapy and to quickly answer relevant questions regarding the design of immunotherapy trials in man, as well as to study questions of toxicity, potential adverse interactions, etc.

The utility of animal models in these regards can be well described by a consideration of animal model studies recently carried out with BCG and its derivatives such as MER and the various cell–wall and cell–wall-skeleton preparations. Animal models have been very useful in studying the effects of BCG and the routes of administration by which these effects are best mediated. Thus, in animal models, BCG can be curative when given intralesionally to treat subcutaneous tumors (Zbar *et al.*, 1972), when given intravenously to treat artificially induced pulmonary metastases (Baldwin and Pimm, 1973*a*), and when given intrapleurally or intravenously to treat pleural metastases of experimental tumors (Pimm and Baldwin, 1975*a*). When given by a variety of routes, including intravenous and intraperitoneal, BCG is capable of augmenting general host resistance so that the development of spontaneous tumors such as AKR leukemia (LeMonde, 1973) or the development of virus- or carcinogen-induced tumors (Schwartz *et al.*, 1971) is blocked. When given by these systemic routes, BCG either alone or in combination with a tumor-cell vaccine can prolong surgery- or chemotherapy-induced remissions of disease. The routes of administration which have proved to be most effective are usually those in thich the BCG is regional or in close approximation to the tumor. Examples include intravenous BCG for pulmonary metastases (Baldwin and Pimm, 1973*a*) or intralesional BCG for tumor nodules in skin or lymph nodes (Zbar *et al.*, 1972). A related approach is to mix BCG organisms directly with tumor cells, either at the time of inoculation or shortly after inoculation at a distant site (Hawrylko and Mackaness, 1973).

The mechanism of BCG action has been studied in great detail. While BCG can augment immunity to weakly immunogenic tumors in mot animal models, the efficacy of BCG is related to the antigenicity of the tumor and is most effective in antigenic tumors (Parr, 1972). Indeed, in some circumstances the growth of weakly antigenic or nonantigenic tumors can be enhanced by the administration of BCG (Chee and Bodurtha, 1974). The mechanism of BCG action is complex. Since each animal model is different, and host defense mechanisms vary from model to model, generalizations are difficult to make. A cretain mechanism of resistance such as that mediated by T lymphocytes may be active in one model, whereas antibody-related mechanisms may be active in another, and macrophage- or histiocyte-related mechanisms may be active in a third. However, there do seem to be three major mechanisms involved in the therapeutic action of BCG. These include augmentation of classical cell mediated immunity (Bansal and Sjögren, 1973), activation of macrophages with subsequent macrophage-mediate killing of tumor cells (Cleveland *et al.*, 1974; Hanna *et al.*, 1973), and cell-mediated and/or humoral immunity to antigens on BCG organisms which cross-react with tumor cells (Minden *et al.*, 1974).

EVAN M. HERSH,
G. M. MAVLIGIT,
J. U. GUTTERMAN,
AND
S. P. RICHMAN

Evidence for the importance of T-cell-mediated immunity includes the fact that, in some animal models, activated T cells are clearly the killer cells and removal of adherent cells does not reduce killer-cell activity. Also, in a number of models, thymectomy or the administration of antilymphocyte serum reduces the immunotherapeutic effect (Chung *et al.*, 1973).

Evidence for the role of macrophages comes from direct histological studies of tumors undergoing necrosis after intralesional BCG (Hanna *et al.*, 1973), the fact that BCG-activated macrophages can selectively kill tumor cells (Cleveland *et al.*, 1974), and the fact that macrophages from animals cured of the guinea pig hepatoma by intralesional BCG kill at an effector–target cell ratio of 10 to 1, whereas lymphocytes from these same animals only kill at a ratio of 10,000 to 1 (Fidler *et al.*, 1977). Direct macrophage lysozome heterocytolysis into tumor cells has been observed (Hibbs, 1974), and histologically one can demonstrate the transfer of lysozomes from macrophages into tumor cells (Hanna *et al.*, 1972, 1973). Furthermore, increased reticuloendothelial system activity with subsequent abolishment of the antigen-induced suppression of delayed hypersensitivity has been demonstrated to be important (Mackaness *et al.*, 1973; Miller *et al.*, 1973).

Since intralesional BCG in the "nude" mouse causes tumor regression but fails to elicit specific tumor resistance (Pimm and Baldwin, 1975*b*), while intralesional BCG in intact animals induces both, we can hypothesize the following complex mechanisms. The administration of BCG regional the tumor causes local activation of macrophages and direct macrophage killing of tumor cells. In the intact animal, a delayed hypersensitivity reaction is induced; lymphocytes produce lymphokines, which activate more macrophages and which kill tumor cells directly. Activated macrophages produce lymphocyte-activating factor, which activates T lymphocytes to produce lymphotoxin, which also kills tumor cells. The BCG–tumor-cell interaction causes localization of tumor antigen in the regional lymph node with subsequent induction of vigorous tumor immunity. This tumor immunity becomes generalized so that subsequent tumor-cell challenge at distant sites results in tumor resistance based on a classical cell-mediated delayed hypersensitivity mechanism.

The development of delayed hypersensitivity and humoral immunity to BCG antigens themselves may also play an important role in the mechanism of BCG action. BCG cross-reactive antigens have been discovered on certain tumor cells, and this may be an important component of the resistance to subsequent tumor-cell challenge. This cross-reactive immunity has been demonstrated in the F91 melanoma of Balb/c mice (Faraci *et al.*, 1975). Immunization with BCG results in specific cell-mediated cytotoxicity to target tumor cells. It has been demonstrated in the line 10 guinea pig heptoma, using anti-BCG antibody and demonstration of specific reactivity by immunoelectronmicroscopy and by a radioimmuno-precipitation assay. It has also been demonstrated in human malignant melanoma and human myelogenous leukemia by these techniques (Bucana and Hanna, 1974).

The optimal conditions for BCG effect have also been established. These
include a high dose of BCG (a low dose being much less effective), the presence of living organisms in most but not all circumstances, the presence of an immunocompetent nonimmunosuppressed host, a small tumor size (tumor enhancement may occur when BCG is given to animals with large tumors), and regional or close approximation of BCG to tumor cells (Zbar *et al.*, 1971). In addition, for the induction of permanent tumor resistance, the tumor must be immunogenic (Baldwin and Pimm, 1973*b*), and an immune response to the BCG is necessary for the effect (Bartlett *et al.*, 1972).

One of the best models which exemplifies these phenomena is the guinea pig hepatoma. This is a carcinogen-induced, transplantable, syngeneic sarcoma in the inbred strain 2 guinea pig (Zbar and Tanaka, 1971). When the primary tumor is inoculated with BCG 7 days after implantation, the primary tumor regresses completely in 60% of the cases. Tumor cells which are present in numbers of approximately 10^5 in the regional lymph nodes never develop into a palpable tumor in these animals. These animals are apparently cured, although recent data indicate that when apparently cured animals are given doses of tumor anitigen, recurrence of tumor may occur (Wainberg, 1977). The suggests the importance of persistence of tumor immunity in the maintenance of remission. The mechanism of tumor rejection at the local site is associated with a heavy infiltration of histiocytes, close approximation of histiocytes and tumor cells, and fusion of histiocytes to tumor cells with subsequent lysis of the latter (Hanna *et al.*, 1972, 1973). If the tumor is large, it does not regress (Zbar *et al.*, 1972). Animals whose tumors do regress are resistant to subsequent potentially lethal tumor-cell challenge at distant sites (Bartlett *et al.*, 1972).

For optimal effect, a large dose of BCG is required. The BCG must be living. There must be close approximation between the BCG organisms and the tumor cells; however, other data indicate that if a vaccine consisting of BCG plus viable or irradiated tumor cells is given at a distant site, on the same day as the primary challenge, cures may also occur (Kronman *et al.*, 1970; Bartlett and Zbar, 1972). Also, if the BCG is administered between the primary tumor and the regional lymph nodes, and the primary tumor is removed several days later, apparent cure of the regional lymph node metastatic disease is observed. The tumor burden is indeed critical, not only because tumors of large size do not regress after intralesional BCG but also because the local effects of BCG and the induction of systemic tumor immunity can be abrogated by the intravenous injection of relatively small numbers (10^3–10^4) of living tumor cells (Hanna and Peters, 1975).

With this model, it is possible to create a biological circumstance which is quite analogous to those human tumors which normally metastasize to regional lymph nodes and in which microscopic foci of tumor cells are frequently found in the regional lymph nodes at the time of removal of the primary tumor. For example, this model has been used to compare the efficacy of different strains and preparations of BCG used by scarification for the prevention of lymph node and distant recurrences after the extirpation of regional lymph node disease (Hanna *et*

442

EVAN M. HERSH,
G. M. MAVLIGIT,
J. U. GUTTERMAN,
AND
S. P. RICHMAN

al., 1977). Fully viable fresh frozen BCG was found to be superior to standard lyophilized preparations, and the Pasteur and Phipps strains were found to be superior to the Tice strain. These observations have formed the basis for a current ongoing study in human melanoma. Also, cure of regional lymph node disease by intralesional treatment of the primary tumor has led to the development of a protocol now being carried out in human melanoma. The primary tumor is inoculated with BCG, and approximately 1 month later the inoculated site is surgically extirpated along with the regional nodes. The hope is that this will lead to cure by a combination of local tumor destruction and induction of systemic tumor immunity. The results of this clinical trial based on a rationale developed in an animal model are awaited with great interest. Another material closely related to BCG which has been studied in a variety of animal models is the methanol extraction residue of BCG, usually referred to as MER (Weiss, 1976). This material is made by methanol extraction of phenol-killed, acid-washed BCG organisms and represents aggregated and particulate, partially delipidated, cell-wall skeletons of the BCG organisms. MER was initially developed as a potential adjuvant to increase resistance to mycobacterial and other infection. Subsequently, it was discovered that it had potent antitumor activity. Basically, the material increases resistance to viral leukemogenesis (Weiss and Yashphe, 1973) and increases resistance to the transplantation of carcinogen-induced tumors in rodents (Weiss *et al.*, 1966). When given to rodents with transplanted carcinogen-induced fibrosarcomas or virus-induced mammary carcinomas, following chemotherapy or radiotherapy, it increases the survival, although it does not usually produce cures (Yron *et al.*, 1973). Administration at sites remote from the tumor is as good as, or superior to, intralesional therapy. Of interest, and in contrast to intact viable BCG, tumor enhancement is usually not observed under any experimental circumstances. The material has been studied by the intradermal, intralesional, subcutaneous, and intraperitoneal routes. The oral and intravenous routes remain to be explored.

The mechanism of action has been studied extensively in rodents. As in the case with other bacterial adjuvants, it is complex. Administration of MER into an extremity increases proliferation of lymphocytes in the regional lymph nodes, but not in the spleen (Gery *et al.*, 1974). Splenic lymphocytes of such animals have increased reactivity to lipopolysaccharide (LPS), while the regional lymph node lymphocytes have increased reactivity to LPS, concanavalin A (Con A), and phytohemagglutinin (PHA) (Gery *et al.*, 1974). This suggests that in different regions of the lymphoid organs selective B-cell or T- and B-cell activation is taking place. These activities may be mediated through macrophages since macrophage activation is regularly observed. There are an increased number of macrophages in the peritoneal space and presumably in other foci (Gery *et al.*, 1974; Yagel *et al.*, 1975). There are increased macrophage lysosomal content and activity and increased production by these activated macrophages of lymphocyte-activating factor (Gery *et al.*, 1974). Most important selective modulation of the immune response can take place as a result of MER administration. Thus—depending on the dose of MER, its timing relationship relative to the time of administration of antigen, and the relative strength of the antigen—augmentation of cell-mediated or humoral immunity, suppression of cell-mediated or humoral immunity, or upward or downward modification of both components of immunity has been observed (Ben-Efraim *et al.*, 1974).

It is obvious from this brief description that the proper manipulation of such an immunoregulatory material may have profound immunotherapeutic potential. Indeed, this has already been observed in the few reported preliminary human experiments. MER has been observed to increase delayed hypersensitivity and lymphocyte blastogenic responses in patients with advanced malignant disease (Moertel *et al.*, 1975). In a small series of patients with metastatic colon carcinoma, regression of metastatic nodules after the administration of MER alone was observed in a minority of cases (Moertel *et al.*, 1975). More important, several studies indicate that when administered between courses of chemotherapy it prolongs remission in acute myelogenous leukemia of the adult (Weiss *et al.*, 1975; Cuttner *et al.*, 1975). Recently, MER administration during remission induction was demonstrated to increase the remission rate in AML (Cuttner *et al.*, 1977). In a comparative study, MER seems to have equivalent activity to BCG in prolongation of remission duration and survival in patients receiving chemotherapy for metastatic breast carcinoma (Hortobagyi, 1977). However, MER appears to have no effect on the remission rate, remission duration, or survival of patients with metastatic colon cancer receiving chemotherapy (Moertel *et al.*, 1977). This material is difficult to administer because of severe local reactions and local abscess formation at higher doses. Because of its great potential, it is obvious that extensive further animal experimentation will be needed before the optimal dose, route, and schedule of administration can be determined.

Animals models have also been very useful in the evaluation of more purified fractions of BCG and other microbial agents. Various purified fractions of BCG have been most extensively investigated. Recently, lipopolysaccharide bacterial extracts (endotoxins) have been used in combination with these mycobacterial fractions. The rationale for this development has been the known activity of BCG, the hope that its toxicity could be avoided by using purified subfractions, and the known antitumor activity of endotoxins. Leadership in this field has been by Edgar Ribi in the United States and by Lederer Chedid and co-workers in France. Progressive fractionation of BCG has led to a series of purified products with increasing activity. These have included BCG cell wall made by lysis of BCG and cell-wall skeleton made by proteolysis and extraction with organic solvents of cell wall (Ribi *et al.*, 1975*a*). The cell-wall skeleton is a peptidoglycolipid (Meyer *et al.*, 1975). Finally, extraction with organic solvents has led to a series of glycolipids including Wax-D and cord factor, a purified subcomponent of which is prepared by microparticulate column chromatography and is a trehalose dimycolate usually referred to as P3 (Ribi *et al.*, 1977). It is not a homogeneous substance since saponization yields four different mycolic acids. In terms of their antitumor potency, the best source of cell-wall skeleton is *Mycobacterium phlei*, while the best source of the P3 fraction is the Aoyma B strain of *Mycobacterium tuberculosis* (Ribi *et al.*, 1977). In regard to the endotoxins (which will be discussed in more detail in

444

EVAN M. HERSH,
G. M. MAVLIGIT,
J. U. GUTTERMAN,
AND
S. P. RICHMAN

another section), while native endotoxin has some activity, the relatively carbohydrate-deficient RE-mutant endotoxins have markedly increased activity (Ribi *et al.*, 1977).

Other mycobacterial products of interest which have not been studied as extensively include water-soluble adjuvants and interphase material. Water-soluble adjuvant (WSA) is made by lysozyme digestion of trypsin-treated delipidated cell walls of *Mycobacterium smegmatis*. It has been observed to increase both cell-mediated and humoral immunity, and the mechanism of action is felt to be increased lymphocyte activity induced by activated macrophages which are themselves induced by the water-soluble adjuvant (Modolell *et al.*, 1974). The active component is now known to be a myramyl dipeptide. To date, no antitumor activity has been demonstrated for this material. However, it may have important activity as an adjuvant in active-specific immunization. Interphase material (IPM) is a complex of carbohydrate, protein and lipid, which is a water-insoluble extract from *M. smegmatis* (Lamensans *et al.*, 1975). It has immunoprophylactic activity against a variety of tumors including L1210 leukemia.

The mycobacterial fractions have been most effectively studied in the previously described guinea pig hepatoma model. The mycobacterial and other extracts outlined above are used to treat this system when combined or bound to the surface of oil droplets with the aid of Tween-80. BCG cell wall is as effective as intact BCG. Cell-wall skeleton alone induces approximately 30% cures, while cell-wall skeleton plus P3 induces 80% regressions, as does RE-endotoxin plus P3. The most active material in this sytem is BCG cell-wall plus P3 plus RE-endotoxin, which cures approximately 95% of the animals (Ribi *et al.*, 1977). These active purified subcomponent combinations are active even 14 days after tumor inoculation, which is not the case for BCG. Also, they are highly active when placed between the primary tumor and the regional draining lymph nodes with subsequent extirpation of the primary tumor at days 7–14 (Ribi *et al.*, 1977). Of interest, P3 alone is inactive. In contrast, cord factor on oil droplets with or without Wax-D has some antitumor activity in that it suppresses the development of urethane-induced lung adenomas in mice (Bekierkunst *et al.*, 1971).

Clinical trials with these purified fractions are now beginning. They obviously offer many advantages to intact BCG in that they can be standardized, they are nonliving, they are likely to be less toxic, and, from the animal model data, they would be predicted to be more effective. BCG cell-wall skeleton has shown great activity in lung cancer, combined either with surgery, with chemotherapy, or with both (Yamamura *et al.*, 1976). Prolongation of remission and survival has been observed. Intralesional therapy with BCG cell wall, cell-wall skeleton, and cell-wall skeleton plus P3 seems to be as active as intralesional therapy with BCG even in patients with advanced tumors (S. P. Richman, J. U. Gutterman, and E. M. Hersh, unpublished observations). These materials certainly warrant intensive further investigation in various human tumors. Clearly there should be a close and continuing interaction between research in animal models and clinical trials of immunotherapy. Discoveries in animal models should result in clinical trials. Clinical problems and certain clinical questions can be solved by appropriately

designed animal model experiments. Questions of mechanism can be asked in
animal models. Also, difficult or dangerous approaches can be worked out first in
animal models, and knowledge gained can be used to develop refined and
scientifically based clinical trials.

6. Active-Nonspecific Immunotherapy

Active-nonspecific immunotherapy—the administration of an adjuvant material
which can boost general immunocompetence, in terms of both cell-mediated and
humoral immunity, and which can activate macrophages—is the most widely
investigated and effective approach to immunotherapy at the current time (Table
2). Most of the active-nonspecific immunotherapeutic agents are intact viable or
killed microorganisms or are extracts of microbial organisms (Ribi *et al.*, 1977).
Some are synthetic chemical substances (Tripodi *et al.*, 1973) or natural products
of mammalian cells (Papermaster *et al.*, 1976a). The most intensively studied
active-nonspecific immunotherapeutic agents include the following: the bacillus
Calmette Guérin (BCG) strain of *Mycobacterium bovis* (Laucius *et al.*, 1974);
derivatives of BCG including methanol extraction residue (MER) (Weiss, 1976),
BCG cell walls, BCG cell-wall skeleton, the cord-factor-related lipid extract of
BCG (P3) (Ribi *et al.*, 1977), and the water-soluble extract derived from BCG
(WSE) (Modolell *et al.*, 1974). Interphase material (IPM) extracted from *M.
smegmatis* is also under investigation (Lamensans *et al.*, 1975). The next most
actively investigated bacterial adjuvant is *Corynebacterium parvum* (Scott, 1974c).
Other active-nonspecific immunotherapeutic reagents include *Pseudomonas* vaccine (Gee and Clarkson, 1977), *Brucella* and pertussis vaccines (Finger *et al.*,
1970), vaccinia virus vaccine (Hunter–Craig *et al.*, 1970), the polysaccharide
extracts of various fungi (Maeda and Chihara, 1973), synthetic or semisynthetic
adjuvants including double-stranded RNA, pyran copolymer, and poly(A)-
poly(U) (Pendergrast *et al.*, 1975). Synthetic lipids such as liposomes and
lysolecithin derivatives also belong to this class of agents. See Table 2 for an outline
of these agents.

It is possible, although not entirely appropriate, to include the chemical
immunorestorative agent levamisole (Tripodi *et al.*, 1973) and products of mammalian cells including lymphokines (Papermaster *et al.*, 1976a), interferon (Grossberg, 1972), and tumor necrosis factor (Carswell *et al.*, 1975) in this category. The
latter three are effector molecules released by lymphocytes, macrophages, and
other cells and might also be included in the adoptive immunotherapy category.
They may be included here in the sense that they are "nonspecific," i.e., not
directly associated with immunity to tumor antigens.

A discussion of active-nonspecific immunotherapy properly begins with a
discussion of Coley's toxin or Coley's mixed bacterial toxins, also called mixed
bacterial vaccine (MBV). This material is a mixture of heat-killed *Streptococcus
pyogenes* and *Serratia marcescens*, and was developed by Coley (1896). It was

EVAN M. HERSH,
G. M. MAVLIGIT,
J. U. GUTTERMAN,
AND
S. P. RICHMAN

TABLE 2

Active-Nonspecific Immunotherapy Agents
Currently in Use or under Investigation

Intact microorganisms
    Mycobacteria
        Baccillus Calmette Guérin (BCG)
        Mycobacterium butesicum
        Other mycobacteria
    Corynebacterium parvum (Cp)
    Mixed bacterial vaccine
    Pertussis vaccine
    OK 432
Microbial subfractions
    Mycobacterial
        Methanol extraction residue (MER)
        Methanol-soluble fraction
        Cell wall
        Cell-wall skeleton
        Cord factor
        P3 (trehalose dimycolate), P4
        Sulfolipid (SL-III)
        Water-soluble adjuvant
        Muramyl dipeptide
    Carbohydrates
        Lentinan
        Pachymaran
        PSK
        Glucan
    Endotoxins
        Pseudomonas
        E. coli
        V. cholerae
        Detoxified endotoxins
Interferon inducers
    Poly(AU)
    Poly(IC)
    Pyran copolymer
    Tylerone
Lipids
    Lysolecithin analogues
    Liposomes

administered to patients with osteogenic and soft tissue sarcomas following surgery. This was based on the observation of an improved survival of sarcoma patients who developed severe infections after surgery. Coley reported that patients receiving at least seven injections of this vaccine in the postsurgical period had a 5-year survival of 36% compared to approximately 18% among patients treated with surgery alone. These results were encouraging enough that a commercial vaccine preparation was made by Parke-Davis. However, Coley's results could not be confirmed, possibly because of decreased vaccine potency or less intensive administration of the vaccine (Nauts, 1975). This represents the first extensive study of active-nonspecific immunotherapy in man. Recent renewed interest in the role of endotoxins in immunotherapy (Ribi *et al.*, 1975*b*) and the demonstration of a similar beneficial effect of infection in lung cancer (Ruckdeschel *et al.*, 1972) tend to support the impression that Coley's original observations were valid. The relationship of Coley's observations to the fever associated with the vaccine and the recent demonstration of the antitumor effects of heat are also of interest in this regard.

The development of effective programs of immunotherapy with BCG was, after a delay of many years from the time of Coley's observation and from the initial animal experiments with BCG, the next major step in immunotherapy, and adequately illustrates the progress of this major approach. Knowledge gained from the development of BCG immunotherapy is the prototype for the development of the other approaches to active-nonspecific immunotherapy. In 1959, after it had been demonstrated that adjuvants such as BCG could protect against infection, their use in prophylaxis against the development of malignant tumors was investigated. It was observed that the administration of a single dose of BCG could reduce the incidence of both virus- and carcinogen-induced tumors (Old *et al.*, 1976). Subsequently, it was demonstrated that BCG immunotherapy could also cause regression of established tumor, when injected either intralesionally or systematically in experimental animals, and could prolong the remission induced by surgery, chemotherapy, or radiotherapy (Laucius *et al.*, 1974). In the 1960s, clinical trials with BCG began, and in the intervening years active-nonspecific immunotherapy has become the most important clinical approach to immunotherapy. The major observed effect is prolongation of remission duration and survival when immunotherapy is added to conventional therapy.

The mechanism of action of active-nonspecific immunotherapy includes augmentation of cell-mediated and humoral immunity and activation of macrophages (Laucius *et al.*, 1974). It has been used in combination with active-specific or adoptive immunotherapy. Active-nonspecific immunotherapeutic agents are mainly bacterial products or bacterial themselves. However, newer synthetic or semisynthetic materials (Pendergrast *et al.*, 1975) are beginning to be investigated and the active subcomponents of the bacterial adjuvants are being defined and purified (Ribi *et al.*, 1977). It is presumed that within the next few years purified and synthesized active components for systemic administration will be available.

The major problems associated with the use of active-nonspecific microbial immunotherapeutic reagents are as follows. For a given agent, there is significant variability of different preparations in terms of biological and immunological characteristics. This is based on differences in methods of preparation, which lead to variability in the number of viable and dead organisms, the number of intact and fragmented organisms, and the amount of the free or soluble antigens in a given preparation. In addition, there are strain variations between different preparations of the same microorganism which result in different biological characteristics. For example the Tice, Pasteur, and Glaxo strains of BCG vary greatly in their ability to stimulate humoral and cell-mediated immunity, as well as in such characteristics as cord factor content, colony size, virulence

EVAN M. HERSH,
G. M. MAVLIGIT,
J. U. GUTTERMAN,
AND
S. P. RICHMAN

(Mackaness *et al.*, 1973). Genetic drift within a strain of microorganisms may also be a problem.

With most of the microbial products, there may be severe local reactions including inflammation and ulceration at the sites of administration in the skin, and, although this is more of a problem during intravenous administration, even cutaneous administration may be associated with severe systemic toxicity includ-ing fever, chills, malaise, nausea, vomiting, acute respiratory complications, and generalized cutaneous eruption (Sparks, 1976). Occasional cases of anaphylaxis have also been observed to be associated with the administration of microbial agents. Since, as will be outlined below, the intravenous route may be the only way to administer a nonspecific active immunotherapeutic agent to activate host defense mechanisms in visceral sites, such as lung and liver, these complications present a severe limitation to the use of these materials in their current state of purification and characterization.

The active-nonspecific immunotherapuetic agents may also depress as well as augment the immune response. This may be via activation of suppressor cells (Geffard and Orbach-Arbouys, 1976). Decline in adjuvant effect and even diminished general immune responsiveness may be seen after long administra-tion and may be associated with antigen overload. Also, certain of the microbial products augment the "wrong" component of the immune system such as antibody, rather than cell-mediated immunity, and this may result in the phenomenon of immunological enhancement (Ter-Grigov and Irlin, 1968).

There are three major routes of administration of active-nonspecific immunotherapeutic reagents. These include local administration directly into the tumor (Rosenberg and Rapp, 1976). The effector cell is the activated macrophage (Hanna *et al.*, 1972, 1973). In this instance, tumor cells are killed by a bystander effect of delayed hypersensitivity. There is probably tumor-cell–adjuvant interac-tion, and this may result in delivery of modified tumor antigen to the regional lymph nodes in a manner which heightens systemic tumor immunity. The second route of administration is regional (see Table 3); and example is administration of

TABLE 3

Regional Immunotherapy of Human Cancer[a]

Histological type of tumor	Stage	Agent	Route	Result
Lung cancer	I	BCG	Intrapleural postoperative	Increased DFI and survival
Lung cancer	II, III	BCG	Intrapleural postoperative	No effect
Lung cancer	III, IV	BCG	Aerosol	No effect
Gastrointestinal cancer	Advanced	BCG	Intraperitoneal	Increased survival
Bladder cancer	Recurrent superficial	BCG	Intravesicular	Decreased recurrent rate

[a] Abbreviations: BCG, bacillus Calmette Guérin; DFI, disease-free interval.

BCG in the deltoid region of the arm in the case where tumor is present or has been recently extirpated from the axillary lymph nodes. In this instance, as in local immunotherapy, there is activation of lymph nodes proximal to the adjuvant injection site which may also include increased antigen trapping and persistence in those nodes. Finally, there is systemic immunotherapy, which, for microbial adjuvants, involves the intravenous route of administration. Local and regional active-nonspecific immunotherapy have their major effects at the regional lymph node level, and systemic tumor immunity results from this interaction (Bast *et al.*, 1976). In contrast, systemic (intravenous) active-nonspecific immunotherapy probably has as its major effect macrophage activation in liver and lungs, which are the major sites of clearance of intravenously administered particles (Halpern *et al.*, 1959).

It is instructive in attempting to understand the development of the clinical field of immunotherapy to review the history of the clinical trials with BCG during the last decade. The first studies done were those of Mathé and co-workers, who administered Pasteur strain BCG alone, or in combination with allogeneic irradiated leukemia cells, to children, with acute lymphocytic leukemia after the termination of chemotherapy (Mathé *et al.*, 1969a). Significant prolongation of disease-free interval and survival was observed in the patients who received BCG alone as well as in the groups receiving BCG plus tumor cells and tumor cells alone (Mathé *et al.*, 1969a) compared to those not receiving immunotherapy. A few years later, Morton *et al.* (1970) observed that the intralesional injection of Glaxo strain BCG into cutaneous nodules of metastatic malignant melanoma resulted in regression of the nodules in patients who were immunocompetent. Regression of uninjected nodules was observed in approximately 20% of the cases. This observation has subsequently been confirmed by several authors, including Mastrangelo *et al.* (1976) and Pinsky *et al.* (1973).

In contrast, attempts to confirm Mathé's observations were unsuccessful. In retrospect, those attempts which failed were associated with a variety of factors that made them different than Mathé's original series, including less intense cytoreductive therapy (Medical Research Council, 1971), the use of a different strain of less virulent BCG (Glaxo) (Medical Research Council, 1971), a lower dose of BCG (Heyn *et al.*, 1975), the use of the intradermal rather than the scarification route of administration (Heyn *et al.*, 1975), and a less intense frequency of administration (Leventhal *et al.*, 1973). This in part led Bluming *et al.* (1972) to do a small but important comparative study of two strains and routes of BCG administration in malignant melanoma. African patients with primary melanoma of the foot received after surgery either repeated intradermal injections of Glaxo BCG or repeated applications of Pasteur strain BCG at a higher dose by the technique of scarification. Only the latter group showed increased disease-free interval and survival compared to controls.

These observations laid the groundwork for several studies in malignant melanoma. BCG alone or in combination with tumor cells was used in two types of studies: repeated administration after surgical extirpation of regional recurrent disease (Gutterman *et al.*, 1973c) or repeated administration before or between

450

EVAN M. HERSH,
G. M. MAVLIGIT,
J. U. GUTTERMAN,
AND
S. P. RICHMAN

courses of systemic chemotherapy for metastatic diseases (Gutterman *et al.*, 1974*a*). Prlongation of the disease-free interval and survival after surgery and increase in the remission rate, remission duration, and survival induced by chemotherapy were noted as a result of this immunotherapy. Attempts to confirm these observations have not been uniformly successful, and the efficacy of BCG immunotherapy in melanoma is still a question. Subsequently, BCG immunotherapy has been used in breast cancer (Hortobagyi, 1977), colon cancer (Mavligit *et al.*, 1976), lung cancer (Pines, 1976), head and neck cancer (Donaldson, 1973; Richman *et al.*, 1976), and acute myelogenous leukemia (Vogler and Chan, 1974). In these diseases, it has been used both after surgical extirpation of evident disease and between courses of chemotherapy for metastatic disease. In both instances, the fundamental effect is that of prolongation of disease-free interval or prolongation of chemotherapy-induced remission with associated prolongation of survival. Recently, regional immunotherapy after surgery for colon cancer (intraperitoneal), and lung cancer (interpleural) has also been suggested to be effective (Falk *et al.*, 1976; McKneally *et al.*, 1976). Effective routes of administration have included the various approaches to immunization in the skin, including intradermal, subcutaneous, multipuncture, Heaf gun, and scarification techniques, oral administration (Falk *et al.*, 1973), intracavitary administration (Falk *et al.*, 1976; McKneally *et al.*, 1976), and even intravenous administration (Whittaker and Slater, 1977).

As outlined above, the administration of viable BCG organisms is associated with a variety of problems. In addition, systemic BCG disease, while extremely rare, has been observed in patients receiving BCG immunotherapy and is a significant potential danger (Rosenberg *et al.*, 1974). Thus it is desirable to use a purified active subcomponent of the whole organism. For this reason, a series of attempts have been made to use fractionated and purified nonviable subcomponents of BCG. Preparations which have been studied fairly extensively include the methanol extraction residue (MER) and BCG cell-wall skeleton coated onto oil droplets in an oil in water suspension, with or without the trehalose dimycolate lipid adjuvant fraction (P3).

MER, developed by Weiss and co-workers, has been shown to have prophylactic and therapeutic antitumor activity in a variety of animal models (Weiss, 1976). MER is an adjuvant which can induce immune responses to usually nonimmunogenic antigens and which can abort immunological tolerance (Ben-Efraim *et al.*, 1977). It can reverse the immunosuppression associated with age or with the administration of cytotoxic drugs or radiotherapy (Weiss and Yashpe, 1973). It can increase the immune response to weak antigens, and it can cause deviation of the immune response to either cell-mediated or humoral immunity, depending on the circumstances of administration (Ben-Efraim *et al.*, 1973). MER has now been investigated in a variety of human tumors. Its administration boosts immunity in man, as measured by *in vitro* lymphocyte blastogenesis and recall delayed hypersensitivity reactions (Moertel *et al.*, 1975), and MER administration prolongs remission duration and survival when administered between courses of chemotherapy for acute leukemia (Weiss *et al.*, 1975). In several recent studies,

however, MER therapy has not added to chemotherapy in the management of
metastatic colon cancer (Moertel *et al.*, 1977). An intradermal route of injection
using multiple sites of 0.1–0.2 mg per site and a total dose of 0.5–1.0 mg repeated
weekly to monthly has been used. In a comparative study in breast cancer, MER
was equivalent in activity in BCG. This is the first evidence that a nonviable BCG
fraction can have activity equivalent to that of living BCG. Problems with MER
administration include usually mild systemic reactions of fever and malaise lasting
less than 48 hr, but, more important, severe local reactions of sterile abscess
formation and ulceration. This is particularly prominent if the MER is administered subcutaneously instead of intradermally.

Important work on BCG subfractions has been carried out by Ribi and
co-workers in this country, and by Lederer, Chedid, and co-workers in France.
The BCG organism has been progressively fractionated, and active fractions
including BCG cell walls, BCG cell-wall skeleton, and a series of lipid extracts
(P1–P4) have been identified (Ribi *et al.*, 1977). Their activity has been investigated
mainly in the line 10 guinea pig hepatoma model (Zbar and Tanaka, 1971). In this
carcinogen-induced transplantable tumor in the inbred strain 2 guinea pig,
intralesional injection of BCG results in regression of the injected tumor and cure
of microscopic metastases in the regional lymph nodes in approximately 60% of
the animals. The cured animals have systemic tumor immunity as evidenced by
resistance to rechallenge with the same tumor. The principles of immunotherapy
for this tumor have been well established. The tumor must be modest in size, and
tumors over a certain size do not respond (Zbar *et al.*, 1972). Certain strains of
BCG may be superior to others (Hanna *et al.*, 1977). The BCG has to be placed into
the tumor or into the regional drainage of the tumor, and BCG placed on the
contralateral side is not effective (Zbar and Tanaka, 1971). The dose of BCG is
critical, and below a certain dose there is no immunotherapeutic effect (Zbar *et al.*,
1971). The BCG organisms must be living, and dead BCG organisms are not
effective (Zbar *et al.*, 1971). The guinea pig must be immunocompetent, and an
immunosuppressed guinea pig will not respond. Under optimal circumstances,
the animals which are treated with intralesional BCG are specifically immune and
are subsequently resistant to rechallenge with the same tumor.

Ribi and co-workers have investigated several subfractions of BCG in this
system. BCG cell walls and cell-wall skeleton with the P3 fraction are at least as
active as intact viable BCG (Ribi *et al.*, 1975a; Meyer *et al.*, 1975). Of interest, some
of these subfractions can be given as late as 14 days after tumor implantation with
results superior to those achieved with intact BCG, which is not effective if
inoculated later than 7 days after tumor implantation. Recently this group has
investigated the activity of endotoxin from mutant salmonella plus the P3 fraction
of BCG coated onto oil droplets in this system, and has found that this material can
cure up to 90% of the animals (Ribi *et al.*, 1977). Thus, highly purified and
partially characterized chemical components of microorganisms may actually be
more effective than the native microorganisms in these systems. BCG cell-wall
skeleton plus P3 is apparently curative upon intralesional injection into oculosquamous carcinoma (a spontaneous malignant squamous cell carcinoma of the

452

EVAN M. HERSH,
G. M. MAVLIGIT,
J. U. GUTTERMAN.
AND
S. P. RICHMAN

nictitating membrane of Hereford cattle) (H. J. Rapp, personal communication). Administration of BCG cell-wall skeleton has recently been shown to prolong survival of patients with various stages of lung cancer when used in a program of local, regional, and/or systematic administration combined with the usual approaches to conventional therapy (Yamamura *et al.*, 1976). These observations illustrate that the development of more sophisticated approaches to immunotherapy based on earlier and cruder work with viable microbial preparations is a realistic objective.

In this section, we have briefly outlined the development of immunotherapy with BCG as an example of the development of an active immunotherapeutic agent and its derivative subcomponents. There are a variety of active-nonspecific immunotherapeutic agents. They include the following: *Corynebacterium parvum*, adjuvant fractions of *C. parvum* (not yet investigated), the various bacterial adjuvants including mixed bacterial toxins, OK 432, *Pseudomonas* vaccine, pertussus vaccine, etc. The various polysaccharide adjuvants include glucan, lentinan, and pachymanan. The various interferon inducers include poly(IC), pyran copolymer, and tylerone, and various lipids such as lysolecithin. The chemical adjuvant levamisole may be included in this category, although it more properly belongs in a separate class of chemical immunorestorative agents. This category might include lymphokines, interferon, and tumor necrosis factor, since they are nonspecific activators of lymphocytes and macrophages, although they may more properly belong in the catregory of adoptive and cellular product immunotherapeutic reagents. Another active-nonspecific immunotherapeutic agent of great interest included in the category of bacterial immunoadjuvants is *C. parvum*. This material is a whole, killed bacterial vaccine consisting of heat-killed formalinized gram-positive rods. Like most other bacterial adjuvants used in cancer immunotherapy, *C. parvum* first came to attention because of its classical adjuvant action in increasing the humoral immune response and in stimulating the reticuloendothelial system (Halpern *et al.*, 1964). In recent years, it has shown very active immunotherapeutic and immunoprophylactic activities in a variety of animal systems and more recently has been shown to have potent antitumor activity in man, either in combination with conventional cancer treatment or even when administered alone. In immunoprophylaxis, *C. parvum* has been demonstrated to increase resistance to a variety of transplantable, virus- and carcinogen-induced tumors (Smith and Scott, 1972), as well as to increase resistance to various experimental leukemias (Mathé *et al.*, 1973a).

True immunotherapy of established tumors can also be achieved with *C. parvum*. Let us first consider systemic immunotherapy. One of the earliest demonstrations was the study by Woodruff and Boak (1966), who reported that the growth rate of murine mammary cancers was delayed when *C. parvum* was administered travenously or intraperitoneally. Subsequently, various fibrosarcomas were also demonstrated to respond to *C. parvum* (Milas *et al.*, 1974a). An important feature of these systems was the fact that while the tumor was implanted subcutaneously, *C. parvum* was active when given intravenously or intraperitoneally. Subsequently, it was demonstrated that *C. parvum* could also retard the course of L1210 leukemia (Mathé *et al.*, 1969b), and, most important, when administered intravenously or intraperitoneally could retard the growth of and reduce the number of artificially produced metastases of various tumors, particularly fibrosarcoma (Milas *et al.*, 1974*b*). Intravenous *C. parvum* was also demonstrated to delay the growth of both subcutaneous and pulmonary metastases of mouse mastocytoma (Scott, 1974*a*). In most of these studies, the effects were transient and incomplete, although a minority of animals were cured. It should be emphasized that in most of these studies, single inoculations of a high dose of *C. parvum* were administered. As will be discussed subsequently, this may be far from the optimal program of administration of *C. parvum* in these experimental systems.

Local or regional immunotherapy with *C. parvum* is also effective (Scott, 1974*b*). Thus the administration of *C. parvum* to regional lymph nodes draining a tumor site can have immunotherapeutic effect. The intravenous administration of *C. parvum* to animals bearing artificial pulmonary metastases might also be considered regional, since the *C. parvum* is cleared mainly by the lung and liver and localizes and persists for long periods of time in lung and liver macrophages (Stiffel *et al.*, 1970). Intralesional *C. parvum* in the mouse mastocytoma model can result in lasting regression of the inoculated tumor, reduction of metastases from this tumor, and increased systemic resistance to subsequent inoculations with the same tumor cells, indicating an active immunotherapeutic effect (Scott, 1974*b*).

Combinations of *C. parvum* immunotherapy with the conventional modalities of cancer treatment have also been demonstrated to be effective in experimental models. Thus, in a variety of solid tumors, treatment with cyclophosphamide followed by treatment with *C. parvum*, or treatment with BCNU followed by *C. parvum*, can increase the remission duration in the treatment of well-established tumors (Woodruff and Dunbar, 1973). In experimental leukemia, the simultaneous adminstration of procarbazine and *C. parvum* also increases the remission rate and remission duration (Amiel and Berardet, 1970). Effective immunotherapy has been demonstrated when established tumors have been treated by surgery, or radiotherapy, followed by *C. parvum* alone or *C. parvum* plus irradiated tumor cells. In one study, for example, subcutaneous tumor responded to some extent to intravenous *C. parvum* alone or to radiotherapy alone, but cures of essentially all animals were achieved by the combination of the two modalities of therapy (Milas *et al.*, 1975).

Certain principles of immunotherapy have been established through the empirical studies of these animal models. First, timing of the administration of *C. parvum* relative to the timing of the administration of the conventional modalities of treatment is critical. In some chemotherapy models, the optimal effect is achieved when chemotherapy is immediately followed by *C. parvum* (Pearson *et al.*, 1972), whereas in others the optimal effect is achieved when there is a delay of a week or more between the chemotherapy and the *C. parvum* (Currie and Bagshawe, 1970). The dose of *C. parvum* is also critical. This has best been demonstrated in intralesional immunotherapy (Scott, 1974*b*) and in the use of *C. parvum* as an adjuvant mixed with tumor cells (Likhite and Halpern, 1973). Low to moderate doses are usually most effective, whereas very low and very high doses

454

EVAN M. HERSH,

G. M. MAVLIGIT,

J. U. GUTTERMAN,

AND

S. P. RICHMAN

are usually less effective. Also, the immune response to a given antigen can be either augmented or suppressed according to the dose and timing of *C. parvum* administration. Finally, the route of administration is quite important. In both animal and human studies, subcutaneous *C. parvum* has not been demonstrated to have major immunological effects, while intravenous *C. parvum* with the proper dose and timing can markedly augment the immune response (Scott, 1974c). No immunological effect of oral *C. parvum* has been demonstrated (Sadler and Castro, 1975). These observations suggest that, for human immunotherapy, empirical studies with appropriate immunological monitoring regarding route, dose, and timing of *C. parvum* administration will be required to achieve an optimal immunotherapeutic effect.

Studies of the mechanism of *C. parvum* action have been carried out. Properly timed doses of *C. parvum* can augment the humoral immune response and can stimulate reticuloendothelial system function (Stiffel *et al.*, 1970; DelGuercio, 1972). *C. parvum* has a macrophage chemotactic and a macrophage-activating effect (Wilkinson *et al.*, 1973). Macrophages from *C. parvum* treated animals have an increased ability to kill tumor cells *in vitro* compared to nonactivated macrophages, and this effect is thymus independent (Ghaffar *et al.*, 1975). Also relevant to macrophage function in antitumor host defense, the systemic administration of *C. parvum* has been demonstrated to increase monocyte and macrophage production by the bone marrow (Wollmark and Fisher, 1974). That the mechanism of antitumor action *in vivo* is at least in part related to macrophage activation and macrophage killing of target tumor cells is suggested by the observations that antitumor action can still be demonstrated in T-cell-deprived mice (Woodruff *et al.*, 1973) and in mice treated with antilymphocyte serum (Hattori and Mori, 1973), and that the antitumor effect of *C. parvum in vivo* is at least partially radioresistant (Bomford and Olivotto, 1974). Such observations indicate that *C. parvum* may be a particularly useful immunotherapeutic agent in subjects with somewhat depressed cell-mediated immunity. They also indicate that if a particular clinical situation calls for a macrophage-activating approach to immunotherapy, *C. parvum* should be considered seriously.

The effects of *C. parvum* on cell-mediated immunity are quite complex. In animal models, large single doses of *C. parvum* markedly suppress cell-mediated immunity. Cell-mediated immune functions which have been depressed by *C. parvum* include delayed-type hypersensitivity (DTH) and graft vs. host response (GVH) *in vivo* (Scott, 1972) and lymphocyte blastogenic responses to PHA and in the MLC *in vitro* (Scott, 1972). In animals, no effect on pokeweed mitogen responses has been observed. Similar observations, that single intravenous doses of *C. parvum* will transiently suppress the blastogenic responses to mitogens and antigens among human peripheral blood lymphocytes collected during the 5 days following the *C. parvum* dose, have also been made in man (E. M. Hersh, unpublished observations). The suppression of delayed hypersensitivity in animals by *C. parvum* depends on the presence of the spleen and can be abolished by splenectomy (Scott, 1974d). This suggests that the effect may be due to some type of suppressor cell activity or to sequestration of effector cells in the spleen. In

contrast to these observations on immunosuppression, lower weekly doses in
animals (comparable to the dose usually used in man of approximately 5 mg/m^2)
lead to an augmentation of the PHA response and delayed hypersensitivity to
sheep red blood cells (Scott and Warner, 1977). Augmentation of DTH in patients
receiving 5 mg/m^2 or larger doses of *C. parvum* weekly has also been observed in
cancer patients (Hersh and Freireich, 1968). In regard to the mechanism of
antitumor action, a positive effect on T-cell-mediated immunity may be quite
important, at least in some of the treatment approaches. Thus local
immunotherapy with *C. parvum* (Scott, 1974b) and the use of *C. parvum* as an
adjuvant when mixed with tumor cells are entirely T-cell dependent (Likhite and
Halpern, 1973). Furthermore, when *C. parvum* is used in such a way that a
bystander effect is required, an immune response to *C. parvum*, at least of the
DTH type, is obviously required. Furthermore, in certain animal tumor systems,
the effect of *C. parvum* relates directly to the immunogenicity of the tumor (Smith
and Scott, 1972). *C. parvum* is also a potent activator of the complement system, by
both the direct and alternate pathways (McBride *et al.*, 1975), and this may account
for at least part of its mechanism of action. Finally, *C. parvum* may contain
antigens which cross-react with tumor cells, but this has not been explored as
intensively as is the case with BCG.

C. parvum has shown activity in human cancer. This area of immunotherapy
research has been pioneered by Lucien Israel. In his original studies, *C. parvum*
was administered at a dose of 4 mg weekly between courses of chemotherapy to
patients with lung cancer and to patients with various solid tumors (Israel, 1974).
A doubling in the survival time was noted, although there were no long-term
survivors. Recently, similar studies have been done by Dimitrov *et al.* (1977) in
lung cancer and by Pinsky *et al.* (1977) in breast cancer, and similar results have
been observed.

C. parvum has also been administered to man intravenously; phase I studies
have shown that doses of up to 5 mg/m^2 are tolerated by younger patients but not
by patients over the age of 60 or with cardiovascular or pulmonary disease (Reed *et
al.*, 1975). Daily intravenous therapy is also being investigated. Patients can
tolerate at least 4 mg i.v. daily for up to several weeks or a month, but further
phase I therapy research must be done before the effectiveness and limits of this
approach can be defined. Daily intravenous *C. parvuum* has been observed itself
to cause regression of pulmonary and hepatic metastatic disease in man (Israel
et al., 1975; Band *et al.*, 1975). This is the first unequivocal example of tumor
regression induced by immunotherapy, with the exception of local immunotherapy.

Recently, we have carried out an important study of immunotherapy with *C.
parvum* (daily for 2 weeks) preceding chemotherapy for metastatic malignant
melanoma (J. U. Gutterman *et al.*, unpublished observations). The short-term
survival was dramatically improved (55–95% at 3 months compared to
chemotherapy alone), and the response rate was also increased. This suggests that
immunotherapy prior to chemotherapy is a new approach which must be explored further.

456

EVAN M. HERSH,
G. M. MAVLIGIT,
J. U. GUTTERMAN,
AND
S. P. RICHMAN

The mechanism of this effect is not known. It may be immunological. Alternatively, the systemic immunotherapy may alter the pharmacology and efficacy of the subsequently administered drug. It is known, for example, that both BCG and *C. parvum* can suppress hepatic microsomal enzyme function (Farquhar *et al.*, 1976; Mosedale and Smith, 1975). This obviously would have a profound effect on the efficacy and toxicity of drugs which are either activated or degraded by this enzyme system.

7. Other Bacterial Adjuvants

A variety of bacterial products in addition to BCG and *C. parvum* have potential for the immunotherapy of human cancer. Considerable work has been done in this area. For example, bacteria such as *Brucella abortus* (Toujas *et al.*, 1977), *B. pertussis* (Fingu *et al.*, 1970), and OK 432 (which is an inactivated *Streptococcus*) all have adjuvant and/or antitumor activity. *Brucella* increases survival in animals bearing L1210 leukemia (Toujas *et al.*, 1977). The mechanism of action is probably based on lipopolysaccharide, since it is known that *B. abortus* lipoplysaccharide increases reistance to infection (Berger *et al.*, 1969). The mechanism of action has been found to include increased antibody response and very important effects on the macrophage and reticuloendothelial system components of the host defense mechanism. Early after the administration of *B. abortus*, there is a shift of stem cells from the bone marrow to the spleen, with early depletion of macrophage stem cells in the marrow. There is subsequent hypertrophy of the reticuloendothelial system in liver and spleen, and increased macrophage colony formation in the bone marrow (Toujas *et al.*, 1977). Pertussis has been shown to have limited antitumor activity in several murine systems (Purnell *et al.*, 1975). Its major effect is to induce marked lymphocytosis (Phanuphak *et al.*, 1972). This is due to a combination of mobilization of lymphocytes into the circulation and proliferation of cells in the lymphoid compartment. While the PHA response is somewhat increased, the main effect is that of a B-cell mitogen and adjuvant. There is a marked increase in antibody response, particularly during the early phases of that response.

OK 432 is an inactivated but viable bacterial product derived from the *Streptococcus* (Oyama *et al.*, 1975). It stimulates both cell-mediated and humoral immunity, and causes regression of established tumor in several animal models (Yasuhara *et al.*, 1974). In man, it also has antitumor activity and can prolong remission duration in patients with solid tumors (Kimura *et al.*, 1976).

Of the various bacterial products, those of greatest interest are the bacterial endotoxins, or lipopolysaccharides. They have long been known to have adjuvant activity. Properly timed doses of bacterial lipopolysaccharides can markedly augment the antibody response (Chisari *et al.*, 1974); however, it is also true that if given late during the antibody response, LPS can actually be immunosuppressive. The mechanism of action is assumed to be that of a B-cell mitogen, increasing the

proliferation of the responding B lymphocytes. The immunosuppressive properties of endotoxins probably relate to their augmentation of cyclic AMP levels
within lymphoid cells through stimulation of adenylyl cyclase (Chisari *et al.*, 1974).
High levels of cyclic AMP within lymphocytes and other immune cells can depress
the antibody response, depress cell-mediated immunity, and depress cell-
mediated cytotoxicity (Braun *et al.*, 1974).

More recently, it has been demonstrated that properly timed doses of endotoxin
can actually stimulate T-cell activity. Using the delayed hypersensitivity model,
augmentation of delayed hypersensitivity and T-cell activity was shown when
endotoxin was given 1–3 days after immunization (LaGrange and Mackaness,
1977). The endotoxin administration had to be regional to the draining lymph
nodes, and was dose dependent. LPS could also depress DTH if given later during
the response, and it was found that this depression was related to an effect on
macrophages (LaGrange and Mackaness, 1977). The stimulatory effect on DTH is
not understood, but endotoxin acts as a mitogenic stimulus or a modifier of the
antibody component of the immune response, allowing better expression of DTH
(Andersson *et al.*, 1977). It may also act through activation or peripheralization of
monocytes and macrophages. The timing and dose effects observed in animals
indicate that the use of LPS in immunotherapy trials must be based on extensive
empirical work in animal systems.

There is already evidence that endotoxin alone can have antitumor activity *in
vivo*. The hemorrhagic necrosis of certain tumors in experimental systems occurs
after the administration of endotoxin, but the endotoxin itself is not cytotoxic to
tumor cells (Carswell *et al.* 1975). However, endotoxin can bind to the tumor-cell
surface, and thereby might sensitize it to other components of host defense.
Recently, two experiments have been carried out which indicate that the use of
endotoxins either directly or indirectly in cancer immunotherapy has great
potential. First, because of the tumor-related effects described above, Ribi and
co-workers have investigated the use of endotoxin in the guinea pig hepatoma
model. They attached endotoxin from *Salmonella* and the P3 fraction of BCG to
oil droplets and used them for intralesional therapy. Regression rates of up to
90% with subsequent tumor resistance were observed (Ribi *et al.*, 1975*b*). There
was no relationship to the toxic activity of endotoxin, and in fact endotoxin from
the relatively nontoxic RE mutant, which is deficient in carbohydrate and rich in
lipid, was most effective. The mechanism of this augmented action is not understood, but perhaps relates to more vigorous granuloma formation and macrophage activation.

In the other major work in this area, Carswell *et al.* (1975) have shown that the
hemorrhagic necrosis induced by endotoxin is due to a circulating substance
known as "tumor necrosis factor." They found that animals which are presen-
sitized with BCG or *C. parvum* and which receive small doses of endotoxin,
develop a factor in their serum that, when injected into tumor-bearing mice with
METH-A tumor, develops rapid necrosis of the tumor. Also, the serum of these
mice can also kill or suppress the growth of tumor cells *in vitro*. The necrosis factor
is a glycoprotein of approximately 150,000 molecular weight which migrates with

458

EVAN M. HERSH,
G. M. MAVLIGIT,
J. U. GUTTERMAN,
AND
S. P. RICHMAN

the α-globulins and is probably produced by the action of endotoxin on activated macrophages (Carswell et al., 1975). The combined action of bacterial adjuvants and endotoxins might prove very useful in immunotherapy. It is also conceivable that tumor necrosis factor could be produced and purified itself and would have activity in cancer therapy. It will be very interesting to determine whether the nontoxic endotoxins also have the property of inducing the generation of tumor necrosis factor. It will also be interesting to determine whether tumor necrosis factor is the basis of the mechanism by which macrophages normally kill tumor cells. It is possible that through the use of materials such as tumor necrosis factor and other products of host defense cells with antitumor activity, we will see the development of a new approach to immunotherapy. This would be the use of specific effector molecules produced by activated host defense cells in the immunotherapy of human cancer.

In addition to bacteria and bacterial products, viruses have been used in immunotherapy. It has been known for many years that viruses can directly or indirectly inhibit tumor growth. Regression of cutaneous and visceral metastases of malignant melanoma has been reported after immunization with or intralesional injection of metastatic nodules (Hunter-Craig et al., 1970). In general, regression was limited to the injected nodules. Recently, a study was performed in which primary melanomas were injected with vaccinia virus and subsequently excised ised (Everall et al., 1974). The disease-free interval and survival were modestly but significantly prolonged in the vaccinia-inoculated group. The mechanism of action is not known. There is probably a component of bystander effect whereby the killing of tumor cells occurs secondary to a DTH response to the virus. There may also be a component of viral oncolysis with subsequent induction of more vigorous tumor immunity by combination of viral with tumor antigen. Thus three mechanisms may be involved: bystander killing related to delayed hypersensitivity to the virus, adjuvant effect of virus–tumor antigen complex, and killing of tumor cells by viral oncolysis (Lindenmann, 1974). This approach warrants further investigation in the future.

Fungi and fungal extracts may also play an important role in active-nonspecific immunotherapy. Early studies using zymosan indicated that it was a potent adjuvant in terms of humoral immunity and could activate the reticuloendothelial system (Martin et al., 1964). More recently, glucan (DiLuzio et al., 1977), lentinan (Haba et al., 1976), and pachymaran (Hamuro et al., 1971), all of which are high molecular weight polysaccharide extracts of fungi, have shown antitumor activity in both immunoprophylaxis and immunotherapy against a variety of animal tumor models, such as sarcoma-180, the Shay chloroleukemia, and B16 melanoma. Each of these materials is a potent stimulator of the humoral immune response, localizes in macrophages, and is a macrophage-activating substance. The mechanism of action of these materials is probably related to a competent T-cell compartment since both neonatal thymectomy and antilymphocyte serum abolished the antitumor activity (Maeda and Chihara, 1973). Glucan has been used in intralesional therapy of human tumors. In a preliminary report on studies in nine patients, intralesional injection of melanoma, lung carcinoma, or breast carcinoma nodules resulted in complete or partial regression (Mansell *et al.*, 1975). Histological study revealed macrophage infiltration with the immunotherapeutic reagent phagocytized by macrophages. Observations on glucan have not yet been confirmed by other investigators. However, the use of a highly purified polysaccharide which is readily metabolized and is potent macrophage activator has great appeal. If such a material could be introduced intravenously, it might activate macrophages extensively both within the reticuloendothelial system and within the tumor itself. This might result in clearance of circulating immunosuppressive factors, such as tumor antigen or antigen–antibody complexes, and also killing of tumor cells by adjacent macrophages.

Another area of considerable interest in active-nonspecific immunotherapy is the use of a variety of synthetic chemicals of different structures which have the common property of being interferon inducers. Since there is some evidence that interferon may have direct antitumor activity (Grossberg, 1972a), or may have adjuvant activity in antitumor systems (Grossberg, 1972a), these compounds are of considerable interest. They include tylerone (Gibson *et al.*, 1977), pyran copolymer (Braun *et al.*, 1970), and synthetic polynucleotides such as poly(AU) and poly(IC) (Drake *et al.*, 1974). A number of these materials have immuno-prophylactic activity and protect animals from subsequent viral and chemical carcinogenesis and from the subsequent implantation of transplantable tumors (Webb *et al.*, 1972). In addition, in experimental leukemias and solid tumors, these materials can prolong remissions induced by chemotherapy (Pearson *et al.*, 1974). The immmunological characteristics of these materials in addition to induction of interferon are augmentation of antibody production (Cone *et al.*, 1971) and activation of macrophages (Alexander and Evans, 1971). However, they have profound immunosuppressive effects on the T-cell system. Thus they induce lymphopenia in normal but not athymic mice, they depress a variety of cell-mediated immune functions, including graft vs. host disease and graft rejection, and when given with appropriate timing after the administration of tumor can accelerate rather than retard tumor growth (Drake *et al.*, 1975). While these materials are of considerable interest, extensive studies must be done in animal models of dose-timing relationships before these materials will be suitable for investigation for immunotherapy in man.

8. Active-Specific Immunotherapy

"Active-specific immunotherapy" may be defined as the administration of tumor cells, modified tumor cells, or tumor-cell surface antigen preparations with the objective of boosting various components of specific tumor immunity and thereby either inducing tumor regression or prolonging tumor remission previously induced by conventional therapy (Table 4). The three classes of tumor-cell surface antigens containing materials which have been used in active-specific immunotherapy include unmodified intact tumor cells, tumor cells modified by

EVAN M. HERSH,
G. M. MAVLIGIT,
J. U. GUTTERMAN,
AND
S. P. RICHMAN

TABLE 4

Some Preparations Used in Active-Specific Immunotherapy[a]

Autochthonous tumor cells
Allogeneic tumor cells
Processing of tumor cells for immunotherapy
   No modification
   Irradiation (X-ray, UV, etc.)
   Coupling to foreign protein with BDB
   Coupled to concanavalin A
   Fixation with iodoacetate, formalin, etc.
Cultured tumor cells used for immunotherapy
   Melanoma cell lines
   Sarcoma cell lines
   Long-term lymphoblastoid lines
     from leukemia patients
   Raji cells
Cell fractions used for immunotherapy
   Crude homogenates
   Viral oncolysates
   KCl extracts of membranes
   Low-frequency sonicates of membranes
   DEAE- and PAGE-purified fractions
Adjuvants used with active specific preparations
   BCG
   BCG-CWS on oil
   Complete Freund's adjuvant

[a] Abbreviations: BDB, bisdiazobenzidine; DEAE, diethyl-aminoethyl; PAGE, polyacrylamide gel electrophoresis.

various physical, chemical or other treatments, and various antigen extracts of the tumor-cell surface.

Methods for tumor-cell modification have been quite varied. They include a variety of physical methods such as simple mechanical disruption, disruption by freezing and thawing, heat treatment, and irradiation by X-rays or ultraviolet light. Chemical modification of the cell surface has been carried out by incubation of the tumor cells with chemicals which attach to SH groups, hydroxyl groups, or amino groups (Prager *et al.*, 1974). Some of these agents include iodoacetate, iodoacetamide, and *N*-ethylmaleimide. The cell surface can also be modified by the chemical attachment of foreign proteins or other substances. One common method is to couple albumin or γ-globulin to the cell surface by the bisdiazotized benzidine (BDB) method. Incubation of tumor cells with concanavalin A also results in the attachment of this material to the tumor cell and therefore the modification of its surface. The tumor-cell surface can also be modified by incubation with neuraminidase (Simmons *et al.*, 1976). This removes terminal sialic acid residues from the glycolipid and glycoproteins of the cell surface, presumably exposing deeper antigenic structures. Other enzymes such as trypsin and hyaluronidase may also be used to treat the tumor-cell surface for the same objective. Finally, the cell surface may be modified by infecting cells with viruses which either bud from the surface and leave the cell intact or cause lysis of the cell, the so-called viral oncolysis method (Lindenmann, 1974).

All of these methods of tumor-cell surface modification are designed to increase the immunogenicity of the tumor cell. Presumably, modification of the surface by attachment of foreign substances or by the chemical modification of certain surface structures will also increase the recognition of the tumor cells as foreign by the host and therefore increase the immune response to the relevant tumor-cell surface antigens as well as to the modifying agent. Enzyme treatment increases immunogenicity, presumably by removing blocking sialic acid and therefore allowing the host immune mechanism to "see" concealed or cryptic relevant tumor antigens which normally would be concealed and would not induce a vigorous immune response. However, the immune reactants generated must be able to "see" these groups in order that there be a functional effector reaction. For each of these approaches to tumor-cell surface modification, there is some evidence that either in immunoprophylaxis or in immunotherapy the modified cells are more effective than analogous unmodified tumor cells.

There are two major methods of tumor-antigen extraction and purification. The first is the hypertonic KCl extraction method (Reisfeld *et al.*, 1971). Cells are incubated in 3 M KCl (other hypertonic chaotropic agents may also be used). The cells and debris are removed by centrifugation, excess protein is removed by ammonium sulfate precipitation, and the supernatant containing presumed tumor antigens may then be concentrated and used in immunotherapy experiments. The other method, which has received wider application in immunotherapy, is the method originally pioneered by Hollinshead and Herberman (Hollinshead, 1975). Cell membranes are prepared by hypotonic lysis of tumor cells; these are then partially purified and concentrated, and are then subjected to low-frequency sonication, which releases tumor antigens. These are then separated from other components (including blocking factors) by polyacrylamide gel electrophoresis. A suitable substitute for the latter is DEAE column chromatography.

Now, there are many examples of immunoprophylaxis using various tumor preparations including intact tumor cells, modified tumor cells, attenuated tumor cells, and tumor antigens. Immunization with these alone or mixed with various adjuvants usually results in increased resistance to subsequent tumor transplantation, particularly in the circumstance of a highly antigenic tumor. However, a particular method which has great activity in immunoprophylaxis may be useless in the immunotherapy setting. Therefore, positive immunoprophylactic effects do not predict for immunotherapeutic effectiveness but simply provide guidance for the development of experimental approaches to be tested in the immunotherapy setting. There have been, however, a limited number of successful approaches or at least suggestive approaches to effective immunotherapy using active specific immunization in animal models. One of the earliest attempts was the study of Mathé *et al.*, (1969*b*), who, a few days after the inoculation of a low dose of L1210 leukemia cells, immunized animals with irradiated tumor cells alone or irradiated tumor cells plus BCG. Increased survival was noted. In the

EVAN M. HERSH,
G. M. MAVLIGIT,
J. U. GUTTERMAN,
AND
S. P. RICHMAN

very important guinea pig hepatoma model, immunization with tumor cells plus BCG on the side contralateral to the primary tumor inoculum will retard tumor growth (Kronman *et al.*, 1970). If the tumor is removed by surgery, tumor-cell plus BCG vaccination can delay or prevent the development of metastatic disease in the regional lymph nodes (Bartlett and Zbar, 1972).

Some of the most encouraging work in animal models relates to the use of neuraminidase-modified tumor cells. This approach has been pioneered by Simmons *et al.*, 1971), who found that mice with established chemically induced fibrosarcomas showed retardation of tumor growth when immunized with neuraminidase-treated tumor cells alone. If neuraminidase-treated cells were combined with BCG, a fraction of the animals showed not only tumor regression but also complete remission with no regrowth of the tumor (Simmons and Rios, 1971). Apparently, neuraminidase injection alone into the tumor itself can result in the same phenomenon. Presumably, the modified tumor cells which develop after neuraminidase treatment can immunize the regional lymph nodes, with resulting augmented tumor immunity and effective antitumor host defense. BCG injection into tumor nodules, which is known to be associated with tumor regression and augmented tumor immunity, conceivably might work by a related method. The use of neuraminidase-treated tumor cells should be approached with caution, however, because in the B16 melanoma model such treatment can also result in tumor enhancement (Froese *et al.*, 1974). Immunotherapy with neuraminidase-treated tumor cells is apparently active in the chemo-immunotherapy setting. Thus both Kollmorgen *et al.* (1974) and Bekesi *et al.* (1976) have treated L1210 leukemia in the mouse with bis-chloroethyl-nitrosourea (BCNU) followed by a single inoculation of neuraminidase-treated tumor cells alone or neuraminidase-treated tumor cells plus BCG. Both of these approaches result in prolongation of the disease-free interval and apparent fractional cure of the treated animals. This approach is also active in AKR leukemia. Thus treatment with BCNU followed by neuraminidase-treated tumor cells produces 180% increase in survival of these animals (Bekesi and Holland, 1974).

Other forms of tumor cell inoculation have also been investigated. Concanavalin A treated tumor cells are as effective as neuraminidase-treated tumor cells in the mouse fibrosarcoma model (Simmons and Rios, 1975). Benjamini *et al.* (1976) have carried out an important experiment in canine lymphoma, in which the animals are treated with chemotherapy followed by repeated immunizations with a 3 M KCl extract of autologous tumor treated by acetylation and mixed with Freund's adjuvant. A prolongation of the remission duration and survival duration after chemotherapy was noted in the immunochemotherapy group, compared to a group of animals receiving chemotherapy alone. Thus, in summary, a variety of approaches to active specific immunotherapy have been encouraging enough in animal models to attempt to translate this experience to experiments in man.

Human active-specific immunization experiments in man have been carried out for some time. Many of the early experiments are difficult to interpret. One of the early intriguing experiments was carried out by Graham and Graham (1962). They made a crude tumor homogenate from autologous tumor in patients with various locally advanced gynecological malignancies. Patients were immunized repeatedly with this homogenate mixed with Freund's adjuvant after surgery. Compared to a group of controls (not well defined for comparability, etc., which makes interpretation of the data difficult), they described significant prolongation of survival. Patients showing maximum effectiveness were those who mounted vigorous inflammatory responses with ulceration at the site of immunization.

There have been a large series of experiments carried out indicating that active-specific immunization can indeed boost specific tumor immunity as measured in man. In malignant melanoma, Ikonopisov et al. (1970) immunized patients with irradiated melanoma cells. These were patients with advanced metastatic disease. None had detectable antibody prior to immunization. However, after immunization, there was a transient 2-week rise in detectable antibody measured by cytotoxicity, immunofluorescence, and inhibition of nucleic acid synthesis within the tumor cells. Currie et al. (1971) from the same group carried these experiments further and demonstrated that autoimmunization could result in boosting of lymphocyte cytotoxicity to target tumor cells. Gercovich et al. (1975) found that immunization with autologous or allogeneic cultured tumor cells led to an increased in vitro blastogenic response against autologous tumor. (Shibata et al. (1976) found that immunization with allogeneic tumor cells increased antibody and increased cytotoxic lymphocyte in immunized melanoma patients. In leukemia, several workers have demonstrated that immunization with autologous leukemia cells can increase the blastogenic response of remission lymphocytes to autologous leukemia cells that had been stored in liquid nitrogen (Gutterman et al., 1973d). Since the level of blastogenic response correlates with prognosis in this disease, these results seem relevant. However, specificity was limited and blastogenic response to mitogens also increased. Carrying these observations further, K. Ezaki et al. (unpublished) studied immunization with pooled allogeneic leukemia cells or pooled allogeneic leukemia antigens prepared by the methods of Hollinshead. A specific increased blastogenic response to autologous leukemia cells was noted and was most striking after the leukemia antigen immunization. There was, however, no increase in delayed hypersensitivity to allogeneic leukemia antigen in the immunized patients beyond that observed to recall antigens. Bekesi and Holland (1974) have immunized patients with neuraminidase-treated tumor cells and found a general increased immunity to leukemia.

In sarcoma, Morton et al. (1971b) showed that immunization with a tumor-cell vaccine mixed with BCG increased antibody to an allogeneic cultured cell line detected by immunofluorescence. Green et al. (1976) immunized patients with an osteogenic sarcoma cell line infected with influenza virus and found increased cytotoxic antibody and increased lymphocyte-dependent, antibody-dependent, cell-mediated cytotoxicity. In lung cancer, Takita et al. (1976) have immunized patients in their immunotherapy trial with autologous tumor cells treated with concanavalin A and neuraminidase. Increased blastogenic responses and increased leukocyte migration inhibition responses to tumor extracts were

464

EVAN M. HERSH,
G. M. MAVLIGIT,
J. U. GUTTERMAN,
AND
S. P. RICHMAN

observed in these immunized patients, in spite of the fact that they had advanced intrathoracic disease. Finally, Rosato *et al.* (1976) showed increased cell-mediated cytotoxicity to autologous tumor in patients with various solid tumors immunized with concanavalin A bound to autologous tumor cells.

Clinical trials of immunotherapy with active-specific immunization have been carried out. However, almost all have been relatively poorly controlled, and almost all are difficult to interpret because of very small numbers of patients. Furthermore, they usually involve relatively heterogeneous groups so that an adequate control becomes even more important.

Several groups have used immunotherapy with coupled tumor cells. Czajkowski *et al.* (1967) have coupled protein to autologous tumor cells by the BDB method. Two of 14 patients with advanced metastatic disease apparently entered remission and remained free of disease. This technique was applied by Cunningham *et al.* (1969) to a heterogeneous group of patients with advanced solid tumors. One out of 36 patients had an objective regression; there were no cures or long-term survivors. Takita *et al.* (1976) have used concanavalin A-treated autologous tumor cells or concanavalin A- and neuraminidase-treated cells in the immunotherapy of patients with locally advanced lung cancer who could not be subjected to complete surgical extirpation of disease. In this study, a highly significant prolongation of survival was noted compared to historical controls, with approximately 40% compared to 0% of patients alive at 1 year. Irradiated tumor cells, or tumor extracts either alone or in combination with BCG, have been used by a number of investigators. One study was reported by Marcove *et al.* (1971) in osteogenic sarcoma. After surgical extirpation of disease, patients were repeatedly immunized with an ultraviolet-irradiated extract of their tumor. Immunizations were repeated until the vaccine became exhausted. There was a highly significant prolongation of disease-free interval and survival among the patients receiving this vaccine compared to historical controls at the same institution. This study has recently been reanalyzed, and the results remain the same after longer follow-up.

In malignant melanoma, several investigators have studied active-specific immunization with irradiated tumor cells mixed with BCG. Currie and McElwain (1975) immunized patients with metastatic disease before and between courses of chemotherapy for metastatic melanoma using irradiated tumor cells mixed with a low dose of BCG. An increased remission rate of approximately 50% was observed compared to the general experience with dimethyl-triazeno-imidazole-carboxamide (DTIC) chemotherapy alone of approximately a 20% response rate. Mastrangelo *et al.* (1975) used irradiated tumor cells plus BCG alone to treat a small number of patients with metastatic melanoma. Several patients showed regression of tumor nodules without any other treatment. However, when Mastrangelo and colleagues extended this observation to a randomized study in which patients with advanced disease were treated with vincristine plus methyl chloroethyl-cyclohexyl-nitrosourea (CCNU) with or without irradiated tumor-cell vaccine mixed with BCG, no effect could be observed. Morton (1977) has been carrying out a study comparing no treatment after surgery to BCG alone or BCG plus allogenic cultured irradiated melanoma cells. There is a prolongation of remission duration and survival in the immunotherapy groups which is not statistically significant, with some advantage to the group receiving active-specific plus active-nonspecific immunotherapy compared to active-nonspecific immunotherapy alone.

A relatively large number of studies with irradiated cells have been carried out in leukemia. In their initial study, Mathé *et al.* (1969*a*) brought pediatric patients with acute lymphatic leukemia (ALL) into complete remission with chemotherapy. Chemotherapy was then stopped on the patients, who were randomized to receive either nothing, BCG, allogeneic irradiated pooled tumor-cell vaccine, or the combination. All forms of immunotherapy prolonged disease-free interval and survival compared to the controls. Subsequent to this, Mathé *et al.* (1973*b*) used the tumor-cell plus BCG vaccine in a variety of studies in which the remission duration and the survival duration have been very long (>5 years). In contrast to other groups, the children do not die of infection or other complications in remission as may be associated with continuing chemotherapy. Powles *et al.* (1973), in a series of studies in acute myelogenous leukemia (AML), have shown that immunization between courses of remission maintenance chemotherapy with BCG plus allogeneic pooled irradiated or even nonirradiated AML cells results in prolongation of survival. This result has recently been confirmed by Reizenstein *et al.* (1977), using a similar experimental design. However, Peto (1977) and Kay (1977), working on AML and ALL, respectively, have not been able to identify an immunotherapeutic benefit using this approach. Also, it must be stated that other workers, using BCG alone, have demonstrated as significant an immunotherapeutic benefit in prolongation of survival as has been observed when BCG was used combined with tumor cells. Therefore, it is questionable that the tumor-cell immunization has added to BCG in the work of Powles, Reizenstein, and their colleagues.

Immunotherapy with tumor cells mixed with BCG vaccine has also been carried out in sarcoma. Townsend *et al.* (1976) repeatedly immunized patients after surgery with allogeneic cultured irradiated tumor cells mixed with BCG. Prolongation of disease-free interval and survival was observed in soft tissue sarcoma but not in osteogenic sarcoma.

Other types of modified tumor cells have been used. Holland and Bekesi (1976) have used repeated immunizations with large doses (up to 10^{10}) of neuraminidase-treated tumor cells between courses of chemotherapy in AML. Prolongation of disease-free interval and survival was observed. Rosato *et al.* (1976) and Cunningham *et al.* (1976) are carrying out similar studies in patients with solid tumors. Boosting of immunity has been observed, but it is too early to determine whether or not there is an immunotherapeutic benefit. Green *et al.* (1976) have carried out a study with repeated immunization of patients with osteogenic sarcoma using an influenza virus-infected sarcoma cell line. A possible improvement in survival of that group of patients having a small tumor burden was observed. The study is too recent and has too few patients for full analysis. Finally, Sauter *et al.* (1977) have carried out a study with a viral oncolysate of AML cells in

EVAN M. HERSH,
G. M. MAVLIGIT,
J. U. GUTTERMAN,
AND
S. P. RICHMAN

patients receiving maintenance chemotherapy for AML. No therapeutic benefit was observed compared to concurrently randomized controls. Purified tumor antigen mixed with complete Freund's adjuvant has been employed by T. H. M. Stewart *et al.* (1976), either alone or in combination with chemotherapy in stage I lung cancer. Some modest prolongation of disease-free interval and a significant prolongation of survival were noted.

In summary, a variety of approaches have been used in animal models to develop the concepts of active-specific immunization for immunotherapy. Unmodified tumor cells, tumor cells modified by a variety of chemical, physical, and biological procedures, and tumor antigens all have immunoprophylactic benefit, as well as some evidence of immunotherapeutic benefit. There are a number of experiments carried out in man in which active-specific immunization has been used. In most, the numbers of patients are too few for a clear-cut determination of therapeutic benefit. In others, immunization with tumor cells has been combined with immunization with BCG or other mycobacterial adjuvants and the relative efficacy of the two modalities in combination has not been sorted out. Therefore, we conclude that active-specific immunization is a modality of immunotherapy worthy of exploration, but, at the moment, the evidence for immunotherapeutic benefit is scanty.

9. Adoptive Immunotherapy with Cells

"Adoptive immunotherapy" can be defined as the transfer from an immune or immunocompetent subject to a nonimmune, hypoimmune, or immunodeficient subject of lymphoid cells, other host defense cells, or their products which would prevent the growth or cause regression of tumor in the recipient. The fundamental basis for the concept of adoptive immunotherapy of cancer is the well-defined transfer of specific immunity, either humoral, cell mediated, or both, from immune to nonimmune syngeneic animals with lymphoid cells from spleen, lymph nodes, peripheral blood, etc. (Moller and Moller, 1975). Adoptive transfer of immunity is at the root of our understanding of the cellular basis of the immune response.

Adoptive immunotherapy of cancer has been studied extensively in animal models. Several different types of studies have been conducted. These include immunoprophylaxis studies in which the immune cells are administered prior to or simultaneous with tumor-cell inoculation, immunotherapy studies in which the tumor is allowed to become established for several days or longer prior to the administration of immune cells, and, finally, studies using or comparing syngeneic, allogeneic, or even xenogeneic immune cells. In the case of allogeneic and xenogeneic cells, the transferred cells are probably eliminated by a host vs. graft reaction, and therefore, either the immunoprophylactic or immunotherapeutic effect is mediated by these cells before they are eliminated, or there is transfer of information or other factors to host cells, which then mediate the effect. This will be dealt with in more detail later in the sections on immune RNA and on transfer factor.

Some of the examples of adoptive immunotherapy experiments in animal models will now be given. Cater and Waldmann (1967) studied protection against the PB8 ascites tumor in mice using lymphocytes from allogeneic animals immunized with tumor cells in complete Freund's adjuvant. These lymphocytes were effective when given before or up to 24 hr after tumor-cell challenge. The growth of 5×10^4 tumor cells could be controlled by 1×10^6 lymphocytes, but not by 2×10^5 lymphocytes. Nonimmune lymphocytes were not effective, nor was serum from immune animals or cells from animals given Freund's adjuvant without tumor cells. Of great interest, active immunization was not so effective as the adoptive transfer system. Wepsic *et al.* (1970) investigated immunoprophylaxis in the guinea pig hepatoma system using the spontaneously regressing line 1 tumor and the progressively growing line 7 tumor. Syngeneic donors were immunized by repeated injection of tumor cells, and peritoneal exudate cells were used for adoptive transfer. Adoptive transfer completely abrogated the subsequent growth of both cell lines. Effective tumor immunity correlated directly with the degree of transfer of delayed hypersensitivity to tumor cells. Transfer of 1.2×10^8 cells was effective, while 1.5×10^6 cells were ineffective. Fractionation of the peritoneal exudate cells showed that the effector cells were lymphocytes and not the macrophages. Recipient animals challenged with tumor as late as 35 days after adoptive transfer still showed delayed hypersensitivity and partial resistance to tumor-cell challenge. Jurin and Suit (1973) studied adoptive immunoprophylaxis in mice using the LP59 tumor derived from C3H fibroblasts. Both syngeneic and allogeneic lymphocytes were protective and increased the minimal tumor cell dose from 10^4 to 10^6 cells. Nonimmune syngeneic or allogeneic cells were not effective. An important immunoprophylactic experiment was carried out by Irvin and Eustace (1970), who studied the effect of immune syngeneic lymphocytes on the growth of an allogeneic implant of EL4 tumor cells in mice. In the allogeneic setting, this tumor grows and then regresses. Lymph node cells from animals immunized 5 days earlier accelerated tumor rejection, while lymph node cells from animals immunized 14 days earlier caused enhanced tumor growth. This indicates that the nature of the transferred cell population may be critical, and that adoptive transfer may be associated with tumor enhancement.

While these immunoprophylactic experiments are of some interest, they add little information to that gained by active-specific immunization experiments, except that they help in characterizing the effective immune cell population. Of greater relevance are those experiments in which true immunotherapy has been applied, i.e., in which adoptive transfer of immune cells is administered after the experimental tumor has been established in the potential recipient animal. The classical experiments in this area have been conducted by Peter Alexander and his co-workers using a chemically induced fibrosarcoma in the rat (Alexander and Delorme, 1971). The tumor is induced by the implantation of a benzpyrene pellet, and treatment is administered when the tumor reaches 1 cm in diameter. Thoracic duct lymphocytes from recently immunized allogeneic or xenogeneic

468

EVAN M. HERSH,
G. M. MAVLIGIT,
J. U. GUTTERMAN,
AND
S. P. RICHMAN

(sheep) animals are effective in a dose of 5×10^8 cells. Approximately half the animals show some inhibition of tumor growth, and approximately 10% show permanent complete regression of tumor. Irradiated cells are as effective as nonirradiated cells, suggesting that nonproliferating lymphoblasts are the mediators of the effect. These studies have been carried out only in immunocompetent animals, and there is likely to be a major contribution of host factors to the effect. Another important model has been described by Glynn et al. (1969), and more recently by Fefer (1971a). Mice are inoculated with a transplantable Moloney lymphoma and are then allowed to go for 3–6 days without treatment, at which time there are both a local tumor and disseminated disease. Animals are then treated with sublethal doses of cyclophosphamide, which prolongs survival from approximately 10–25 days but produces no long-term survivors. Both allogeneic histocompatible and syngeneic immune cells, if administered following chemotherapy, markedly prolong survival and lead to a fractional cure rate. Nonimmune cells are not effective. Irradiation completely abolishes the effect. Immune cells alone without cyclophosphamide also have no effect. This suggests that adoptive immunotherapy will be most effective when preceded by effective cytoreduction. Borberg et al. (1972) studied adoptive immunotherapy of an established chemically induced fibrosarcoma in mice, the so-called METH-A ascites tumor. Intravenous injection of lymph node cells from immunized Balb/C, C57BL/6×AF1 mice, or even from immunized sheep induced regression or inhibition of established grafts of this tumor in syngeneic animals. This confirms the observations on allogeneic and xenogeneic adoptive immunotherapy made by Fefer and Alexander. The effective dose of lymph node cells was $1–3 \times 10^9$, given in divided doses daily for 7 days between days 7 and 14 after tumor implantation. Only syngeneic cells produced complete regression, while allogeneic and xenogeneic cells slowed tumor growth only up to four fold.

A variant of adoptive immunotherapy which has been investigated in animal systems is the so-called graft vs. leukemia. In experimental leukemias in mice, spleens of animals inoculated with leukemia could not transfer leukemia to secondary recipients if removed 10 days after irradiation and injection of allogeneic spleen cells (Branic, 1970). The disappearance of the leukemia was thought to be on the basis of graft vs. host disease killing leukemic cells. Bortin et al. (1973) studied graft vs. leukemia in a transplanted AKR system in the mouse. Animals were treated with whole-body irradiation to eliminate host immunological participation against leukemia, and to prevent rejection of the transplanted immunocompetent allogeneic cells. Twenty-four hours later, 2×10^7 bone marrow cells and 10^7 lymph node cells were administered. Cells were then transferred to secondary recipients, and 40–90% cures were observed, depending on the leukemia blast cell inoculation to the primary AKR animals. There is one clinical experiment, to be described below, which suggests that the transfer of allogeneic leukocytes into immunosuppressed leukemia patients can also have a therapeutic benefit, and this could be based on the graft vs. leukemia principle.

A number of interesting although incompletely controlled and hard to interpret experiments involving adoptive immunotherapy with intact immune or competent cells have been done in man. The first study was reported by Woodruff and Nolan (1963), who administered spleen cells from normal allogeneic donors to recipients with solid tumors and observed some regressions of tumor. However, interpretation is difficult because of concomitant therapy with other agents. A series of studies were reported by Nadler and Moore (1969) using the cross-grafting cross-transfusion approach. Pairs of patients were selected with matching histological type of tumor and were cross-grafted with each other's tumor. After tumor rejection, they were given repeated transfusions of their partner's peripheral blood leukocytes. At least 10^{10} lymphocytes were administered. Usually no other therapy was given, and no major side effects were noted. Patients generally had advanced metastatic disease. Most had malignant melanoma, but patients with breast cancer, colon cancer, sarcoma, and other tumors were also treated. A total of 23 of 118 patients studied were reported to have an objective response, and three patients were reported to have complete remission. This observation was confirmed by Krementz and Samuels (1967), who observed benefit in two of 20 melanoma patients, and by Curtis *et al.* (1969), who noted complete remission in one of 12 melanoma patients so treated. It has also been confirmed by Brandes *et al.* (1971) in one of two patients. Cross-immunized patients have also been studied by Humphrey *et al.* (1971), with similar results. They observed seven objective regressions in 38 treated patients. However, Enneking and co-workers, in a similar study in postsurgical patients with osteogenic sarcoma, gave $2-11 \times 10^9$ lymphocytes from immunized cancer-bearing donors and failed to observe an effect in 32 patients compared to historical controls. This approach has not been followed aggressively because it is extremely tedious and time consuming, patients with accessible transplantable tumor are not usually available, and there are a variety of theoretical objections including the problem of immunization against histocompatibility antigens. However, it must be concluded that the effect is real.

The original observation of Woodruff regarding normal nonimmune cells has also been followed up to some extent. Symes and Riddell (1968) studied nine patients with malignant melanoma who received normal allogeneic spleen cells, at a dose of $2-4 \times 10^9$. One objective response was noted. Schwarzenberg *et al.* (1966) administered allogeneic leukocytes from patients with chronic myelogenous leukemia (CML) at a dose of $6-120 \times 10^{10}$ cells. These collections should have contained normal numbers of normal lymphocytes. Nine relatively complete remissions were observed in 21 treated patients.

Moore and Gerner (1970) established lymphoblastoid cell lines from the peripheral blood of patients with malignant melanoma. From 1 to 600 g of these was administered over a period of several weeks. Six patients were treated with allogeneic cell line cells, and six patients were treated with autologous cell line cells. Two objective responses were observed, with an intense inflammatory reaction around the tumor with necrosis of tumor cells. Frenster (1976) also used a form of adoptive immunotherapy with autologous cells. In his study, lymphocytes were collected and activated *in vitro* with phytohemagglutinin. They were then reinfused. Among five patients, three with pulmonary metastases showed objec-

470

EVAN M. HERSH,
G. M. MAVLIGIT,
J. U. GUTTERMAN,
AND
S. P. RICHMAN

tive regression of tumor. Cheema and Hersh (1972) used *in vitro* PHA-activated lymphocytes for intralesional therapy in malignant melanoma. Patients' tumors were inoculated either with PHA-activated lymphocytes, nonactivated lympho-cytes, or saline. Objective regression of the majority of nodules injected with activated lymphocytes was observed. These three studies indicate that autologous lymphoblastoid cells have the capacity to kill tumor cells, either on systemic administration or on intralesional injection. This presumably relates to the release of lymphokines such as lymphotoxin.

These scanty results are essentially all the work that has been done with adoptive immunotherapy of human cancer with intact lymphoid cells. This field has not progressed rapidly, for several reasons. First, to precisely mimic the optimal animal model conditions, one would require syngeneic donors, which are not available. Second, allogeneic donors can only be other cancer patients with metastatic disease, and these would be unsuitable because of their immuno-incompetence. It is also questionable whether one should remove lymphocytes from patients with metastatic cancer. It is also felt that repeated doses of allogeneic cells would sensitize to HLA antigens and these cells would then be rapidly removed by the reticuloendothelial system. Many obvious criticisms can be raised against the use of intact xenogeneic cells. Finally, the cell-collection and cell-transfer techniques are very tedious, time consuming, and expensive. For these reasons, investigations of adoptive immunotherapy at present and in the future will almost certainly emphasize the use of subcomponents of immune cells such as transfer factor and immune RNA.

10. Immune RNA in Cancer Therapy

Because of the above outlined problems associated with the systemic transfer of intact immune cells, considerable interest has developed in adoptive immunotherapy using subcellular fractions. The subcellular fraction which has received the most attention is the so-called immune or immunogenic RNA. Work in this area was initiated in 1967 by Alexander and co-workers. They speculated that a subcellular fraction must be involved in adoptive immunotherapy, since they achieved positive results with allogeneic and even xenogeneic lymphocytes, which they speculated could not survive in the recipient (Alexander and Delorme, 1971). At that time, a number of studies indicated that systemic immunity could be transferred with RNA extracts of immune lymphoid cells (Fishman, 1964). It was speculated that this achieved information transfer, although later it was demon-strated that this effect was probably due to antigen–RNA complex or so-called superantigen (Wilson and Wecker, 1966). In their initial experiment, Alexander *et al.* (1967) extracted RNA by the hot phenol method from the efferent lymph nodes of sheep locally stimulated with rat tumor, or from the thoracic duct lymphs of rats immunized with allogeneic rat tumor. Lymphoid cells were collected 3 days after immunization, and animals with 15–25 mg tumors were treated repeatedly with 0.5 mg of RNA, representing approximately 0.5 g of lymphoid cells. In four

out of ten rats treated for primary carcinogen-induced fibrosarcoma with sheep
RNA and in three out of five treated with allogeneic rat RNA, significant tumor
regression lasting up to 80 days was observed, with permanent cure of one animal.
Subsequently, Londner *et al.* (1968) demonstrated that immune RNA, but not
normal RNA, had an immunoprophylactic effect in retarding tumor growth in a
transplantable rat fibrosarcoma. Rigby (1969) demonstrated that immune RNA
prolonged the survival of mice bearing Ehrlich ascites tumor when syngeneic
spleen cells incubated immune RNA were administered to tumor-bearing mice.
Ramming and Pilch (1970*a*) demonstrated that the growth of tumor isografts in
inbred mice was inhibited by the intraperitoneal injection of syngeneic spleen
cells, incubated *in vitro* with RNA extracts from guinea pig lymphocytes
immunized with the same mouse tumor. Partial tumor specificity was observed
and ribonuclease treatment of the RNA extract abolished the response.

Pilch and his co-workers have subsequently done most of the work in this field.
In an early study, they incubated nonimmune guinea pig lymphocytes with
immune RNA from syngeneic guinea pigs immunized against a guinea pig
liposarcoma (Ramming and Pilch, 1970*b*). This conferred cytotoxic reactivity
upon these lymphocytes when examined in an *in vitro* cytotoxicity assay. The
reactivity was specific for the immunizing tumor, nonimmune RNA was inactive,
ribonuclease abolished the activity, and incubation of lymphocytes with antigen
did not confer cytotoxicity upon them. Subsequently, this group extended their
studies of the activity of immune RNA *in vitro* in tumor cytotoxicity studies to
include both syngeneic and xenogeneic immune RNA in mouse and rat tumor
systems (Pilch and Ramming, 1970).

The next step was to demonstrate that immune RNA could have immunoprophylactic activity *in vivo*. The experimental design was to incubate lymphocytes with immune RNA and to administer these cells to animals and to subsequently administered tumor cells. Retardation of tumor growth or decreased
tumor takes were demonstrated in these animals (Pilch *et al.*, 1971; Deckers and
Pilch, 1971*a*). Both syngeneic and xenogeneic immune RNA appeared to be
active in a rat fibrosarcoma system. Nonspecific RNA was not active. RNA from
nonimmune lymphocytes was not active, and dextran sulfate, a powerful inhibitor
of ribonuclease, augmented the activity (Deckers and Pilch, 1971*b*). Similar
observations were made ultilizing xenogeneic guinea pig immune RNA in a
mouse benzpyrine-induced tumor system (Ramming and Pilch, 1971). Ribonuclease destroyed the reactivity, while pronase and DNase had no effect. RNA from
animals immune to normal tissue or to an antigenically distinct syngeneic tumor
was not effective. Of interest, graft vs. host disease was not observed in these
animals. Next, using another benzpyrene-induced tumor in the mouse, it was
demonstrated that simultaneous administration of immune RNA-incubated
lymphocytes and tumor cells also was associated with growth retardation and
decreased tumor takes (Deckers and Pilch, 1972).

Recently, immune RNA has been shown to have activity in a true
immunotherapy setting (Pilch *et al.*, 1976*a*). Using a transplantable syngeneic

472

EVAN M. HERSH,
G. M. MAVLIGIT,
J. U. GUTTERMAN,
AND
S. P. RICHMAN

spontaneous rat mammary carcinoma, it was demonstrated that when excision at 18 days after implantation was followed by treatment with specific immune RNA, either syngeneic or xenogeneic, 50–90% of animals were disease free at 180 days, compared to all animals dead between 70 and 100 days in the control and surgery-alone groups. Some confirmation of this observation has come from the work of Schlager *et al.* (1975), who showed that a combination of immune RNA, normal lymphocytes, and tumor antigen, when inoculated intralesionally into a 5-day-old line 10 tumor in the guinea pig, caused regression of that tumor and of the tumor placed at the same time at a distant site. Use of nonspecific immune RNA or RNA from nonimmune cells was ineffective, as was deletion from the experiment of any of the three components.

Very recently, Pilch and co-workers have also begun clinical studies. They first demonstrated that human lymphocytes became cytolytic to cultured human colon, breast, or melanoma cell lines after incubation with sheep or guinea pig specific immune RNA at a dose of 5 mg/ml for 30 min. This was first demonstrated with normal human lymphocytes (Veltman *et al.*, 1974) and then to a limited extent with the lymphocytes of melanoma and gastric carcinoma patients (Veltman *et al.*, 1974). A clinical trial has now been started (Pilch *et al.*, 1976*b*). Cancer patients' lymphocytes are incubated with immune RNA made in sheep by weekly immunization with appropriate histological type of tumor cells in Freund's adjuvant, for weekly immunizations. Ten days later, spleen and lymph node cells are collected, immune RNA is made, and it is administered intradermally at doses of 1–12 mg/week. Among patients with advanced disseminated malignant diseases, there have been 0 out of 12 responses in malignant melanoma, three out of 12 partial remissions in hypernephroma, and one out of three partial remissions in sarcoma. No other therapy was administered. Trials are also ongoing in patients with minimal residual disease to see if prolongation of disease-free interval and survival or increased time to recurrence will be observed.

While considerable skepticism exists regarding immune RNA in cancer treatment, there have been some confirmatory experiments of the immunological observations. Thus both Thor and Schlossman (1969) and Paque *et al.* (1975) have demonstrated that immune RNA from strain 2 guinea pigs immune to DNP-poly-L-lysine can confer specific immunological reactivity to the usually nonresponder strain 13 animals. They also demonstrated that immune RNA from various human and animal immune lymphocyte sources could confer PPD, histoplasmin, coccidioidin, and tumor-antigen reactivity-measured migration inhibition on normal nonimmune guinea pig lymphocytes (Paque *et al.*, 1975). Schlager *et al.* (1974), in an important study using an arsenic-containing antigen, demonstrated that the immune RNA contained no detectable antigen. Paque and Dray (1974) demonstrated that monkey immune RNA could transfer delayed hypersensitivity to KLH, measured by migration inhibitory factor (MIF) *in vitro*, to nonimmune human lymphocytes. Finally, Han (1973), in an *in vivo* study in man, demonstrated that the intradermal inoculation of immune RNA could transfer *in vivo* delayed-type hypersensitivity reactivity to PPD, varidase, and candidin from normal immune donors to patients with Hodgkin's disease.

In summary, there is evidence from several laboratories that immune RNA can specifically confer various types of immunological reactivity on the lymphocytes of nonimmune subjects. This reactivity can include tumor immunity, and recipients can be cancer-bearing individuals. Most of the animal work has been done in an immunoprophylaxis setting; however, there is one experiment suggesting that true immunotherapy in animal models can result from the use of immune RNA. Very preliminary studies in man suggest that immunity can be transferred, and clinical trials have been initiated by one investigator. This area of investigation is promising, but needs broader confirmation by additional investigators.

11. Transfer Factor

The discovery and development of transfer factor were based on the observation in animal systems that transfer of immunity from immune to nonimmune animals could be achieved with lymphocytes (Lawrence, 1974, 1976). This has been demonstrated using a variety of inbred animal species, and immunity to a variety of antigens including bacterial, protein, and tissue antigens can be transferred. It was also observed that such transfer can occur in outbred animals. This led to many attempts, mostly unsuccessful, to transfer immunity between animals with subcellular fractions. A few attempts were made to transfer immunity with leukocytes between normal human individuals (Lawrence, 1949). It was observed that immunity to tuberculin could be transferred with peripheral blood leukocytes from strongly positive but not weakly positive donors. The immunity was evaluated in donor and recipient by cutaneous delayed hypersensitivity measurement. Transfer was also observed after the transfusion of 1 unit of whole blood from tuberculin-positive donor to tuberculin-negative recipient (Mohr et al., 1969). It was also observed that renal transplant recipients would sometimes develop delayed hypersensitivity reactions characteristic of the kidney donor (Kirkpatrick et al., 1964). Finally, the transfer was entirely specific for the specific antigen immunity of the donor, and was achieved with the non-glass-adherent fraction of peripheral blood cells, assumed to be mainly composed of lymphocytes.

The original experiments with transfer factor carried out by Sherwood Lawrence (1976) involved the use of peripheral blood leukocyte lysates. Both the retentate and the dialysate had activity in this regard. The original antigen used was PPD, but, as will be described below, transfer of immunity has occurred to many other antigens which have been used subsequently. The basic biological characteristics of transfer factor, as discovered mainly during investigations carried out by Lawrence (1976), are as follows: transfer factor is a dialyzable, lyophilizable, heat-stable substance with a molecular weight of approximately 1000. It can resist repeated freezing and thawing, and can be stored in the frozen state for many months. It is resistant to enzyme treatment with DNase, RNase, and various proteolytic enzymes. Its activity cannot be neutralized with antigen

474

EVAN M. HERSH,
G. M. MAVLIGIT,
J. U. GUTTERMAN,
AND
S. P. RICHMAN

(Lawrence and Pappenheimer, 1977) and recent studies suggest that it is a combination of nucleic acid and polypeptide (Hitzig and Grob, 1974). There is a definite dose–response relationship associated with successful transfer. Recipients can express delayed hypersensitivity in 24 hr or less after administration of transfer factor, and the ability to express donor-type delayed hypersensitivity persists in the recipient for up to 2 years. Serial transfer of delayed hypersensitivity is possible (Lawrence, 1976). Thus actively immunized subject A can donate leukocytes for transfer factor to unimmunized recipient B, whose lymphocytes can then be used to transfer the same specific immunological reactivity to unimmunized recipient C. Only delayed hypersensitivity and other manifestations of cell-mediated or cell-associated immunity are transferred. There is no evidence for transfer of antibody production even when the transfer factor donor has strong humoral immunity and a high antibody titer to the antigen (Lawrence, 1976).

The fundamental characteristic of transfer factor is that it is antigen specific. If the donor does not have delayed hypersensitivity to the antigen, then the transfer factor recipient will not develop it. Some of the antigens to which *in vivo* delayed hypersensitivity or other *in vivo* manifestations of cell-mediated immunity have been transferred from donor to recipient include the following: PPD, varidase (streptokinase-streptodornase), and streptococcal M protein; the fungal antigens coccidioidin, histoplasmin, dermatophytin, and candidin; diphtheria toxoid; the purified or synthetic antigens keyhole limpet hemocyanin (KLH), dinitrochlorobenzene (DNCB), orthochlorobenzoyl chloride (OCBC), and chemically modified heterologous albumin; histocompatibility antigens (as evaluated by transfer of accelerated skin graft rejection), and various tumor antigens including melanoma and sarcoma (see below; see also Table 5 for a list of antigens).

TABLE 5

Antigens to Which Immunity Has Been Specifically Transferred in Vivo with Dialyzable Transfer Factor[a]

Bacterial	Viral	Fungal	Other	Malignant
Tuberculin	Mumps	Candidin	DNCB	Melanoma
Varidase	Measles	Histoplasmin	OCBC	Sarcoma
Diptheria	Herpes	Coccidioidin	KLH	Nasopharyngeal carcinoma
	Vaccinia	Blastomycin	Modified albumin	Wilms' tumor[b]
	EB virus	Dermatophytin	Histocompatibility antigens	Renal cell carcinoma[b]
				Adeno carcinoma of colon[b]
				Lymphoma[b]
				Neuroblastoma[b]

[a] Abbreviations: DNCB, dinitrochlorobenzene; OCBC, orthochlorobenzoyl chloride; KLH, keyhole limpet hemocyanin.
[b] These are designated because there is some evidence based indirectly on a therapeutic response to transfer factor in these disease categories.

While originally transfer factor was evaluated only *in vivo* by means of delayed hypersensitivity skin testing or by evaluation of skin graft rejection, the *in vivo* administration of transfer factor may now also be evaluated by a number of *in vitro* studies. These include lymphocyte blastogenic responses to the antigens to which the donor is sensitive (Spitler *et al.*, 1973) and to which the recipient should become reactive, leukocyte migration inhibition or macrophage migration inhibition responses to these antigens (Kirkpatrick *et al.*, 1972), lymphocyte cytotoxicity to target tumor cells, non-antigen-specific reactions including chemotaxis (Gallin and Kirkpatrick, 1974), lymphocyte blastogenic responses to T-cell mitogens such as PHA (Kirkpatrick, 1975), and the number of circulating T-cell rosettes (Wyman *et al.*, 1973). There is evidence for some degree of nonspecificity or general immunocompetence-boosting activity associated with transfer factor. Thus it has not been possible to transfer delayed hypersensitivity from immunized donors to nonimmune recipients to synthetic antigens such as the amino acid copolymer of glutamic acid, lysine, and tryrosine (GLT) (Kirkpatrick, 1975). In a number of cases, conversion of skin tests in transfer factor recipients has occurred to antigens to which the donor was not sensitive (Levin *et al.*, 1970). Transfer factor has been demonstrated to have other types of activity such as chemotactic activity (Gallin and Kirkpatrick, 1974). Transfer factor can stimulate the synthesis of cyclic GMP in a number of different types of leukocytes (Kirkpatrick, 1975). The PHA response, the number of circulating T-cell rosettes, and the mixed lymphocyte response (MLC) have been observed to increase in recipients after administration of transfer factor (Kirkpatrick, 1975). In addition, transfer factor has been observed to be associated with immunosuppressive events both *in vitro* and *in vivo*. Thus there is evidence of decline in delayed hypersensitivity after the administration of transfer factor (Kirkpatrick and Gallin, 1975) and of decline in blastogenic responses when transfer factor is added to cells *in vitro* (Kirkpatrick and Gallin, 1975), and there is one case in which hemolytic anemia has developed concurrent with the administration of transfer factor (Ballow *et al.*, 1973). Thus the material we currently call "transfer factor" is complex and contains multiple factors, some of which transfer specific cell-mediated immunity and others which are nonspecific or even may be immunosuppressive.

Attempts have been made to clarify our understanding of transfer factor by the use of animal models. Initially, many attempts to use transfer factor in animal systems have failed. However, there are now a number of examples in which either dialyzable or nondialyzable lymphocyte extracts from immune animals can confer specific immunity on allogeneic or even xenogeneic recipients. Thus transfer of delayed hypersensitivity *in vivo* or of cell-mediated immunity measured *in vitro* has been demonstrated after *in vivo* transfers from man to guinea pigs (Salaman, 1974), from monkey to man (Baram and Condoulis, 1970), from monkey to monkey (Baram and Condoulis, 1970; Maddison *et al.*, 1972), from man to monkey (Baram and Condoulis, 1974), among rats (Berger *et al.*, 1972), and among guinea pigs (Berger *et al.*, 1972), using antigens such as PPD, KLH, DNCB, and OCBC. It seems reasonable to assume that the characteristics of transfer factor will be worked out in detail in animal systems in the next few years.

476

EVAN M. HERSH,
G. M. MAVLIGIT,
J. U. GUTTERMAN,
AND
S. P. RICHMAN

It is also important that transfer factor or transfer factor-like substances are active in animal systems since this puts this long-questioned phenomenon on a broader and sounder scientific basis.

Extensive studies on purification of transfer factor are being conducted at present. Using a variety of chromatographic and other separatory methods, highly purified peaks of activity can be separated from the complex mix of substances obtained after lymphocytes are subjected to repeated freezing and thawing and dialysis. This material contains substances which can transfer specific immunity, substances which can be of a general immunostimulating nature, and substances which can also inhibit lymphocyte function (Kirkpatrick, 1975). While beyond the scope of this chapter, it appears that transfer factor is a low molecular weight substance which consists of a nucleic acid and a peptide unit connected by a sugar molecule (Hitzig and Grob, 1974). Most investigators now believe that transfer factor does not contain superantigen. The various biochemical data have led Novelli to hypothesize that there is a relationship between transfer factor and immune RNA, that immune RNA is the larger, more complete transfer molecule, and that transfer factor is the subcomponent which contains the specific immunological information (Novelli, 1976).

Transfer factor has been used to treat a wide variety of diseases (Table 6). Usually, dialyzable transfer factor is made by a method similar to that originally described by Lawrence, and a dose equivalent to approximately 10^9 lymphocytes is administered weekly, every several weeks, or monthly. A number of immunodeficiency diseases have been treated with transfer factor. For example, Levin et al. (1970) and Spitler et al. (1973) treated patients with the Wiskott–Aldrich syndrome. They observed the development of delayed hypersensitivity to antigens to which the donor was sensitive. There was also some increased in vitro lymphocyte blastogenic reactivity, or increased numbers of circulating T-cell rosettes and associated clinical improvement. Other investigators have also attempted to treat ataxia telangiectasia, Swiss-type agammaglobulinemia, combined immunodeficiency disease, and various not clearly classified immunodeficiency syndromes

TABLE 6

Diseases or States in Which Transfer Factor Has Shown Some Evidence for Therapeutic Activity

Immunodeficiency	Infectious	Malignant
Congenital	Mucocutaneous	Breast cancer
Wiskott-Aldrich	candidiasis	Malignant melanoma
Ataxia telangiectasia	Herpes zoster	Sarcoma
Combined	Herpes simplex	Nasopharyngeal
	Measles	carcinoma
Aquired	Subacute sclerosing	Laryngeal
Common variable	panencephalitis	papillomatosis
Sarcoid	Leprosy	Wilms' tumor
Nutritional deficiency	Tuberculosis	Renal cell carcinoma
	Coccidioidomycosis	Adenocarcinoma colon
		Lymphoma
		Neuroblastoma

(Hitzig and Grob, 1974; Marshall, 1972). Some claim has been made that these immunodeficiency syndromes also respond clinically to transfer factor, although they are very poorly documented. In addition, in none of these circumstances can a clear cause-and-effect relationship between the administration of transfer factor and clinical changes in the patient be documented.

A number of investigators have also tended to treat infectious diseases with transfer factor. These include measles, subacute sclerosing panencephalitis, herpes zoster, herpes simplex, mucocutaneous candidiasis, leprosy, and disseminated tuberculosis (Hitzig and Grob, 1974; Marshall, 1972). In each instance, transfer factor was obtained from individuals manifesting *in vivo* delayed hypersensitivity to the antigens of the infectious agent in question. Evidence for development of delayed hypersensitivity in the recipient and clinical improvement have been noted in these cases.

Because of the energy which is often seen in cancer patients, and because a decline in specific immunological reactivity may be associated with progression of malignancy, a number of attempts have been made to treat human malignant diseases with transfer factor. First, a series of studies have been done whose objective was to demonstrate that one could transfer delayed hypersensitivity to common antigens from normal immune donors to anergic cancer-bearing recipients (Table 5). Successful transfer of specific immunity to antigens such as PPD and candidin has been achieved regularly in patients with solid tumors (Soloway *et al.*, 1968), and in patients with non-Hodgkin's lymphoma (Soloway *et al.*, 1968), but generally, with the exception of the work of one author (Khan *et al.*, 1975), not in patients with Hodgkin's disease (Muftuoglou and Balkur, 1967). Thus immunotherapy of cancer with transfer factor seems possible. Two types of donors have been used: (1) relatives or close personal contacts who can be demonstrated to have specific immunity to the potential recipient's tumor, and (2) donors who either do not have or who have not been tested for specific tumor immunity, but have good general immunocompetence. In a few instances, a third type of donor who has recently been actively immunized against the tumor is available. For example, Brandes *et al.* (1971) and Morse *et al.* (1973) have immunized melanoma patients or other cancer patients with melanoma tissue, have collected their leukocytes and prepared transfer factor, and have administered it to melanoma-bearing recipients. Both groups of investigators observed transient regression of melanoma nodules in the transfer factor recipients. This type of donor must be selected carefully and is generally not available, and one might even question the safety of removing lymphocytes from cancer-bearing donors.

What is the evidence for a role for transfer factor in cancer? LoBuglio *et al.* (1973) identified relatives of a patient with immunity to alveolar soft part sarcoma. They made transfer factor from the lymphocytes and demonstrated that an unresponsive tumor-bearing recipient developed *in vitro* manifestations of blastogenic response to tumor after *in vivo* transfer factor. Spitler *et al.* (1972) made transfer factor from relatives of patients who had evidence of melanoma immunity, administered this in combination with BCG to patients with metastistic

478

EVAN M. HERSH,
G. M. MAVLIGIT,
J. U. GUTTERMAN,
AND
S. P. RICHMAN

melanoma, and observed remissions of disease in two out of six patients. Byers *et al.* (1976) and Fudenberg (1976) carried out similar studies in patients with sarcoma. Repeated doses of transfer factor were administered from relatives and contacts with evidence of immunity (cell-mediated cytotoxicity). Stabilization and even some regression of disease were noted. Goldenberg and Brandes (1972) gave immunotherapy with transfer factor from donors with previous infectious mononucleosis to recipients with nasopharyngeal carcinoma. The rationale was based on the observation that nasopharyngeal carcinoma is possibly caused by the Epstein–Barr virus, which is the known cause of infectious mononucleosis. In one patient, regression of tumor was observed after the administration of this transfer factor. Oettgen *et al.* (1974) made transfer factor from a pool of lymphocytes of normal women over the age of 40 years and administered this repeatedly in high doses to five patients with metastatic breast cancer. Some stabilization of disease was noted in each of these patients. One patient had clear-cut complete regression of tumor. The donors were selected on the basis of having no history of tumor and therefore were presumed to contain at least a subpopulation who had resisted the development of this common malignancy. Quick *et al.* (1975) treated two patients with laryngeal papillomatosis with weekly doses of transfer factor. The donor for the first patient was the child's mother, the donor for the second was a 19-year-old female who had had a remission of this disease at puberty. Significant clinical response with reduction in the disease was noted in both patients.

The most extensive study of transfer factor immunotherapy to date has been carried out by Vetto *et al.* (1976). They made transfer factor by the vacuum dialysis method. Donors were family members who had had a long physical association with the cancer patients and could be referred to as cohabitants. One unit of transfer factor, equivalent to 10^9 leukocytes, was administered every 2 weeks subcutaneously. Seven out of 35 patients with various solid tumors not receiving any other therapy showed objective regression of disease. This included three complete remissions, two in melanoma and one in rhabdomyosarcoma, and 50% or greater regression in additional cases with malignant melanoma, adenocarcinoma of the colon, lymphosarcoma, and neuroblastoma. Several other patients were reported to have manifested arrest of tumor growth.

One extensive trial of transfer factor has been carried out in malignant melanoma. M. Schwarz (unpublished observations) administered transfer factor from the immunocompetent relatives of melanoma patients to patients with metastatic malignant melanoma receiving chemoimmunotherapy with DTIC and BCG. Sixty-four patients received transfer factor every 3 weeks, and 15 patients received transfer factor weekly. While there was evidence that recipients could express donor immunity after transfer factor, there was no evidence for an increased remission rate, remission duration, or survival in these patients.

In summary, there seems no doubt that transfer factor can confer donor immunity on cancer patients who have manifestations of anergy. The mechanism of action, the site of action, and the biochemical characteristics of transfer factor are not well understood at this time. A number of preliminary clinical studies, mostly not controlled, and mostly carried out in small numbers of patients, have demonstrated that transfer factor can induce tumor regression in a fraction of the patients. Extensive work is in progress on the biochemical and physiological characterization of transfer factor. Extensive studies of its nature and use in animal models are also ongoing. Immunorestoration with transfer factor is an appealing approach to immunotherapy since immunodeficiency in cancer patients may be correctable with its use and it can transfer specific immunity into cancer patients with it. It may be active itself, and may augment immunotherapy with other agents such as active-nonspecific immunotherapy or specific immunization with tumor antigen. The proper place for transfer factor in the scheme of immunotherapy is not known at this time and will await further basic experiments as well as empirical well-controlled clinical trials in large enough numbers of patients for proper interpretation.

12. Interferon and Interferon Inducers

The interferon system is a complex mechanism of cellular defense or immunity which involves the release of substances from cells infected with viruses. These substances subsequently show the ability to inhibit the proliferation of certain cells and to either augment or suppress other host defense mechanisms (Grossberg, 1972a). Since interferon and interferon inducers apparently have direct and possibly also indirect antitumor activity, and since certain human tumors are probably caused by and may also be reinduced after remission by viruses, these substances are of significant current interest. The interferons are a remarkably heterogeneous family of glycoproteins ranging in molecular weight from 20,000 to 120,000 or greater. They are remarkably heat, acid, and alkali stable, and while they have been purified by a variety of methods with a marked increase in specific activity, they still are felt to be impure by workers in this field (Grossberg, 1972a). In general, interferon is partially species specific in that the interferon of one species usually has less than 10% of its homologous activity in another species (Grossberg, 1972a). The mechanism of action is apparently the production of a polypeptide repressor substance which acts on RNA to prevent new viral nucleic acid and protein synthesis.

In vivo, interferon can be induced by a wide variety of agents. These include many viruses, including the usual infectious viruses. Newcastle disease and Sendai viruses are used *in vivo* and *in vitro* to specifically induce interferon (Henle *et al.*, 1959). Inactivated viruses apparently also can induce interferon. A number of bacteria (Grossberg, 1963), protozoa (Freshman *et al.*, 1966), and fungi (Lackovic *et al.*, 1970) can also induce interferon, as can extracts of these organisms such as endotoxins (Ho, 1964) and the fungal extract statalon. Finally, a number of synthetic chemical substances which presumably mimic virus–cell interaction are active interferon inducers. These include the synthetic polynucleotides such as poly(IC) (Hilleman, 1970), and poly(AU) (Drake *et al.*, 1974), other synthetic polymers including maleic anhydride copolymers such as pyran (Pearson *et al.*,

480

EVAN M. HERSH,
G. M. MAVLIGIT,
J. U. GUTTERMAN,
AND
S. P. RICHMAN

1974), and low molecular weight ethylamines such as tylerone (Mayer and Krueger, 1970).

Interferon has a wide variety of inhibitory activities. It inhibits the proliferation of most RNA and DNA viruses (Grossberg, 1972a). It also has been demonstrated to interfere with the proliferation of protozoal, bacterial, and fungal organisms (Grossberg, 1972), and, finally, it has been demonstrated to inhibit the proliferation of malignant cells *in vitro* (Gresser *et al.*, 1970). While the mechanism of action of the last is not known, this activity is definitely associated with the classical interferon molecules (W. E. Stewart *et al.*, 1976).

There are many sources of interferon. *In vivo*, it is probably produced by lymphoid cells and macrophages, and there is also some evidence for its production by spleen, liver, lung, and thymus (Grossberg, 1972a). *In vitro*, interferon has been produced by lymphoid cells, including peripheral blood leukocytes and peritoneal exudate cells, by lymphoblastoid cell lines, and by various tissue culture lines, particularly fibroblasts (Grossberg, 1972a).

Clinically, interferon and interferon inducers have a variety of immunological effects. Interferon itself can augment cell-mediated cytotoxicity to target cells (Grossberg, 1972a), but most of the observations on its function have been that it is immunosuppressive. Thus the *in vivo* administration of interferon in mice can suppress the expression of delayed-type hypersensitivity to sheep red blood cells (DeMayer *et al.*, 1975), and to picryl chloride (DeMayer *et al.*, 1975) when the interferon is administered within 24 hr of the application of the skin test. Interferon can also inhibit the acute inflammatory response to carrageenin (Koltai and Mees, 1973) and suppress the antibody response of mice to sheep red blood cells (Brodeur and Morigan, 1974). *In vitro*, interferon has been demonstrated to suppress the mixed lymphocyte culture reactions (Lindahl–Magnusson and Gresser, 1972) and to suppress the proliferative response of rabbit lymph node cells to antigens such as diphtheria (Thorbecke *et al.*, 1974). Presumably, all of these effects are mediated by the antiproliferative activity of interferon on lymphoid cells. It is hypothesized that the energy associated with viral infection may be due to this mechanism. It might also be speculated that if the release of virus is a component of the malignant process, the release of interferon may explain some of the immunosuppression associated with malignancy.

In contrast, a number of interferon inducers have been observed to be powerful adjuvants. Thus poly(AU) administration can result in increased phagocytic activity (Braun, 1974), increase in the antibody response to primary and secondary antigens (Schmidtke and Johnson, 1971), and increase in delayed hypersensitivity or graft vs. host reactions (Cone and Johnson, 1971). In addition, the administration of poly(AU) can restore suppressed T-cell function and can lead to maturation of T-cells with improvement in lymphocyte proliferative responses to low doses of mitogens, but with decreased lymphocyte proliferative responses to high doses of mitogens (Chess *et al.*, 1972). Poly(AU) has been studied to some extent clinically, and is associated with quite variable effects on host defense mechanisms (Wanebo *et al.*, 1976). In contrast, the administration of poly(IC) to

AML patients has been associated with a transient but marked suppression of the PHA response (McIntyre et al., 1977).

The complexity of the action of the synthetic interferon inducers is exemplified by studies of tylerone. Tylerone can increase macrophage function and phagocytosis (Munson et al., 1970) and increase the RES clearance of particulate materials (Munson et al., 1972). It is a B-cell stimulant and can increase the antibody response of mice (Munson et al., 1972). However, it is a T-cell suppressor and decreases delayed-type hypersensitivity reactions, increases skin graft survival, and can suppress the PHA response (Levine et al., 1974).

Interferon and interferon inducers have antitumor effects not only on virus induction of tumors, and not only on virus-induced tumors, but also on other experimental tumors. The characteristics of the effects of interferon itself and interferon inducers are similiar. Thus interferon retards the development of Friend leukemia virus diseases after inoculation of Friend leukemia virus (Wheelock and Larke, 1968). It can also block the development of leukemia after the inoculation of Rauscher leukemia virus (Gresser et al., 1968). In both instances, interferon is inoculated at approximately the same time as the virus. However, in animals with established Friend leukemia virus leukemia, prolongation of life occurs on repeated inoculation with interferon (Wheelock and Larke, 1968). Interferon administration also prolongs the life of animals bearing transplantable tumors. These inlude the transplantable RC19 leukemia, which originated from a Rauscher leukemia virus system (Gresser et al., 1969), L 1210 leukemia (Gresser et al., 1968), and the EL4 lymphoma (Gresser et al., 1969). Interferon also delays the development of pulmonary metastases in the Lewis lung carcinoma (Gresser and Bourali-Mawry, 1972). For these effects, interferon must be given at high doses and must be administered frequently.

The classical interferon inducers are, of course, viruses, and it has been observed that virus infection or virus administration with, for example, the lymphocytic choriomeningitis virus or with Sendai virus can inhibit L2C leukemia and the development of Rauscher leukemia (Grossberg, 1972b).

The interferon inducer tylerone has been studied fairly extensively. The development of Friend leukemia, the growth of Ehrlich ascites tumor, and the growth of Lewis lung carcinoma are all inhibited by tylerone. The mold extract statalon, which is a potent interferon inducer, can prevent or delay the development of Friend leukemia virus, and can prolong the life of animals with established tumors of this type (Rhim et al., 1969). Poly(AU) delays the development of leukemia or lymphoma in AKR mice and decreases the rate of development of spontaneous mammary cancers in mice. However, at certain doses and schedules, the reverse can occur. Poly(AU) also retards the development of transplantable leukemia (Wanebo et al., 1976). Poly(IC) has been used to treat animals with established tumors. It prolongs survival in L1210 leukemia and in a mouse tumor induced by the human adeno type 12 virus, and can induce complete remission when administered simultaneously with Moloney sarcoma virus (Levy et al., 1969). In the last instance, treated animals have tumors which grow and regress while

EVAN M. HERSH,
G. M. MAVLIGIT,
J. U. GUTTERMAN,
AND
S. P. RICHMAN

482

untreated animals have progressively growing tumors. Pyran copolymer can delay the development of Friend leukemia virus disease (Chirigos *et al.*, 1969).

In contrast, probably because of their immunosuppressive properties, several of the interferon inducers have been associated with tumor enhancement. If animals are pretreated with one to three doses of certain interferon inducers, and are subsequently inoculated with a variety of tumors, augmentation of tumor growth can occur (Regelson, 1976). This has been observed with poly(IC) and tylerone, and with the injection of Newcastle disease virus.

Based on these observations, and on the known efficacy of interferon in certain selected human infectious diseases of viral origin, several clinical trials with interferon or interferon inducers have been carried out or are currently under way. Regelson (1976) has carried out several phase I studies of tylerone therapy of human cancer. Patients received tylerone either daily or weekly and showed some regression of metastatic malignant melanoma or breast cancer. However, these observations could not be confirmed by the Eastern Cooperative Oncology Group, and these studies have now been terminated (Regelson, 1976). McIntyre *et al.* (1977) have studied the remission duration and survival of patients who received a single dose of poly(IC) 3 months after the onset of treatment for acute myelogenous leukemia. No clinical effect was observed, although transient suppression of the PHA response was seen. It seems unlikely that a single dose of any antitumor agent would have a measurable effect in this circumstance. Habif (1975) has given intralesional interferon to four patients with breast cancer and apparently has observed regression in two. Strander (1975) has treated one patient with stage IV Hodgkin's disease with 5×10^6 units of interferon daily for 6 months, and has noted lymph node regression and clearing of pulmonary involvement.

The most extensive study in man has been carried out by Strander *et al.* (1975) in osteogenic sarcoma. Fourteen postsurgical patients were treated with 3×10^6 units of human leukocyte interferon 3 times a week for $1\frac{1}{2}$ years. Only one out of 14 patients in the treated group relapsed, compared to 15 out of 33 historical controls. This study obviously warrants further patient accrual and confirmation by other investigators.

In summary, "interferon" refers to a family of proteins which have a variety of biological effects, including the inhibition of viral proliferation, inhibition of cellular proliferation, modulation of the immune response, and antitumor activity. Some modestly encouraging animal experiments of interferon inducer therapy of malignancy have been made. Clearly, these observations have to be extended to other tumor systems, dose–response and schedule studies need to be more extensively done, and relative efficacy alone or in combination with other modalities of treatment needs to be investigated. There are a few extremely preliminary clinical observations regarding the use of interferon in human malignancy. They have been somewhat encouraging, and the use of both interferon and interferon inducers must be much more extensively studied before its proper role, if any, in the immunotherapy of cancer is defined.

During the last 10 years, we have come to recognize that delayed-type hypersensitivity reactions are one of the important components of antitumor host defense (Golub, 1975) and that these reactions are associated with the release from antigen-stimulated lymphocytes of protein substances which can act, at least over a short distance, to augment and mediate the delayed-type hypersensitivity reaction (Bloom, 1969). The mediators or lymphokines include macrophage and leukocyte migration inhibitory factors, macrophage-activating factors, lymphotoxins, lymphocyte blastogenic factors, and chemotactic factors (Bloom, 1969). These products of stimulated lymphocytes are intimately associated with the recruitment, localization, and activation of the inflammatory cells which mediate delayed hypersensitivity responses.

One of the important mediators or group of mediators is the so-called macrophage-activating factor or factors (Fowles *et al.*, 1973), which can influence macrophage adherence, macrophage phagocytosis, macrophage spreading and motility, and the oxidative metabolism of the macrophage. Such activated macrophages are known to selectively recognize and kill tumor cells and leave nontumor cells relatively unaffected (Hibbs *et al.*, 1972). During the last several years, it has also been recognized that tumors can be heavily infiltrated by macrophages (Alexander *et al.*, 1976) and that tumor immunity is mediated in a major way by activated macrophages. The major mechanism of action by which the intralesional BCG effect is mediated is by activation of macrophages and killing of tumor by these activated cells (Kaplan and Morohan, 1976). The mechanism of local immunotherapy with a variety of products including bacterial adjuvants and antigens to which the individual is sensitive is by a bystander effect of delayed hypersensitivity. Activated macrophages are very important in this.

Now, since there is a defect in lymphocyte-mediated immunity in cancer patients (Hersh *et al.*, 1975; Hersh and Freireich, 1968), a failure of effector mechanism against tumor may relate to the failure of release of lymphokines. Also, it is conceivable that lymphokine-inhibiting substances may be present in tumors. It is theoretically possible that by the systemic (presumably intravenous) administration of lymphokines, which could nonspecifically activate macrophages and the reticuloendothelial system, a major immunotherapeutic effect could be achieved.

Several investigations support this possibility. First, the products of stimulated lymphocytes can induce inflammatory responses in the skin of both animal and human subjects (Papermaster *et al.*, 1976*b*). These inflammatory responses show a mixed cell population of granulocytes, lymphocytes, eosinophils, and activated macrophages. Holterman *et al.* (1975) described the injection of the supernatant of concanavalin A-stimulated lymphocyte cultures into human tumors. Regression of tumor nodules was observed. Subsequently, Papermaster and co-workers observed that a product found in the supernatant of long-term normal lymphoblastoid cell lines contained a substance or group of substances between 10,000 and 100,000 molecular weight which had lymphotoxin, macrophage-activating, and

484

EVAN M. HERSH,
G. M. MAVLIGIT,
J. U. GUTTERMAN,
AND
S. P. RICHMAN

skin reactive factor activities (Papermaster *et al.*, 1976*b*; McDaniel *et al.*, 1976). This material was subsequently used for immunotherapy (Papermaster *et al.*, 1976*c*). Repeated injections were made into the tumor nodules of patients with metastatic tumors, including breast cancer, reticulum cell sarcoma, mycosis fungoides, squamous cell carcinoma of the skin, and adenocarcinoma. Regression greater than 80% was seen in 16 out of 30 injected nodules with one particular active column fraction of the lymphoblastoid cell line supernatant.

The future of this area lies in purification of the macrophage-activating factor, dose–response studies of its intralesional effect, and attempts to use it systemically. This obviously must be based on appropriate animal model studies. If an active macrophage-activating factor could be developed that is tolerated clinically and effective systemically, resultant activation of macrophages within tumor and activation of the reticuloendothelial system might have profound therapeutic effects, including tumor regression. Obviously, considerable biochemical purification as well as animal model work must be done before this will become a viable clinical possibility.

14. Thymic Hormones in Immunotherapy

Since the demonstration of the role of the thymus in cell-mediated and humoral immunity (Miller and Osoba, 1967) and since the demonstration that thymic grafts or thymus placed in diffusion chambers could restore the immunocompetence of thymectomized animals (Levey *et al.*, 1963), considerable work has been done to identify and characterize the presumed thymic hormones (Table 7). At present, a number of laboratories have identified factors extractable from the thymus or present in the serum which have activity identifiable as associated with normal thymic function. The first steps along these lines were taken by White, Goldstein, and their collaborators, who were able to extract from bovine thymus a substance which would induce lymphocytosis in rats and mice (Roberts and White, 1949; Klein *et al.*, 1965). Subsequently, they partially purified a substance which has a variety of *in vitro* and *in vivo* thymus-associated biological functions (Goldstein *et al.*, 1972) and which has recently been introduced into clinical trials in patients with immunodeficiency diseases and in cancer patients.

Both Allan Goldstein and his collaborators (Hooper *et al.*, 1975) and Bach *et al.* (1975) have demonstrated that the level of thymic hormone activity declines in the blood with increasing age, and is particularly low in patients with certain malignancies. This has resulted in the hypothesis that diminished thymic hormone activity and associated deficiencies in cell-mediated immunity may be associated with development and/or progression of certain human malignancies. If this is the case, then the administration of thymic hormone should correct these abnormalities in cell-mediated immunity and improve host resistance to tumor. One approach would be to identify patients with defined defects in cell-mediated immunity, to demonstrate that at least certain of these defects could be corrected

TABLE 7

Study Subjects and Biological Functions Influenced by Thymic
Factors

Prethymosin manipulation in test animals
   Neonatal thymectomy
   Adult thymectomy
   Immunosuppression
     Chemical
     Radiotherapy
     Antilymphocyte serum treated
   NZB mice
   Tumor bearing
   Normal
Patient subjects for study and treatment
   Immunodeficiency disease
     DiGeorge syndrome
     Nezelof syndrome
     Wiskott-Aldrich syndrome
     Ataxia telangiectasia
     Cellular immunodeficiency with immunoglobulins
     Thymicx hypoplasia syndromes
   Malignancies with cellular immunodeficiency
     Advanced metastatic malignancies
     Lung cancer
     Head and neck cancer
     Malignant lymphoma
   Autoimmune disease with cellular immunodeficiency
     (hypothetical)
   Normal (*in vitro* studies only)
Tests for cell surface markers
   θ antigen
   TL antigen
   Sheep red blood cell receptor
In vitro lymphocyte function
   NDA synthesis in unstimulated lymphocytes
   PHA, Con A, OWM, and other blastogenic responses
   Mixed lymphocyte response
   T- and B-cell cooperation studies
In vivo lymphocyte function
   Graft vs. host reaction
   T- and B-cell cooperation
   Suppressor cell activity
   Thymus-dependent antibody response
   Antitumor host defense

by addition of hormone or extract to their lymphocytes *in vitro*, and then attempt a trial *in vivo*.

The material prepared by Goldstein and co-workers is referred to as "thymosin." Thymosin is purified through a series of steps as follows. Saline extraction is followed by acetone precipitation, the supernatant of which is precipitated by ammonium sulfate, resuspended, and fractionated sequentially on Sephadex G25, DEAE-cellulose, Sephadex G50, and polyacrylamide gel electrophoresis (Hooper *et al.*, 1975). Fraction V contains a mixture of approximately 12 polypep-

EVAN M. HERSH,
G. M. MAVLIGIT,
J. U. GUTTERMAN,
AND
S. P. RICHMAN

TABLE 8

Characteristics of Selected Thymic Factors[a]

Factor	Source	Molecular weight	Biological activity: level of immune factor or function modified				
			Cell markers induced	*In vitro* mitogen responses	*In vivo* effects	GVH	NMTB
Thymosin fraction V	Thymus	1000–15,000	+	+	+	+	−
Thymosin fraction α_1	Thymosin	3354	+	+	+	ND	−
Thymopoietin	Thymus	5562	+	±	−	−	+
Ubiquitin	Many tissues	8451	+	±	−	−	−
Thymic humoral factor	Thymus	3220	+	+	+	+	−
Thymic factor	Serum	>1000	+	+	+	ND	−

[a] Abbreviations: GVH, graft vs. host disease; NMTB, neuromuscular transmission blockade.

tides varying in molecular weight from 1000 to 15,000 (Table 8). After a variety of other procedures, including isoelectric focusing, a highly purified fraction known as "thymosin in α_1" is obtained, with a molecular weight of 3400 and consisting of 28 amino acids (Hooper *et al.*, 1975). It is now undergoing sequencing.

Thymosin fraction V has been demonstrated to partially restore the immunocompetence of cells from NZB mice, neonatally thymectomized mice, adult thymectomized mice, and nude mice, when added *in vitro*, and to also partially restore various immune functions when administered *in vivo* (Hooper *et al.*, 1975). Immune functions or levels restored include the percentage or level of T-cell rosettes, the mixed lymphocyte response, and the lymphocyte blastogenic response to phytohemagglutinin and concanavalin A (Hooper *et al.*, 1975). When administered to NZB mice, thymosin can restore the level of suppressor cells to normal and can reduce the production of autoantibodies such as antinuclear or anti-DNA antibodies (Hooper *et al.*, 1975). Thymosin can also increase the expression of θ and TL antigens in various lymphocyte populations from thymus-deprived as well as normal mice and can restore lymphocyte reactivity of mice in terms of graft vs. host reactivity measured by the spleen weight assay (Hooper *et al.*, 1975).

Another series of studies on thymic hormones has been carried out by Gideon Goldstein and co-workers. He has extracted two closely related polypeptides referred to as "thymopoietin 1" and "thymopoietin 2" from bovine thymus by saline extraction, heating, molecular sieving, absorption chromatography, and hydroxylapatite and ion exchange chromatography (Goldstein, 1974). Antibody raised against these hormones has demonstrated their presence only in thymic epithelial cells. Subnanogram amounts of thymopoietins 1 and 2 have been demonstrated to result in T-cell differentiation so that θ and TL surface markers are increased and can also marginally increase the blastogenic response of mouse

lymphocytes to PHA and Con A (Basch and Goldstein, 1975). In contrast to most
of the other thymic factors, thymopoietin does not increase the level of T-cell
rosettes. Another characteristic of thymopoietin is that it produces neuromuscular blockade when injected in mice *in vivo* (Goldstein and Hoffman, 1969). The
property has been used to monitor purification of the hormone. Goldstein (1975)
has extracted a third polypeptide from the thymus, which is also extractable from
a variety of other tissues. It has the property of inducing maturation of both T and
B lymphocytes, but has no neuromuscular blockade activity. It is referred to as
"ubiquitous immunopotentiating polypeptide" or "ubiquitin." Thymopoietins 1
and 2 have not yet been used in tumor models or *in vivo* in animals, and have not
been administered to humans. Bach *et al.* (1975) have obtained what they refer to
as "thymic factor" from serum of animals and man. It is produced by molecular
sieving, has a molecular weight of approximately 1000, is a polypaptide, and has a
neutral pH. In contrast to thymosin and thymopoietin, this material is very heat
labile, and its activity even disappears after a few hours at 37°C. Thymic factor
diminishes in the serum with age both in mice and in man (Bach *et al.*, 1975). It is
diminished in mice with autoimmune diseases, disappears after thymectomy, and
reappears with thymic grafting (Bach *et al.*, 1975). It is best detected by a modified
rosette assay. It is purified by dialysis, ultrafiltration, Sephadex G25 column
chromatography, CM cellulose chromatography, thin-layer chromatography,
and electrophoresis. Bach and Dardenne (1973) have also identified a circulating
serum thymic factor inhibitor with a molecular weight greater than 100,000.
Biological tests which have been demonstrated thymic factor activity include
increased levels of θ-bearing cells, increased levels of rosette-forming cells,
increased blastogenic response to Con A but not to PHA, and decreased cell
surface steroid receptors. These have been demonstrated both on addition of
thymic factor *in vitro* and *in vivo* in thymectomized mice.

Another thymic factor somewhat similar to that described by Bach is "thymic
humoral factor," described by Trainin *et al.* (1967). This material is extracted from
mouse or calf thymus homogenates and purified by dialysis. It is found in the
dialysate and has a molecular weight of approximately 3000. It can restore the
graft vs. host reactivity of lymphocytes from neonatally thymectomized animals,
and can increase mouse lymphocyte reactivity in the MLC (Trainin *et al.* (1975).
Trainin *et al.* (1975) have demonstrated that thymic humoral factor action is
associated with an obligatory increase in adenylyl cyclase and cyclic AMP with
subsequent transient arrest in proliferation and induction of protein synthesis in
thymic lymphocytes. It protein synthesis is clocked, evidence for maturation of T
cells is not observed. Of interest, none of the thymic factors seems to be species
specific, and bovine or even human thymic factors can be demonstrated to have
biological activity in mice.

Several investigators have demonstrated that thymic hormones have activity in
various tumor systems. Bach *et al.* (1975) have demonstrated that thymic factor
increases resistance of thymectomized animals to Moloney sarcoma virus-induced
sarcomas. If thymic factor is administered simultaneously with virus, tumors
develop but regress compared to progressive tumor growth in thymectomized

EVAN M. HERSH,
G. M. MAVLIGIT,
J. U. GUTTERMAN,
AND
S. P. RICHMAN

animals. Serrou *et al.* (1975) have demonstrated that a thymic extract increases survival and decreases tumor size in thymectomized animals bearing the Lewis lung tumor. The effect is also seen in nonthymectomized animals. A. L. Goldstein (personal communication) has demonstrated that the administration of thymosin alone without other treatment can induce remissions and prolong life in certain experimental leukemias.

In man, there are a number of observations which suggest that thymic factors might play a role in cancer. Using a radioimmunoassay, Hooper *et al.* (1975) have demonstrated that there is a progressive decline in the level of thymosin with increasing age, and that thymosin levels are also low in patients with lymphomas and chronic leukemia. Using a rosette assay, Bach *et al.* (1975) demonstrated in man that there is approximately a 50% reduction in thymic factor by the age of 30 years and a 75% reduction by the age of 40 years, and that thymic factors are also depressed in patients with systemic lupus erythematosus. The presence of a correctable thymic hormone deficiency has been demonstrated in man by studies in which thymosin has been added to lymphocytes *in vitro*. In a variety of immunodeficiency diseases including the Nezelof syndrome, the DiGeorge syndrome, ataxia telangiectasia, the Wiskott-Aldrich syndrome, and common variable immunodeficiency, the addition of thymosin increases the percentage of T-cell rosettes (Goldstein *et al.*, 1976). In cancer patients, the *in vitro* addition of thymosin to peripheral blood lymphocytes has increased the level of active T cells or total T cells as reported by Wybran *et al.* (1975) and Kenady *et al.* (1977) and has increased the baseline *in vitro* lymphocyte proliferation and the mixed lymphocyte reactivity as reported by Schafer *et al.* (1976).

Thymosin has now been used clinically in the treatment of patients with immunodeficiency diseases. The disease categories treated are those mentioned above and also severe combined immunodeficiency disease. Most patients have been treated with approximately 40 mg subcutaneously weekly. In the majority of patients, except those with severe combined immunodeficiency disease, there has been some evidence for immunorestoration. Immunological parameters which have improved or increased in immunodeficiency disease patients receiving thymosin include the level of E rosettes, the lymphocyte blastogenic response to PHA. Con A, and pokeweed mitogen, or, in the MLC, delayed-type-hypersensitivity responses to recall antigens, the lymphocyte count, and the level of normal immunoglobulin, as well as the levels of various isoantibodies (Goldstein *et al.*, 1976). In one patient, there was a diminution in the level of abnormal protein associated with a gamopathy (Goldstein *et al.*, 1976). Immunological changes in these patients have not been uniform. Most patients show an increase in the level of rosette-forming cells, but many do not show increases in blastogenic responses, or changes in serum immunoglobulins. Clinically, there has been a variable degree of improvement. Approximately half of the patients, excluding those with severe combined immunodeficiency disease, have improved, and this has included diminished hospitalization time, diminished frequency of infection, cessation of diarrhea, clearing of skin rash, and pronounced weight gain (Goldstein *et al.*, 1976).

Several groups have carried out phase I clinical trials with cancer. Several hundred patients with solid tumors, malignant lymphomas, and leukemias have been treated (Goldstein *et al.*, 1976; Schafer *et al.*, 1976). In general, patients with immunodeficiency have shown improvement in the levels of T-cell rosettes, of delayed hypersensitivity to recall antigens, and of *in vitro* blastogenic responses or baseline *in vitro* lymphocyte proliferation. Doses of thymosin have ranged from 1 mg/m² per week to up to 200 mg/m² per week (Goldstein *et al.*, 1976; Schafer *et al.*, 1976). No severe untoward side effects have been observed, although approximately 20% of the patients had a local inflammatory response at the site of injection.

Thymosin doses from 20 to 60 mg/m² per week are now in phase II trial in patients with malignant melanoma, head and neck cancer, and lung cancer. An extremely important observation has been made in malignant melanoma (Y. Patt, unpublished observations). In this trial, thymosin immunotherapy was added to BCG or DTIC-BCG therapy for the prevention of recurrence of stage IIIB disease (regional lymph node metastases) after surgery. No overall beneficial effect was observed in approximately 40 patients, and indeed the previously demonstrated beneficial effect of BCG appeared to be abolished. On careful analysis of the immunological data, it was found that immunocompetent patients receiving a high dose of thymosin and immunoincompetent patients receiving a low dose of thymosin did not benefit, while immunoincompetent patients receiving a high dose of thymosin or immunocompetent patients receiving a low dose of thymosin did seem to benefit. Thus there may be risk involving in administering an immunorestorative agent such as thymosin or levamisole to already immunocompetent subjects.

In summary, there is evidence in animals and in man that thymic deficiency may be corrected by the administration of thymic factors. There is some evidence that thymic deficiency is associated with malignancy. Therefore, immunotherapy of the immunorestorative type with agents like thymosin or levamisole seems to be indicated. Administration of thymosin to cancer patients can improve their immunological function. Phase I and II trials are now in progress. There is some evidence that administration of thymosin to immunocompetent patients may be dangerous. Progress in this area will depend on the following: more complete definition and charization of T-cell deficiencies in cancer patients, development of simple techniques for ongoing evaluation of T-cell-associated host defense in cancer, complete purification and characterization of thymic hormones, definitive phase I trials in immunodeficient cancer patients, and well-designed and controlled phase II trials of efficacy in appropriate disease categories.

15. Levamisole

A unique immunological reagent which has already shown some activity in immunotherapy of animal and human tumors is levamisole. This imidazole

EVAN M. HERSH,
G. M. MAVLIGIT,
J. U. GUTTERMAN,
AND
S. P. RICHMAN

compound is likely to be the prototype of a class of immunorestorative and immunopotentiating agents which, via their action on biochemical mechanisms of host defense cells, restore or augment general host defense mechanisms and therefore improve host defense against tumors. Levamisole has been used for a number of years as an antihelminthic agent (Thienpont et al., 1966). It was then discovered to increase the antibody response to a variety of antigens in experimental animals (Renoux and Renoux, 1973). The first observation in man was that the administration of levamisole increased tuberculin and DNCB reactivity among immunodeficient individuals and had essentially no effect on the immunological reactivity of immunologically normal individuals (Tripodi et al., 1973). This has now been observed in patients with a variety of solid tumors (Verhaegen et al., 1973) and lymphomas (Ramot et al., 1976), and involves various measures of host defense including DTH, lymphocyte blastogenesis, and T-cell numbers. On this basis, immunotherapeutic trials have been started in a number of these tumor categories in experimental animals and in man, and effective immunotherapy for breast cancer (Rojas et al., 1976) and lung cancer (Amery, 1976) has already been reported.

In vitro, levamisole has been demonstrated to increase lymphocyte blastogenic responses to a variety of antigens and mitogens including PHA, PPD, candidin, and measles virus, and in the MLC (Pabst and Crawford, 1974). These effects have been described for experimental animal and human lymphocytes. In addition, baseline proliferation of unstimulated human and mouse spleen lymphocytes has been described (Pabst and Crawford, 1974). These effects are seen at low doses of levamisole, and high doses may suppress spontaneous and mitogen or antigen-induced lymphocyte proliferation. Recent studies by Sunshine et al. (1977) have indicated that the mechanism of this effect is through the cyclic nucleotide system and may be similar to the well-known effects of imidazole in this system. Lympho-cyte cyclic AMP phosphodiesterase levels are increased while cyclic GMP phos-phodiesterase levels are decreased, and this results in increased levels of cyclic GMP and decreased levels of cyclic AMP, thus facilitating their proliferation.

Levamisole has a number of other related and unrelated effects. Thus it can increase the number of T-cell rosettes when added to lymphocyte suspensions from T-cell-deficient subjects in vitro (Ramot et al., 1976), it can restore and stabilize the number of rosette-forming cells in mice receiving azathioprine therapy (Van Ghinckel and Hoebeke, 1977) and it can increase suppressor-cell activity (Sampson and Lui, 1975). It has effects on other systems as well, in that it increases carbon particle clearance by the reticuloendothelial system (Hoebeke and Franchi, 1973), increases leukocyte motility (Douglas et al., 1976), and increase chemotaxis and phagocytosis by monocytes (Gallin and Wolfe, 1975). While not studied, the mechanisms here may also be mediated through the cyclic nucleotide system.

In vivo administration of levamisole has a variety of immunological effects. Thus the original observation that the in vivo administration of levamisole to patients increases delayed hypersensitivity responses to PPD and DNCB has been widely confirmed. In T-cell-deficient individuals, the administration of levamisole *in vivo* increases the numbers of circulating T-cell rosettes, and peripheral blood lymphocytes of these patients have increased *in vitro* responsiveness to PHA and other mitogens and antigens (Ramot *et al.*, 1976). These observations have been made in individuals without known diseases as well as in individuals with malignant and autoimmune diseases.

Levamisole has been studied in several animal tumor models. In an early study, Renoux and Renoux (1972) reported that the administration of levamisole cured a fraction of animals with the Lewis lung carcinoma. This has not been confirmed by other workers, and most studies in animal tumor models have not shown significant antitumor activity for levamisole used alone as the only antitumor agent (Potter *et al.*, 1974). However, in a study by Spreafico *et al.* (1975), levamisole was shown to be capable of reducing the number of pulmonary metastases of the Lewis lung tumor without increasing the mean survival time. Levamisole is also apparently capable of reducing pulmonary metastases in herpesvirus type I-induced tumores in hamsters (Thiry *et al.*, 1977). The mechanism probably does not involve direct antitumor activity but rather augmented host control of small foci of metastatic disease or host prevention of the metastatic event. In contrast to these generally negative resuts on direct antitumor activity, levamisole has been more convincingly shown to be effective in a variety of animal models when combined with other modalities of treatment. For example, in methylcholanthrene-induced mouse sarcoma, if cytoxan chemotherapy is followed by levamisole immunotherapy, prolonged survival is observed compared to chemotherapy alone (Chirigos *et al.*, 1974). The immune response to the tumors increases concomitantly. In the Lystra leukemia, cures are achieved at a higher rate of one dose of levamisole is given following BCNU chemotherapy than if levamisole is not given (Perk *et al.*, 1975). In L1210 leukemia, if immunotherapy with irradiated tumor cells and levamisole are given concurrently, an increased mean survival time is observed (Spreafico *et al.*, 1975). If nitrosourea chemotherapy for the Lewis lung tumor is followed by a single dose of levamisole approximately 7 days later, an increased mean survival time and an increased cure rate are observed (Spreafico *et al.*, 1975). In contrast, no effects of levamisole have been associated with its addition to other modalities of immunotherapy for the rat fibrosarcoma (Hopper *et al.*, 1975), and in one study, when levamisole was given for treatment of L1210 leukemia in the allogeneic setting, enhancement of tumor growth rather than an immunotherapeutic effect was observed (Mantovani and Spreafico, 1975).

In man, there are now several relevant observations. In nonmalignant disease, levamisole has been shown to induce remission in both rheumatoid arthritis and systemic lupus (Gordon and Keenan, 1975). The mechanism here is felt to be activation of suppressor cells with a restoration of the immune balance, the disturbance of which is felt to be fundamental to the expression of these diseases. A variety of infectious diseases in man, in which impaired cell-mediated immunity is thought to be the main host defense problem, have also responded to levamisole. These include aphthous stomatitis (Symdens and Brugmans, 1974) and recurrent herpes labialis (Kint and Verlinden, 1974), in which a decline of

EVAN M. HERSH,
G. M. MAVLIGIT,
J. U. GUTTERMAN,
AND
S. P. RICHMAN

cell-mediated immunity to the herpesvirus, as measured by leukocyte migration inhibition, immediately precedes the recurrent episode. If levamisole is administered for 3 days every 2 weeks, the frequency and severity of these recurrent episodes are markedly reduced.

In human cancer, there are several cases of cutaneous metastases of solid tumors which have been observed to regress after the administration of levamisole alone without any other therapy. There is one case reported in which immunoblastic lymphadenopathy entered a good partial remission for a period of 2 years after the institution of levamisole therapy (Bensa *et al.*, 1976). Finally there are two clinical trials, one in breast cancer and the other in lung cancer, in which levamisole has been demonstrated to have what appears to be a striking immunotherapeutic effect. In the first study, patients with stage I lung cancer received 150 mg of levamisole in three divided doses per day for 3 consecutive days, repeated every 2 weeks starting 3 days prior to surgery (Amery, 1976). There was significant improvement in survival, and reduced recurrence in patients under 70 kg in weight who had primary tumors at least 4 cm in diameter. Patients with smaller tumors showed no difference compared to a placebo matched control. A total of 69 patients were treated with levamisole and 79 were treated with placebo. Intrathoracic relapses were not significantly reduced by the administration of levamisole, whereas distant metastases were significantly reduced. In the other study, 43 patients with inoperable stage III breast carcinoma were placed on a similar regimen of levamisole after being rendered clinically free of disease by radiotherapy (Rojas *et al.*, 1976). Twenty-three patients were in the control group and 20 patients were in the levamisole group. There was significant prolongation of the median disease-free interval from 9 to 25 months, and there was prolongation of survival in the levamisole-treated group compared to the control. In the control, 35% were alive at 30 months, compared to 90% of the levamisole-treated patients. In both of these studies, associated investigations of delayed hypersentivity revealed its boosting in the patients receiving levamisole. In neither study was major toxicity of levamisole observed. However, it is known that higher doses of this compound are associated with modest toxicity including nausea, vomiting, anorexia, and a variety of mild and transient neurological and emotional symptoms. Finally, in our clinic, levamisole immunotherapy has been added to actinomycin D chemotherapy for advanced refractory malignant melanoma (S. Hall, unpublished observations). A prolongation of survival but no effect on the marginal response rate (9%) was observed.

Thus the use of levamisole in immunotherapy is of great promise. It is a simple chemical compound taken by mouth with few if any severe side effects. Its immunological effects can be measured quite accurately. There is reasonable evidence to suggest that it is active in restoring immunity in immunologically depressed individuals. The use of this compound opens a new and exciting chapter in the field of immunotherapy. However, precautions with its use must be exercised. Higher doses may be immunosuppressive, and tumor enhancement has been demonstrated in animal systems. It seems likely that one of the major uses of levamisole will be the restoration of immunocompetence so that the

immunodeficient or immunodepressed patient will respond more effectively to
active-specific immunotherapy and to active-nonspecific immunotherapy with
immunopotentiating and macrophage-activating agents such as BCG, MER and
C. parvum.

493
IMMUNOTHERAPY
OF HUMAN
CANCER

16. Passive Immunotherapy

The term "passive immunotherapy" implies the administration of serological
components which might have direct or indirect antitumor activity. While, in
general, the concept of serotherapy is restricted to antibody, it might also include
other components such as complement, circulating lymphokines, or other circulating factors with antitumor activity. Passive immunotherapy is the least well
developed and least completely explored component of immunotherapy. This is
because most emphasis in cancer has been placed on various aspects of cell-
mediated immunity, and, in addition, only a limited number of animal experiments have been done in which the role of antibody as a component of antitumor
host defense has been intensively investigated. The potential for passive
immunotherapy is further complicated by the observation that certain antitumor
antibody preparations can contain enhancing activity, i.e., activity which accelerates rather than retards tumor growth (Kaliss, 1962). Since the nature of this
enhancing activity, the *in vitro* correlative of which is blocking of cell-mediated
immunity or blocking factors (Hellström *et al.*, 1968, 1971), is not well understood,
the enthusiasm of laboratory or clinical investigators to work in this area is further
reduced. In spite of this, there are some data regarding passive immunotherapy
with various antibody preparations, and this approach, while still highly experimental, may eventually play an important role in clinical immunotherapy.

The basis for antibody-associated passive serum immunotherapy is that one can
demonstrate antibody activity against tumors *in vitro*. Thus antibody from
specifically immunized allogeneic or xenogeneic (Fefer, 1971*b*) animals, from
specifically immunized syngeneic animals (Hellström and Hellström, 1974), and
from animals whose tumors have regressed either spontaneously or because of a
variety of types of therapy (Hellström and Hellström, 1974) can kill cells *in vitro* in
the presence of complement. Antibody can also arm various leukocytes, including
lymphocytes and macrophages, by attaching via the Fc component of the
immunoglubin molecule, and these armed cells can then kill or inhibit the growth
of tumor cells (Pollack *et al.*, 1972). Antibody can also coat target tumor cells and
make them susceptible to the activity of lymphocytes or macrophages with the
specific ability to recognize and selectively kill them. This is referred to as
"antibody-dependent cell-mediated cytotoxicity" (Skurzak *et al.*, 1972). Finally,
serum either from immunized animals or from animals with regressing tumors
can have deblocking activity. It can reverse the blocking effect of so-called
progressor serum from animals with progressively growing tumors on cell-
mediated cytotoxicity to tumor cells *in vitro* (Bansal and Sjögren, 1972).

EVAN M. HERSH,
G. M. MAVLIGIT,
J. U. GUTTERMAN,
AND
S. P. RICHMAN

The major reservation relating to passive immunotherapy is that allogeneic and xenogeneic antitumor antibody produced by immunization can cause tumor enhancement or the accelerated take or growth of transplanted tumor cells (Kaliss, 1962). This has been demonstrated in several animal models, and is one of the earliest observations made in the field of tumor immunology. The presence of enhancing activity relates to the method of antibody induction, the dose and timing of the antibody, and the immunoglobulin class (Hellström and Möller, 1965). Most, but not all, studies indicate that enhancing activity is the IgG fraction, while inhibitory activity is in the IgM fraction (Hellström and Möller, 1965). Recent analogous studies in tissue transplantation in mice have indicated that it is the IgG_1 subclass of immunoglobulin which contains this enhancing activity. Obviously, before an antiserum is used in a clinical experiment it should be characterized for this type of activity. At present, appropriate *in vitro* assays for this activity do not exist.

In animal experiments, serotherapy or passive immunotherapy has been most active in immunoprophylaxis, and has shown less activity in true immunotherapy. In animals with tumors less than 1 week after implantantation, there is some evidence that antiserum alone can cause significant regression of tumor and even prolong tumor-free intervals in approximately 20% of cases (Gorer, 1956). The tumors that have shown responses to passive immunotherapy in animal systems include the EL4, L1210, Friend leukemia virus-induced, and Moloney leukemia virus-induced tumors in mice, Moloney lymphoma in rats, AKR leukemia in mice, and polyoma- and SV40-induced fibrosarcomas in hamsters (Wright *et al.*, 1976). Experimental ovarian carcinomas and experimental malignant melanomas have also shown some response (Hill and Littlejohn, 1971).

Another type of passive immunotherapy involves the coupling of radioactive isotopes, drugs, or toxins to antitumor antibody (Davies and O'Neal, 1976). These antibodies then deliver the antitumor agent directly to the tumor. There are a number of experiments in which the drug or the antitumor antibody alone has little effect on the tumor, while the combination has a dramatic effect, clearly indicating synergism. For example, Reif *et al.* (1976) made specific antibody to L1210 leukemia and to EL4 lymphoma by immunizing with tumor cells and at the same time administering antibody to normal cellular components. An alkylating agent was coupled to this highly purified antibody, and the complex of antibody and drug was effective, while the drug complexed to normal γ-globulin was ineffective. However, in this experiment, administration of drug and antibody simultaneously but separately was also effective. Ghose *et al.* (1967) coupled the drug chlorambucil or high specific activity ^{131}I to antibody made in another species to either EL4 lymphoma or B16 melanoma. Antitumor activity and prolongation of survival were demonstrated by the complex but not by either reagent alone. Scanning of treated tumor-bearing animals showed that the isotope localized the tumor 5 times more than it localized in other tissues. Molton *et al.* (1976) have studied the effects of passive immunotherapy with antiserum to SV40-induced tumor-cell surface antigens coupled to various toxins in hamster lymphomas. Toxins that have been studied or that are currently under study include diphtheria toxin, phospholipase C, ribonuclease, and ricin, which is a plant extract with activity similar to that of diphtheria toxin. With diphtheria toxin coupled antibody in a transplantable tumor system, there is moderate and acceptable systemic toxicity and a 50% regression rate, 20% of which is permanent.

There have been a very limited number of studies of passive immunotherapy in man. None of these studies has been controlled, none has been carried out with adequate numbers of patients, and none has been carried out with highly purified well-characterized immunoglobulin components. Therefore, none is really useful in evaluating the potential for passive immunotherapy. Furthermore, none has come to grips with the major problem regarding passive immunotherapy with heterologous antiserum, which, of course, is the danger of allergic reactivity developing to the therapeutic reagent itself. Early in this century, Lindstrom (1927) used rabbit antisera made to AML cells and induced some degree of remission by administering this antiserum plus radiotherapy and chemotherapy to four out of 11 patients with AML. Hueper and Russell (1932) made a rabbit antibody to CML and treated one patient, with resultant decrease in peripheral blood count and diminution in spleen size. De Carvalho (1963) made a horse antiserum to leukemia cells, administered this to 15 patients, and claimed some degree of objective remission in 11 of these. Murry (1958) made antisera in horses to breast cancer tissue, treated a relatively large number of patients, and claimed decreased pain, decreased pleural effusion, decreased size of lung metastases, and recalcification of tumor. It is unclear what ancillary therapy these patients may have also received.

More recently, Lazlo et al. (1968) and Herberman et al. (1969) used antiserum made against normal leukocytes (presumably anti-HLA antibody) in allogeneic subjects and administered this to patients with chronic lymphocytic leukemia. Both investigators observed transient diminution in peripheral blood counts without any other significant changes. Also, Skurkovich et al. (1969) reported prolongation of remission duration in acute leukemia patients receiving repeated transfusions of autologous plasma and autologous leukocytes. It is impossible in the last study to sort out which of the agents had the therapeutic benefits. In Burkitt's lymphoma, there have been two reports of the administration of serum from patients in remission to patients with active disease (Ngu, 1967; Burkitt, 1967). Large amounts of serum were administered, and objective tumor regression was observed. However, Fass et al. (1970), using much smaller amounts of serum from apparently cured patients, could not confirm this observation in five cases.

There is also some hint of activity in solid tumors for passive immunotherapy. Sumner and Foraker (1960) and Teimoorian and McCune (1963), in separate experiments administered serum from patients free of disease to patients with metastatic disease. Both investigators observed single instances of regression of tumor. There is also a report of regression of metastatic renal cell cancer after transfusion of serum from an apparently cured relative who previously had the same histological type of tumor (Horn and Horn, 1971). Since none of these studies was controlled in any way, it is impossible to evaluate them adequately.

EVAN M. HERSH,
G. M. MAVLIGIT,
J. U. GUTTERMAN,
AND
S. P. RICHMAN

Recently, there has been some limited experience with treatment of human tumors with drug coupled to antibody. Ghose *et al.* (1976) have treated a group of melanoma patients with chlorambucil-bound heterologous antimelanoma antibody and compared the results to those from treatment of patients in a conventional manner with DTIC. In the group receiving the drug–antibody complex, there were two complete remissions and an improvement in survival compared to the patients receiving DTIC. In a patient subsequently showing recurrent tumor, the tumor had a diminution of those surface markers recognized by the heterologous antibody. This suggested that antibody may modulate the tumor-cell surface and that a type of antibody resistence may result. Also, there are no data concerning whether the groups of patients were comparable in any way, and therefore this study is very difficult to interpret.

Recently, there has been a great deal of interest in leukopheresis or other plasma or serum reduction techniques with or without serum or plasma transfusion. A number of investigators have demonstrated improved immunological antitumor reactivity by this maneuver (Isbister *et al.*, 1975), and one investigator has claimed therapeutic benefit (Hesey *et al.*, 1976). Whether this approach is due to the removal of blocking factors or whether it is due to the administration of some absent normal component in the transfused plasma is not known at this time.

In summary, a minimal amount of work has been done on passive immunotherapy. In animal models, there is some evidence that heterologous antibody can cause tumor regression or can prolong remission. However, this is complicated by the potential and actual demonstration of enhancing effects. In man, there are more than 20 studies claiming some activity for passive immunotherapy with antiserum. However, all of these studies are on small numbers of patients, are poorly controlled, or have other defects which make interpretation extremely difficult. All that can be stated at this time is that there is some evidence that in isolated cases tumor regression can be induced in man by either heterologous antiserum, allogenic antiserum, or serum obtained from patients who have gone into remission as a result of conventional therapy. Future work in animals should be directed toward careful characterization of antitumor antibodies either spontaneous or induced in syngeneic, allogeneic, or xenogeneic subjects. The *in vitro* activity of these antibodies should be carefully characterized in terms of whether they are cytotoxic, can cooperate with lymphoid cells or macrophages, have deblocking activity, etc. Then careful, clinically relevant animal model experiments should be done in which dose and timing features are investigated. Finally, purified classes of immunoglobulins should be investigated with particular reference to using subcomponents of immunoglobulin which might not be immunogenic. The role of complement and other serum components also should be investigated. Work in man should be directed toward the development of highly specific antitumor antibody, the characterization of this antibody *in vitro*, the use of nonimmunogenic immunoglobulin subcomponents, adequate dose–response studies, and studies of combination of passive serum immunotherapy with other modalities of cancer treatment. The work with cytotoxic substances, drugs, radioisotopes, or toxins also warrants further study.

"Local immunotherapy" is really a misnomer, because the local or regional treatment of a malignant tumor with an immunotherapeutic reagent often has a systemic effect and usually depends on systemic immunocompetence for local efficacy. Local immunotherapy is the application of an immunotherapeutic reagent in the region of a primary or metastatic tumor or into the tumor itself. There are three broad types of local immunotherapy. The first is topical or epilesional treatment, which can be used in the case of an intradermal tumor. The immunotherapeutic reagent is placed directly over the tumor on the surface of the skin or is introduced into the skin by techniques such as scarification (Richman *et al.*, 1975) and intradermal injection (Klein *et al.*, 1976). The second is true intratumoral or intralesional inoculation, in which the immunotherapeutic agent is injected directly into the tumor. This is usually applied to intradermal or subcutaneous tumors (Morton *et al.*, 1970). The third, which may be classified as a form of local immunotherapy, is regional immunotherapy. This refers to placement of an immunotherapeutic reagent in the region of a primary or metastatic tumor, either before or after that tumor is removed surgically or treated locally with radiotherapy (McKneally *et al.*, 1976). There is then interaction between the agent and the tumor cell or tumor antigen in the lymphatic drainage and/or in the regional lymph node.

The essential feature of local immunotherapy is a delayed hypersensitivity reaction to the adjuvant at the site of the tumor and killing of tumor cells by a bystander effect of delayed hypersensitivity. There is compelling evidence from the animal model and suggestive evidence in man that the effector cell is the activated macrophage (Alexander *et al.*, 1976). The second major feature, as yet poorly understood, is some type of direct or indirect interaction between the immunotherapeutic agent and either the tumor cells or tumor antigens. This results in either the introduction of modified tumor antigen into the lymph node or some modification of the distribution in or presentation of the antigen to the lymph node (Alexander *et al.*, 1976). At any rate, what results is a much more vigorous sensitization of the host and the development of systemic tumor immunity so that the host is resistant to challenge with tumor cells at another site, or even so that distant metastases regress (Zbar and Tanaka, 1971). The prime requisites for effective local immunotherapy include a modest size of the tumor (large tumors do not respond) (Zbar *et al.*, 1972) and immunocompetence on the part of the host (Bartlett *et al.*, 1972). The one exception to this may be the use of lymphokines, which may directly attract and activate macrophages or other host defense cells in local immunotherapy (Papermaster *et al.*, 1976a). However, even in this case, a normal monocyte macrophage system may be required.

The immunotherapeutic agents which have been active in local immunotherapy include the following (Table 9): intact viable or killed microbial agents, including BCG (Morton *et al.*, 1970), *C. parvum* (Scott, 1974a), and vaccinia virus (Everall *et al.*, 1975); derivatives of microbial agents, including the BCG cell-wall skeleton (Yamamura *et al.*, 1975) and MER (Weiss, 1977); purified

EVAN M. HERSH,
G. M. MAVLIGIT,
J. U. GUTTERMAN,
AND
S. P. RICHMAN

TABLE 9

Topical and Intratumoral Immunotherapy[a]

Histological type of tumor	Stage	Agent(s)	Route	Result
Basal cell carcinoma	Primary	TEIB DNCB	Topical	Cure in 95%
Mycosis fungoides	Cutaneous	TEIB DNCB	Topical	Regression in immunocompetent patients
Various solid tumors	Cutaneous metastases	DNCB TEIB	Topical	Regression in immunocompetent patients
Malignant melanoma	Cutaneous metastases	Vaccinia virus	Intralesional (IL)	Partial to complete remission in about 50%
Malignant melanoma	Primary	Vaccinia virus	IL followed by surgery	Increased DFI and survival
Malignant melanoma	Cutaneous metastases	BCG	IL	Regression of injected nodules in 30–80%
Various solid tumors	Cutaneous metastases	BCG	IL	Regression of injected nodules in about 50%
Various solid tumors	Cutaneous metastases	PHA-activated lymphocytes	IL	Regression of injected nodules in 90%
Various solid tumors	Cutaneous metastases	Lymphokines	IL	Regression of injected nodules in 50%
Various solid tumors	Cutaneous metastases	Glucan + humoral recognition factor	IL	Regression of injected nodules in 90%
Prostatic cancer	Stage D	BCG	IL	Regression of mass in 5/7
Glioblastoma	Recurrent intracerebral	Autologous lymphocytes	IL	Regression or improvement in about 35%

[a] Abbreviations: TEIB, triethyleneiminobenzoquinone; DNCB, dinitrochlorobenzene; IL, intralesional; BCG, bacillus Calmette Guérin; DFI, disease-free interval; PHA, phytohemagglutinin.

or semipurified antigens, such as DNCB (Klein and Holterman, 1972), TEIB (Stjernsward and Levin, 1971), PPD (Klein *et al.*, 1975), and streptokinase-streptodornase (Klein *et al.*, 1975); drugs such as nitrogen mustard (Waldorf *et al.*, 1967) and 5-fluoruracil (Litwin *et al.*, 1975); and, more recently, a whole spectrum of newer drugs including nitrosoureas and adriamycin (Borsos *et al.*, 1976); and, finally, lymphokines, the products of activated lymphocytes. In the case of local immunotherapy with drugs, increased specific immune activation by drug–tumor-antigen complex or by tumor antigen released from dying tumor cells might be hypothesized as one of the mechanisms of action.

Animal models in which local immunotherapy has been shown to be effective include the guinea pig hepatoma (Zbar and Tanaka, 1971), hamster melanoma

(Paslin *et al.*, 1974), and, more recently, oculosquamous cell carcinoma of
Hereford cattle (H. J. Rapp, personal communication). Local immunotherapy of
both metastatic disease and primary tumors has been shown to be effective in man.
Early studies by Morton *et al.* (1970) and by Klein *et al.* (1976) showed that
malignant melanoma nodules would regress when directly injected with BCG and
that metastatic breast cancer lesions as well as primary skin cancer lesions would
clear completely when painted with DNCB, nitrogen mustard, or 5-fluorouracil
(FU) (Litwin *et al.*, 1975). PPD and DNCB are also effective, but only in previously
sensitized subjects who can manifest delayed hypersensitivity (Klein *et al.*, 1975).
Recently, it has been demonstrated that delayed hypersensitivity also develops to
topical nitrogen mustard and topical FU (Waldorf *et al.*, 1967; Litwin *et al.*, 1975).
There is a good correlation between the development of delayed hypersensitivity
to FU and the response of the local lesion. Therefore, it can be assumed that these
drugs are acting through an immunological mechanism. This has recently been
confirmed by studies in the guinea pig hepatoma, in which a variety of
chemotherapeutic agents have been used for intralesional chemotherapy. Animals which show complete regression of tumor after intralesional chemotherapy
are resistant to subsequent tumor challenge, indicating activation of systemic host
defense mechanisms and immunological memory to tumor antigens (Zbar and
Tanaka, 1971). This is also demonstrated by the fact that most workers in this field
at the clinical level have found that a small but significant fraction of non-locally
treated tumors will also regress in patients receiving local immunotherapy to some
but not all of their tumor nodules (Rosenberg and Rapp, 1976).

A number of studies have also been reported in which local or regional
immunotherapy is being used to treat early cancer. Primary squamous skin
tumors respond to topical agents such as DNCB (Klein *et al.*, 1975). The injection
of the primary malignant melanoma lesions with vaccinia virus prior to excision
has delayed the recurrence and prolonged the survival (Everall *et al.*, 1975).
Intravesicular BCG is reported to reduce the incidence or the rate of development
of primary recurrent bladder cancers (Eidinger and Moralis, 1976), and intrapleural BCG after surgical extirpation of stage I lung cancer is associated with a
striking prolongation of disease-free interval and survival compared to concurrent controls (McKneally *et al.*, 1976). The topical application of DNCB to the
cervix in sensitized women has delayed the appearance of primary cervical cancer
after the appearance of malignant cells in the pap smear (Guthrie and Way, 1975).

These data suggest several important principles and avenues for investigation
in the future. Local lesions, if small and superficial, should be treated by local
immunotherapy if possible. If the host is immunocompetent, a variety of antigenic
materials as described above may be used. If the host is immunoincompetent, the
use of lymphokines may be effective, as reported in one small series by Papermaster *et al.* (1976*a*). In addition to curing the local lesion, these local approaches may
heighten systemic tumor immunity. Most important, the animal studies and the
limited clinical data indicate the need to investigate primary intralesional therapy
of a variety of malignant tumors prior to their surgical extirpation. It is conceivable that the ideal approach to the therapy of malignant solid tumors in man is

500

EVAN M. HERSH,
G. M. MAVLIGIT,
J. U. GUTTERMAN,
AND
S. P. RICHMAN

direct intralesional injection of an active-nonspecific immunotherapeutic agent such as BCG or one of its purified derivatives, a chemotherapeutic agent, or a haptene, which may modify the antigenicity and immunogenicity of cells of the primary tumor. A period of time would then be allowed to pass, during which interaction of adjuvant and tumor cells would occur, the host would mount an immune response at the local site, and systemic tumor immunity would develop. The primary tumor or its residual would then be excised completely, and the host, with markedly heightened regional and systemic tumor immunity, would not develop recurrence of disease, even in poor-prognosis disease categories. Such trials are now beginning in several centers.

18. Immunotherapy of Various Disease Categories in Man

18.1. Immunotherapy of Malignant Melanoma

The biological characteristics of malignant melanoma make it an excellent candidate for immunotherapeutic approaches, and it indeed has served as a model for the development of some of the principles of immunotherapy. The disease most frequently starts in the skin, travels by means of regional lymphatics to regional lymph nodes, and disseminates either from there or from second or third lymph node groups hematogeneously to organs such as brain, lungs, and liver. Thus the disease has periods when it is localized, when it is regional, and when it is widely metastatic. There is also considerable evidence (beyond the scope of this chapter) that malignant melanoma is under host control and that specific immunity of both the humoral and cell-mediated types develop to it in the tumor-bearing patient. The presence of this host control and its presumed breakdown in the patient who disseminates also make this disease an ideal candidate for immunotherapy. Finally, at every stage of the disease—i.e., when it is primary, when it is metastatic to the regional lymph nodes, or even in selected circumstances when it is metastatic to distant organs—the patients can be brought into a state of no clinically evident disease by surgery. Thus even patients with widely disseminated disease can have the tumor burden reduced to a minimum and therefore can become excellent candidates for immunotherapy.

Immunotherapy has been studied fairly extensively in melanoma (Table 10). There are three major approaches to immunotherapy based on the location and extent of disease. Intralesional therapy, i.e., the injection directly into the tumor nodule of an immunoreactive reagent, can be used in cases of cutaneous or subcutaneous metastatic nodules. It is also beginning to be investigated for treatment of the primary tumors. The second approach is after surgical extirpation of regional or distant disease, when the patient is in a state of no evident disease. The third is in patients with widely metastatic disease.

Intralesional therapy for metastatic disease has already been discussed in detail in the section on local immunotherapy. Intralesional therapy with BCG, vaccinia, other microbial adjuvants, activated lymphocytes, or lymphokines has been

TABLE 10
Immunotherapy of Malignant Melanoma[a]

Stage (Anderson)	Evident Disease	Immunotherapy	Concurrent Chemotherapy	Result
I	Yes	Vaccinia IL then surgery	No	Increased DFI and S
I	Yes	BCG IL then surgery	No	Too early
I	No	BCG (cutaneous)	No	Too early
IV	No	BCG (cutaneous)	No	Increased DFI and S
III	No	BCG plus allo. irr. cultured TC	No	Increased DFI and S
IVA	No	BCG (cutaneous)	No	Increased DFI and S
IVB	Yes	BCG (cutaneous)	Yes	Increased remission duration and S
IVB	Yes	BCG plus autolo. irr. TC	No	Regression in 40%
IVB	Yes	BCG plus allo. irr. TC	Yes	Remission in 60%
IVB	Yes	*C. parvum* i.v. for 14 days	Yes	Increased remission rate, duration, and S
IVB	Yes	BCG (oral)	No	Tumor regression and S
IVB	Yes	Cross-grafting and cross-leukocyte transfusion	No	Tumor regression in 26/123
IVB	Yes	Transfer factor	No	Tumor regression in about 20%
IVB	Yes	Transfusion of remission serum	No	Tumor regression
IVB	Yes	Tranfusion of anti-body-bound drug	Yes	Increased remission rate
IVB	Yes	Levamisole	Yes	Increased survival

[a] Abbreviations and definitions: stage I, primary III, regional lymph node metastases; IVA, distant metastases but no evident disease; IVB, distant metastases, evident disease; IL, intralesional; DFI, disease-free interval; S, survival; allo., allogeneic; autolo., autologous; irr., irradiated; TC, tumor cells, i.v., intravenous.

effective in eradicating local tumor nodules. Under such circumstances, noninjected nodules usually do not regress, but regression has been described in from 0% to 20% of uninjected nodules. Nodule regression is most common in cutaneous and less common in subcutaneous nodules. Regression is more common in small than in large nodules and is seen more commonly in immunocompetent patients and only rarely in immunoincompetent patients. Intralesional therapy may induce an increase in specific tumor immunity which might benefit the host–tumor interaction in general. However, no clinical study has ever been done in which nodule injection has been combined with other forms of treatment in an interpretable way to determine whether nodule injection with active-nonspecific immunotherapeutic or other reagents could improve the overall response rate, response duration, or survival found with conventional therapy. Intralesional therapy is beginning to be explored now for primary tumor. The primary tumor is injected, and subsequently, after a vigorous immune response has developed, the

502

EVAN M. HERSH,
G. M. MAVLIGIT,
J. U. GUTTERMAN,
AND
S. P. RICHMAN

injected primary tumor is removed. This has been carried out with the vaccinia virus, and prolongation of the disease-free interval after the removal of the primary tumor has been observed (Everall *et al.*, 1975). Intralesional therapy is currently under investigation with BCG (Rosenberg and Rapp, 1976).

The most extensive studies of immunotherapy in malignant melanoma have been done to prevent recurrence after extirpation of regional metastatic disease. The experimental design in general is that either at the time of primary surgery, when prophylactic regional lymph node dissection is done, or subsequently, when metastatic disease presents itself clinically in the regional lymph node area, lymphadenectomy is carried out, after which the patient is subjected to immunotherapy. We refer to these as "stage IIIB patients." For patients with one positive lymph node, there is approximately a 55% cure rate by this surgery. For patients with two or more positive lymph nodes, the cure rate is under 20%. Therefore, adjuvant treatment of some kind is obviously required.

The major approach has been the use of BCG. Studies have been carried out by Morton *et al.* (1974), Siegler *et al.* (1976), Gutterman *et al.* (1973c, 1974a), Grant *et al.* (1974), Ikonopisov (1975), and Berreta (1977), to name just a few. The results basically show that the addition of BCG immunotherapy will prolong the remission and survival of at least certain subgroups of patients with this malignant melanoma. Not all studies have been positive, and those by Pinsky *et al.* (1976), Cunningham *et al.* (1977), and Simmons (1977) utilizing BCG alone or in combination with tumor cells and by Spitler *et al.* (1977) utilizing levamisole have shown no difference from the appropriate controls. Detailed discussion of some of these studies is indicated.

Morton *et al.* (1974) have administered BCG alone by multipuncture plate in patients who had had lymph node metastases of melanoma removed by prophylactic lymph node dissection. High doses of Tice strain BCG were administered simultaneously in the axillary and inguinal drainage bilaterally, and over the primary site. Regardless of the location of the primary site, these patients have shown prolongation of disease-free interval and survival. In their first study, which utilized historical controls from their own institution, and from other institutions, approximately a doubling of the disease-free interval was observed. This group has subsequently initiated a randomized trial comparing no further treatment to BCG alone and BCG plus an allogenic cultured tumor-cell vaccine in the same stage of patients (Spitler *et al.*, 1977). Treatments are approximately weekly for the first 3 months, and then monthly. The prolongation of the disease-free interval by either BCG or BCG plus tumor cells is at the borderline of significance at this time.

Our group has done extensive studies with BCG immunotherapy of malignant melanoma. Patients with regional lymph node metastases which had presented clinically are rendered free of disease by surgery and then are placed on BCG by scarification to the four proximal extremities by rotation. Treatment is weekly for 3 months, and then every other week. We have not given BCG over the primary site. In a study comparing low and high doses of BCG, only the high dose had broad immunotherapeutic effectiveness (Morton, 1977). Patients who originally had trunk or extremity primaries benefited, while there was no effect after metastatic disease had been removed if the primary had been in the head and neck area. This probably related to the lack of placement of BCG in the regional lymph node drainage. Several strains of BCG, including lyophilized Tice strain and fully viable suspension-grown Pasteur strain, have been utilized, and both are effective. However, low doses of BCG are usually without effect or even may produce tumor enhancement.

The observation of therapeutic efficacy of BCG has been confirmed by Ikonopisov and by Berreta, but has not been confirmed by Pinsky *et al.* (1976), Cunningham *et al.* (1977), Simmons (1977). A number of these nonconfirmatory studies suffer from several defects, including the use of a low dose of BCG and a failure to put the BCG in the drainage of the primary tumor. The general observation in the positive studies is that the disease-free interval and survival are approximately doubled; however, the majority of patients still relapse and progress. Therefore, BCG immunotherapy with or without tumor-cell vaccine must be considered as a preliminary first step in the development of effective immunotherapy for regional lymph node metastases of malignant melanoma.

Metastatic disease which cannot be removed surgically has been treated very ineffectively with chemotherapy alone. The most effective chemotherapy agents such as DTIC or the nitrosoureas produce approximately a 15–20% response rate, a median response duration of about 4 months, and an overall median survival of less than 7 months. We have observed that the addition of BCG immunotherapy between courses of chemotherapy, where the DTIC chemotherapy is given on days 1–5 and the BCG on days 7, 12, and 17 of each 21-day cycle, increases the remission rate among elderly patients and increases the remission duration and survival of responding patients compared to historical controls (Gutterman *et al.*, 1974*a*). This observation has also been made by Ikonopisov (1975). However, this observation could not be confirmed by Costanzi (1977), although the study was carried out with a different chemotherapy and therefore the studies are not directly comparable. Negative studies of adjuvant immunotherapy for metastatic melanoma have also been carried out by Presant *et al.* (1977). He combined chemotherapy with intravenous *C. parvum* on days 8 and 15 after chemotherapy at a dose of 5 mg/m^2 without benefit either on remission rate, remission duration, or survival.

Other approaches to immunotherapy of metastatic melanoma have been investigated with some promise. Mastrangelo *et al.* (1975) carried out a preliminary study in which they immunized patients with irradiated tumor cells mixed with BCG as the only treatment. A number of patients were observed to have regression of metastatic disease. Subsequently, Mastrangelo *et al.* (1977) carried out a definitive study in which patients were randomized to receive either chemotherapy with nitrosourea and vincristine or the same plus tumor-cell BCG vaccine. No effect on remission rate, remission duration, and survival duration was observed. Currie and McElwain (1975) immunized patients with irradiated tumor cells plus BCG before and between courses of DTIC chemotherapy. In a relatively small group of patients, they observed a 50% response rate, which was

504

EVAN M. HERSH,
G. M. MAVLIGIT,
J. U. GUTTERMAN,
AND
S. P. RICHMAN

much higher than had been observed by any other group using DTIC chemotherapy alone. Recently, Newlands *et al* (1976) attempted to confirm this observation by immunizing patients repeatedly with relatively low doses of tumor cells between courses of chemotherapy. No benefit was observed. Therefore, active specific immunotherapy in malignant melanoma needs further investigation before it can be fully evaluated.

Several investigators, including Vetto *et al.* (1976) and Spitler *et al.* (1972), have treated patients with transfer factor alone for metastatic malignant melanoma, and have observed patients who responded with tumor regression, sometimes complete. However, in a recent study, we added transfer factor immunotherapy (1×10^9 lymphocyte equivalent) monthly or weekly between courses of DTIC plus BCG (M. Schwarz, unpublished observations). While there was improvement in immunological reactivity, there was no benefit compared to DTIC-BCG alone without transfer factor immunotherapy. Thus the possible role of transfer factor in immunotherapy of melanoma remains unclear and requires further investigation. Adoptive immunotherapy with lymphocytes from actively immunized donors (Nadler and Moore, 1969) and passive immunotherapy (Wright *et al.*, 1976) have been sporadically carried out in malignant melanoma. None of these studies, however, can be considered extensive or definitive at this time.

A recent advance in systemic adjuvant immunotherapy, however, is worthy of note. We have treated a group of 64 patients having advanced metastatic disease with 2 weeks of *C. parvum* intravenously daily in doses escalating from 0 to 2 mg/m^2 followed by chemotherapy with DTIC or DTIC plus actinomycin D and subcutaneous *C. parvum* between courses. In addition, the 2 weeks of intraveneous *C. parvum* have been repeated every 3 months. We have observed a complete and partial remission rate of 43% in these patients (compared to the 27% on DTIC-BCG) and a marked improvement in remission duration and survival, with over 90% of patients alive at 6 months (J. U. Gutterman *et al.*, unpublished observations). We presume that this result is related to macrophage activation within the tumor, and to activation of the reticuloendothelial system. Thus systemic immunotherapy may be a major breakthrough in malignant melanoma. This observation was based on the findings of Band *et al.* (1975) and Israel *et al.* (1975), who showed that *C. parvum* immunotherapy alone could cause regression of pulmonary and liver metastases.

At present, we can conclude that for patients brought into a state of no evident disease by surgery, microbial adjuvant immunotherapy is beneficial and should be administered. For patients with metastatic melanoma, BCG immunotherapy added to chemotherapy has had some modest effect. A new breakthrough involving administration of 2 weeks of intensive immunotherapy prior to the start of intermittent chemotherapy may open a new pathway, not only to the treatment of malignant melanoma but for other malignant diseases as well.

18.2. Immunotherapy of Lung Cancer

Lung cancer is one of the most common as well as one of the most serious and highly fatal of the human malignancies. In spite of this, it is one of the most

TABLE 11
Immunotherapy of Lung Cancer[a]

Stage	Evident disease	Immunotherapy	Concurrent chemotherapy	Result
I	No	BCG, intrapleural	No	Increased DFI
II, III	No	BCG, intrapleural	No	No effect
I–II	No	BCG, cutaneous	No	Increased DFI and S
I–IV	No, yes	BCG–CWS–oil, multiple routes	Yes	Increased survival
III	Yes	BCG water extract	No	Partial remission
III, IV	Yes	*C. parvum* (SC)	Yes	Increased survival
III, IV	Yes	OK 432	Yes	Increased survival
II, III	Yes	Modified auto. TC + CFA	No	Increased survival
I	No	PAGE-purified tumor antigen + CFA	Yes	Increased DFI
I	No	Levamisole	No	Increased DFI and S
II, III	No	Levamisole	No	No effect

[a] Abbreviations: BCG, bacillus Calmette Guérin; DFI, disease-free interval; S, survival; CWS, cell-wall skeleton; PAGE, polyacrylamide gel electrophoresis; CFA, complete Freund's adjuvant; TC, tumor cells.

encouraging with regard to immunotherapy (Table 11). Lung tumors have been shown to contain tumor-associated antigens, and immunological reactivity to lung cancer cells or lung cancer antigens has been demonstrated in man. Most of the reports concerning immunotherapy in lung cancer for both minimal residual and advanced disease have been positive. There are several reports that the cutaneous administration of BCG repeatedly following surgery modestly prolongs the disease-free interval and the survival (Pines, 1976). However, this approach does not seem to offer much promise. In contrast, with regard to systemic immunotherapy, the intensive use of a systemic adjuvant such as *C. parvum* seems to offer considerable promise. It has already been demonstrated that intravenous *C. parvum* can cause regression of pulmonary metastases of other types of tumors, and this approach should certainly be investigated in lung cancer patients. One of the problems is the pulmonary toxicity of *C. parvum*, which may limit its use under the circumstance of the postoperative lung cancer patient. However, this would indicate the need for the use of a less toxic systemic adjuvant.

An experiment of nature has led to the development of what is currently the most exciting approach to immunotherapy of lung cancer. Ruckdeschel *et al.* (1972) carried out a retrospective study of lung cancer patients with postoperative empyema. The overall 5-year survival rate for the empyeme group of 18 patients was 50% compared to a 5-year survival of 18% in a control group of patients who did not have empyema but who were comparable in all other ways. Based on this observation, McKneally *et al.* (1976) began a study of intrapleural BCG in lung cancer following surgical extirpation of the primary tumor. Ninety-five patients were entered into the prospective study, which was stratified and randomized. Using a single injection of 10^7 viable units of Tice strain BCG, they observed a marked reduction in the incidence of recurrent cancer and a prolongation of the disease-free interval and survival in patients with stage I disease. More patients

EVAN M. HERSH,
G. M. MAVLIGIT,
J. U. GUTTERMAN,
AND
S. P. RICHMAN

have to be studied in stage II disease before the results can be interpreted since they are equivocal at this time. In stage III disease, intrapleural postoperative BCG was not beneficial. The median duration of the follow-up in this study is 20 months, at this time. Among 26 BCG-treated stage I patients, there have been two recurrences compared to nine among 32 controls not receiving BCG. We have already seen that regional immunotherapy is effective in malignant melanoma, and this is another example of effective regional immunotherapy. This experiment is currently being repeated in a number of clinics around the country with various additions of other approaches to immunotherapy, or other approaches to multimodality therapy with hopes of improving the results still further.

Japanese workers under the leadership of Professor Yamamura have been utilizing BCG cell-wall skeleton for the treatment of lung cancer (Yamamura *et al.*, 1976). Their approach is to instill the BCG cell-wall skeleton intrapleurally when that is possible, to inject it intralesionally at the time of surgery for inoperable disease, and to give the BCG cell-wall skeleton repeatedly intradermally between courses of chemotherapy for more advanced disease. This historically controlled study has shown positive beneficial effects in all stages of lung cancer, most interpretable in patients with stage III and IV disease. Thus in stage III disease the 50% survival in the control group is approximately 9 months, and it is at 20 months in patients receiving cell-wall skeleton. There are 56 treated patients compared to 72 controls. In stage IV disease, while all patients eventually die, the median survival of 30 patients treated with BCG cell-wall skeleton is 15 months compared to 3 months in 43 control patients. BCG cell-wall skeleton appears to have certain advantages because it can be better quantitated than BCG, and it can be administered by a variety of routes including intralesional and intracavitary without the danger of systemic BCG disease. These observations with cell-wall skeleton must be confirmed in large numbers of patients and by other groups.

A number of investigators are currently exploring the use of other adjuvant immunotherapy in more advanced lung cancer. For example, Dimitrov *et al.* (1977) have conducted a study in which patients receive adrimycin chemotherapy every 3 weeks plus weekly subcutaneous *C. parvum*. This was an extension of the original work with subcutaneous *C. parvum* carried out by Israel (1974). In both studies, it appears to have no effect on the remission rate; however, the remission duration and particularly the survival appear to be prolonged. The statistical significance is borderline.

Other approaches to immunotherapy of lung cancer are also showing potentially beneficial effects. One of these is immunorestorative therapy with levamisole. Amery (1976) in a multiinstitutional double-blind prospectively randomized study administered levamisole 50 mg by mouth, 3 times a day for 3 days every 2 weeks starting before surgery and continuing for 1 year. Among patients under 70 kg in weight, there was a statistically significant reduction in distant metastases and prolongation of survival in the treated compared to the placebo-controlled group. The benefit was most pronounced for patients who had relatively large tumors at the time of surgery. This study is currently being expanded with more carefully defined staging and with administration of levamisole according to the patient's weight, rather than according to a fixed dose. It has not yet been confirmed.

There are also two important studies of active-specific studies of lung cancer. In the first, Stewart *et al.* (1976) immunized patients with lung cancer in stages I and II after surgery with a purified tumor antigen preparation in complete Freund's adjuvant. Patients received three injections over approximately 3 months; there were three groups, patients treated with high-dose methotrexate or left untreated, patients given immunotherapy alone, or patients given immunotherapy plus high-dose methotrexate. Among 24 stage I controls, there have been six deaths, and an additional two patients have developed distant metastases. Among 11 patients receiving immunotherapy, one patient has developed distant metastases and three have developed local recurrence. Among 11 patients treated with immunochemotherapy, there has been one death, and no other patients had recurrence or developed a distant metastasis. The survival of the treated group is significantly longer than that of the control patients, with a *P* value of 0.001 at this time. This study is very promising and will be continued with larger numbers of patients. Takita *et al.* (1976) have carried out a study of active-specific immunotherapy in patients with locally far-advanced lung cancer that is conventionally inoperable. They observed 30 patients who underwent maximum tumor reduction by surgery, but who had residual tumor. Patients were divided postoperatively into one group which received adjuvant immunotherapy and the other group which served as a control. Adjuvant immunotherapy consisted of autologous tumor cell vaccine prepared by concanavalin A and neuraminidase treatment. This was administered in complete Freund's adjuvant on the day of surgery, and at 2-week intervals usually for three inoculations. Subsequently, the patients received 0.02 mg of Glaxo strain BCG intradermally in both deltoid regions for four doses. BCG was then continued every 6 weeks for several years. At present, seven of the 15 treated patients are alive, with a median survival estimated at 34 months, while only three of the 15 controls are alive, with a median survival of 12 months. This difference is statistically significant, with a *P* value of 0.05.

In summary, in spite of its poor prognosis, most studies of immunotherapy in lung cancer have led to suggestively positive results. These include active-nonspecific immunotherapy given for its systemic adjuvant effect, active-nonspecific immunotherapy given locally or regionally, immunorestorative immunotherapy with levamisole, and active-specific imunotherapy with tumor-cell or tumor-antigen vaccine. Certainly, more extensive well-controlled studies of immunotherapy in lung cancer are indicated, particularly since the results with adjuvant chemotherapy to prevent recurrence of this disease and of chemotherapy for advanced metastatic disease are not very encouraging.

18.3. Immunotherapy of Leukemia

There have been more than 20 trials of immunotherapy in human leukemia reported (Table 12). At least in AML, the majority have demonstrated at a

EVAN M. HERSH,
G. M. MAVLIGIT,
J. U. GUTTERMAN,
AND
S. P. RICHMAN

TABLE 12

Immunotherapy of Leukemia[a,b]

Histological type	Immunotherapy		Concurrent chemotherapy	Result
	Nonspecific	Specific		
ALL	BCG	Allo. irr. TC	No	Increased DFI and S
ALL	*B. pertussis*	None	Yes	Increased DFI
AML	BCG	Allo. irr. TC	Yes	Increased DFI and S
AML	BCG	None	Yes	Increased S.
AML	MER	None	Yes	Increased DFI and S and remission rate
AML	*Pseudomonas* vaccine	None	Yes	Increased DFI and S
AML	None	Allo. neuraminidase-treated TC	Yes	Increased DFI and S
CML	BCG	Allo. irr. cultured lymphoid cell line	No	Increased S
CLL	None	Antiallotype serum	No	Hematological improvement

[a] Abbreviations: ALL, acute lymphatic leukemia; AML, acute myelogenous leukemia; CML, chronic myelogenous leukemia; CLL, chronic lymphatic leukemia; BCG, bacillus Calmette Guérin; allo., allogeneic; irr., irradiated; TC, tumor cells; MER, methanol extraction residue; DFI, disease-free interval; S, survival.
[b] In ALL, most attempts at immunotherapy have not been effective; see text.

minimum prolongation of survival. Active-nonspecific and active-specific approaches have been used separately or in combination. In AML, the prolongation of survival has been significant enough so that it is our feeling that the majority of patients with this disease will benefit from immunotherapy and should receive it. While immunotherapy results are encouraging, it is unclear that long-term survival is being significantly improved, and therefore additional approaches to immunotherapy, as well as to chemotherapy and combined-modality approaches, are clearly indicated.

The classical study of Mathé *et al.* (1969a) was the first report of immunotherapy of acute leukemia in the modern era. This study has been referred to repeatedly in the body of this text and therefore the results will not be reiterated in detail here. It should be pointed out that subsequent to Mathé's report, there have been several attempts by various investigators to confirm his observations in childhood ALL which have not succeeded. However, in none of these has there been an attempt to exactly reproduce his experimental design, and therefore these studies cannot be evaluated in a comparable fashion. For example, the British Medical Research Council (1971) attempted to administer the BCG to patients in remission by multipuncture plate. They used the Glaxo rather than the Pasteur strain of BCG, the dose of BCG was lower, no tumor cells were given, and no therapeutic benefit was seen. Heyn *et al.* (1975) carried out a similar study with low doses of BCG in children in remission. Patients were randomized to receive no further therapy, BCG, or biweekly methotrexate. BCG results were the same as no therapy and were shorter than that for chemotherapy maintenance. In another recently reported study, Leventhal *et al.* (1973) gave either maintenance

chemotherapy alone or 4-month cycles of chemotherapy alternating with 2
months of intermittent Pasteur strain BCG administered by multipuncture plate.
They also administered irradiated allogeneic cells from a single ALL donor
intradermally. There was no significant difference in the relapse rate, with 59% of
all patients in remission at 30 months in both groups. In our studies of BCG
immunotherapy in adult leukemia, while we were able to demonstrate benefit for
patients with AML, we were unable to demonstrate benefit for patients with ALL
(Gutterman et al., 1974b).

In contrast to these results in lymphocytic leukemia, there seems to be reasonably good evidence that immunotherapy is active in myelogenous leukemia. Either BCG alone or BCG plus allogeneic tumor cells seems to have activity. Thus Vogler and Chan (1974) randomized 41 AML patients in remission after chemotherapy to receive either Tice strain BCG by multipunctute plate, followed by maintenance methotrexate therapy, or maintenance methotrexate therapy alone. In their initial report, they demonstrated a prolongation of remission duration in the immunotherapy group. In their recent update of these data, remission duration is longer, but not significantly so, and survival is significantly longer in the immunotherapy group (Vogler et al., 1977). In our own studies, BCG immunotherapy using liquid Pasteur BCG was administered by scarification approximately weekly between courses of remission maintenance chemotherapy (Gutterman et al., 1974b). Initially, we observed prolongation of remission duration. In our recent update, significant prolongation of survival duration is observed in the BCG-treated patients compared to historical controls. However, it should be pointed out that when a similar regimen was extended to the Southwest Oncology Group with relatively large numbers of patients, these results were not confirmed (Hewlett, 1977). In contrast, Whittaker and Slater (1977) using BCG immunotherapy in AML by the intravenous route, and Cuttner et al. (1977), utilizing the cutaneous administration of MER, have shown prolongation of survival duration or prolongation of remission and survival as well as a possible increase in the remission rate in patients with AML.

One other approach to immunotherapy of the active-nonspecific type has been reported by Clarkson et al. (1975) and recently updated by Gee and Clarkson (1977). Patients were randomized during remission induction to receive Pseudomonas vaccine as a prevention of infection or not to receive it. There was a striking prolongation of the disease-free interval among the patients receiving Pseudomonas vaccine compared to the controls. A new study has been initiated.

The other major approach to immunotherapy of acute myelogenous leukemia has been the administration of BCG plus allogeneic irradiated tumor cells. In a large series of studies initiated by the late Gordon Hamilton-Fairley (1975) and recently updated by Powles et al. (1973), patients with AML brought into remission by chemotherapy received intermittent chemotherapy and between cycles received BCG plus pooled allogeneic irradiated tumor cells at approximately weekly intervals. Two and one-half years after the entry of the last patient into this program, there is a highly significant prolongation of survival in the immunotherapy group compared to controls, although eventually most patients

510

EVAN M. HERSH,
G. M. MAVLIGIT,
J. U. GUTTERMAN,
AND
S. P. RICHMAN

do relapse. The prolongation of survival is mainly accounted for by prolongation of the survival subsequent to relapse, and there is no significant difference in the remission duration of the immunotherapy compared to the control patients. This result has recently been confirmed by Reizenstein *et al.* (1977) in a similar study. However, a number of attempts to confirm this observation have been unsuccessful (Peto, 1977).

An impressive study of active-specific immunotherapy has been conducted by Holland and Bekesi and (1976), who immunized patients with AML in remission with frequent large doses of neuraminidase-treated tumor cells alone. Injections were at multiple sites on upper and lower extremities and trunk. This study does not include the addition of BCG immunotherapy. The results indicate a significant prolongation of the disease-free interval and survival by this approach to immunotherapy added to maintenance chemotherapy.

A number of other investigators have used active-specific immunotherapy in patients with myelogenous leukemia. Thus Skurkovich *et al.* (1969) have done a series of studies in which they included passive cyclic immunization with autologous plasma, and autologous leukocytes early in remission or active immunization with viable allogeneic leukemic cells. Significant prolongation of remission and survival was reported in patients receiving this immunotherapy compared to controls. In another recent study, although no clinical effect was observed, some important data regarding immunotherapy were generated. Gutterman *et al.* (1974*c*) have observed that the Raji lymphoma cell line shares antigens with acute leukemias. The antigen was the target for cytotoxicity reactions, and immunized patients could generate antibody. Based on this observation, patients in the second remission with advanced AML were randomly assigned to receive chemotherapy alone or chemotherapy plus immunotherapy with the cell line (Thomas *et al.*, 1975). Remission duration in both groups was identical; however, complement-dependent cytotoxic antibody developed in a number of the immunized patients and in none of the controls. This suggested that this approach to immunotherapy should be further explored.

Sokal *et al.* (1973) have reported that patients with uncomplicated Philadelphia chromosome positive CML have prolonged remission duration and survival when vaccinated repeatedly after the termination of chemotherapy with BCG and irradiated allogeneic cultured cells. The cultured cells are a lymphoblastoid cell line derived originally from a CML patient. Sokal *et al.* (1976) have recently observed that less intensive immunizations carry a greater immunotherapeutic benefit than more intensive immunization schedules, suggesting that excessive immunotherapy might be detrimental. We have some evidence that tends to confirm this. Thus when we added tumor cell immunization to our BCG immunotherapy program, utilizing viable nonirradiated autologous leukemia cells, we observed an abrogation of the immunotherapeutic benefit (Gutterman *et al.*, 1976).

In summary, there is little evidence that immunotherapy is beneficial in acute lymphocytic leukemia. The reasons for this are complex, and may relate to experimental design of studies subsequent to Mathé's. However, the overwhelming body of evidence indicates prolongation of survival and perhaps of remission in myelogenous leukemia treated with immunotherapy either with BCG, other microbial adjuvants, or various types of modified tumor cells. Intensive investigation of more aggressive approaches to immunotherapy is clearly indicated in this disease.

18.4. Immunotherapy of Other Human Tumors

There have been a modest number of additional reports that various approaches to immunotherapy can benefit patients with a variety of other malignancies. These will be briefly reviewed in this section (Table 13). In breast cancer, Klein *et al.* (1975) first demonstrated that intralesional or topical immunotherapy with microbial products of various types or with topical DNCB could cause the regression of local lesions. In metastatic breast cancer, our group has demonstrated that the addition of BCG by the scarification method to combination chemotherapy with FU, adriamycin, and cytoxan can improve the remission duration at the borderline of significance and can significantly improve survival, particularly of responders (Hortobagyi, 1977). We have subsequently observed

TABLE 13
Immunotherapy of Other Malignant Diseases[a]

Histological type	Stage	Evident disease	Immunotherapy	Concurrent chemotherapy	Result
Hodgkin's	I–IV	No	BCG	No	Increased DFI
Non-Hodgkin's lymphoma	III–IV	No	BCG	No	Increased DFI
Osteogenic sarcoma	I	No	TC homogenate	No	Increased DFI and S
Osteogenic sarcoma	I	No	BCG plus allo. irr. cultured TC	No	No effect
Osteogenic sarcoma	Advanced	Yes	Transfer factor	Yes, no	Stabilization
Soft tissue sarcoma	I	No	BCG plus allo. irr. cultured TC	Yes, no	Increased DFI and S
Breast cancer	II	No	BCG	Yes	Increased DFI and S
Breast cancer	III	No	Auto. irr. TC	No	Increased S
Breast cancer	III	No	Levamisole	No	Increased DFI and S
Breast cancer	IV	Yes	Transfer factor	No	Partial remission
Breast cancer	IV	Yes	BCG or MER	Yes	Increased remission duration and S
Colon Cancer	Dukes' C	No	BCG or FU-BCG	Yes	Increased DFI and S
Colon cancer	Dukes' D	Yes	BCG or MER	Yes	No effect
Head and neck cancer	Advanced	Yes	BCG	Yes	Increased remission rate or survival
Renal cancer	Advanced	Yes	BCG	No	Partial remission in 40%

[a] Abbreviations: BCG, bacillus Calmette Guérin; DFI, disease-free interval; S, survival; allo., allogeneic; irr., irradiated; TC, tumor cells; auto., autologous; MER, methanol extraction residue; FU, 5-fluorouracil.

512

EVAN M. HERSH,
G. M. MAVLIGIT,
J. U. GUTTERMAN,
AND
S. P. RICHMAN

that the effect on survival is equivalent if BCG is substituted by MER (Hortobagyi, 1977). In a small uncontrolled study, Cuttner et al. (1976) observed that the addition of MER immunotherapy to a five-drug combination chemotherapy program produced surprisingly long remission and survival durations. Recently, Pinsky et al. (1977) have utilized active-nonspecific immunotherapy with C. parvum given subcutaneously between courses of combination chemotherapy for metastatic disease and have observed prolongation of remission duration and survival, compared to the remission and survival for concurrent controls treated with chemotherapy alone. Thus active-nonspecific immunotherapy can prolong drug-induced therapeutic effects in breast cancer, although it cannot improve the remission rate according to the methods by which it has been administered to date (see Table 12 for details).

There has also been a small report that adoptive immunotherapy is active in breast cancer. Oettgen et al. (1974) repeatedly administered pooled transfer factor from the lymphocytes of normal women to patients with metastatic breast cancer. One out of four patients appeared to have a significant regression of tumor and therefore an immunotherapy-induced remission. Immunorestoration may also be active in breast cancer. Rojas et al. (1976) reported that patients with inoperable breast cancer had marked prolongation of survival after radiotherapy if they received levamisole. All the above outlined studies need confirmation and extension before we can unequivocally conclude that immunotherapy is active in breast cancer.

In colon cancer, Mavligit et al. (1976) have done an important study in which Duke's class C patients were randomized to receive BCG alone or FU plus BCG following surgery. The disease-free interval and survival of these patients were compared to those of a carefully selected historical control group. A striking prolongation of disease-free interval and survival was observed, so that the natural history of the treated Duke's class C patients was similar to that of untreated Duke's class B patients. Several investigators, including Moertel et al. (1977) and Engstrom et al. (1977), have attempted to use active-nonspecific immunotherapy in combination with chemotherapy for metastatic colon cancer. Neither BCG nor MER in the doses and schedules used appeared to have any effect on the response to chemotherapy.

Historically, the treatment of sarcoma with immunotherapy was one of the earliest areas in which positive results were reported in this field. Coley (1896), using mixed bacterial toxins, found that postsurgical immunotherapeutic treatment could prolong disease-free interval and survival and that in patients with residual disease this treatment could even induce remissions. However, it should be pointed out that the science of clinical observation was not well developed at the time that Coley did his pioneering experiments and that the staging and classification of sarcomas were also in a primitive state. Therefore, the interpretation of these very important historical data is somewhat difficult. However, there are at least two important studies which have been done in recent years. Marcove et al. (1971), as already mentioned above, treated patients having osteogenic sarcoma with an ultraviolet-irradiated homogenate of autologous tumor, repeatedly inoculated after surgery. Striking prolongation of disease-free interval was observed. Similarly, Townsend *et al.* (1976) used a cultured allogeneic sarcoma cell line plus BCG in the postsurgical treatment of patients with sarcoma. Patients with soft tissue sarcoma had prolongation of disease-free interval and survival, whereas patients with osteogenic sarcoma did not benefit.

In a number of other tumors, benefit from immunotherapy has also been described. For example, in superficial recurrent bladder carcinomas, Eidinger and Morales (1976) have described the fact that the intravesicular installation of BCG reduces the rate of appearance of new primary tumors. Donaldson (1973) and Richman *et al.* (1976) observed that the addition of BCG immunotherapy to methotrexate chemotherapy or to combination chemotherapy prolonged the survival of patients with metastatic head and neck cancer compared to that of controls treated with chemotherapy alone. Klein and co-workers have firmly established the fact that skin cancer can be induced into complete remission by topical or intralesional treatment, and apparently, in some patients with multiple skin cancer, topical immunotherapy of some lesions can have antitumor effects on other primary tumors at distal sites or can delay the appearance of subsequent new primary tumors. Finally, Sokal *et al.* (1974) and Hoerni *et al.* (1976) have described the fact that BCG immunotherapy added to radiotherapy or chemotherapy can improve the survival of patients with malignant lymphomas. Very recently, Jones (1977) has reported that BCG given between courses of remission–induction therapy can increase the remission rate in lymphoma.

In summary, immunotherapy appears to be developing into the fourth major modality of cancer treatment. The development of immunotherapy is based on observations of tumor-associated antigens in human malignancies, immune responses to these antigens, and a relationship between general immunocompetence and the level of specific tumor immunity and prognosis of the cancer patient. In a variety of animal models, none of which is an exact duplicate of human tumors, various immunotherapeutic maneuvers can either induce remissions or prolong remissions induced by conventional therapy. There are a variety of approaches to immunotherapy, including active-specific, active-nonspecific, adoptive, immunorestorative, passive, local, and combinations. Some of these have shown immunotherapeutic effects in human malignancies. In most immunotherapy studies reported to date, the number of patients studied has been small and the immunotherapeutic benefit is modest. It appears unequivocal, however, that immunotherapy is of significant benefit. However, the modest effect is such that the future of the field will depend on the development of either more potent approaches to immunotherapy or better alternative approaches to cytoreductive therapy, which will bring the tumor burden into a state where the current relatively weak effects of immunotherapy may be most important. Very recently, the use of systemic adjuvant immunotherapy by the intravenous route has suggested that more potent immunotherapeutic effects are possible. There are many exciting leads in the area of immunotherapy, but a good number of years of extensive clinical trials will be necessary before this field is firmly established.

EVAN M. HERSH,
G. M. MAVLIGIT,
J. U. GUTTERMAN,
AND
S. P. RICHMAN

ACKNOWLEDGMENTS

This work was supported by Grant CA-05831 and Contract N01-CB-33888 from the National Cancer Institute, National Institutes of Health, Bethesda, Maryland. Drs. Gutterman and Mavligit are recipients of Public Health Research Career Development Awards 1-K04-CA-71007 and 1-K04-CA-00130, respectively, from the National Institutes of Health, Bethesda, Maryland. Dr. Richman is the recipient of Junior Faculty Award 321, from the American Cancer Society, New York, New York.

19. References

ALEXANDER, P., AND DELORME, E. J., 1971, The use of irradiated immune lymphoid cells for immunotherapy of primary tumors in rats, *Israel J. Med. Sci.* **7**:239.

ALEXANDER, P., AND EVANS, R., 1971, Endotoxin and double-stranded RNA render macrophages cytotoxic, *Nature (London)* **232**:76.

ALEXANDER, P., DELORME, E. J., HAMILTON, L. D. G., *et al.*, 1967, Effect of nucleic acids from immune lymphocytes on rat sarcomata, *Nature (London)* **213**:569.

ALEXANDER, P., ECCLES, S., AND GAUCI, C. L. L., 1976, The significance of macrophages in human and experimental tumors, *Ann. N.Y. Acad. Sci.* **276**:124.

ALLISON, A. C., BERMAN, L. D., AND LEVY, R. H., 1967, Increased tumor induction by adenovirus type 12 in thymectomized mice and mice treated with anti-lymphocyte serum, *Nature (London)* **125**:185.

AMERY, W. K., 1976, Double-blind levamisole trial in resectable lung cancer, *Ann. N.Y. Acad. Sci.* **277**:216.

AMIEL, J. L., AND BERARDET, M., 1970, An experimental model of active immunotherapy preceded by cytoreductive chemotherapy, *Eur. J. Cancer* **6**:557.

ANDERSON, J., SJÖBERG, O., AND MOLLER, G., 1972, Mitogens as probes for immunocyte activation and cellular cooperation, *Transplant Rev.* **11**:131.

BACH, J. F., AND DARDENNE, M., 1973, Studies on thymus products. II. Demonstration and characterization of a circulating thymic hormone, *Immunology* **25**:353.

BACH, J. F., DARDENNE, M., PLEAU, J. M., *et al.*, 1975, Isolation, biochemical characteristics, and biological activity of a circulating thymic hormone in the mouse and in the human, *Ann. N.Y. Acad. Sci.* **249**:186.

BALDWIN, R. W., AND PIMM, M. V., 1973*a*, BCG immunotherapy of pulmonary growths from intravenously transferred rat tumour cells. *Br. J. Cancer* **27**:48.

BALDWIN, R. W., AND PIMM, M. V., 1973*b*, BCG immunotherapy of rat tumors of defined immunogenicity, *Natl. Cancer Inst. Monogr.* **39**:11.

BALLOW, M., DUPONT, B., AND GOOD, R. A., 1973, Autoimmune hemolytic anemia in Wiscott–Aldrich syndrome during treatment with transfer factor, *J. Pediat.* **83**:772.

BALNER, H., AND DERSJANT, H., 1969, Increased oncogenic effect of methylcholantherene after treatment with anti-lymphocyte serum, *Nature (London)* **224**:376.

BAND, P. R., JAO-KING, C., AND URTASUN, R. C., 1975, Phase I study of *Corynebacterium parvum* in patients with solid tumors, *Cancer Chemother. Rep.* **59**:1139.

BANSAL, S. C., AND SJÖGREN, H. O., 1972, Counter action of the blocking of cell-mediated tumor immunity by inoculation of unblocking sera and splenectomy: Immunotherapeutic effects on primary polyoma tumors in rats, *Int. J. Cancer* **9**:490.

BANSAL, S. C., AND SJÖRGEN, H. O., 1973, Effects of BCG on various facets of the immune response against polyoma tumors in rats, *Int. J. Cancer* **11**:162.

BARAM, P., AND CONDOULIS, W., 1970, The *in vitro* transfer of delayed hypersensitivity to rhesus monkey and human lymphocytes with transfer factor obtained from rhesus monkey peripheral white blood cells, *J. Immunol.* **104**:769.

BARAM, P., AND CONDOULIS, W., 1974, Studies on rhesus monkey non-dialyzable and dialyzable transfer factor, *Transplantation Proc.* **6**:209.

BARTLETT, G. L., AND ZBAR, B., 1972, Tumor-specific vaccine containing *Mycobacterium bovis* and tumor cells: Safety and efficacy, *J. Natl. Cancer Inst.* **48**:1709.

BARTLETT, G. L., ZBAR, B., AND RAPP, H. J., 1972, Suppression of murine tumor growth by immune reaction to the bacillus Calmette Guérin strain of *Mycobacterium bovis, J. Natl. Cancer Inst.* **48**:245.

BASCH, R. S., AND GOLDSTEIN, G., 1975, Antigenic and functional evidence for the in vitro inductive actvity of thymopoietin (thymin) on thymocyte precursors, *Ann. N.Y. Acad. Sci.* **291**:290.

BAST, R. C., BAST, B. S., AND RAPP, H. J., 1976, Critical review of previously reported animal studies of tumor immunotherapy with non-specific immunostimulants, *Ann. N.Y. Acad. Sci.* **277**:60.

BEKESI, J. G., AND HOLLAND, J. F., 1974, Combined chemotherapy and immunotherapy of transplantable and spontaneous murine leukemia in DBA/2 HA and AKR mice, *Recent Results Cancer Res.* **47**:357.

BEKESI, J. G., ROBOZ, J. P., AND HOLLAND, J. F., 1976, Therapeutic effectiveness of neuraminidase treated tumor cells as an immunogen in man and experimental animals with leukemia, *Ann. N.Y. Acad. Sci.* **277**:313.

BEKIERKUNST, A., LEVIJ, I. S., AND YARKONI, E., *et al.*, 1971, Suppression of urethane-induced lung adenomas in mice treated with trehalose-6,6-dimycolate (core factor) and living bacillus Calmette Guérin, *Science* **174**:1240.

BEN-EFRAIM, S., CONSTANTINI-SOUROJON, M., AND WEISS, D. W., 1973, Potentiation and modulation of the immune response of guinea pigs to poorly immunogenic protein haptene conjugates by pre-treatment with the MER fraction of attenuated tubercle bacilli, *Cell. Immunol.* **7**:370.

BEN-EFRAIM, S., TEITELBAUM, R., OPHIR, R., *et al.*, 1974, Non-specific modulation of immunological responsiveness in guinea pigs and mice by the tumor protective methanol extraction residue (MER) mycobacterial fraction, *Israel J. Med. Sci.* **10**:972.

BEN-EFRAIM, S., OPHIR, R., TEITELBAUM, R., *et al.*, 1977, Effect of the MER tubercle bacillus fraction on the tolerance threshold of mice to T-independent polysaccharide antigens, submitted for publication.

BENJAMINI, E., THEILEN, G. H., TORTEN, M., *et al.*, 1976, Tumor vaccines for immunotherapy of canine lymphosarcoma, *Ann. N.Y. Acad. Sci.* **277**:305.

BENSA, J. C., FOURE, J., MARTIN, H., *et al.*, 1976, Levamisole in angioimmunoblastic lymphadenopathy, *Lancet* **1**:1081.

BERETTA, A., 1977, Controlled study for prolonged chemotherapy, immunotherapy, and chemotherapy plus immunotherapy as adjuvant to surgery, in: *Immunotherapy of Cancer: Present Status of Trial in Man* (W. TERRY AND D. WINDHORST, eds.), in press.

BERGER, D. R., VETTO, R. M., AND MALLEY, A., 1972, Transfer factor from guinea pigs sensitive to dinitrochlorobenzene: Absence of supra-antigen properties, *Science* **185**:1473.

BERGER, F M., FUKUI, G. M., LUDWIG, B. J., *et al.*, 1969, Increased host resistance to infection solicited by lipopolysaccharides from *Brucella abortus, Proc. Soc. Exp. Biol.* **131**:1376.

BLACK, M. M., SPEAR, S. P., AND OPLER, S. R., 1956, Structural representations of tumor host relationship in mammary carcinoma: Biologic and prognostic significance, *Amer. J. Clin. Pathol.* **26**:250.

BLOOM, B. R., 1969, Elaboration of effector molecules by activated lymphocytes, in: *Mediators of Cellular Immunity* (H. S. LAWRENCE AND M. LANDY, eds.), pp. 249–319, Academic Press, New York.

BLUMING, A. Z., VOGEL, C. L., ZIEGLER, J. L., *et al.*, 1972, Immunological effects of BCG in malignant melanoma: Two modes of administration compared, *Ann. Intern. Med.* **76**:405.

BOMFORD, R., AND OLIVOTTO, M., 1974, The mechanism of inhibition by *Corynebacterium parvum* of the growth of lung nodules from intravenously injected tumor cells, *Int. J. Cancer* **14**:226.

BORBERG, H., OETTGEN, H. F., AND CHOUDRY, K., 1972, Inhibition of established transplants of chemically induced sarcomas in syngeneic mice by lymphocytes from immunized donors, *Int. J. Cancer* **10**:539.

BORSOS, T., BAST, R. C., O'HANIAN, S. H., *et al.*, 1976, Induction of tumor immunity by intratumoral chemotherapy, *Ann. N.Y. Acad. Sci.* **276**:560.

BORTIN, M. M., RIMM, A. A., AND SALTZSTEIN, E. C., 1973, Graft versus leukemia: Quantification of adoptive immunotherapy in murine leukemia, *Science* **179**:811.

BRANDES, L. J., GALTON, D. A. G., AND WILTSHA, W., 1971, New approaches to immunotherapy of melanoma, *Lancet* **2**:293.

EVAN M. HERSH,
G. M. MAVLIGIT,
J. U. GUTTERMAN,
AND
S. P. RICHMAN

BRANIC, M., 1970, Transplantability of leukemia from leukemic mice after irradiation and injection of allogeneic spleen cells, *Eur. J. J. Clin. Biol. Res.* **15:**104.

BRAUN, W., 1974, Regulatory factors in the immune response, in: *Cyclic AMP, Cell Growth and the Immune Response* (W. BRAUN *et al.*, eds.), pp. 4–23, Springer-Verlag, New York.

BRAUN, W., REGELSON, W., YAJIMA, Y., *et al.*, 1970, Stimulation of antibody formation by pyran copolymer, *Proc. Soc. Exp. Biol. Med.* **133:**171.

BRAUN, W., LICHTENSTEIN, L. M., AND PARKER, C. W., 1974, in: *Cyclic AMP, Cell Growth and the Immune Response*, Springer-Verlag, New York.

BRODEUR, B. R., AND MARIGAN, T. C., 1974, Suppressive effect of interferon on the humoral immune response to sheep red blood cells in mice, *J. Immunol.* **113:**1319.

BUCANA, C., AND HANNA, M. G., 1974, Immunoelectron microscopic analysis of surface antigens common to *Mycobacterium bovis*, BCG and tumor cells , *J. Natl. Cancer Inst.* **53:**1313.

BULLOUGH, W. S., AND LAURENCE, E. B., 1968, Melanocyte chalone and mitotic control in melanomata, *Nature (London)* **220:**137.

BURKITT, D., 1967, Clinical evidence suggesting the development of an immunological response against African lymphoma, in: *Treatment of Burkitt's Tumor* (J. H. BURCHENAL AND D. P. BURKITT, eds.), pp. 197–203, Springer-Verlag, New York.

BURNETT, F. M., 1970, The concept of immunological surveillance, *Prog. Exp. Tumor Res.* **13:**1.

BYERS, V. S., LEVIN, A. S., LECAM, L., *et al.*, 1976, Tumor-specific transfer factor therapy in osteogenic sarcoma, *Ann. N.Y. Acad. Sci.* **277:**621.

CARSWELL, E. A., OLD, L. J., KASSEL, R. L., *et al.*, 1975, An endotoxin-induced serum factor that causes necrosis of tumors, *Proc. Natl. Acad. Sci. USA* **72:**3666.

CATALONA, W. J., TARPLEY, J. L., CHRETIEN, P. B., *et al.*, 1974, Lymphocyte stimulation in urologic cancer patients, *J. Urol.* **112:**373.

CATER, D. B., AND WALDMANN, H., 1967, The effects on the growth of PB/8 ascites tumor in C3H, C57, F1, or C3H mice of lymphocyte preparations from C57 mice injected with PB/8 cells and Freund's adjuvant, *Br. J. Cancer* **21:**124.

CHEE, D. O., AND BODURTHA, A. J., 1974, Facilitation and inhibition of B16 melanoma by BCG *in vivo* and by lymphoid cells from BCG-treated mice *in vitro*, *Int. J. Cancer* **14:**137.

CHEEMA, R. A., AND HERSH, E. M., 1972, Local tumor immunotherapy with *in vitro* activated autochthonous lymphocytes, *Cancer* **29:**982.

CHESS, L., LEVY, M., SCHMUKLER, K., *et al.*, 1972, The effect of synthetic polynucleotides on immunologically induced treated thymidine incorporation, *Transplantation* **14:**748.

CHIRIGOS, M. A., TURNER, W., PIERSON, J., *et al.*, 1969, Effective anti-viral therapy of two murine leukemias with an interferon-inducing synthetic carboxylate copolymer, *Int. J. Cancer* **4:**267.

CHIRIGOS, M. A., PIERSON, J. W., AND FUHRMAN, F. S., 1974, Effect of tumor load reduction on successful immunostimulation, *Proc. Am. Assoc. Cancer Res.* **15:**116.

CHISARI, F. V., NORTHRUP, R. S., AND CHEN, L. C., 1974, The modulating effect of cholera enterotoxin on the immune response, *J. Immunol.* **113:**729.

CHUNG, E. B., ZBAR, B., AND RAPP, H. J., 1973, Tumor regression mediated by *Mycobacterium bovis* (strain BCG): Effects of isonicotinic acid hydrazide, cortisone acetate, and anti-thymocyte serum, *J. Natl. Cancer Inst.* **51:**241.

CLARKSON, B. C., DOWLING, M. D., GEE, T. S., *et al.*, 1975, Treatment of acute leukemia in adults, *Cancer* **36:**775.

CLEVELAND, R. P., MELTZER, M. S., AND ZBAR, B., 1974, Tumor cytotoxicity *in vitro* by macrophages from mice infected with *Mycobacterium bovis* strain BCG, *J. Natl. Cancer Inst.* **52:**1887.

COLEY, W. B., 1896, The therapeutic value of the mixed toxins of the *Streptococcus* of erysipelas and *Bacillus prodigiosus* in the treatment of inoperable tumors with a report of 160 cases, *Amer. J. Med. Sci.* **112:**251.

CONE, R. E., AND JOHNSON, A. G., 1971, Regulation of the immune system by synthetic polynucleotides: Action on antigen reactive cells of thymic origin, *J. Exp. Med.* **133:**665.

COSTANZI, J. J., 1977, Chemotherapy and BCG in the treatment of disseminated malignant melanoma: A Southwest Group Study, In: *Immunotherapy of Cancer: Present Status of Trials in Man* (W. TERRY AND D. WINDHORST, eds.), in press.

CUNNINGHAM, T. J., OLSON, K. B., LAFFIN, R., *et al.*, 1969, Treatment of advanced cancer with active immunization, *Cancer* **24:**932.

CUNNINGHAM, T. J., ANTENANN, R., AND PAONESSA, D., 1976, Adjuvant immuno- and/or chemotherapy with neuraminidase treated autogenous tumor vaccine and bacillus Calmette Guérin for head and neck cancers, *Ann. N.Y. Acad. Sci.* **277:**339.

CUNNINGHAM, T. J., SCHOENFELD, D., WALTERS, J., et al., 1977, A controlled study of adjuvant therapy (BCG–BCG–DTIC) with stage I and II melanoma, in: *Immunotherapy of Cancer: Present Status of Trials in Man* (W. TERRY AND D. WINDHORST, eds.), in press.

CURRIE, G. A., AND BAGSHAWE, K. D., 1970, Active immunotherapy with *Corynebacterium parvum* and chemotherapy in murine fibrosarcomas, *Br. Med. J.* 1:541.

CURRIE, G. A., AND McELWAIN, T. J., 1975, Active immunotherapy as an adjunct to chemotherapy in the treatment of disseminated malignant melanoma: A pilot study, *Br. J. Cancer* 31:143.

CURRIE, G. A., LEJEUNE, F., AND FAIRLEY, G. H., 1971, Immunization with irradiated tumor cells and specific lymphocyte cytotoxicity in malignant melanoma, *Br. Med. J.* 2:305.

CURTIS, J. E., HERSH, E. M., AND FREIREICH, E. J., 1969, Transfer of immunity in man with peripheral blood leukocytes (PBL), *Proc. Am. Assoc. Cancer Res.* 10:17.

CUTTLER, S. J., AND HEISE, H. W., 1969, Efficacy of current treatment methods of cancer of the breast, *Cancer* 24:1117.

CUTTNER, J., HOLLAND, J. F., BEKESI, J. G., et al., 1975, Chemoimmunotherapy of acute myelocytic leukemia, *Proc. Am. Soc. Clin. Oncol.* 16:264.

CUTTNER, J., BEKESI, J. G., AND HOLLAND, J. F., 1976, Chemoimmunotherapy of acute leukemia using MER, *Proc. Am. Assoc. Cancer Res.* 17:196.

CUTTNER, J. GLIDWELL, O., AND HOLLAND, J. F., 1977, A comparative study of the value of immunotherapy with MER as adjuvant to induction and two maintenance chemotherapy programs in acute myelocytic leukemia, in: *Immunotherapy of Cancer: Present Status of Trials in Man* (W. TERRY AND D. WINDHORST, eds.), in press.

CZAJKOWSKI, N. P., ROSENBLATT, M., WOLFE, P. L., et al., 1967, A new method of active immunization to autologous human tumor tissue, *Lancet* 2:905.

DAVIES, D. A. L., AND O'NEAL, G. J., 1976, Specific cancer therapy by drugs attached to tumor-specific antibodies, *Ann. N.Y. Acad. Sci.* 277:670.

DE CARVALHO, S., 1963, Preliminary experimentation with specific immunotherapy of neoplastic disease in man. I. Immediate effects of hyperimmune equine gammaglobulin, *Cancer* 16:306.

DECKERS, P. J., AND PILCH, Y. H., 1971a, RNA-mediated transfer of tumor immunity: A new model for the immunotherapy of cancer, *Cancer* 28:1219.

DECKERS, P. J., AND PILCH, Y. H., 1971b, Transfer of immunity to tumor isografts by the systemic administration of xenogeneis immune RNA, *Nature (London)* 231:181.

DECKERS, P. J., AND PILCH, Y. H., 1972, Mediation of immunity to tumor-specific transplantation antigens by RNA inhibition of isograft growth in rats, *Cancer Res.* 32:839.

DELGUERCIO, P., 1972, Adjuvant effects and antibody production against a haptenic determinant: Alternative collaboration between T and B, or B and B lymphocytes, *Nature (London)* 238:213.

DEMAYER, E., DEMAYER, J., AND VANDEPUTTE, M., 1973, Inhibition by interferon of delayed type hypersensitivity in the mouse, *Proc. Natl. Acad. Sci. (USA)* 72:1753.

DILUZIO, N. R., HOFFMAN, E. O., COOK, J. A., et al., 1977, Glucan-induced enhancement in host resistance to experimental tumors, *Natl. Cancer Inst. Monogr.* (in press).

DIMITROV, M. V., CONROY, J., SUHRLAND, L. G., et al., 1977, Combination therapy with *C. parvum* and adriamycin in patients with lung cancer, in: *Immunotherapy of Cancer: Present Status of Trials in Man* (W. TERRY AND D. WINDHORST, eds.), in press.

DIZON, Q. S., AND SOUTHAM, C. M., 1963, Abnormal cellular response to skin abrasions in cancer patients, *Cancer* 16:1288.

DONALDSON, R. C., 1973, Chemoimmunotherapy for cancer of the head and neck, *Am. J. Surg.* 126:507.

DOUGLAS, S. G., SCHMIDT, M. E., AND DAUCHADAY, C. C., 1976, Effect of levamisole on monocyte macrophage immunoprotein receptors and *in vitro* functions, *Fed. Proc.* 35:335.

DRAKE, W. P., CIMINO, E. F., MARDINEY, M. R., et al., 1974, Prophylactic therapy of sponatenous leukemia in AKR mice by polyadenylic-polyuridylic acid, *J. Natl. Cancer Inst.* 52:941.

DRAKE, W. P., PENDERGRAST, W. J., KRAMER, R. E., et al., 1975, Enhancement of spontaneous C3H/HeJ mammary tumorigenesis by long-term polyadenylic-polyuridylic acid therapy, *Cancer Res.* 35:3051.

DUPONT, B., BALLOW, M., HANSEN, J. A., et al., 1974, Effect of transfer factor on mixed lymphocyte culture reactivity, *Proc. Natl. Acad. Sci. (USA)* 71:867.

EIDINGER, D., AND MORALES, A., 1976, Treatment of superficial bladder cancer in man, *Ann. N.Y. Acad. Sci.* 277:239.

EILBER, F. R., AND MORTON, D. L., 1970, Impaired immunological reactivity and recurrence following cancer surgery, *Cancer* 25:362.

EVAN M. HERSH,
G. M. MAVLIGIT,
J. U. GUTTERMAN,
AND
S. P. RICHMAN

EILBER, F. R., NIZZE, J. A., AND MORTON, D. L., 1975, Sequential evaluation of general immune competence in cancer patients: Correlation with clinical course, *Cancer* **35**:660.

ELTRINGHAM, J. R., AND KAPLAN, H. S., 1973, Impaired delayed hypersensitivity: Delayed responses in 154 patients with untreated Hodgkin's disease, *Natl. Cancer Inst. Monogr.* **36**:107.

ENGSTROM, P. F., PAUL, A. R., CATALANO, R. B., *et al.*, 1977, Fluorouracil versus fluorouracil plus bacillus Calmette Guérin in colorectal adenocarcinoma, in: *Immunotherapy of Cancer in Man: Present Status of Trials in Man* (W. TERRY AND D. WINDHORST, eds.), in press.

EVERALL, J. D., O'DONERTY, C. J., WAND, J., *et al.*, 1975, Treatment of primary melanoma by intralesional vaccinia before excision, *Lancet* **2**:583.

FALK, R. E., MANN, P., AND LANGER, B., 1973, Cell-mediated immunity to human tumors: Abrogation by serum factors and non-specific effects of oral BCG therapy, *Arch. Surg.* **107**:261.

FALK, R. E., MacGREGOR, A. D., LANDI, S., *et al.*, 1976, Immunostimulation with intraperitoneally administered bacillus Calmette Guérin for advanced malignant tumors of the gastrointestinal tract, *Surg. Gynecol. Obstet.* **152**:363.

FARACI, R. P., BARONE, J., AND SCHOUR, L., 1975, BCG induced protection against malignant melanoma: Possible immunospecific effect in a murine system, *Cancer* **35**:372.

FARQUHAR, D., LOO, T. L., GUTTERMAN, J. U., HERSH, E. M., *et al.*, 1976, Inhibition of drug metabolizing enzymes in the rat after bacillus Calmette Guérin treatment, *Biochem. Pharmacol.* **25**:1529.

FASS, L., HERBERMAN, R. B., ZIEGLER, J., *et al.*, 1970, Evaluation of the effect of remission plasma on untreated patients with Burkitt's lymphoma, *J. Natl. Cancer Inst.* **44**:145.

FEFER, A., 1971*a*, Adoptive chemoimmunotherapy of a Moloney lymphoma, *Int. J. Cancer* **8**:364.

FEFER, A., 1971*b*, Experimental approaches to immunotherapy of cancer, *Recent Results Cancer Res.* **36**:182.

FIDLER, I. J., BUDMEN, M. B., AND HANNA, M. G., 1977, Characterization of *in vitro* reactivity of BCG-treated guinea pigs to syngeneic line 10 hepatocarcinoma, *Cancer Immunol. Immunother.* (in press).

FINGER, H., EMMERLING, P., AND BRUSS, E., 1970, Variable adjuvant activity of *Bordetella* pertussis with respect to the primary and secondary immunization of mice, *Infect. Immun.* **1**:251.

FISHER, B., CARBONE, P., ECONOMOU, S. G., *et al.*, 1975, L-Phenylalanine mustard (L-PAM) in the management of primary breast cancer: A report of early findings, *N. Engl. J. Med.* **292**:117.

FISHMAN, M. J., 1964, Antibody formation by normal mouse spleen cell cultures exposed in vitro to RNA from immune mice, *Science* **146**:934.

FLANNERY, G. R., CHALMERS, P. J., ROLLAND, J. N., AND NAIRN, R. C., 1973, Immune response to a syngeneic rat tumor: Evolution of serum cytotoxicity and blockade, *Br. J. Cancer* **28**:293.

FLETCHER, G. H., JESSE, R. H., LINDBERG, R. D., *et al.*, 1970, Radiation therapy in management of carcinoma of supraglottic larynx, *Am. J. Roentgenol.* **108**:19.

FOWLES, R. E., FAJARDO, I. M., LEIBOWITCH, J. L., *et al.*, 1973, The enhancement of macrophage bacteriostasis by products of activated lymphocytes, *J. Exp. Med.* **138**:952.

FRENSTER, J. H., 1976, Phytohemagglutinin activated autochtonous lymphocytes for systemic immunotherapy of human neoplasms, *Ann. N.Y. Acad. Sci.* **277**:45.

FRESHMAN, M. M., MERIGAN, T. C., REMINGTON, J. S., *et al.*, 1966, *In vitro* and *in vivo* anti-viral action of an interferon-like substance induced by *Toxoplasma gondii*, *Proc. Soc. Exp. Biol. Med.* **123**:862.

FROESE, G., BERCZI, I., AND ASEHON, A. C., 1974, Neuraminidase induced enhancement of tumor growth in mice, *J. Natl. Cancer Inst.* **52**:1905.

FUDENBERG, H. H., 1976, Dialyzable transfer factor in the treatment of human osteosarcoma an analytical review, *Ann. N.Y. Acad. Sci.* **277**:545.

GALLIN, J. I., AND KIRKPATRICK, C. H., 1974, Chemotactic activity in dialyzable transfer factor, *Proc. Natl. Acad. Sci. (USA)* **71**:498.

GALLIN, J. I., AND WOLFE, S. M., 1975, Leukocyte chemotaxis—Physiological considerations and abnormalities, *Clin. Haematol.* **4**:567.

GEE T. S., AND CLARKSON, B. D., 1977, *Pseudomonas aeruginosa* vaccine in a treatment protocol for adult patients with acute non-lymphoblastic leukemia: A preliminary report, in: *Immunotherapy of Cancer: Present Status of Trials in Man* (W. TERRY AND D. WINDHORST, eds.), in press.

GEFFARD, M., AND ORBACH-ARBOUYS, S., 1976, Enhancement of T-suppressor activity in mice by high doses of BCG, *Cancer Immunol. Immunother.* **1**:41.

GERCOVICH, F. G., GUTTERMAN, J. U., MAVLIGIT, G. M., AND HERSH, E. M., 1975, Active-specific immunization in malignant melanoma, *Med. Pediat. Oncol.* **1**:277.

GERY, I., BAER, A., STUPP, Y., AND WEISS, D. W., 1974, Further studies on the effects of the methanol extraction residue fraction of tubercle bacilli on lymphoid cells in macrophages, *Israel J. Med. Sci.* **10**:984.

GHAFFAR, A., CULLEN, R. T., AND WOODRUFF, M. F. A., 1975, Further analysis of the antitumor effect *in vitro* of peritoneal exudate cells from mice treated with *Corynebacterium parvum*, *Br. J. Cancer* **31**:15.

GHOSE, S. E. T., TAI, J., GUCLU, A., *et al.*, 1976, Antibodies as carriers of radionuclides and cytotoxic drugs in the treatment and diagnosis of cancer, *Ann. N.Y. Acad. Sci.* **277**:671.

GHOSE, T., CERINI, M., CARTER, M., *et al.*, 1967, Immunoradioactive agent against cancer, *Br. Med. J.* **1**:90.

GIBSON, J. P., MEGEL, H., CAMYRE, K. P., *et al.*, 1977, Effect of tylerone hydrochloride on the lymphoid and interferon responses of athymic mice, submitted.

GLYNN, J. P., HALPERN, B. L., AND FEFER, A., 1969, An immunochemotherapeutic system for the treatment for the transplanted Moloney virus-induced lymphoma in mice, *Cancer Res.* **29**:515.

GOLDENBERG, B. J., AND BRANDES, L. J., 1972, Immunotherapy of nasopharyngeal carcinoma with transfer factor from donors with previous infectious mononucleosis, *Clin. Res.* **20**:947.

GOLDSTEIN, A. L., ASANUMA, Y., BATTISTO, J. R., *et al.*, 1970, Influence of thymosin on cell-mediated and humoral immune responses in normal and immunologically deficient mice, *J. Immunol.* **104**:359.

GOLDSTEIN, A. L., GUHA, A., ZATZ, M. M., *et al.*, 1972, Purification of biological properties of thymosin: A hormone of the thymus gland, *Proc. Natl. Acad. Sci. (USA)* **69**:1800.

GOLDSTEIN, A. L., COHEN, G. H., ROSSIO, J. L., *et al.*, 1976, Use of thymosin in the treatment of primary immunodeficiency diseases and cancer, *Med. Clin. N. Am.* **60**:591.

GOLDSTEIN, G., 1974, Isolation of bovine thymin, a polypeptide hormone of the thymus, *Nature (London)* **247**:11.

GOLDSTEIN, G., 1975, The isolation of thymopoietin (thymin), *Ann. N.Y. Acad. Sci.* **249**:177.

GOLDSTEIN, G., AND HOFFMAN, W. W., 1969, Endocrine function of the thymus affecting neuromuscular transmission, *Clin. Exp. Immunol.* **4**:181.

GOLUB, S H , 1975, Host immune response to human tumor antigens, in: *Cancer: A Comprehensive Treatise*, Vol. 4 (F. BECKER, ed.), pp. 259–302, Plenum Press, New York.

GORDON, B. L., AND KEENAN, J. P., 1975, The treatment of systemic lupus erythematosus (SLE) with the T-cell immunostimulant drug levamisole: A case report, *Ann. Allergy* **35**:343.

GORER, P. A., 1956, Some recent work on tumor immunity, *Adv. Cancer Res.* **4**:149.

GRAHAM, J. B., AND GRAHAM, R. M., 1962, Autogenous vaccine in cancer patients, *Surg. Gynecol. Obstet.* **114**:1.

GRANT, R. M., COCHRAN, A. J., AND HOYLE, D., 1974, Results of administry of BCG to patients with melanoma, *Lancet* **2**:1096.

GREEN, A. A., PRATT, C., WEBSTER, R. G., *et al.*, 1976, Immunotherapy of osteosarcoma patients with virus modified tumor cells, *Ann. N.Y. Acad. Sci.* **277**:396.

GRESSER, I., AND BOURALI-MAURY, I., 1972, Inhibition by interferon preparations of a solid malignant tumor and pulmonary metastases in mice, *Nature (London)* **236**:78.

GRESSER, I., BERMAN, L., DETHE, G., *et al.*, 1968, Interferon and murine leukemia. V. Effect of interferon preparations on the evolution of Rauscher disease in mice, *J. Natl. Cancer Inst.* **41**:505.

GRESSER, I., BOURALI, C., LEVY, J. P., *et al.*, 1969, Increased survival in mice inoculated with tumor cells and treated with interferon preparations, *Proc. Natl. Acad. Sci.* **63**:51.

GRESSER, I., BROUTY-BOYE, D., THOMAS, M. T., *et al.*, 1970, Interferon in cell division. I. Inhibition of the multiplication of mouse L-1210 leukemia cells *in vitro* by interferon preparations, *Proc. Natl. Acad. Sci. (USA)* **66**:1052.

GROSSBERG, S. E., 1963, Interferon as a metabolic agent of host resistance, in: *Conceptual Advances in Immunology and Oncology*, pp. 116–136, Harper and Row, New York.

GROSSBERG, S. E., 1972a, The interferons and their inducers: Molecular and therapeutic considerations, *N. Engl. J. Med.* **287**:13.

GROSSBERG, S. E., 1972b, The interferons and their inducers. Molecular and therapeutic considerations. *N. Engl. J. Med.* **287**:122.

GUTHRIE, D., AND WAY, S., 1975, Immunotherapy of non-clinical vaginal cancer, *Lancet* **2**:1242.

GUTTERMAN, J. U., ROSSEN, R. D., BUTLER, W. T., *et al.*, 1973a, Immunoglobulin on tumor cell and tumor-induced lymphocyte blastogenesis in human acute leukemia, *N. Engl. J. Med.* **288**:169.

GUTTERMAN, J. U., HERSH, E. M., MAVLIGIT, G. M., *et al.*, 1973b, BCG stimulation of immune responsiveness in patients with malignant melanoma, *Cancer* **11**:521.

520

EVAN M. HERSH,
G. M. MAVLIGIT,
J. U. GUTTERMAN,
AND
S. P. RICHMAN

GUTTERMAN, J. U., MAVLIGIT, G. M., McBRIDE, C. M., et al., 1973c, Active immunotherapy with BCG for recurrent malignant melanoma, Lancet 1:1208.

GUTTERMAN, J. U., MAVLIGIT, G. M., McKREDIE, K. B., et al., 1973d, Autoimmunization with acute leukemia cells: Demonstration of increased lymphocyte responsiveness, Int. J. Cancer 11:521.

GUTTERMAN, J. U., MAVLIGIT, G. M., GOTTLIEB, J. A., et al., 1974a, Chemoimmunotherapy of disseminated malignant melanoma with dimethyl imidazole carboxamide and bacillus Calmette Guérin, N. Engl. J. Med. 291:592.

GUTTERMAN, J. U., RODRIGUEZ, V., MAVLIGIT, G. M., et al., 1974b, Chemoimmunotherapy of adult acute leukemia: Prolongation of remission in myeloblastic leukemia with BCG, Lancet 2:1405.

GUTTERMAN, J. U., HERSH, E. M., MAVLIGIT, G. M., et al., 1974c, Cell-mediated and humoral immune response to acute leukemia cells and soluble leukemia antigen-relationship to immunocompetence and prognosis, Recent Results Cancer Res. 47:97.

GUTTERMAN, J. U., MAVLIGIT, G. M., BURGESS, M. A., et al., 1976, Immunotherapy of breast cancer, malignant melanoma, and acute leukemia with BCG: Prolongation of disease-free interval and survival, Cancer Immunol. Immunother. 1:99.

GUTTERMAN, J. U, HERSH, E. M., AND MAVLIGIT, G. M., 1977, BCG immunotherapy for recurrent metastatatic melanoma: Study of dose, strain, site of administration, degree of residual disease and immunocompetence, J. Natl. Cancer Inst. (in press).

HABA, S., HAMAOKA, T., AND TAKATSU, K., 1976, Selective suppression of T-cell activity in tumor-bearing mice and its improvement by lentinan, a potent antitumor polysaccharide, Natl. J. Cancer 18:93.

HALPERN, B. N., BIOZZI, G., STIFFEL, C., et al., 1959, Effect of the stimulation of the reticuloendothelial system by the inoculation of baccilus Calmette Guérin on the development of the atypical T8 lymphoma in the rat, C. R. Soc. Biol. (Paris) 153:919.

HALPERN, B. N., PREVOT, A. R., BIOZZI, G., et al., 1964, Stimulation of the phagocytic activity of the reticuloendothelial system provided by Corynebacterium parvum, J. Reticuloendothel. Soc. 1:77.

HAMILTON-FAIRLEY, G., 1975, Immunotherapy in the management of leukemia, Br. J. Haematol. 31:181.

HAMURO, J., MAEDA, Y. Y., ARAI, Y., et al., 1971, The significance of the higher structure of the polysaccharides lentinan and pachymaran with regard to their antitumor activity, Chem. Biol. Interact. 3:69.

HAN, T., 1973, Immune RNA-mediated transfer of delayed skin reactivity in patients with Hodgkin's disease, Clin. Exp. Immunol. 14:213.

HANNA, M. G., AND PETERS, L. C., 1975, Efficacy of intralesional BCG therapy in guinea pigs with disseminated tumor, Cancer 36:1298.

HANNA, M. G., ZBAR, B., AND RAPP, H. J., 1972, Histopathology of tumor regression after intralesional injection of Mycobacterium bovis. I. Tumor growth and metastasis, J. Natl. Cancer Inst. 48:1441.

HANNA, M. G., SNODGRASS, M. J., AND ZBAR, B., 1973, Histologic and ultrastructural studies of tumor regression in inbred guinea pigs after intralesional injection of Mycobacterium bovis (BCG), Natl. Cancer Inst. Monogr. 38:71.

HANNA, M. G., PETERS, L. C., GUTTERMAN, J. U., AND HERSH, E. M., 1977, An evaluation of BCG administered by scarification for immunotherapy of metastatic hepatocarcinoma in the guinea pig, J. Natl. Cancer Inst. 56:1013.

HATTORI, T., AND MORI, A., 1973, Antitumor activity of anaerobic Corynebacterium isolated from the human bone marrow, Gann 64:15.

HAWRYLKO, E., AND MACKANESS, G. B., 1973, Immunopotentiation with BCG. III. Modulation of the response to a tumor-specific antigen, J. Natl. Cancer Inst. 51:1677.

HELLSTRÖM, I., HELLSTRÖM, K. E., Pierce, G. E., AND YANG, G. P. S., 1968, Cellular and humoral immunity to different types of human neoplasms, Nature (London) 220:1352.

HELLSTRÖM, I., SJÖGREN, H. O., WARNER, G. A., AND HELLSTRÖM, K. E., 1971, Blocking of cell-mediated tumor immunity by sera from patients with growing neoplasms, Int. J. Cancer 7:226.

HELLSTRÖM, K. E., AND HELLSTRÖM, I., 1974, Lymphocyte-mediated cytotoxicity in serum activity to tumor antigens, Adv. Immunol. 18:209.

HELLSTRÖM, K. E., AND MÖLLER, G., 1965, Immunological and immunogenetic aspects of tumor transplantation, Prog. Allergy 9:158.

HENLE, W., HENLE, G., AND DEINHARDT, F., 1959, Studies on persistent infections in tissue cultures. IV. Evidence for the production of an interferon in MCN cells by myxovirus, J. Exp. Med. 110:525.

HERBERMAN, R. B., ROGENTINE, G. N., AND OREN, M. E., 1969, Bioassay of antitumor effects of human allo antisera, *Clin. Res.* **17**:328.

HERSEY, P., ISBISTER, J., EDWARDS, A., *et al.*, 1976, Antibody-dependent cell-mediated cytotoxicity against melanoma cells induced by plasmaphoresis, *Lancet* **1**:825.

HERSH, E. M., AND FREIREICH, E. J., 1968, Host defense mechanisms and their modification by cancer chemotherapy, in: *Methods in Cancer Research*, Vol. 4 (H. BUSCH, ed.), pp. 355–451, Academic Press, New York.

HERSH, E. M., GUTTERMAN, J. U., MAVLIGIT, G. M., *et al.*, 1974, Serial studies of immunocompetence of patients undergoing chemotherapy for acute leukemia, *J. Clin. Invest.* **54**:401.

HERSH, E. M., GUTTERMAN, J. U., AND MAVLIGIT, G. M., 1975, Cancer and host defense mechanisms, in: *Pathobiology Annual* (H. L. IOACHIM, ed.), pp. 133–168, Appleton-Century-Crofts, New York.

HERSH, E. M., GUTTERMAN, J. U., MAVLIGIT, G. M., *et al.*, 1976a, Immunocompetence, immunodeficiency, and prognosis in cancer, *Ann. N.Y. Acad. Sci.* **276**:386.

HERSH, E. M., GUTTERMAN, J. U., MAVLIGIT, G. M., MCBRIDE, C. M., AND BURGESS, M. A., 1976b, Immunostimulation with different BCG preparations during immunochemotherapy of melanoma, *Am. Soc. Clin. Oncol.* **17**:246.

HEWLETT, J. S., BALCERZAK, S., AND GUTTERMAN, J. U., 1977, Remission induction in adult acute leukemia by a ten-day continuous infusion of ara-C plus Oncovin and prednisone: Maintenance with and without BCG, in: *Immunotherapy of Cancer: Present Status of Trials in Man* (W. TERRY AND D. WINDHORST, eds.), in press.

HEYN, R. M., JOO, P., KARON, M., *et al.*, 1975, BCG in the treatment of acute lymphatic leukemia, *Blood* **46**:431.

HIBBS, J. B., 1974, Heterocytolysis by macrophages activated by bacillus Calmette Guérin lysozome exocytosis into tumor cells, *Science* **184**:468.

HIBBS, J. B., LAMBERT, L. H., AND REMINGTON, J. S., 1972, Possible role of macrophage-mediated non-specific cytotoxicity in tumor resistance, *Nature (London)* **235**:48.

HILL, G. J., AND LITTLEJOHN, K., 1971, B16 melanoma in C57 black 6J mice: Kinetics and effects of heterologous serum, *J. Surg. Oncol.* **3**:1.

HILLEMAN, N. R., 1970, Double-stranded RNAs in the prevention of viral infections, *Arch. Intern. Med.* **126**:109.

HITZIG, W. H., AND GROB, P. J., 1974, Therapeutic uses of transfer factor, *Prog. Clin. Immunol.* **2**:69.

HO, M., 1964, Interferon-like viral inhibitor in rabbit after intravenous administration of endotoxin, *Science* **146**:1472.

HOEBEKE, J., AND FRANCHI, G., 1973, Influence of tetramazole and its optical isomers on the mononuclear phagocytic system: Effect on carbon clearance in mice, *J. Reticuloendothel. Soc.* **14**:317.

HOERNI, B., CHAUVERGNE, J., HOERNI-SIMON, G., *et al.*, 1976, BCG in the immunotherapy of Hodgkin's disease and non-Hodgkin's lymphoma, *Cancer Immunol. Immunother.* **1**:109.

HOLLAND, J. F., AND BEKESI, J. G., 1976, Immunotherapy of human leukemia with neuraminidase modified cells, *Med. Clin. N. Am.* **60**:539.

HOLLINSHEAD, A. C., 1975, Analysis of soluble melanoma cell membrane antigens in metastatic cells of various organs and further studies of antigens present in primary melanoma, *Cancer* **36**:1282.

HOLLINSHEAD, A. C., STEWART, T. H. M., AND HERBERMAN, R. B., 1974, Delayed hypersensitivity reactions to soluble membrane extracts of human malignant lung cells, *J. Natl. Cancer Inst.* **52**:327.

HOLTERMAN, O. A., PAPERMASTER, B. W., ROSNER, D., MILGROM, H., AND KLEIN, E., 1975, Regression of cutaneous neoplasma following delayed type hypersensitivity challenge reactions to microbial antigens or lymphokines, *J. Med.* **6**:157.

HOOPER, J. A., MCDANIEL, M. C., THURMAN, G. B., *et al.*, 1975, Purification of properties of bovine thymosin, *Ann. N.Y. Acad. Sci.* **249**:125.

HOPPER, D. G., PIMM, M. V., AND BALDWIN, R. W., 1975, Levamisole treatment of local and metastatic growth of transplanted rat tumors, *Br. J. Cancer* **32**:345.

HORN, L., AND HORN, H. L., 1971, An immunological approach to therapy of cancer, *Lancet* **2**:466.

HORTOBAGYI, G. N., 1977, Chemoimmunotherapy of advanced breast cancer with BCG and MER, in: *Immunotherapy of Cancer: Present Status of Trials in Man* (W. TERRY AND D. WINDHORST, eds.), in press.

HUEPER, W. C., AND RUSSELL, M., 1932, Some immunological aspects of leukemia, *Arch. Intern. Med.* **49**:113.

HUMPHREY, J. L., JEWELL, W. R., MURRAY, D. R., *et al.*, 1971, Immunotherapy for the patient with cancer, *Ann. Surg.* **173**:47.

EVAN M. HERSH,
G. M. MAVLIGIT,
J. U. GUTTERMAN,
AND
S. P. RICHMAN

HUNTER-CRAIG, I., NEWTON, K. A., WESTBURY, G., et al., 1970, Use of vaccinia virus in the treatment of malignant melanoma, Br. Med. J. **2**:512.

HYNES, R. O., 1973, Alteration of cell-surface proteins by viral transformation and by proteolysis, Proc. Natl. Acad. Sci. (USA) **70**:3170.

IKONOPISOV, R. L., 1975, The use of BCG in the combined treatment of malignant melanoma, in: International Symposium on Immunological Reactions to Melanoma, Antigens, pp. 206–214, Behring-werke, Hanover.

IKONOPISOV, R. L., LEWIS, M. G., HUNTER-CRAIG, I. D., et al., 1970, Autoimmunization with irradiated tumor cells in human malignant melanoma, Br. Med. J. **2**:752.

IRVIN, G. L., AND EUSTACE, J. C., 1970, The enhancement and rejection of tumor allografts by immune lymph node cells, Transplantation **5**:55.

ISBISTER, W. H., NOONAN, F. P., HALLIDAY, W. J., et al., 1975, Human thoracic duct cannulation: Manipulation of tumor-specific blocking factors in a patient with malignant melanoma, Cancer **35**:1465.

ISRAEL, L., 1974, Clinical results with corynebacteria, in: Recent Results in Cancer Research: Investigations and Stimulation of Immunity in Cancer Patients (G. MATHÉ AND R. WEINER, eds.), p. 486, Springer-Verlag, New York.

ISRAEL, L., EDELSTEIN, R., DePIERRE, A., et al., 1975, Brief communication: Daily intravenous infusion of Corynebacterium parvum in twenty patients with disseminated cancer. A preliminary report of clinical and biological findings, J. Natl. Cancer Inst. **55**:29.

JONES, S. E., 1977, Chemoimmunotherapy of non-Hodgkin's lymphoma, in: Immunotherapy of Cancer: Present Status of Trials in Man (W. TERRY AND D. WINDHORST, eds.), in press.

JOSE, D. G., AND SESHADRI, R., 1974, Circulating immune complexes in human neuroblastoma direct assay and role in blocking specific cellular immunity, Int. J. Cancer **13**:824.

JURIN, M., AND SUIT, H. D., 1973, Transfer of resistance to tumor with lymphoid cells from immunized allogeneic donors, Texas Rep. Biol. Med. **31**:29.

KALISS, N., 1962, The elements of immunological enhancement: Consideration of mechanisms, Ann. N.Y. Acad. Sci. **101**:64.

KAPLAN, A. M., AND MORAHAN, P. S., 1976, Macrophage-mediated tumor cell cytolysis, Ann. N.Y. Acad. Sci. **276**:134.

KAY, H., 1977, Five year follow-up of the Medical Research Council's Concord Trial of ALL immunotherapy, in: Immunotherapy of Cancer: Present Status of Trials in Man (W. TERRY AND D. WINDHORST, eds.), in press.

KENADY, D. E., POTVIN, C., SIMON, R. M., et al., 1977, Thymosin modulation of T-cell levels in vitro in cancer patients, Cancer (in press).

KHAN, A., HILL, J. M., MACLELLAN, A., et al., 1975, Improvement in delayed hypersensitivity in Hodgkin's disease with transfer factor, Cancer **36**:86.

KIMURA, I., OHNOSHI, T., AND YASUHARA, S., 1976, Immunotherapy in human lung cancer using a streptococcal agent OK432, Cancer **37**:2201.

KINT, A., AND VERLINDEN, L., 1974, Levamisole for recurrent herpes labialis, N. Engl. J. Med. **291**:308.

KIRKPATRICK, C. H., 1975, Properties and activities of transfer factor, J. Allergy Clin. Immunol. **55**:411.

KIRKPATRICK, C. H., AND GALLIN, J. I., 1975, Suppression of cellular immune responses following transfer factor: Report of a case, Cell. Immunol. **15**:470.

KIRKPATRICK, C. H., WILSON, W. E. C., AND TALMADGE, D. W., 1964, Immunologic studies in human organ transplantation. I. Observation and characterization of suppressed cutaneous reactivity in uremia, J. Exp. Med. **119**:727.

KIRKPATRICK, C. H., RICH, R. R., AND SMITH, P. K., 1972, Effect of transfer factor on lymphocyte function in anergic patients, J. Clin. Invest. **51**:2948.

KLEIN, E., AND HOLTERMAN, O. A., 1972, Immunotherapeutic approaches to the management of neoplasms, Natl. Cancer Inst. Monogr. **35**:279.

KLEIN, E., HOLTERMAN, O. A., HELM, F., et al., 1975, Immunological approaches to the management of primary and secondary tumors involving the skin and soft tissues: Review of a ten year program, Transplant. Proc. **7**:297.

KLEIN, E., HOLTERMAN, O., MILGROM, H., et al., 1976, Immunotherapy for accessible tumors utilizing delayed hypersensitivity reactions and separated components of the immune system, Med. Clin. N. Am. **60**:389.

KLEIN, J. J., GOLDSTEIN, A. L., AND WHITE, A., 1965, Enhancement of in vivo incorporation of labelled precursors in DNA and total protein of mouse lymph nodes after administration of thymic extracts, Proc. Natl. Acad. Sci. (USA) **53**:812.

KOLLMORGEN, G. M., KILLION, J. J., AND SANSING, W. A., 1974, Combination chemotherapy and immunotherapy of transplantable murine leukemia, in: *The Cell Cycle in Malignancy and Immunity* (J. C. HAMPTON, ed.), NTIS, Springfield, Mass.

KOLTAI, M., AND MECS, E., 1973, Inhibition of the acute inflammatory response by interferon inducers, *Nature (London)* **242**:525.

KREMENTZ, E. T., AND SAMUELS, M. S., 1967, Tumor cross-transplantation and cross-transfusion in the treatment of advanced malignant disease, *Bull. Tulane Univ. Med. School* **26**:263.

KRONMAN, B. S., WEPSIC, H. T., CHURCHILL, W. H., et al., 1970, Immunotherapy of cancer: An experimental model in syngeneic guinea pigs, *Science* **168**:258.

LACKOVIC, V., BORECKY, L., SIKL, D., et al., 1970, Stimulation of interform production by mannans, *Proc. Soc. Expl. Biol. Med.* **134**:874.

LaGRANGE, P. H., and MACKANESS, G. B., 1977, Effect of bacterial lypopolysaccharide on the induction and expression of cell-mediated immunity. II. Stimulation of the efferent arc, submitted.

LAMENSANS, A., CHEDID, L., LEDERER, E., et al., 1975, Enhancement of immunity against murine syngeneic tumors by a fraction extracted from a non-pathogenic *Mycobacterium*, *Proc. Natl. Acad. Sci. (USA)* **72**:3656.

LAUCIUS, J. F., BODURTHA, A. J., MASTRANGELO, M. J., et al., 1974, Bacillus Clamette guérin in the treatment of neoplastic disease, *J. Reticuloendothel. Soc.* **16**:347.

LAW, K. K., DUDRICK, S. J., AND ABDOU, N. I., 1973, Immunocompetence of patients with protein calorie malnutrition, *Ann. Intern. Med.* **79**:545.

LAWRENCE, H. S., 1974, Transfer factor in cellular immunity, *The Harvey Lectures Series*, pp. 239–350, Academic Press, New York.

LAWRENCE, H. S., 1976, Transfer factor, in: *Advances in Immunology* (F. J. DICKSON AND H. G. KUNKLE, eds.), pp. 195–266, Academic Press, New York.

LAWRENCE, H. S., 1949, The cellular transfer of cutaneous hypersensitivity to tuberculin in man, *Proc. Soc. Exptl. Biol.* **71**:516.

LAWRENCE, H. S., AND PAPPENHEIMER, A. M., JR., 1956, Transfer of delayed hypersensitivity to diphtheria toxin in man, *J. Exp. Med.* **104**:321.

LAZLO, J., BUCKLEY, C. E., AND AMOS, D. B., 1968, Infusion of isologous immune plasma in chronic lymphocytic leukemia, *Blood* **31**:104.

LEE, A. K. Y., ROWLEY, M., AND MACKAY, I. R., 1970, Antibody-producing capacity in human cancer, *Br. J. Cancer* **24**:454.

LeMONDE, P., 1973, Protective effect of BCG and other bacteria against neoplasia in mice and hamsters, *Natl. Cancer Inst. Monogr.* **39**:21.

LEVENTHAL, B. G., LePOURHEIT, A., HALTERMAN, R. H., et al., Immunotherapy in previously treated acute lymphatic leukemia, *Natl. Cancer. Inst. Monogr.* **39**:177.

LEVEY, R. H., TRAININ, N., AND LAW, L. W., 1963, Evidence for function of thymic tissue in diffusion chambers implanted into neonatally thymectomized mice: Preliminary report, *J. Natl. Cancer Inst.* **31**:199.

LEVIN, A. S., SPITLER, L. E., STITES, D. P., et al., 1970, Wiskott-Aldrich syndrome: A genetically determined cellular immunological deficiency: Clinical and laboratory responses to therapy with transfer factor, *Proc. Natl. Acad. Sci. (USA)* **67**:821.

LEVINE, S., GIBSON, J. P., AND MEGEL, H., 1974, Selective depletion of thymus-dependent areas in lymphoid tissue by tylerone, *Proc. Soc. Expl. Biol. Med.* **146**:245.

LEVY, H. B., LAW, L. W., AND RABSON, A. S., 1969, Inhibition of tumor growth by polyinosinic-polycytidylic acid, *Proc. Natl. Acad. Sci. (USA)* **62**:357.

LIKHITE, V. V., AND HALPERN, B. N., 1973, The delayed rejection of tumors formed from the administration of tumor cells mixed with killed *Corynebacterium parvum*, *Int. J. Cancer* **12**:699.

LINDAHL-MAGNUSSON, P., AND GRESSER, I., 1972, Interferon inhibits DNA synthesis induced in mouse lymphocyte suspensions by phytohemagglutinin or by allogeneic cells, *Nature (London)* **237**:120.

LINDENMANN, J., 1974, Viruses as immunological adjuvants in cancer, *Biochim. Biophys. Acta* **355**:79.

LINDSTROMM, B. A., 1927, An experimental study of myelotoxic sera: Therapeutic attempts in myeloid leukemia, *Acta Med. Scand. Suppl.* **22**:1.

LITWIN, M. S., KREMENTZ, E. T., MANSELL, P. W., et al., 1975, Topical chemotherapy of lentigo muligna with 5-fluorouracil, *Cancer* **35**:721.

LoBUGLIO, A. F., NEIDHART, J. A., HILBERG, R. W., et al., 1973, The effect of transfer factor therapy on tumor immunity in alveolar soft part sarcoma, *Cell. Immunol.* **7**:159.

LONDNER, M. V., MORINI, J. C., FONT, M. T., et al., 1968, RNA-induced immunity against the rat sarcoma, *Experientia* **24**:596.

524

EVAN M. HERSH,
G. M. MAVLIGIT,
J. U. GUTTERMAN,
AND
S. P. RICHMAN

MACKANESS, G. B., AUCLAIR, D. J., AND LaGRANGE, P. H., 1973, Immunopotentiation with BCG. I. Immune response to different strains and preparations, *J. Natl. Cancer Inst.* **51**:1655.

MADDISON, S. E., HICKLIN, M. D., CONWAY, B. P., *et al.*, 1972, Transfer factor: Delayed hypersensitivity to schistosoma mansoni and tuberculin in *Macaca mulatta*, *Science* **178**:757.

MAEDA, Y. Y., AND CHIHARA, G., 1973, The effects of neonatal thymectomy on the antitumor activity of lentinan carboxymethyl pachymaran and zymosan, and their effects on various immune responses, *Int. J. Cancer* **11**:153.

MANSELL, P. W. A., ICHINOSE, H., AND REED, R. J., 1975, Macrophage-mediated destruction of human malignant cells *in vivo*, *J. Natl. Cancer Inst.* **54**:571.

MANTOVANI, A., AND SPREAFICO, F., 1975, Allogeneic tumor enhancement by levamisole: A new immunostimulatory compound, *Eur. J. Cancer* **11**:537.

MARCOVE, R. C., SOUTHAM, C. M., LEVIN, A., *et al.*, 1971, A clinical trial of autogenous vaccine in osteogenic sarcoma in patients under the age of twenty-five, *Surg. Forum* **22**:434.

MARSHALL, W. H., 1972, Transfer of immune responsiveness, *Med. Clin. N. Am.* **56**:465.

MARTIN, D. S., HAYWORTH, P., AND FUGMANN, R. A., 1964, Combination therapy with cyclophosphamide and zymosan on a spontaneous mammary cancer in mice, *Cancer Res.* **24**:652.

MASTRANGELO, M. J., BELLET, R. E., AND BERKELHAMMER, J., 1975, Regression of pulmonary metastatic disease associated with intralesional BCG therapy of intracutaneous melanoma metastases, *Cancer* **36**:1305.

MASTRANGELO, M. J., SULIT, H. L., PREHN, L. M., *et al.*, 1976, Intralesional BCG in the treatment of metastatic malignant melanoma, *Cancer* **37**:684.

MASTRANGELO, M. J., BELLET, R. E., AND BERD, D., 1977, A randomized prospective trial comparing MECCNU plus vincristine to MECCNU plus vincristine plus BCG plus allogeneic tumor cells in patients with metastatic malignant melanoma, in: *Immunotherapy of Cancer: Present Status of Trials in Man* (W. TERRY AND D. WINDHORST, eds.), in press.

MATHÉ, G., AMIEL, J. L., SCHWARZENBERG, L., SCHNEIDER, M., *et al.*, 1969a, Active immunotherapy for acute lymphoblastic leukemia, *Lancet* **1**:697.

MATHÉ, G., GOUILLART, P., AND LAPEYRAQUE, F., 1969b, Active immunotherapy of L-1210 leukemia applied after the graft of tumor cells, *Br. J. Cancer* **23**:814.

MATHÉ, G., KAMEL, M., AND DEZFULIAN, M., 1973a, An experimental screening for systemic adjuvants of immunity applicable in cancer immunology, *Cancer Res.* **33**:1987.

MATHÉ, G., WEINER, R., POUILLART, P., *et al.*, 1973b, BCG in cancer immunotherapy: Experimental and clinical trials of its use in treatment of leukemia minimal and/or residual disease, *Natl. Cancer Inst. Monogr.* **39**:165.

MAVLIGIT, G. M., GUTTERMAN, J. U., BURGESS, M. A., *et al.*, 1976, Prolongation of post-operative disease-free interval and survival in human colorectal cancer by BCG or BCG plus 5-fluorouracil, *Lancet* **1**:871.

MAYER, G. D., AND KRUEGER, R. F., 1970, Tylerone hydrochloride and orally active antiviral agent, *Science* **169**:1213.

McBRIDE, W. H., WEIR, D. M., KAY, A. B., *et al.*, 1975, Activation of the classical and alternate pathways of complement by *C. parvum*, *Clin. Expl. Immunol.* **19**:143.

McDANIEL, M. C., LAUDICO, R., AND PAPERMASTER, B. W., 1976, Association of macrophage activation factor from a human cultured lymphoid cell line with albumin and alpha-2-macroglobulin, *Clin. Immunol. Immunopathol.* **5**:91.

McINTYRE, O. R., RAI, K., GLIDEWELL, O., *et al.*, 1977, Poly-I–poly-C as an adjunct to remission maintenance therapy in acute myelogenous leukemia, in: *Immunotherapy of Cancer: Present Status of Trials in Man* (W. TERRY AND D. WINDHORST, eds.), in press.

McKNEALLY, M. F., MAVER, C., AND KAUSEL, H. W., 1976, Regional immunotherapy of lung cancer with intrapleural BCG, *Lancet* **1**:377.

MEDICAL RESEARCH COUNCIL, 1971, Treatment of acute lymphoblastic leukemia, *Br. Med. J.* **4**:189.

MEYER, T. J., RIBI, E., AND AZUMA, I., 1975, Biologically active components from mycobacterial cell walls. V. Granuloma formation in mouse lungs and guinea pig skin, *Cell. Immunol.* **16**:11.

MILAS, L., HUNTER, N., AND BASIC, I., 1974a, Complete regressions of an established murine fibrosarcoma induced by systemic application of *Corynebacterium granulosum*, *Cancer Res.* **34**:2470.

MILAS, L., GUTTERMAN, J. U., BASIC, I., HERSH, E. M., *et al.*, 1974b, Immunoprophylaxis and immunotherapy for a murine fibrosarcoma with *C. granulosum* and *C. parvum*, *Int. J. Cancer* **14**:493.

MILAS, L., HUNTER, N., AND WITHERS, H. R., 1975, Combination of local irradiation with systemic application of anaerobic corynebacteria in therapy of a murine fibrosarcoma, *Cancer Res.* **35**:1274.

MILLER, J. F. A. P., AND OSOBA, D., 1967, Current concepts of the immunological function of the thymus, *Physiol. Rev.* **47**:437.

MILLER, T. E., MACKANESS, G. B., AND LaGRANGE, P. H., 1973, Immunopotentiation with BCG. II. Modulation of the response to sheep red blood cells, *J. Natl. Cancer Inst.* **51**:1669.

MINDEN, P., McCLATCHY, J. K., WAINBERG, M., AND WEISS, D. W., 1974, Shared antigens between *Mycobacterium bovis* (BCG) and neoplastic cells, *J. Natl. Cancer Inst.* **53**:1325.

MODOLELL, M., LUCKENBACH, G. A., PARANT, M., et al., The adjuvant activity of a mycobacterial water soluble adjuvant (WSA) *in vitro*, *J. Immunol.* **113**:395.

MOERTEL, C. G., RITTS, R. E., SCHUTT, A. J., et al., 1975, A phase I study of methanol extraction residue of BCG (MER-BCG), *Proc. Am. Assoc. Cancer Res.* **16**:143.

MOERTEL, C. G., O'CONNELL, M. J., RITTS, R. E., et al., 1977, A controlled evaluation of combination immunotherapy (MER-BCG) and chemotherapy for advanced colorectal cancer, in: *Immunotherapy of Cancer: Present Status of Trials in Man* (W. TERRY AND D. WINDHORST, eds.), in press.

MOHR, J. A., KILLEBREW, L., MUCHMORE, H. G., et al., 1969, Transfer of delayed hypersensitivity: The role of blood transfusions in humans, *J. Am. Med. Assoc.* **207**:517.

MOLLER, G., AND MOLLER, E., 1975, Considerations of current concepts in cancer research, *J. Natl. Cancer Inst.* **55**:755.

MOOLTEN, F., ZAJEDEL, S., AND COOPERBAND, S., 1976, Immunotherapy of experimental animal tumors with antitumor antibodies conjugated to diphtheria toxin or ricin, *Ann. N.Y. Acad. Sci.* **277**:690.

MONARD, D., SOLOMAN, F., RENTSCH, M., AND GYSIN, R., 1973, Glia-induced morphological differentiation in neuroblastoma cells, *Proc. Natl. Acad. Sci. (USA)* **70**:1894.

MOORE, G. E., AND GERNER, R. E., 1970, Cancer immunity: Hypothesis and clinical trial of lymphocytotherapy for malignant disease, *Ann. Surg.* **172**:733.

MORSE, P. A., DERAPS, G. D., SMITH, G. V., et al., 1973, Transfer factor therapy of human cancer, *Clin. Res.* **21**:71.

MORTON, D. L., 1977, Clinical trial comparing no further therapy to BCG or BCG plus allogeneic cells in stage II melanoma, in: *Immunotherapy of Cancer: Present Status of Trials in Man* (W. TERRY AND D. WINDHORST, eds.), in press.

MORTON, D. L., EILBER, F. R., MALMGREN, R. A., et al., 1970, Immunological factors which influence response to immunotherapy in malignant melanoma, *Surgery* **68**:158.

MORTON, D. L., EILBER, F. R., AND MALMGREN, R. A., 1971a, Immune factors in human cancer: Malignant melanomas, skeletal and soft tissue sarcomas, *Prog. Exp. Tumor Res.* **14**:25.

MORTON, D. L., HOLMES, E. C., EILBER, F. R., et al., 1971b, Immunological aspects of neoplasia: A rational basis for immunotherapy, *Ann. Intern. Med.* **74**:587.

MORTON, D. L., EILBER, F. R., HOLMES, E. C., et al., 1974, BCG immunotherapy of malignant melanoma: Summary of seven years experience, *Ann. Surg.* **180**:635.

MOSEDALE, B., AND SMITH, M. A., 1975, *Corynebacterium parvum* and anesthetics, *Lancet* **1**:168.

MUFTUOGLOU, A. U., AND BALKUR, S., 1967, Passive transfer of tuberculin sensitivity to patients with Hodgkin's disease, *N. Engl. J. Med.* **277**:126.

MUNSON, A. E., REGELSON, W., AND WOOLES, W., 1970, Tissue localization studies in evaluating the functional role of the reticuloendothelial system, *J. Reticuloendothel. Soc.* **7**:366.

MUNSON, A. E., MUNSON, J. A., REGELSON, W., et al., 1972, Effect of tylerone hydrochloride and cogenes on reticuloendothelial system: Tumors, and the immune response, *Cancer Res.* **32**:1397.

MURRAY, G., 1958, Experiments in immunity in cancer, *Can. Med. Assoc. J.* **79**:249.

NADLER, S. H., AND MOORE, G. E., 1969, Immunotherapy of malignant disease, *Arch. Surg.* **99**:376.

NAUTS, H. C., 1975, *Osteogenic Sarcoma: End Results Following Immunotherapy with Bacterial Vaccines, 165 Cases, or Following Bacterial Infections Inflammation or Fever, 41 cases*, Monograph No. 15, Cancer Research Institute, New York.

NEWLANDS, E. S., OON, C. J., ROBERTS, J. T., et al., 1976, Clinical trial of combination chemotherapy and specific active immunotherapy in disseminated melanoma, *Br. J. Cancer* **34**:174.

NGU, V. A., 1967, Clinical evidence of host defenses in Burkitt's tumor, in: *Treatment of Burkitt's Tumor* (J. H. BURCHENAL AND D. P. BURKITT, eds.), pp. 204–208, Springer-Verlag, New York.

NOVELLI, D., 1976, A biochemist's view of the mediators of cellular immunity with special reference to application, in: *Transfer Factor: Basic Properties and Clinical Application* (M. S. ASCHER, A. GOTTLIEB, AND C. H. KIRKPATRICK, eds.), pp. 723–739, Academic Press, New York.

OCCHINO, J. C., GLASGOW, A. H., AND COOPERBAND, S. R., 1973, Isolation of an immunosuppressive peptide fraction from human plasma, *J. Immunol.* **110**:685.

OETTGEN, H. F., OLD, L. J., FARROW, J. H., et al., 1974, Effect of dialyzable transfer factor in patients with breast cancer, *Proc. Natl. Acad. Sci. (USA)* **71**:2319.

EVAN M. HERSH,
G. M. MAVLIGIT,
J. U. GUTTERMAN,
AND
S. P. RICHMAN

OLD, L. J., CLARK, D. A., AND BENACERRAF, B., 1959, Effective bacillus Calmette Guérin infection on transplanted tumors in the mouse, *Nature* **184**:291.

OYAMA, K., TAKAGAKI, Y., NIKI, R., *et al.*, 1975, Studies on the interrelation between clinical effects and immune response of a streptococcal antitumor agent OK432. I. Immunological findings in animals sensitized with OK432, *Jpn. J. Clin. Cancer* **21**:253.

PABST, H. F., AND CRAWFORD, J. A., 1974, Enhancement of *in vitro* cellular immune response by L-tetramizole, *Pediat. Res.* **8**:416.

PAPERMASTER, B. W., HOLTERMAN, O. A., MCDANIEL, M. C., *et al.*, 1976a, Effect of supernatants from long-term lymphoid cell lines on metastatic cutaneous tumors following local injection, *Ann. N.Y. Acad. Sci.* **276**:584.

PAPERMASTER, B. W., HOLTERMAN, O. A., AND KLEIN, E., 1976b, Lymphokine properties of a lymphoid culture cell supernatant fraction active in promoting tumor regression, *Clin. Immunol. Immunopathol.* **5**:48.

PAPERMASTER, B. W., HOLTERMAN, O. A., KLEIN, E., *et al.*, 1976c, Preliminary observations on tumor regressions induced by local administration of a lymphoid cell culture supernatant fraction in patients with cutaneous metastatic lesions, *Clin. Immunol. Immunopathol.* **5**:31.

PAQUE, R. E., AND DRAY, S., 1974, Transfer of delayed hypersensitivity to nonsensitive human leukocytes with rhesus monkey lymphoid RNA extracts, *Transplant. Proc.* **6**:203.

PAQUE, R. E., ALI, M., AND DRAY, S., 1975, RNA extracts of lymphoid cells sensitized to DNP-oligolysines convert non-responder lymphoid cells to responder cells which release migration inhibitory factor, *Cell. Immunol.* **16**:261.

PARR, I., 1972, Response of syngeneic murine lymphomata to immunotherapy in relation to the antigenicity of the tumor, *Br. J. Cancer* **26**:174.

PASLIN, D., DIMITROV, N. V., AND HEATON, C., 1974, Regression of transplantable hamster melanoma by intralesional injections of *C. granulosum*, *J. Natl. Cancer Inst.* **52**:571.

PEARSON, J. W., PEARSON, G. R., GIBSON, W. T., *et al.*, 1972, Combination chemoimmuno stimulation therapy against murine leukemia, *Cancer Res.* **32**:904.

PEARSON, J. W., CHIRIGOS, M. A., AND CHAPARAS, S. V., 1974, Combined drug and immunostimulation therapy against a syngeneic murine leukemia, *J. Natl. Cancer Inst.* **52**:463.

PENDERGRAST, W. J., DRAKE, W. P., AND MARDINEY, M. R., 1975, The dependence of successful immunotherapy on adequate tumor burden as shown by the treatment of AKR leukemia with poly-A, poly-U, *J. Natl. Cancer Inst.* **55**:1223.

PENN, I., AND STARZL, T. E., 1972, Malignant tumors *de novo* in immunosuppressed organ transplant recipients, *Transplantation* **14**:407.

PENNY, R., CASTALDI, P. A., AND WHITSED, H. M., 1971, Inflammation and hemostasis in para-proteinemias, *Brit. J. Haematol.* **20**:35.

PERK, K., CHIRIGOS, M. A., FUHRMAN, F., *et al.*, 1975, Some aspects of host response to levamisole after chemotherapy in a murine leukemia, *J. Natl. Cancer Inst.* **54**:253.

PETO, R., 1977, Immunotherapy of acute myeloid leukemia, in : *Immunotherapy of Cancer: Present Status of Trials in Man* (W. TERRY AND D. WINDHORST, eds.), in press.

PHANUPHAK, P., MOORHEAD, J. W., AND CLAMAN, H. N., 1972, Immunological activities of pertussis treated lymphocytes, *Int. Arch. Allergy Appl. Immunol.* **43**:305.

PIESSENS, W. F., LACHAPELLE, F. L., LEGROS, N., *et al.*, 1970, Facilitation of rat mammary tumour growth by BCG, *Nature (London)* **228**:1210.

PILCH, Y. H., AND RAMMING, K. P., 1970, Transfer of tumor immunity with ribonucleic acid, *Cancer* **26**:630.

PILCH, Y. H., RAMMING, K. P., AND DECKERS, P. J.: Transfer of immunity to transplantation and tumor-specific antigens by RNA from lymphoid organs of xenogeneic, allogeneic, and syngeneic animals, *Transplant. Proc.* **3**:566.

PILCH, Y. H., VELTMAN, L. L., AND KERN, D. H., 1974, Immune cytolysis of human tumor cells mediated by xenogeneic immune RNA, *Arch. Surg.* **109**:30.

PILCH, Y. H., FRITZE, D., AND KERN, D. H., 1976a, Immune RNA in the immunotherapy of cancer, *Med. Clin. N. Am.* **60**:567.

PILCH, Y. H., FRITZE, D., DEKERNION, J. B., *et al.*, 1976b, Immunotherapy of cancer with immune RNA in animal models and cancer patients, *Ann. N.Y. Acad. Sci.* **277**:592.

PIMM, M. V., AND BALDWIN, R. W., 1975a, BCG therapy of pleural and peritoneal growth of transplanted rat tumors, *Int. J. Cancer* **15**:260.

PIMM, M. B., AND BALDWIN, R. W., 1975*b*, BCG immunotherapy of rat tumors in athymic "nude" mice, *Nature (London)* **254**:77.

PINES, A., 1976, A five-year controlled study of BCG and radiotherapy for inoperable lung cancer, *Lancet* **1**:380.

PINSKY, C. M., HIRSHAUT, Y., AND OETTGEN, H. F., 1973, Treatment of malignant melanoma by intratumoral injection of BCG, *Natl. Cancer Inst. Monogr.* **39**:225.

PINSKY, C. M., HIRSHOUT, Y., WANEBO, H., *et al.*, 1976, Randomized trial of bacillus Calmette Guérin (percutaneous administration) as surgical adjuvant: Immunotherapy for patients with stage II melanoma, *Ann. N.Y. Acad. Sci.* **277**:187.

PINSKY, M., DEJAGER, R. L., KAUFMAN, R. J., *et al.*, 1977, *Corynebacterium parvum* as adjuvant to combination chemotherapy in patients with advanced breast cancer: Preliminary results of a prospective randomized trial, in: *Immunotherapy of Cancer: Present Status of Trials in Man* (W. TERRY AND D. WINDHORST, eds.), in press.

POLLACK, S., HEPPNER, G., BRAUN, R. J., *et al.*, Specific killing of tumor cells *in vitro* in the presence of normal lymphoid cells and sera from hosts immune to the tumor antigens, *Int. J. Cancer* **9**:316.

POTTER, C. W., CARR, I., JENNINGS, R., *et al.*, 1974, Levamisole inactive in treatment of four animal tumors, *Nature (London)* **249**:567.

POWLES, R., CROWTHER, D., BATEMAN, C. T. J., *et al.*, 1973, Immunotherapy for acute myelogenous leukemia, *Br. J. Cancer* **28**:365.

PRAGER, M. D., RIBBLE, R. J., AND MEHTA, J. M., 1974, Aspects of the immunology of the tumor host relationship and responsiveness to modified lymphoma cells, *Recent Results Cancer Res.* **47**:379.

PRESANT, C. A., BARTOLUCCI, A., SMALLEY, R., *et al.*, 1977, Effect of *C. parvum* (Cp) on combination chemotherapy of metastatic malignant melanoma, in: *Immunotherapy of Cancer: Present Status of Trials in Man* (W. TERRY AND D. WINDHORST, eds.), in press.

PURNELL, D. M., KREIDER, J. W., AND BARTLETT, G. L., 1975, Evaluation of antitumor activity of *Bordetella pertussis* in two murine tumor models, *J. Natl. Cancer Inst.* **55**:123.

QUICK, C. A., BEHRENS, H. W., DARNELL, M. B., *et al.*, 1975, Treatment of papillomatosis of the larynx with transfer factor, *Ann. Otolaryngol.* **84**:607.

RAMMING, K. P. AND PILCH, Y. H., 1970*a*, Mediation of immunity to tumor isografts in mice by heterologous ribonucleic acid, *Science* **168**:492.

RAMMING, K. P., AND PILCH, Y. H., 1970*b*, Transfer of tumor-specific immunity with RNA: Demonstration by immune cytolysis of tumor cells *in vitro*, *J. Natl. Cancer Inst.* **45**:543.

RAMMING, K. P., AND PILCH, Y. H., 1971, Transfer of tumor-specific immunity with RNA: Inhibition of growth of murine tumor isografts, *J. Natl. Cancer Inst.* **46**:735.

RAMOT, B., BINIAMINOV, M., SHOHAM, C., *et al.*, 1976, Effect of levamisole on E-rosette forming cells *in vivo* and *in vitro* in Hodgkin's disease, *N. Engl. J. Med.* **294**:809.

REED, R. C., GUTTERMAN, J. U., MAVLIGIT, G. M., *et al.*, 1975, *Corynebacterium parvum*: Preliminary report of a phase I clinical and immunological study in cancer patients, in: *Corynebacterium parvum* (B. N. HALPERN, ed.), pp. 349–366, Plenum Press, New York.

REGELSON, W., 1976, Clinical immunoadjuvant studies with tylorone, *Ann. N.Y. Acad. Sci. (USA)* **277**:269.

REIF, A. E., ROBINSON, C. M., AND SMITH, P. J., 1976, Preparation and therapeutic potential of rabbit antisera with directed specificities for mouse leukemias, *Ann. N.Y. Acad. Sci.* **277**:647.

REISFELD, R. A., PELLEGRINO, M. A., AND KAHAN, B. D., 1971, Salt extraction of soluble HLA antigens, *Science* **172**:1134.

REIZENSTEIN, P., BRENNING, G., ENGSTEDT, L., *et al.*, 1977, Effective immunotherapy on survival and remission duration in acute non-lymphatic leukemia, in: *Immunotherapy of Cancer: Present Status of Trials in Man* (W. TERRY AND D. WINDHORST, eds.), in press.

RENOUX, G., AND RENOUX, M., 1972, Levamisole inhibits and cures a solid malignant tumor and its pulmonary metastases in mice, *Nature (London)* **240**:217.

RENOUX, G., AND RENOUX, M., 1973, Stimulation of anti-brucella vaccination in mice by tetramisole, a phenyl-imidothiazole salt, *Infect. Immun.* **8**:544.

RHIM, J. S., HUEBNER, R. J., AND GISIN, S., 1969, Effect of statolon on acute and persistent murine leukemia and sarcoma virus infections, *Proc. Soc. Exp. Biol. Med.* **130**:181.

RIBI, E., MEYER, T. J., AZUMA, I., *et al.*, 1975*a*, Biologically active components from mycobacterial cell walls. Protection of mice against aerosol infection with virulent *Mycobacterium tuberculosis*, *Cell. Immunol.* **16**:1.

528

EVAN M. HERSH,
G. M. MAVLIGIT,
J. U. GUTTERMAN,
AND
S. P. RICHMAN

RIBI, E., GRANGER, D. L., MILNER, K. C., *et al.*, 1975*b*, Tumor regression caused by endotoxins and mycobacterial fractions, *J. Natl. Cancer Inst.* **55**:1253.

RIBI, E., MILNER, K., KELLY, M. T., *et al.*, 1977, Structural requirements of microbial agents for immunotherapy of the guinea pig line-10 tumor, in: *Present Status of BCG in Cancer Immunotherapy*, in press.

RICHMAN, S. P., MAVLIGIT, G. M., WOLK, R., *et al.*, 1975, Epilesional scarification: Preliminary report of a new approach to local immunotherapy with BCG, *J. Am. Med. Assoc.* **234**:1233.

RICHMAN, S. P., LIVINGSTON, R. B., GUTTERMAN, J. U., *et al.*, 1976, Chemotherapy versus chemo-immunotherapy of head and neck cancer: Report of a randomized study, *Cancer Treat. Rep.* **60**:535.

RIGBY, P. G., 1969, Prolongation of survival of tumor-bearing animals by transfer of immune RNA with DEAE dextran, *Nature (London)* **221**:968.

ROBERTS, S., AND WHITE, A., 1949, Biochemical characterization of lymphoid tissue proteins, *J. Biol. Chem.* **178**:151.

ROJAS, A. F., MICKIEWICZ, E., FEIERSTEIN, J. N., *et al.*, 1976, Levamisole in advanced human breast cancer, *Lancet* **1**:211.

SCHLAGER, S. I., DRAY, S., AND PAQUE, R. E., 1974, Atomic spectroscopic evidence for the absence of a low molecular weight antigen in RNA extracts shown to transfer delayed type hypersensitivity *in vitro*, *Cell. Immunol.* **14**:104.

SCHMIDTKE, J. R., AND JOHNSON, A. G., 1971, Regulation of the immune system by synthetic polynucleotides. I. Characteristics of adjuvant action on antibody synthesis, *J. Immunol.* **106**:1191.

SCHWARTZ, D. B., ZBAR, B., GIBSON, W. T., AND CHIRIGOS, M. A., 1971, Inhibition of murine sarcoma virus oncogenesis with living BCG, *Int. J. Cancer* **8**:320.

SCHWARZENBERG, L., MATHÉ, G., SCHNEIDER, M., *et al.*, 1966, Attempted adoptive immunotherapy of acute leukemia by leukocyte transfusions, *Lancet* **2**:365.

SCOTT, M. T., 1972, Biological effects of the adjuvant *Corynebacterium parvum*: inhibition of PHA, mixed lymphocytes, and GVH reactivity, *Cell. Immunol.* **5**:459.

SCOTT, M. T., 1974*a*, *Corynebacterium parvum* as a therapeutic antitumor agent in mice I. Systemic effects from intravenous injection, *J. Natl. Cancer Inst.* **53**:855.

SCOTT, M. T., 1974*b*, *Corynebacterium parvum* as a therapeutic antitumor agent in mice. II. Local injection, *J. Natl. Cancer Inst.* **53**:861.

SCOTT, M. T., 1974*c*, *Corynebacterium parvum* as an immunotherapeutic anti-cancer agent, *Sem. Oncol.* **1**:367.

SCOTT, M. T., 1974*d*, Depression of delayed type hypersensitivity by *Corynebacterium parvum*: Mandatory role of the spleen, *Cell. Immunol.* **13**:251.

SCOTT, M. T., 1974*e*, *Corynebacterium parvum* as an immunotherapeutic anti-cancer agent, *Sem. Oncol.* **1**:367.

ROSATO, F. E., MILLER, E., ROSATO, E. F., *et al.*, 1976, Active-specific immunotherapy of human solid tumors, *Ann. N.Y. Acad. Sci.* **277**:332.

ROSENBERG, E. B., KANNER, S. P., SCHWARTZMAN, R. J., *et al.*, 1974, Systemic infection following BCG therapy, *Arch. Intern. Med.* **134**:769.

ROSENBERG, S. A., AND RAPP, H. J., 1976, Intralesional immunotherapy of melanoma with BCG, *Med. Clin. N. Am.* **60**:419.

RUCKDESCHEL, J. C., CODISH, S. D., STRANAHAN, A., *et al.*, 1972, Post-operative empyema improved survival in lung cancer: Documentation and analysis of a natural experiment, *N. Engl. J. Med.* **287**:1013.

SADLER, T. E., AND CASTRO, J. E., 1975, Lack of immunological and antitumor effects of orally administered, *Corynebacterium parvum* in mice, *Br. J. Cancer* **31**:359.

SALAMAN, N. R., 1974, Studies on the transfer factor of delayed hypersensitivity, *Immunology* **26**:1069.

SAMPSON, D., AND LUI, A., 1975, The effect of levamisole on cell-mediated immunity and suppressor cell function, *Cancer Res.* **36**:952.

SAUTER, C., CAVALLI, F., AND LINDENMANN, J., 1977, Viral oncolysis: Its application in maintenance treatment of acute myelogenous leukemia, in: *Immunotherapy of Cancer in Man: Present Status of Trials in Man* (W. TERRY AND D. WINDHORST, eds.), in press.

SCHAFER, L. A., GOLDSTEIN, A. L., GUTTERMAN, J. U., AND HERSH, E. M., 1976, *In vitro* and *in vivo* studies with thymosin in cancer patients, *Ann. N.Y. Acad. Sci.* **277**:609.

SCHLAGER, S. I., AND DRAY, S., 1975, Tumor regression at an untreated site during immunotherapy of an identical distant tumor, *Proc. Natl. Acad. Sci.* **72**:3680.

SCOTT, M. T., AND WARNER, S. L., 1976, The accumulated effects of repeated systemic or local injections of low doses of *C. parvum* in mice, *Cancer Res.* **36**:1335.

SERROU, B., REME, T., AND SENELAR, R., 1975, T-lymphocyte maturation and antitumor effect of a thymic extract obtained from a stimulated model, *Ann. N.Y. Acad. Sci.* **249**:328.

SIEGLER, H. F., BUCKLEY, C. E., AND SHEPPARD, L., 1976, Adoptive transfer and specific active immunization with patients with malignant melanoma, *Ann. N.Y. Acad. Sci.* **277**:522.

SIMMONS, R. L., 1977, Comparison of chemotherapy to chemotherapy plus VCN treated autologous tumor cells in stage II and III melanoma, in: *Immunotherapy of Cancer: Present Status of Trials in Man* (W. TERRY AND D. WINDHORST, eds.), in press.

SIMMONS, R. L., AND RIOS, A., 1971, Immunotherapy of cancer, immunospecific rejection of tumors in recipients of neuraminidase-treated tumor cells plus BCG, *Science* **174**:591.

SIMMONS, R. L., AND RIOS, A., 1975, Comparative immunotherapeutic effect of concanavalin-A and neuraminidase-treated cancer cells, *Transplant. Proc.* **7**:247.

SIMMONS, R. L., RIOS, A., RAY, P. K., *et al.*, 1971, Effect of neuraminidase on growth of a 3-methylcholantherene-induced fibrosarcoma in normal and immunosuppressed syngeneic mice, *J. Natl. Cancer Inst.* **47**:1087.

SIMMONS, R. L., RIOS, A., AND TRITES, P., 1976, Modified tumor cells in the immunotherapy of solid mammary tumors, *Med. Clin. N. Am.* **60**:551.

SHIBATA, H. R., JERRY, L. M., LEWIS, M. G., *et al.*, 1976, Immunotherapy of human malignant melanoma with irradiated tumor cells, oral bacillus Calmette Guérin, and levamisole, *Ann. N.Y. Acad. Sci.* **277**:355.

SKURKOVICH, S. V., MAKHONOVA, F. M., AND REZNICHENKI, G. I., *et al.*, 1969, Treatment of children with acute leukemia by passive cyclic immunization with autoplasma and auto-leukocytes operated during the remission period, *Blood* **33**:186.

SKURZAK, H. M., KLEIN, E., YOSHIDA, T. O., *et al.*, 1972, Synergistic or antagonistic effect of different antibody concentrations on *in vitro* leukocyte cytotoxicity in the Moloney sarcoma virus system, *J. Exp. Med.* **135**:997.

SMITH, S. E., AND SCOTT, M. T., 1972, Biological effects of *Corynebacterium parvum* III. Amplification of resistance and impairment of active immunity to murine tumors, *Br. J. Cancer* **26**:361.

SOKAL, J. E., AUNGST, C. W., AND GRACE, J. T., 1973, Immunotherapy in well-controlled chronic myelocytic leukemia, *N.Y. State J. Med.* **73**:1180.

SOKAL, J. E., AUNGST, C. W., AND SCHNEIDERMAN, M., 1974, Delay in progression of malignant lymphoma after BCG vaccination, *N. Engl. J. Med.* **291**:1226.

SOKAL, J. E., AUNGST, C. W., SCHNEIDERMAN, M., *et al.*, 1976, Immunotherapy of chronic myelocytic leukemia: Effects of different vaccination schedules, *Ann. N.Y. Acad. Sci.* **277**:367.

SOLOWAY, A. C., RAPPAPORT, F. T., AND LAWRENCE, H. S., 1968, Cellular studies in neoplastic disease, in: *Histocompatibility Testing* (E. S. CURTIN *et al.*, eds.), pp. 75–78, Munksgaard, Copenhagen.

SPARKS, F. C., 1976, Hazrds and complications of BCG immunotherapy, *Med. Clin. N. Am.* **60**:499.

SPITLER, L. E., LEVIN, A. S., STITES, D. E., *et al.*, 1972, The Wiskott-Aldrich syndrome: Results of transfer factor therapy, *J. Clin. Invest.* **51**:3216.

SPITLER, L. E., LEVIN, A. S., AND FUDENBERG, H. H., 1973, Human lymphocyte transfer factor, *Methods Cancer Res.* **8**:59.

SPITLER, L. E., SAGEBIEL, R., WONG, P., *et al.*, 1977, A randomized double-blind trial of adjuvant therapy with levamisole in patients with malignant melanoma, in: *Immunotherapy of Cancer: Present Status of Trials in Man* (W. TERRY AND D. WINDHORST, eds.), in press.

SPREAFICO, F., VECCHI, A., MANTOVANI, A., *et al.*, 1975, Characterization of the immunostimulants levamisole and tetramizole, *Eur. J. Cancer* **11**:555.

STERN, K., 1960, The reticuloendothelial system and neoplasia, in: *The Reticuloendothelial System Structure and Function* (J. H. HELLER, ed.), pp. 233–258, Ronald Press, New York.

STEWART, T. H. M., HOLLINSHEAD, A. C., HARRIS, J. E., *et al.*, 1976, Immunochemotherapy of lung cancer, *Ann. N.Y. Acad. Sci.* **277**:436.

STEWART, W. E., GRESSER, I., TOVEY, M. G., *et al.*, 1976, Identification of the cell multiplication inhibitory factors in interferon preparations as interferons, *Nature (London)* **262**:300.

STIFFEL, C., MOUTON, D., AND BOUTHILLIER, Y., *et al.*, 1970, Response of RES to *Mycobacterium tuberculosis* BCG and to *Corynebacterium parvum* in mice of different strains, *J. Reticuloendothel. Soc.* **7**:280.

STJERNSWARD, J., AND LEVIN, A., 1971, Delayed hypersensitivity induced regression of human neoplasms, *Cancer* **28**:628.

530

EVAN M. HERSH,
G. M. MAVLIGIT,
J. U. GUTTERMAN,
AND
S. P. RICHMAN

STRANDER, H., 1975, in: *International Workshop on Interferon in the Treatment of Cancer* (M. CRIM, A. S. LEVINE, T. C. MERRIGAN, AND J. VILCEK, eds.), submitted.

STRANDER, H., CANTELL, K., CARLSTROM, G., *et al.*, 1975, Clinical and laboratory investigations in man: Systemic administration of potent interferon to man, *J. Natl. Cancer Inst.* **51**:733.

SUMNER, W. C., AND FORAKER, A. G., 1960, Spontaneous regression of human melanoma: Clinical and experimental studies, *Cancer* **13**:79.

SUNSHINE, G., LOPEZ-CORRALES, E., HADDEN, E. M., *et al.*, 1977, Levamisole and imidazole *in vitro* effects in mouse and man and their possible mediation by cyclic nucleotides, *Fogarty Int. Cent. Proc.* **28**:31.

SYMDENS, J., AND BRUGMANS, J., 1974, Treatment of recurrent aphthous stomatitis and herpes infections with levamisole, *Br. Med. J.* **2**:592.

SYMES, M. O., AND RIDDELL, A. G., 1968, Immunologically competent cells in the treatment of malignant disease, *Lancet* **1**:1054.

TAKITA, H., MINOWADA, J., HAN, T., *et al.*, 1976, Adjuvant immunotherapy in bronchogenic carcinoma, *Ann. N.Y. Acad. Sci.* **277**:345.

TEIMOORIAN, B., AND McCUNE, W. S., 1963, Surgical management of malignant melanoma, *Am. Surg.* **29**:515.

TER-GRIGOROV, V. S., AND IRLIN, I. S., 1968, The stimulating effect of complete Freund's adjuvant on tumor induction by polyoma virus in mice and by Rous sarcoma virus in rats, *Int. J. Cancer* **3**:760.

THIENPONT, D., VANPARIJS, O. F. J., RAEYMAEKERS, A. H. M., *et al.*, 1966, Tetramisole (R-8299), a new, potent broad spectrum anthelmintic, *Nature (London)* **209**:1084.

THIRY, L., GOLDBERGER, S., TACK, L., *et al.*, 1977, Comparison of the immunogenicity of hamster cells transformed by adenovirus and herpes simplex virus, *Cancer Res.* (in press).

THOMAS, E. D., STORB, R., CLIFT, R. A., *et al.*, 1975, Bone marrow transplantation, *N. Engl. J. Med.* **292**:832.

THOR, D. E., AND SCHLOSSMAN, S., 1969, Transfer of the cellular immune response in guinea pigs with RNA extracts, *Fed. Proc.* **28**:629.

THORBECKE, G. J., FRIEDMAN-KIEN, A. E., AND VILCEK, J., 1974, Effect of rabbit interferon on immune responses, *Cell. Immunol.* **11**:290.

TOUJAS, L., SABOLOVIC, D., DAZORD, L., 1972, The mechanism of immunostimulation induced by inactivated *Brucella abortus*, *Rev. Eur. Etud. Clin. Biol.* **17**:267.

TOWNSEND, C. M., EILBER, F. R., AND MORTON, D. L., 1976, Skeletal and soft tissue sarcomas, *J. Am. Med. Assoc.* **236**:2187.

TRAININ, N., BERGER, M., AND KAYE, A., 1967, Some characteristics of a thymic humoral factor determined by assay *in vivo* of DNA synthesis in lymph nodes of thymectomized mice, *Biochem. Pharmacol.* **16**:711.

TRAININ, N., KOOK, A. I., UMIEL, T., *et al.*, 1975, The nature and mechanism of stimulation of immune responsiveness by thymus extracts, *Ann. N.Y. Acad. Sci.* **249**:349.

TRIPODI, D., PARKS, L. C., AND BRUGMANS, J., 1973, Drug-induced restoration of cutaneous delayed hypersensitivity in anergic patients with cancer, *N. Engl. J. Med.* **289**:354.

VAN GHINCKEL, R. F., AND HOEBEKE, J., 1977, Effect of levamisole on spontaneous rosette-forming cells in murine spleen, *Eur. J. Immunol.* (in press).

VELTMAN, L. L., KERN, D. H., AND PILCH, Y. H., 1974 Immune cytolysis of human tumor cells mediated by xenogeneic immune RNA, *Cell. Immunol.* **13**:367.

VERHAEGEN, H., DeCREE, J., DeCOCK, W., *et al.*, 1973, Levamisole and the immune response, *N. Engl. J. Med.* **289**:1148.

VETTO, R. M., BERGER, D. R., AND NOLTE, J. E., 1976, Transfer factor therapy in patients with cancer, *Cancer* **37**:90.

VOGLER, W. R., AND CHAN, Y. K., 1974, Prolongation of remission in myeloblastic leukemia by Tice strain bacillus Calmette Guérin, *Lancet* **2**:128.

VOGLER, W. R., BARTOLUCCI, A. A., AND OMURA, G. A., 1977, A randomized clinical trial of BCG in myeloblastic leukemia conducted by the Southeastern Cancer Study Group, in: *Immunotherapy of Cancer: Present Status of Trials in Man* (W. TERRY AND D. WINDHORST, eds.), in press.

WAINBERG, M. A., AND MARGOLESE, R. G., 1977, Desentization of effective anti-tumor immunity in guinea pigs, *Eur. J. Med.* (in press).

WALDORF, D. S., HAYNES, H. A., AND VAN SCOTT, E. J., 1967, Cutaneous hypersensitivity and desensitization to mechlorethamine in patients with mycosis fungoides lymphoma, *Ann. Intern. Med.* **67**:282.

WALDMANN, T. A., STROBER, W., AND BLAESE, R. M., 1972, Immunodeficiency disease and malignancy: Various immunological deficiencies of man and the role of immune processes in the control of malignant disease, *Ann. Intern. Med.* **77**:605.

WANEBO, H. J., KENENY, M., PINSKY, C. M., *et al.*, 1976, Influence of poly-A poly-U on immune responses in cancer patients, *Ann. N.Y. Acad. Sci.* **277**:288.

WEBB, D., BRAUN, W., AND PLESCIA, O. J., 1972, Antitumor effect of polynucleotide and theophylline, *Cancer Res.* **32**:1814.

WEISS, D. W., 1976, MER and other mycobacterial fractions in the immunotherapy of cancer, *Med. Clin. N. Am.* **60**:473.

WEISS, D. W., 1977, Neoplastic disease and tumor immunology from the prospective of host parasite relationships, in: *International Symposium on the Spontaneous Regression of Cancer*, NCI Monograph, in press.

WEISS, D. W., AND YASHPHE, D. J., 1973, Non-specific stimulation of anti-microbial and antitumor resistance and of immunological responsiveness by MER fraction of tubercle bacilli, in: *Dynamic Aspects of Host Parasite Relationships*, Vol. 1 (N. ZUCKERMAN AND D. W. WEISS, eds.), pp. 163–223, Academic Press, New York.

WEISS, D. W., BONHAG, R. S., AND LESLIE, P., 1966, Studies on the heterologous immunogenicity of methanol insoluble fraction of attenuated tubercle bacilli BCG. II. Protection against tumor isografts, *J. Exp. Med.* **124**:1039.

WEISS, D. W., STUPP, Y., MANNY, N., *et al.*, 1975, Treatment of acute myelocytic leukemia (AML) patients with the MER tubercle bacillus fraction: A preliminary report, *Transplant. Proc.* **7**:545.

WEIS, D. W., KUPERMAN, O., FATHALLAH, N., *et al.*, 1976, Mode of action of mycobacterial fractions in antitumor immunity, *Ann. N.Y. Acad. Sci.* **276**:536.

WEPSIC, H. T., ZBAR, B., RAPP, H. J., *et al.*, 1970, Systemic transfer of tumor immunity: Delayed hypersensitivity and suppression of tumor growth, *J. Natl. Cancer Inst.* **44**:955.

WHEELOCK, E. F., AND LARKE, R. P. B., 1968, Efficacy of interferon in the treatment of mice with established Friend virus leukemia, *Proc. Soc. Exp. Biol. Med.* **127**:230.

WHITTAKER, J. A., AND SLATER, A. J., 1977, The immunotherapy of acute myelogenous leukemia using intravenous BCG, in: *Immunotherapy of Cancer: Present Status of Trials in Man* (W. TERRY AND D. WINDHORST, eds.), in press.

WILKINSON, P. C., O'NEAL, G. J., McINROY, R. J., *et al.*, 1973, Chemotaxis of macrophages: The role of a macrophage-specific cytotoxan from anaerobic corynebacteria and its relation to immunopotentiation *in vivo*, *CIVA Found. Symp. Immunopotentiation* **18**:120.

WILSON, D. B., AND WECKER, E. E., 1966, Quantitative studies on the behavior of sensitized lymphoid cells *in vitro*. III. Conversion of normal lymphoid cells to an immunologically active status with RNA derived from isologous lymphoid tissue of specifically immunized rats, *J. Immunol.* **47**:512.

WOLLMARK, N., AND FISHER, B., 1974, The effect of a single and repeated administration of *Corynebacterium parvum* on bone marrow macrophage colony production in syngeneic tumor-bearing mice, *Cancer Res.* **34**:2869.

WOODRUFF, M. F. A., AND BOAK, J. L., 1966, Inhibitory effect of injection of *Corynebacterium parvum* on the growth of tumor transplants in isogenic hosts, *Br. J. Cancer* **20**:345.

WOODRUFF, M. F. A., AND DUNBAR, N., 1973, The effect of *Corynebacterium parvum* and other reticuloendothelial stimulants on transplanted tumors in mice, *CIBA Found. Symp. Immunopotentiation* **18**:287.

WOODRUFF, M. F. A., AND NOLAN, B., 1963, Preliminary observations on treatment of advanced cancer by injection of allogeneic spleen cells, *Lancet* **2**:426.

WOODRUFF, M. F. A., DUNBAR, N., AND CHAFFAR, A., 1973, The growth of tumors in T-cell deprived mice and their resonse to treatment with *Corynebacterium parvum*, *Proc. R. Soc. London Ser. B* **184**:97.

WRIGHT, P. W., HELLSTRÖM, K. E., HELLSTRÖM, I., *et al.*, 1976, Sera therapy of malignant disease, *Med. Clin. N. Am.* **60**:607.

WYBRAN, J., LEVIN, A. S., SPITLER, L. E., AND FUDENBERG, H. H., 1973, Rosette-forming cells, immunological deficiency diseases, and transfer factor, *N. Engl. J. Med.* **288**:710.

WYBRAN, J., LEVIN, A. S., FUDENBERG, H. H., *et al.*, 1975, Thymosin effects in normal human blood T-cells, *Ann. N.Y. Acad. Sci.* **249**:300.

YAGEL, S., GALLILY, R., AND WEISS, D. W., 1977, Effect of treatment of MER fraction of tubercle bacilli on hydrolytic lysozomal enzyme activity of mouse peritoneal macrophages, *Cell. Immunol.* **19**:381.

YAMAMURA, Y., YOSHIZAKI, K., AZUMA, I., *et al.*, 1975, Immunotherapy of human malignant melanoma with oil-attached BCG cell wall skeleton, *Gann* **66**:355.

EVAN M. HERSH,
G. M. MAVLIGIT,
J. U. GUTTERMAN,
AND
S. P. RICHMAN

YAMAMURA, Y., AZUMA, I., TANIYAMA, T., *et al.*, 1976, Immunotherapy of cancer with cell wall skeleton of *Mycobacterium bovis* bacillus Calmette Guérin, *Ann. N.Y. Acad. Sci.* **277**:209.

YASUHARA, S., KIMURA, I., AND ONOSHI, T., 1974, Antitumor activity of peritoneal exudate cells of the mouse administered with OK432, *Med. Biol.* **89**:375.

YRON, I., WEISS, D. W., ROBINSON, E., COHEN, D., ADELBERG, M. G., MEKORI, T., AND HABER, M., 1973, Immunotherapeutic studies in mice with the methanol extraction residue (MER) fraction of BCG: Solid tumors, *Natl. Cancer Inst. Monogr.* **39**:33.

ZBAR, B., AND TANAKA, T., 1971, Immunotherapy of cancer: Regression of tumors after intralesional injection of living *Mycobacterium bovis*, *Science* **172**:271.

ZBAR, B., BERNSTEIN, I. D., AND RAPP, H. J., 1971, Suppression of tumor growth at the site of infection with living BCG, *J. Natl. Cancer Inst.* **46**:831.

ZBAR, B., BERNSTEIN, I. D., AND BARTLETT, G. L., 1972, Immunotherapy of cancer: Regression of intradermal tumors and prevention of growth of lymph node metastases after intralesional injection of living *Mycobacterium bovis*, *J. Natl. Cancer Inst.* **49**:119.

Index

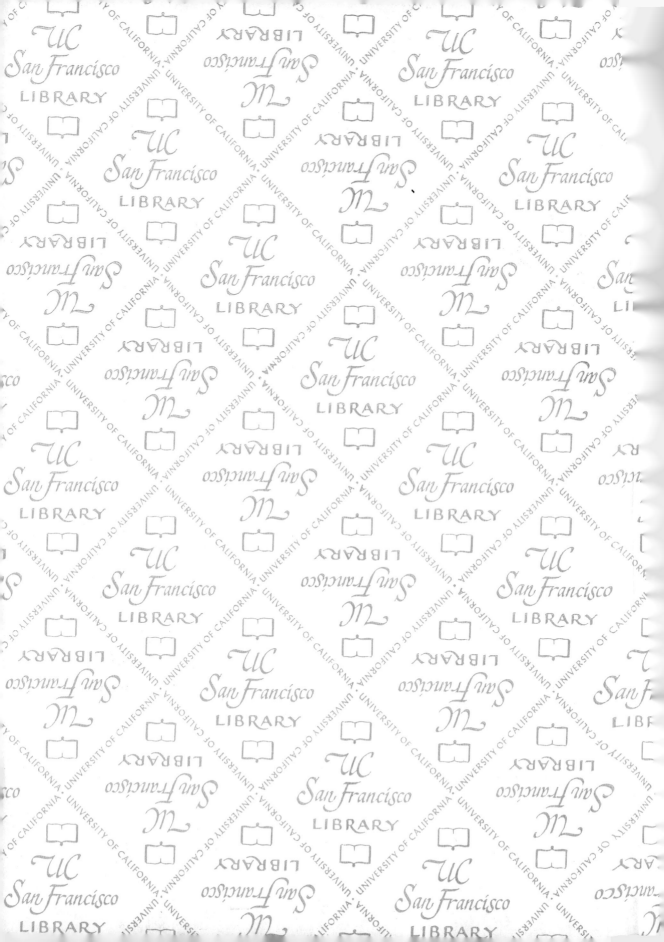